ACCOMPANYING SOFTWARE

in the back of the book

Anthropometric Standards

A. Roberto Frisancho is Thurnau Professor of Anthropology and Research Professor at the Center for Human Growth and Development at the University of Michigan.

Anthropometric Standards: An Interactive Nutritional Reference of Body Size and Body Composition for Children and Adults

A. Roberto Frisancho

Ann Arbor

The University of Michigan Press

Copyright © by the University of Michigan, 1990, 2008
Published in the United States of America by
The University of Michigan Press
Manufactured in the United States of America

♾ Printed on acid-free paper

2011   2010   2009   2008   4   3   2   1

A CIP catalog record for this book is available from the British Library.

U.S. CIP data applied for.

ISBN 13: 978-0-472-11591-4
ISBN 10: 0-472-11591-X

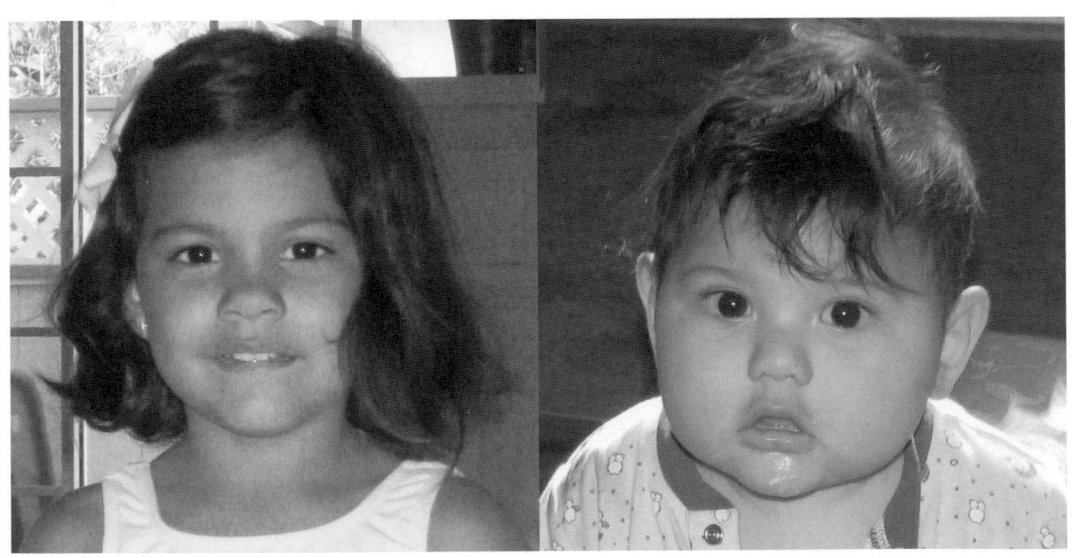

To my grandchildren
Lauren Victoria and Andrew Michael Frisancho
who brought a great deal of joy to our family

INTRODUCTION AND PREFACE

Anthropometry is the single most universally applicable non-invasive technique for assessing both health and nutritional status of clinical and non-clinical samples. The previous anthropometric reference (Frisancho, 1993) provided information assessing growth and nutritional status on individuals ranging in age from 2 to 75 years of age. However, throughout the world, and especially in the industrialized populations during the last decade, the demographic profile has changed drastically. For example, in the 1970s less than 5% of the population was older than 65 years of age, but at present more than 13% of the population is older than 65 years of age. *These changes emphasize the need for anthropometric standards that are contemporary.* Furthermore, the previous reference did not include values for individuals younger than 2 years of age. For this reason, the present anthropometric reference provides information for assessing growth and nutritional status of individuals ranging in age from 2 months to 90 years. In addition, data on prenatal growth derived from established anthropometric studies has also been included in the present anthropometric reference.

In auxology the term **standard** implies that the growth curves depicted on the chart reflect desirable growth, while a **reference** chart reflects the growth pattern of the children who were selected as the source sample for the charts, and no judgment of desirability is placed against their growth. Yet, in studies of anthropometry and nutrition and growth, the terms **standard** and **reference** are used interchangeably. The reason for this practice is that current growth charts have been developed through a series of studies that included cross-sectional and longitudinal samples that were in good health and were raised under good socio-economic conditions, but without judgment of desirability or optimality of growth. The present anthropometric reference has been developed using statistical approaches that converted otherwise skewed anthropometric data into normally distributed information that excludes the excessively fat or overweight individuals. Therefore, the present reference is suitable and appropriate for the evaluation of growth and anthropometric nutritional status of children and adults. The contents of this monograph are oriented to practicing professionals such as pediatricians, family practice physicians, nutritionists, dieticians, epidemiologists, and human biologists that need to define nutritional status of children and adults.

The book is divided into six chapters. Chapter I presents a succinct description of the methods and measurement techniques used for obtaining anthropometric information of children and adults. Chapter II considers the anthropometric reference for the evaluation of nutritional status during pregnancy and prenatal growth. Chapter III presents a summary of the non-smoothed anthropometric reference based on the third National Health and Nutrition Examination Survey (NHANES III) conducted during 1994-1998 of the US civilian population, upon which this reference is based. Chapter IV focuses on the statistical approaches used in the development of the normalized anthropometric reference. This chapter also gives the anthropometric indices in tabular and graphic form for the evaluation of growth and nutritional status of children and adults ranging in age from 2 to 90 years of age derived from NHANES III. The present anthropometric reference is very applicable to surveys where the age of participants is rounded to the nearest year or where the age of the participants exceeds 20 years, but for studies where the age of children is rounded to the nearest month there is a need for a more precise reference. For this reason, Chapter V presents in tabular and graphic form: (a) the growth standard for children ranging in age from 2 months to 240 months (20 years) developed by the Centers for Disease Control (CDC); and (b) the growth standard for children ranging in age from 2 months to 5 years published by the World Health Organization (WHO). Chapter VI concentrates on the actual process of anthropometric evaluation of nutritional status of children and adults, which where appropriate is applicable to all three anthropometric references.

COMPACT DISC (CD) FOR A COMPUTER ASSISTED EVALUATION OF NUTRITIONAL ANTHROPOMETRY

In addition, a compact disc (CD) is available for a computer assisted evaluation of nutritional anthropometry to determine the individual's percentile and Z-score of the measurements of body size and body composition. It is divided into two sections: One is based on the Anthropometric data source derived from the third National Health and Nutrition Examination Survey (NHANES III) conducted during 1994-1998 developed specifically for the present reference and hereafter referred to as BASED ON NHANES III. The other section is based on the information of weight, height, and body mass index for children ranging in age from 2 to 240 months (20 years) developed by the Centers for Disease Control (CDC), hereafter referred to as BASED ON CDC. The third section is based on the information of weight and length for children ranging in age from birth to 5 years developed by the World Health Organization (WHO), hereafter referred to as BASED ON WHO.

(a). Anthropometric Reference of Growth and Body Composition for children and adults ranging in age from 2 months to 90 years of age. This reference is used to determine percentile and Z-score of children and adults ranging in age from 2 months to 90 years of age with reference to measurements of body size and body composition developed specifically for the present reference and hereafter is referred to as Comprehensive reference.

(b). Anthropometric Reference for children ranging in age from 2 to 240 months (20 years) developed by the Centers for Disease Control (CDC). This reference is used to determine the percentile and Z-score of children with reference to weight, stature, and body mass index and hereafter is referred to as CDC reference.

(c). Anthropometric Reference for children ranging in age from birth to 5 years of age developed by the World Health Organization (WHO). This reference is used to determine the percentile and Z-score of children with reference to weight, length, stature, and body mass index and hereafter is referred to as WHO reference.

These three references are presented in Excel spreadsheets (Excel of Microsoft Excel and accessible to either Macintosh or PC), formatted with equations that allow the calculation of age- and sex-specific Z-scores and percentiles directly without the need of additional computer programs or software. The calculation of Z-scores and percentiles can be done using either metric (kg, cm) or non-metric (pounds and inches) systems.

Acknowledgments

Dr. Niko Maceroti, Research Scientist of the Center for Human Growth and Development of the University of Michigan, provided valuable advice regarding the development of the computer-assisted program for calculating Z-scores and percentiles using the Excel program, and Mr. Andrew Peterson, a computer science major, set the code protection for these Excel files. Ms. Amy Mangieri, Mr. Adam Janosko, Ms. Emily Mathias, and Mr. Thomas George, undergraduate students, provided diligent assistance in the proofreading of the manuscript.

CONTENTS

CHAPTER I
ANTHROPOMETRIC METHODS FOR OBTAINING ANTHROPOMETRIC MEASUREMENTS FOR THE EVALUATION OF NUTRITIONAL STATUS OF CHILDREN AND ADULTS

MEASUREMENTS OF BODY SIZE AND BODY COMPOSITION
Weight
Height
Rohrer Index
Body Mass Index
Head Circumference
Sitting Height
Sitting Height Index
Upper Leg (Thigh) Length
Knee Height
Indices of Relative Leg Length
Biacromial Breadth
Bi-iliac (Bitrochanteric) Breadth
Waist (Abdominal) Circumference
Hip (Buttocks) Circumference
Waist-To-Hip (W/H) Ratio
Mid-Upper Arm Circumference
Mid-Thigh Circumference
Skinfolds
Range of Tolerance of Skinfold Measures
Triceps Skinfold Thickness
Subscapular Skinfold Thickness
Suprailiac Skinfold
Mid-Thigh Skinfold
Sum of Skinfold Thickness
Upper Arm Muscle, Fat Area, and Arm Fat Index
No-Correction of Muscle Area for Size of Bone in Adults
Limitation of Measurements of Upper Arm Muscle Area
Elbow Breadth
Wrist Breadth

MEASUREMENTS OF BIOELECTRIC IMPEDANCE
Fat-Free Mass and Percent Body Fat
Fat-Free Mass and Fat Mass Indices

RELIABILITY OF ANTHROPOMETRIC MEASUREMENTS

LITERATURE CITED

CHAPTER I
ANTHROPOMETRIC METHODS FOR OBTAINING ANTHROPOMETRIC MEASUREMENTS FOR THE EVALUATION OF NUTRITIONAL STATUS OF CHILDREN AND ADULTS

The evaluation and interpretation of anthropometric data require standardized measurement procedures, trained personnel, the use of appropriate, regularly calibrated instruments, and the collection of reliable data. This chapter focuses on the techniques and procedures for obtaining anthropometric measurements of children and adults. These procedures follow the guidelines described in previous publications (1-3).

MEASUREMENTS OF BODY SIZE AND BODY COMPOSITION

The anthropometric variables included in this section are given in **Table I.1**.

Weight

The weight of children under 2 years of age is measured on a leveled pan scale with a beam and movable weight. A quilt is left on the scale at all times and the scale is calibrated to zero. The scale should be calibrated every month using objects with known weight. When the scale is not in use, the beam should be locked in place to reduce wear. The infant, with or without a diaper, is placed on the scale, making sure the weight is distributed equally on each side of the center of the pan (see **Figure I.1a**). Weight is recorded to the nearest 10 grams. If a diaper is worn, to obtain a nude weight, the diaper's weight is subtracted from the observed weight of the infant. (In cases in which infants cannot be weighed alone on the pan scale, they can be weighed with their mother on the platform weight scale.)

For subjects older than 2 years, the body weight should be measured using a platform-beam scale with movable weights or an instrument of equivalent accuracy (see **Figure I.1b**). The beam of the platform scale must be graduated so that it can be read from both sides.

The calibration of the scale should also be done every month using objects with known weight. The subjects stand still over the center of the platform with a body weight evenly distributed between both feet. Light indoor clothing such as hospital gowns or shorts can be worn. Do not subtract the weight of the clothing when comparing to the weights given in the present monograph because the weights are given with light clothing but without shoes. Weight is recorded to the nearest 100 grams.

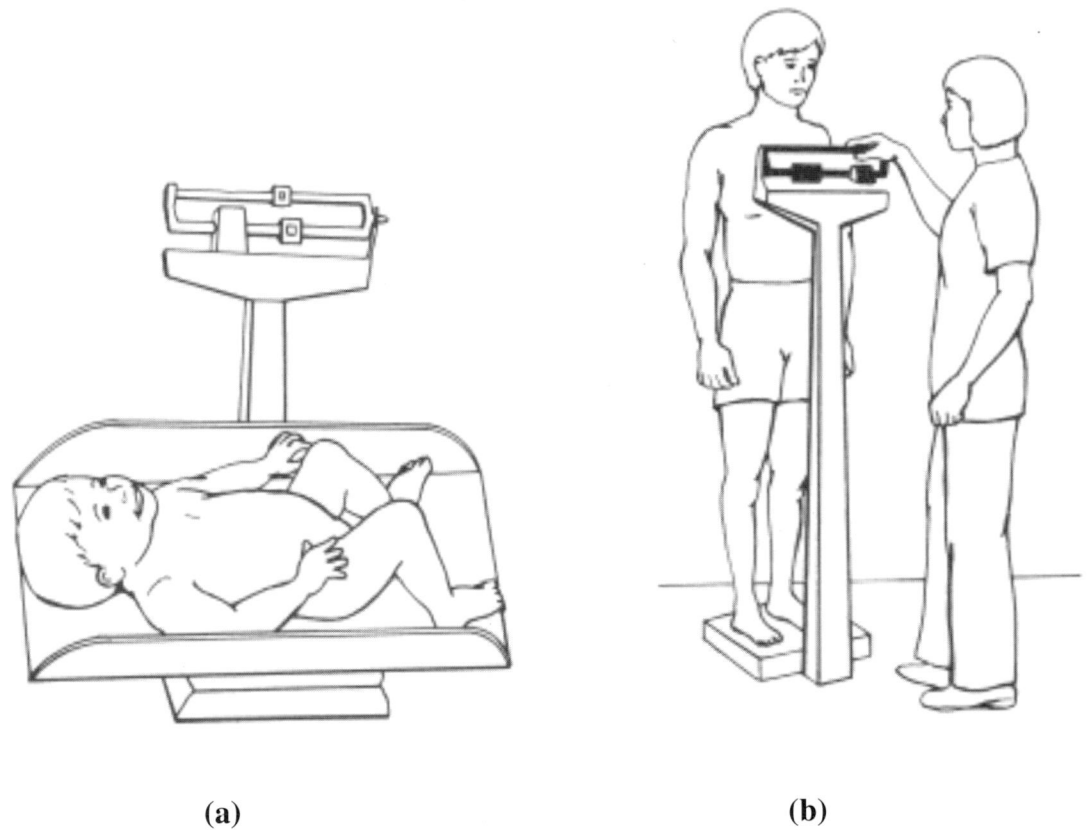

(a)   **(b)**

Figure I.1. Measurement of Weight in Infants Less Than 2 Years of Age (a) and in Subjects Older Than 2 Years of Age (b). Infants are weighed while lying down naked on a pan pediatric scale and older subjects are weighed with shorts or standard gown on a platform-beam scale. From refer. #1: Frisancho (1990).

Height

In children under 2 years of age, length should be obtained in the recumbent position while individuals older than 3 years of age are measured standing.

Recumbent Length. In children under 2 years of age, length should be obtained in the recumbent position using an infantometer. An infantometer is a device that consists of a flat board with a fixed headboard and a movable footboard, both of which are perpendicular to the table surface. The device has a fixed measuring tape marked off in millimeters or inches with its zero end at the edge of the headboard. Infant length is recorded as the distance between the headboard and footboard. To obtain accurate measurements two people are required (see **Figure I.2**). The assistant stands at the head of the table and holds the infant's head so the infant looks vertically upward with the crown of the head against the headboard. The examiner straightens the infant's legs, holding the feet with toes pointed directly up, and moves the footboard against the feet. The measurement is indicated by the position of the footboard and is recorded to the nearest 0.1 cm.

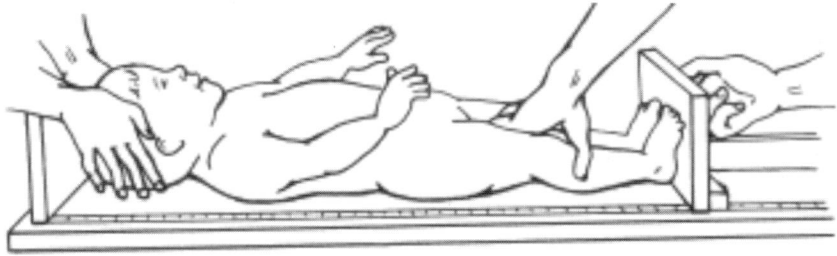

Figure I.2. Measurements of Recumbent Length. Infants less than 2 years of age are measured with an infantometer. From refer. #1: Frisancho (1990).

Stature. The length of subjects older than 3 years of age is measured, without shoes, with a stadiometer (see **Figure I.3**). A stadiometer consists of a metric tape affixed to a vertical surface, such as a wall or a rigid free-standing measuring device, and a movable block, attached to the vertical surface at a right angle, that can be brought down to the crown of the head. In the absence of a stadiometer, height can be measured on a platform scale, but this device is less accurate than the stadiometer. In either case, the subject should stand with heels together and back as straight as possible; the heels, buttocks, shoulders, and head should touch the wall or the vertical surface of the measuring device as shown in **Figure I.3**. The weight of the subject is distributed evenly on both feet and the head is positioned in the Frankfort horizontal plane. The arms hang freely by the sides with the palms facing the thighs. The subject should be asked to inhale deeply and maintain a fully erect position. The movable block is brought down until it touches the head, making sure to put sufficient pressure to compress the hair. The measurement is recorded to the nearest 0.1 cm. Two measurements are taken and if the difference between both readings is less than 1 cm, the mean measurement is recorded.

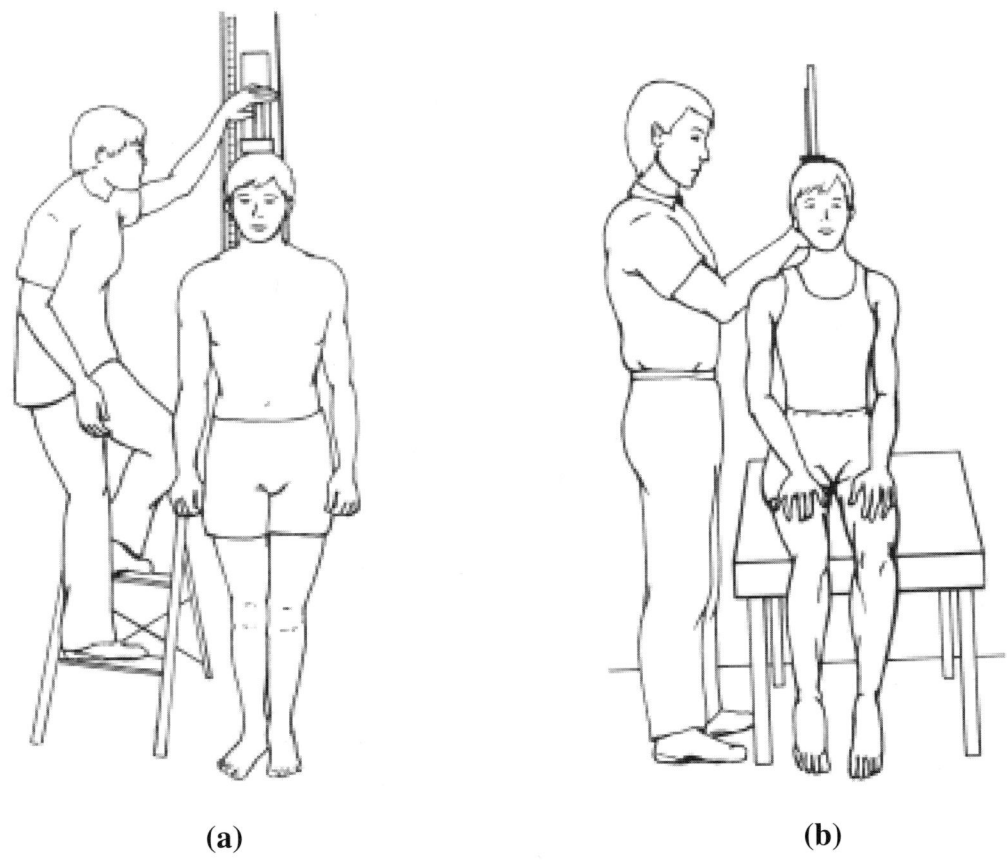

(a)   (b)

Figure I.3. Measurements of Stature (a) and of Sitting Height (b). Subjects older than 2 years of age are measured standing using a stadiometer. Sitting height is measured with an anthropometer while the subject sits on a measuring table. From refer. #1: Frisancho (1990).

Rohrer Index

The Rohrer index (grams/cm^3) is derived by computation as the quotient of weight in kilograms divided by recumbent length in centimeters cubed, multiplied by 100:

Rohrer Index (RI) = (Weight, g/recumbent length, cm^3) x 100

Table I.1. Anthropometric Dimensions and Indices Presented in This Book

Weight	Rohrer Index
Recumbent Length	Weight-for-Height or Weight-for-Length
Height or Stature	Body Mass Index
Head Circumference	Sitting Height
Sitting Height Index	Upper Leg (Thigh) Length
Knee Height	Relative Total Length
Relative Lower Leg Length	Biacromial Breadth
Bi-iliac or Bitrochanteric Breadth	Waist (Abdominal) Circumference
Hip (Buttocks) Circumference	Waist-Hip (Buttock) Index
Thigh Circumference	Mid-upper Arm Circumference
Triceps Skinfold Thickness	Mid-upper Arm Muscle Area
Subscapular Skinfold Thickness	Suprailiac Skinfold Thickness
Thigh Skinfold Thickness	Body Fat Distribution
Upper Body Fat Distribution	Elbow and Wrist Breadth

Body Mass Index

The body mass index (kg/m^2), also known as the Quetelet index, is a measure of weight per unit of height. It is expressed as kilograms of weight, per square meter of body height. As it is a relative measure, the BMI allows for a comparison of weight, taking into account height. That is, some people can be of low weight simply because they are short. Conversely, some people can be heavy simply because they are tall. In general, the BMI is highly correlated with body fat, but in some cases, it is not. For example, many people have a high body mass index without being fat because they are muscular. The body mass index (kg/m^2) is derived by computation as the quotient of weight in kilograms divided by height in meters squared:

Body Mass Index (kg/m^2) = Weight/Height ^{2}

If the measurements have been recorded in English units, BMI can be obtained by dividing the weight in pounds by height, and dividing by the square of stature in inches, and then multiplying the product by 703:

Body Mass Index (BMI, kg/m^2) = [Weight/(Height/Height)] x 703

Although it is preferable and more accurate to calculate, **Table I.2** gives the BMI that corresponds to a given height and weight.

Table I.2. Table to Derive Body Mass Index (kg/m^2) from Measurements of Height in Feet and Inches and Weight in Pounds

Height	19	20	21	22	23	24	25	26	27	28	29	30	31	32	33	34	35
							Weight (in pounds)										
4'10"(58")	91	96	100	105	110	115	119	124	129	134	138	143	148	153	158	162	167
4'11"(59")	94	99	104	109	114	119	124	128	133	138	143	148	153	158	163	168	173
5'0"(60")	97	102	107	112	118	123	128	133	138	143	148	153	158	163	168	174	179
5'1"(61")	100	106	111	116	122	127	132	137	143	148	153	158	164	169	174	180	185
5'2"(62")	104	109	115	120	126	131	136	142	147	153	158	164	169	175	180	186	191
5'3"(63")	107	113	118	124	130	135	141	146	152	158	163	169	175	180	186	191	197
5'4"(64")	110	116	122	128	134	140	145	151	157	163	169	174	180	186	192	197	204
5'5"(65")	114	120	126	132	138	144	150	156	162	168	174	180	186	192	198	204	210
5'6"(66")	118	124	130	136	142	148	155	161	167	173	179	186	192	198	204	210	216
5'7"(67")	121	127	134	140	146	153	159	166	172	178	185	191	198	204	211	217	223
5'8"(68")	125	131	138	144	151	158	164	171	177	184	190	197	203	210	216	223	230
5'9"(69")	128	135	142	149	155	162	169	176	182	189	196	203	209	216	223	230	236
5'10"(70")	132	139	146	153	160	167	174	181	188	195	202	209	216	222	229	236	243
5'11"(71")	136	143	150	157	165	172	179	186	193	200	208	215	222	229	236	243	250
6'0"(72")	140	147	154	162	169	177	184	191	199	206	213	221	228	235	242	250	258
6'1"(73")	144	151	159	166	174	182	189	197	204	212	219	227	235	242	250	257	265
6'2'(74")	148	155	163	171	179	186	194	202	210	218	225	233	241	249	256	264	272
6'3'(75")	152	160	168	176	184	192	200	208	216	224	232	240	248	256	264	272	279

Head Circumference

Head circumference is done on children 2 months to 7 years of age with a metric tape (see **Figure I.4**). Place the tape across the frontal bones just above the eyebrows, around the head above the ears on each side, and over the occipital prominence at the back of the head.

Meanwhile, the child either sits in the parent's lap, on the footstool, or stands. The examiner holds the tape snugly around the head. The tape is moved up and down over the back of the head to locate the maximal circumference of the head. The tape should be perpendicular to the long axis of the face and should be pulled firmly to compress the hair and underlying soft tissues. **Note**: Make sure that hair ornaments and braids are removed prior to the measurement. Record the measurement to the nearest 0.1 cm.

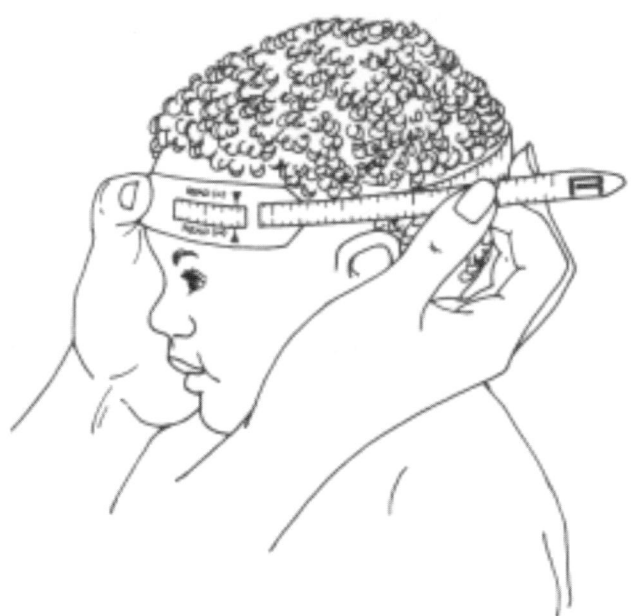

Figure I.4. Measurements of Head Circumference of Infants. From refer. #1: Frisancho (1990).

Sitting Height

Sitting height is measured with an anthropometer. The subject sits erect on a 30 x 40 x 50 cm box. The subject sits on the table or box with the legs hanging unsupported over the edge and the hands resting on the thighs (see **Figure I.3b**). The subject sits as erect as possible, with the head in the Frankfort horizontal plane and the eyes also in a horizontal plane looking straight ahead. The head, shoulders, and buttocks should touch the vertical surface of the measuring device. The subject should be asked to inhale deeply and maintain a fully erect position and the measurement is made just before the subject exhales. The movable block is brought down until it touches the head. The knees are directed straight ahead while the subject sits fully erect with the head in the same position as for the measurement of stature. Sufficient pressure is applied to compress the hair. The measurement is recorded to the nearest 0.1 cm. Two measurements are taken and if the difference between both readings is less than 1 cm, the mean is then recorded.

Sitting Height Index

The sitting height index (%), also known as the Cormic index, is derived by computation as the ratio of sitting height to stature times 100:

Sitting Height Index (%) = (Sitting height, cm/stature, cm) x 100

Upper Leg (Thigh) Length

The subject sits straight on the measuring box with the right knee bent at a 90° angle. Upper leg length is measured from the midpoint of the inguinal ligament to the proximal edge of the patella (see **Figure I.5**). A non-stretchable tape measure is used. No pressure is to be applied at the inguinal crease; however, folds of fat tissue may have to be lifted on some obese subjects to measure at the crease. The exam gown should be lifted and the pants slightly pulled to smooth out gathers.

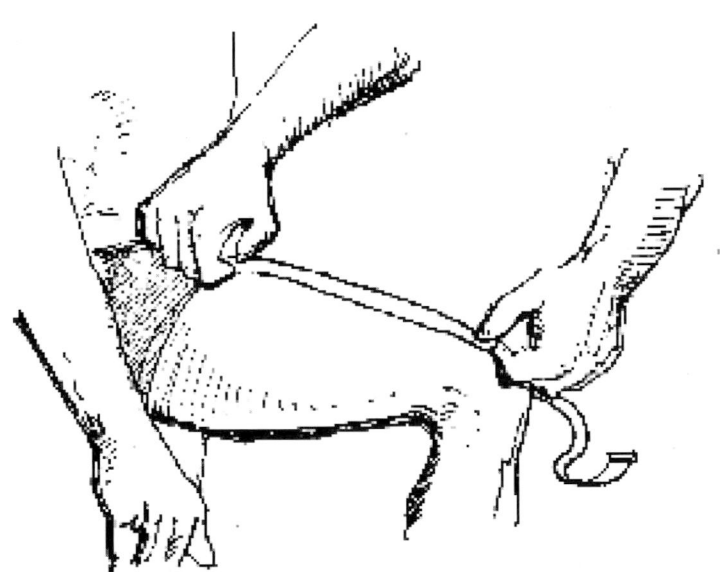

Figure I.5. Measurements of Upper Leg (thigh) Length. Upper leg (thigh) length is measured with non-stretchable tape. From refer. # 3: Lohman et al. (1988).

Knee Height

Knee height is only measured on adults 60 years of age and older. To obtain the measurement, the subject sits on the examination table with both legs dangling. The examinee may require the assistance of the examiner to help him onto the table. The knee height is measured with a sliding broad-blade caliper. As shown in **Figure I.6a** and **b,** while lying supine the subject being measured bends the knee and ankle to a 90° angle. The fixed blade of the caliper is placed under the heel of the foot, and the other blade is placed over the anterior surface of the thigh over the condyle of the femur. The shaft of the caliper is held parallel to the shaft of the tibia, and pressure is applied to compress the tissue.

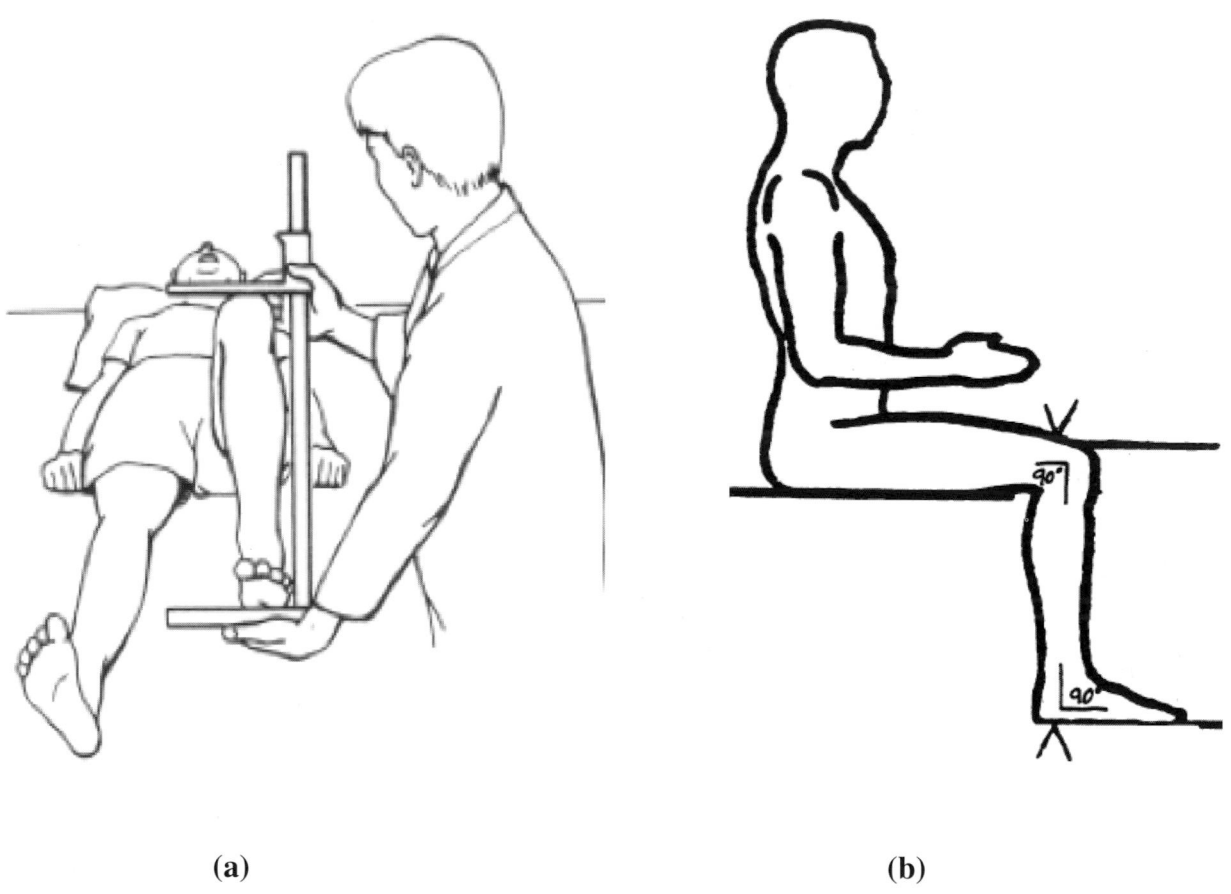

(a)   **(b)**

Figure I.6. Measurements of Knee Height. Knee height can be measured in either a (a) recumbent or (b) sitting position with a broad-blade caliper.

Indices of Relative Leg Length

Two indices of leg length are computed:

Total Leg Length Index (%) = (total leg length, cm - stature, cm) x 100

Where Total Leg Length = stature - sitting height

Lower Leg Length Index (%) = (lower leg length, cm/stature, cm) x 100

Where Lower Leg Length = total leg length - upper leg length

Biacromial Breadth

The examinee sits on the body measurement table that is approximately chair height. The examinee is asked to sit erect with the arms hanging freely at the sides. The examiner stands behind the examinee with the sliding calipers. The examiner checks the posture of the examinee, making sure that the shoulders are neither too far back nor forward, and that there is a noticeable curvature in the lower back. The objective is to have the examinee relaxed with the shoulders downward and slightly forward so that the reading is maximal. The sleeves of the exam gown are pulled up towards the neck, rather than pulling the gown down over the shoulders. The examiner then locates the acromial process. The caliper rests firmly between the thumb and forefinger of the examiner. This allows the examiner to palpate the bony ridges with his other fingers. The examiner locates the lateral border of the acromial process on each shoulder. The arms of the sliding caliper are placed directly on the skin next to the lateral border of each acromial process. Pressure is applied to compress the soft tissue over the acromial processes without hurting the examinee (see **Figure I.7a**). The maximum breadth across the lateral borders of the acromial processes is measured to the nearest 0.1 cm.

Bi-iliac (Bitrochanteric) Breadth

The measurement of bi-iliac breadth is also referred to as bitrochanteric breadth. To measure the bitrochanteric breadth, the subject stands with the heels together and the arms folded over the chest. An anthropometer with straight blades is used. The examiner stands behind the subject (see **Figure I.7b**). The maximum distance between the trochanter is measured and is recorded to the nearest 0.1 cm. Considerable pressure must be applied with the anthropometer blades to compress the soft tissues.

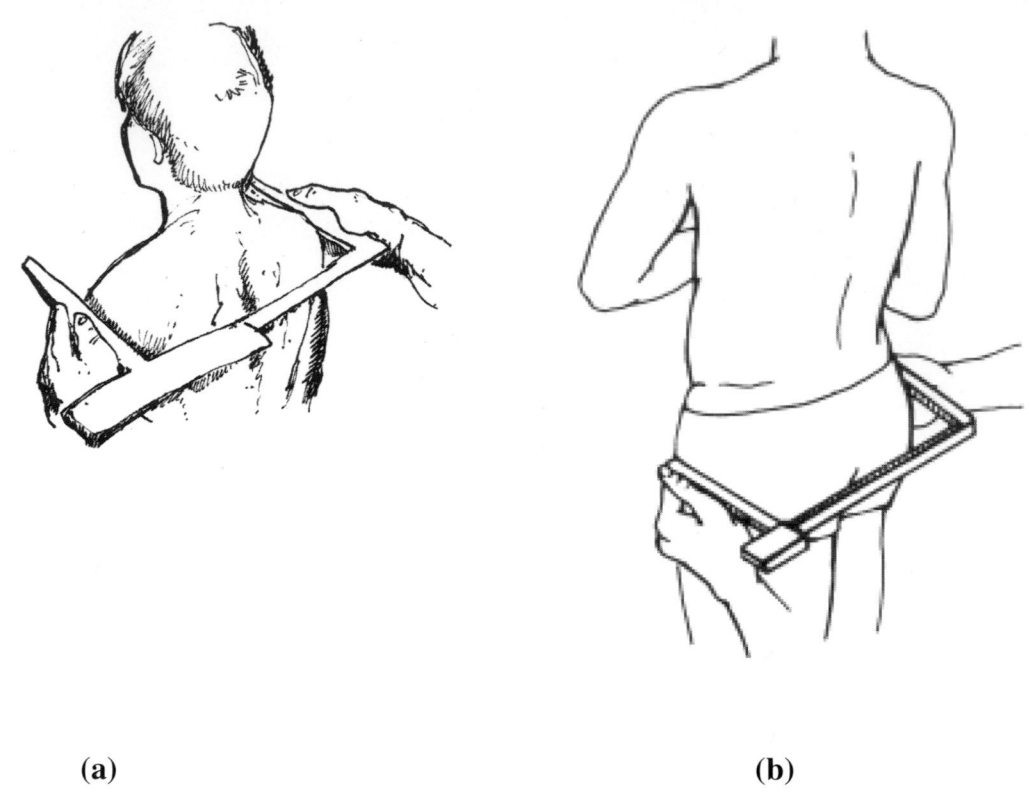

(a)   (b)

Figure I.7. Measurements of Biacromial Breadth (a) and Bitrochanteric Breadth (b). From refer. #3: Lohman et al. (1988).

Waist (Abdominal) Circumference

The pants and underclothing of the subject must be lowered slightly for the examiner to palpate directly on the hip area for the iliac crest. The subject wears little clothing. The subject stands erect with the abdomen relaxed, the arms at the sides and the feet together. The examiner faces the subject and places a non-stretchable tape around the subject, in a horizontal plane, *at the level of the natural waist.* This is the narrowest part of the torso, as seen from the anterior aspect (see **Figure I.8a**). This level is usually, but not always, at the level of the umbilicus, especially during pregnancy and in the obese. The measurement should be taken at the end of a normal expiration, without the tape compressing the skin. It is recorded to the nearest 0.1 cm.

Hip (Buttocks) Circumference

The subject wears only nonrestrictive clothing. The subject stands erect with arms at the sides and feet together. The measurer squats at the side of the subject so that the level of maximum extension of the buttocks can be seen. The tape is placed at the maximum extension of the buttocks (see **Figure I.8b**), making sure that the plane of the tape is horizontal. An assistant is needed to help position the tape on the opposite side of the subject's body. The zero end of the tape should be below the measurement value. The tape is in contact with the skin but does not indent the soft tissues. The measurement is recorded to the nearest 0.1 cm.

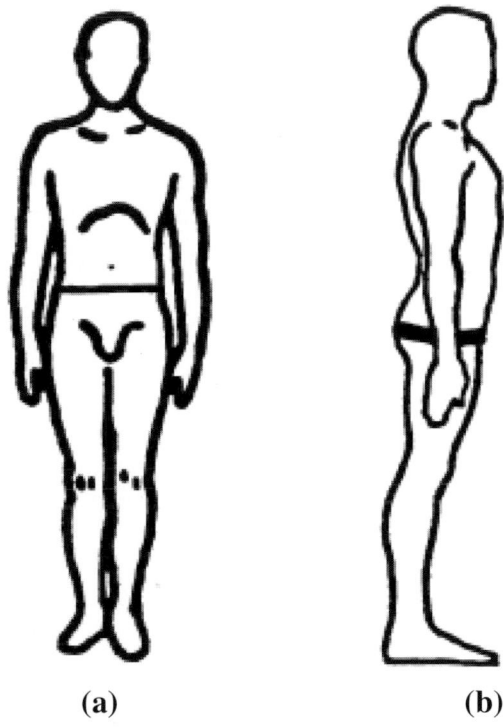

(a)   (b)

Figure I.8. Tape Position for Measuring (a) Waist (abdominal) and (b) Hip (buttocks) Circumference. From refer. #2: National Center for Health Statistics (1996).

Waist-To-Hip (W/H) Ratio

Variation in waist circumference reflects mainly change in subcutaneous and visceral fat, whereas variation in hip circumference incorporates variation in bone structure (pelvic width), gluteal muscle, and subcutaneous gluteal fat. Therefore, the waist-to-hip ratio may provide an effective measure of adiposity and fat distribution (5). If the W/H ratio is **less** than 1 (i.e., the waist circumference is smaller than the circumference of the hip as it occurs in women), the distribution corresponds to lower fat distribution. If W/H ratio is **greater** than 1 (i.e., the waist circumference is greater than the hip circumference), this indicates a relative abundance of abdominal fat and a relative lack of gluteal muscle (decreased hip circumference). Several reports from Asia also indicate that waist-to-height ratio (W/Ht) greater than 0.51 is associated with an increased risk of overweight and obesity (6). Therefore, the waist-to-height ratio may provide an additional measure of adiposity and different aspects of body composition and fat distribution.

Mid-Upper Arm Circumference

To obtain the mid-upper arm circumference, the subject's right arm is bent at the elbow at a 90° angle, with the upper arm held parallel to the side of the body. Then, using either a metallic tape or an insert tape, measure the distance between the acromion (the bony protrusion on the posterior of the upper shoulder) and the olecranon process of the elbow (tip of the elbow) (see **Figure I.9a**). Mark the midpoint between these two landmarks with indelible ink. (If an insert tape is used, the same number should appear at the top of the shoulder and the elbow, and the midpoint is given by the mark on the tape.) The subject's right arm should then be relaxed and hanging loosely at his or her side (see **Figure I.9b**). Position the metric tape around the upper arm at the previously marked midpoint. Make sure the tape is snug, but not so tight as to cause skin indentation or pinching. The circumference is recorded to the nearest 0.1 cm.

Mid-Thigh Circumference

The examinee is standing with the right leg just in front of the left leg and the weight shifted back to the left leg. This instruction should be demonstrated by the examiner. The edge of the examining table may be used for the examinee to hold onto, to maintain his balance. The examiner stands on the examinee's right side and the measuring tape is placed around the mid-thigh at the point that is already marked by a (+). The tape is positioned perpendicular to the long axis of the thigh with the zero end of the tape held below the measurement value (see **Figure I.10**). The tape rests firmly on the skin without compressing the skin. The recorder checks to make sure the tape is positioned correctly. The thigh circumference is measured to the nearest 0.1 cm.

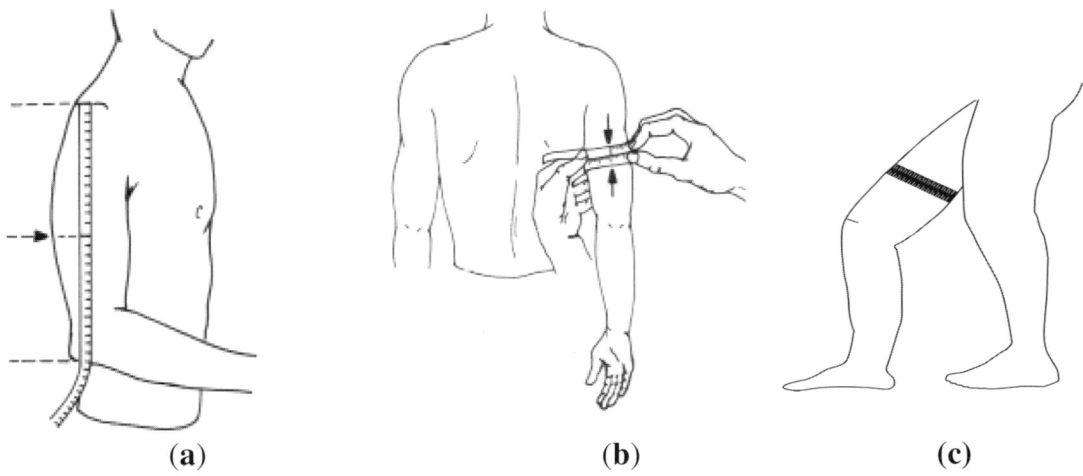

Figure I.9. Measurement of Midpoint (a) and Circumference (b) of the Upper Arm, and (c) Mid-Thigh Circumference. From refer. #1: Frisancho (1990).

Skinfolds

The skinfolds are measured either with a Lange skinfold caliper or a Holtain skinfold caliper. The measurements are taken on the *right* side of the body. The fold of skin and underlying subcutaneous adipose tissue should be *firmly* grasped between the examiner's left thumb and *bent* forefingers. The amount of skin and subcutaneous fat to be elevated depends on the thickness of the subcutaneous fat at the site. The thicker the fat layer, the larger should be the separation between thumb and index finger when the anthropometrist begins to elevate the skinfold. The examiner grasps enough skin and adipose tissue to form a distinct fold that separates from the underlying muscle. The sides of the fold should be roughly parallel. The skinfold is grasped 2.0 cm above the place the measurement is to be taken and is held gently with the thumb and forefinger. The jaws of the calipers are placed at the marked level, perpendicular to the length of the fold, and the skinfold thickness is measured to the nearest 0.1 mm while the *fingers continue* to hold the skinfold. The actual measurement is read from the caliper about 3 seconds after the caliper tension is released. All skinfolds are recorded to the nearest 0.1 mm. It is recommended that all sample measurements be practiced until good measurement reliability is obtained (see section on reliability and interpretation of measurements).

Range of Tolerance of Skinfold Measures

In NHANES III skinfold thickness was measured at four different anatomic body sites: triceps, subscapular, suprailiac, and thigh. Independent measures were taken at each body site by two technicians, resulting in a minimum of two skinfold observations for each site. If the difference between the two measurements at a given site was within a pre-specified tolerance limit, no further measurements were taken at that site. The tolerance limits increased by 2 mm for every 10 mm measured. For the first two measures, the first measure represents the base. Thus, from 0–10 mm, observations were acceptable if they differed from the base measurement by 2 mm or less; from 10–20 mm, observations were acceptable if they differed from the base measurement by 4 mm or less; from 20–30 mm, observations were acceptable if they differed from the base measurement by 6 mm or less, and so on. If the difference between the wo measurements at a given site did exceed the tolerance limit, each technician repeated and recorded a second measurement, resulting in a total of four measurements at that skinfold site. The tolerance was defined using the base skinfold measure. For the third and fourth measures, the third measure represents the base.

If base > 0 and base ≤ 10, then tolerance is 2 mm

If base > 10 and base ≤ 20, then tolerance is 4 mm

If base > 20 and base ≤ 30, then tolerance is 6 mm

If base > 30 and base ≤ 40, then tolerance is 8 mm

If base > 40, then tolerance is 10 mm

The value reported was the mean of all available skinfold measurements at that site.

Triceps Skinfold Thickness

Triceps skinfold thickness is measured with a skinfold caliper (see **Figure I.10**). Skinfold thickness is measured at the previously marked midpoint of the right upper arm (posterior or back side). The subject should stand with right arm hanging loosely by his or her side. The examiner should palpate the subject's measuring site to familiarize himself with soft tissues. Then the examiner should grasp a vertical pinch of skin and subcutaneous fat between thumb and forefinger about 1 cm above the previously marked midpoint. The skinfold should be gently pulled away from underlying muscle. The skinfold caliper should be placed on the skinfold at the midpoint marked, while maintaining a grasp of the skinfold. Three readings should be taken in quick succession, and the average of the three recorded in millimeters. Each reading should be taken as soon as the jaws of the caliper come into contact with the skin and the dial reading stabilizes.

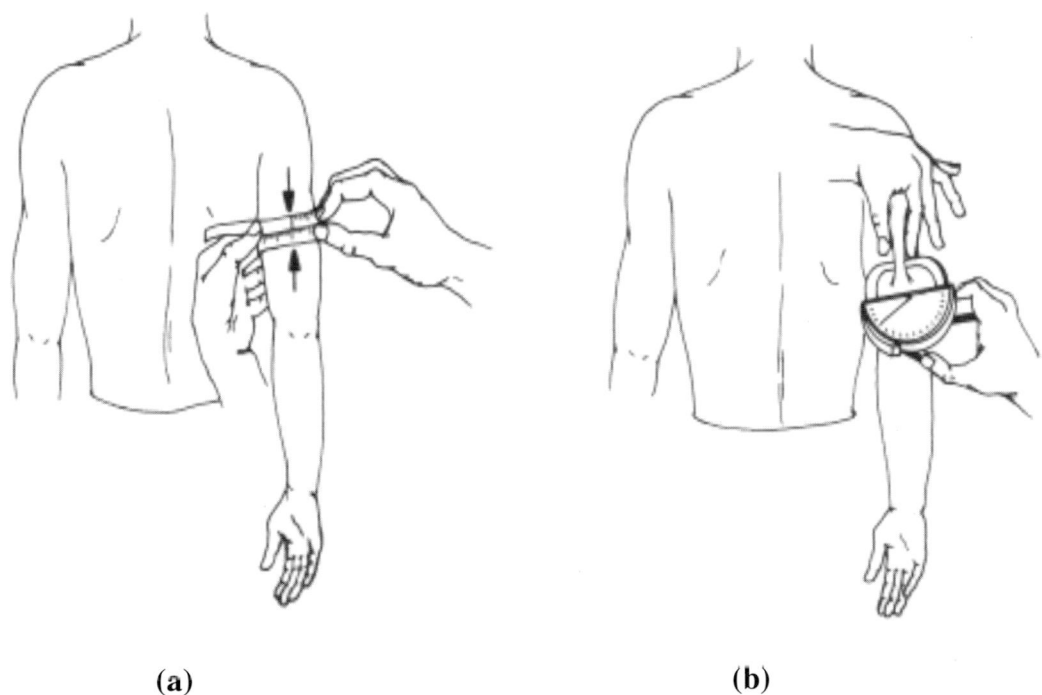

(a)   **(b)**

Figure I.10. Measurements of Upper Arm Circumference (a) and Triceps Skinfold Thickness (b). From refer. #1: Frisancho (1990).

Subscapular Skinfold Thickness

The subscapular skinfold is picked up on a diagonal, inclined infero-laterally approximately 45° to the horizontal plane in the natural cleavage lines of the skin. The site is just below the inferior angle of the scapula (see **Figure I.11a**). The subject stands comfortably erect with the hands relaxed at the sides of the body. The examiner palpates the subject's scapula to locate the inferior border of the scapula. The examiner should grasp a horizontal pinch of skinfold at about 1 cm below the inferior angle of the right scapula (shoulder blade). The examiner holds tightly and raises the skinfold. Then the jaws of the caliper are applied 1 cm above the thumb and finger. The average of the three readings is recorded in millimeters.

Suprailiac Skinfold

The examinee stands and holds the right side of the examining gown up so that the right hip area is exposed. It may be necessary to lower the exam pants slightly to expose the area. The iliac crest had already been marked from previous measurements. The examiner places his/her left thumb on the intersecting marks and picks up the skinfold with the thumb and fingers. The skinfold should slope downward and forward at a 45° angle, extending toward the pubic symphysis (**Figure I.11b**). The caliper is placed perpendicular to the skinfold about 2.0 centimeters medial to the fingers, and the skinfold is measured to the nearest 0.1 mm.

Mid-Thigh Skinfold

The thigh skinfold is measured in the midline of the anterior aspect of the right thigh. This level has already been marked from the thigh circumference measurement. The examinee stands with his weight shifted back on the left leg with the right leg forward, knee slightly flexed, foot flat on the floor. Some examinees will need to hold onto the edge of the table to maintain their balance in this position. This is the same position used for measuring the thigh circumferences. A fold of skin and subcutaneous tissue is grasped in the midline about 2.0 cm above the marked point. The jaws of the skinfold calipers are placed perpendicular to the length of the fold and the shaft of the thigh over the marked point (see **Figure I.11c**). Skinfolds are recorded to the nearest 0.1 mm.

Sum of Skinfold Thickness

The sum of skinfold thickness was derived from body sites two and four:

Two-Site Sum of Skinfold Thickness (mm) = triceps + subscapular skinfold thickness

Four-Site Sum of Skinfold Thickness (mm) = triceps + subscapular skinfold + suprailiac + thigh thickness.

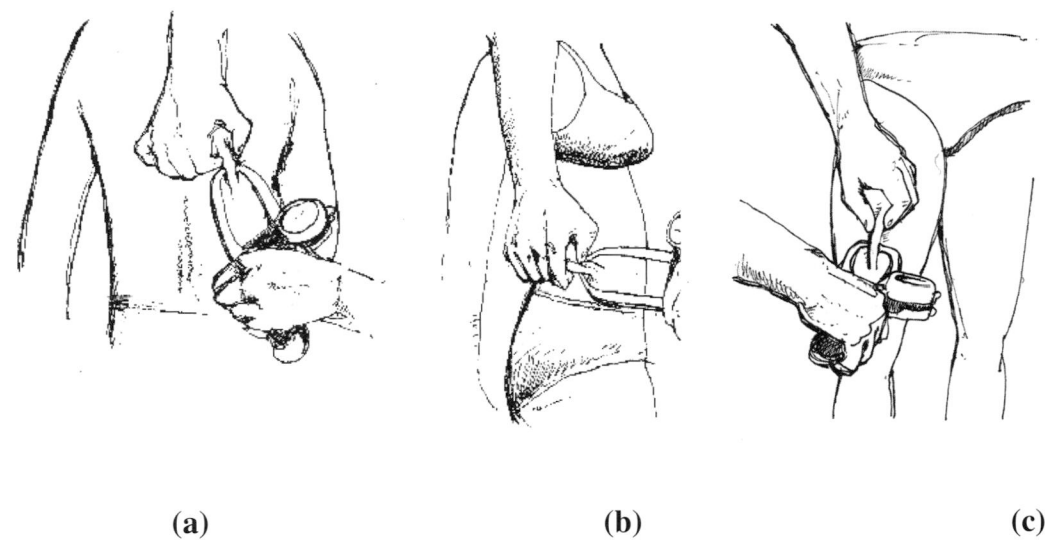

(a)   **(b)**   **(c)**

Figure I.11. Measurement of Subscapular (a) and Suprailiac (b) Skinfold Thickness, and (c) Mid-Thigh Skinfold Thickness.

Upper Arm Muscle, Fat Area, and Arm Fat Index

Upper Arm Muscle Area. Calculations of upper arm muscle and fat areas are based on measurements of the upper arm circumference and triceps skinfolds (see **Figure I.12**). The technique of computing upper arm areas using brachium radiographic shadow was originally used by Baker and associates (7), who assumed that the upper arm and its constituents are cylindrical. Since then, this approach has been applied to determine upper arm muscle and fat areas and circumferences from measurements of upper arm circumference and skinfold thickness (1,8,9). This technique assumes that the upper arm and its constituents are cylindrical, hence the corresponding areas of cross section are computed from the formula that yields the areas of a circle from its circumference. Letting C equal the circumference of the upper arm, the total area is calculated as:

Total Upper Arm Area (TUA) = $(C^2)/(4 \times \pi)$ (7)

Similarly, letting Ts equal the triceps skinfold thickness, the upper arm muscle area equals

Upper Arm Muscle Area (UMA) = $[C - (Ts \times \pi)]^2/(4 \times \pi)$ (8)

Then the upper arm fat area is calculated by subtraction

Upper Arm Fat Area (UFA) = (Total Upper Arm Area - Upper Arm Muscle Area)   (9)

Arm Fat Index (%) = (Upper arm fat area/Total upper arm area) x 100   (10)

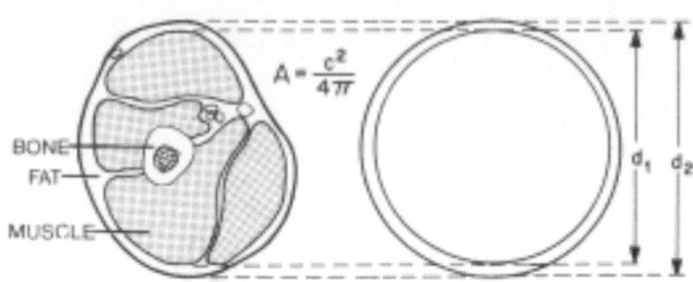

Figure I.12. Cross-Sectional View of the Upper Arm Tissue Areas, Derived from Measurements of Upper Arm Circumference (**Figure I.11a**) and Triceps Skinfold Thickness (**Figure I.11b**).

Example 1: A 12-year-old male had the following measurements:

Mid-Upper Arm Circumference (C) = 23.1 cm

Triceps Skinfold Thickness = 10.5 mm (or 1.5 cm)

Total Upper Arm Area (TUA) = $(C^2) \div (4 \times \pi)$

TUA = $(23.1^2/12.57) = 42.45$ cm^2

Upper Arm Muscle Area (UMA) (cm^2) = $(C - (3.1416 \times \text{Triceps Skinfold})^2)/12.57$

UMA = $(23.1 - (3.1416 \times 1.5)^2/12.57 = 28.90$ cm^2

Upper Arm Fat Area (FA) (cm^2) = Total Upper Arm Area (TUA) - Upper Arm Muscle Area (UMA)

FA = 42.45 - 28.90 = 13.55 cm^2

Arm Fat Index (AFI) (% Fat Area) = (13.55/42.45) x 100 = 31.92%

Example 2: A 21-year-old female had the following measurements:

Mid-Upper Arm Circumference (C) = 28.5 cm

Triceps Skinfold Thickness = 20 mm (or 2.0 cm)

Total Upper Arm Area (TUA) = $(C^2)/(4 \times \pi)$

TUA = $(28.5^2)/12.57 = 64.64$ cm^2

Upper Arm Muscle Area (UMA) (cm^2) = $(C - (3.1416 \times \text{Triceps Skinfold})^2)/12.57$

UMA = $(28.5 - 3.1416 \times 2.0)^2/12.57 = 39.27$ cm^2

Upper Arm Fat Area (FA) (cm^2) = Total Upper Arm Area (TUA) - Upper Arm Muscle Area (UMA)

FA = 64.64 - 39.27 = 25.37 cm^2

Arm Fat Index (AFI) (% fat area) = (25.37/64.64 x 100) = 39.25%

No-Correction of Muscle Area for Size of Bone in Adults

In previous publications the estimates of arm muscle area (UMA) in individuals older than 18 years were corrected for the area of the bone (9) by subtracting a constant from the muscle area of males and females (e.g., 10.0 cm^2 from the estimate of males and 6.5 cm^2 from the estimate of females). *However, because the bone area is not constant across individuals, these corrections distort the reference, the values of muscle area are not adjusted for size of bone.*

Limitation of Measurements of Upper Arm Muscle Area

As inferred from comparative studies, arm muscle area estimated by anthropometry overestimates the arm muscle area determined by CAT (computerized axial tomography) scans, and the degree of overestimation varies directly with the degree of adiposity (10). As a result, an anthropometric estimate of muscle area, especially among the obese or those whose triceps skinfold thickness exceeds the 85th age- and sex-specific percentiles, can give an excessive estimate of body muscle. For this reason, evaluation of nutritional status among the obese based upon anthropometric estimates of muscle area should be done with great caution. Similarly, evaluations of UAMA with reference to biochemical markers of muscle storage have been made. These evaluations indicate that estimates of fat-free mass, derived from anthropometric equations incorporating measurements of triceps and subscapular skinfolds, proved to be good predictors for muscularity before puberty in healthy children and are on par with the similarly easy-to-obtain UAMA during puberty (10,11).

Elbow Breadth

To measure elbow breadth, two instruments are available: (a) an anthropometric sliding caliper and (b) the frameter. *Sliding Caliper* (**Figure I.13b**). A broad faced sliding caliper is recommended for measuring elbow breadth. The subject's right arm is raised forward to the horizontal and the forearm is flexed to a right (90°) angle at the elbow, with the dorsum of the hand facing the examiner. The examiner stands in front, facing the subject, palpates the lateral and medial epicondyles of the humerus, and then places the caliper jaws parallel to, or slightly at a slant to, these two sites. The examiner then measures the greatest bony width across the elbow joint (see **Figure I.13b**). Obtaining accurate measurements of elbow breadth with the sliding

21

caliper requires expertise in measurement techniques. Erroneous information can be obtained because of difficulties in locating the anatomical landmarks and positioning the caliper jaws on the subject's arms. When this occurs, use the frameter instead. *Frameter* (**Figure I.13a**). The elbow breadth can also be measured with a frameter, which includes components that accurately measure the distance between the bony landmarks that demarcate elbow breadth, the medial and lateral epicondyles of the humerus. Direct the subject to extend his or her right arm and bend the forearm towards the shoulder at a 90° angle, turning the palm of the hand toward his or her body (see **Figure I.13a**). Place the subject's elbow on the baseboard against the fixed end board, making sure that the fixed end board is to the subject's left and the mobile board is to his or her right. Then slide the mobile board against the right side of the subject's elbow as firmly as possible, and read the actual elbow breadth measurement and the corresponding frame size for his or her sex.

Wrist Breadth

The examinee stands and extends the right arm, keeping the arm straight and near the side of the chest. The examiner stands to the right side of the examinee and guides the blades of the small sliding caliper with the thumb and first finger of each hand. The examiner palpates the most prominent aspect of the ulna styloid process with the middle or index finger of the right hand and slides the right blade of the caliper on to this landmark (see **Figure I.13c**). The most prominent aspect of the radial styloid process is located with the middle or index finger of the left hand. Firm pressure is applied and the breadth is recorded to the nearest 0.1 cm. Analysis of the data from the Fells Longitudinal Study indicates that wrist and biacromial breadths are more related to total body bone mineral content (BMQ), bone mineral density (BMD), and fat-free mass (FFM) than other measures of frame size, such as elbow and knee breadths (13). Furthermore, elbow breadth is probably more related to stature than it is to amounts of lean or fat tissue or bone (13).

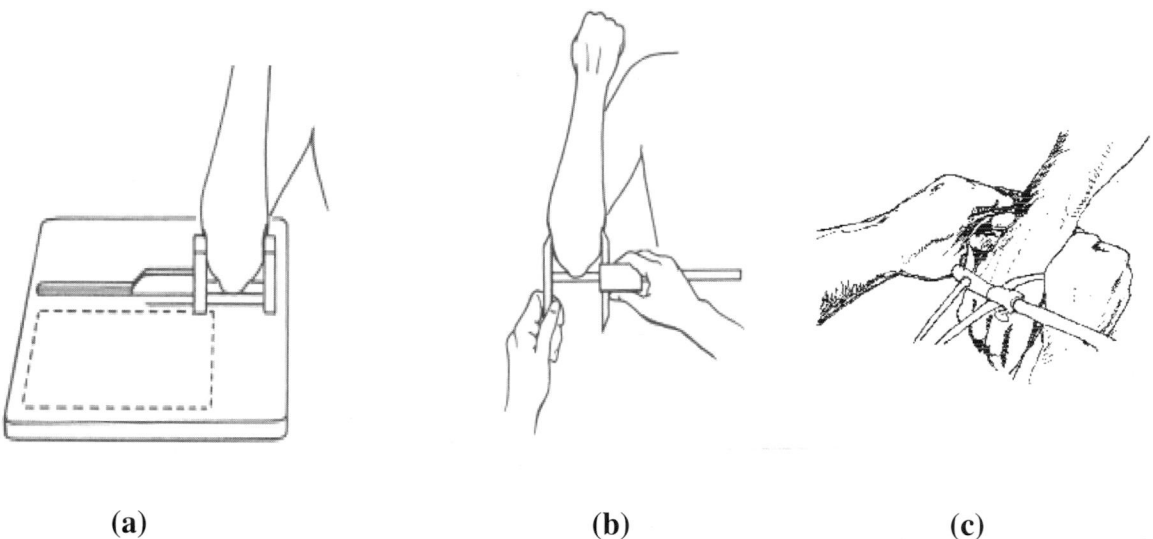

(a)   (b)   (c)

Figure I.13. Measurements of Elbow and Wrist Breadth. Elbow breadth with the frameter (a), with the sliding caliper (b), and (c) wrist breadth with the sliding caliper.

MEASUREMENTS OF BIOELECTRIC IMPEDANCE

To supplement the information derived from direct anthropometry, several approaches have been used to derive estimates of body composition employing various instruments. These include hydrostatic (underwater) weighing, plethysmograph, determination of total body water, total body potassium, total body nitrogen, dual-photon absorptiometry, and detecting the electrical conductivity and impedance of the body. These methods consider the body to be composed of either two or four compartments. The four-compartment model divides the body into four chemical groups: water, protein, minerals, and fat; whereas the two-compartment model assumes that the total body mass is composed of body fat and the fat-free mass. The estimates of percent body fat reported in this monograph were obtained using bioelectrical impedance techniques. This technique is based upon the principle that fat-free mass and body fat differ in their abilities to conduct an alternating electric current at low frequencies. For example, the fat-free mass, composed largely of electrolyte-containing water, will readily conduct an applied electric current, whereas fat is a poor conductor. The difference in the conductivity of these body constituents is a reflection of differences in their water and electrolyte concentrations.

At present, there are three types of instruments designed for measuring the flow of electricity through (a) the whole body (**Figure I.14a**), (b) the upper body (**Figure I.14b**), and (c) the lower body (**Figure I.14c**). Bioelectrical impedance (BI) measures the electrical property known as impedance, using a weak current of electricity passed through the body between electrodes on the wrist and ankle. Electrical impedance is the opposition of a material to the flow of an alternating electrical current that is frequency dependent, corresponding to the true resistance in a direct current. Electrical impedance is also equal to the sum of resistance and the reactance, which is the opposition to the flow of an alternating electric current made by an inductance coil or a condenser. In practice only bioelectric resistance (R) is measured. This is because the reactance of the human body, which is produced by the capacitant effects of tissue interfaces and cell membranes, is quite small and the value of bioelectric resistance is highly correlated with bioelectric impedance. From Ohm's Law, electrical impedance is proportional to the length of the conductor—a distance that is usually a function of the height of the subject—and indirectly proportional to the cross-sectional area. Equivalently, the impedance is proportional to the square of the length of the conductor/subject, divided by its volume.

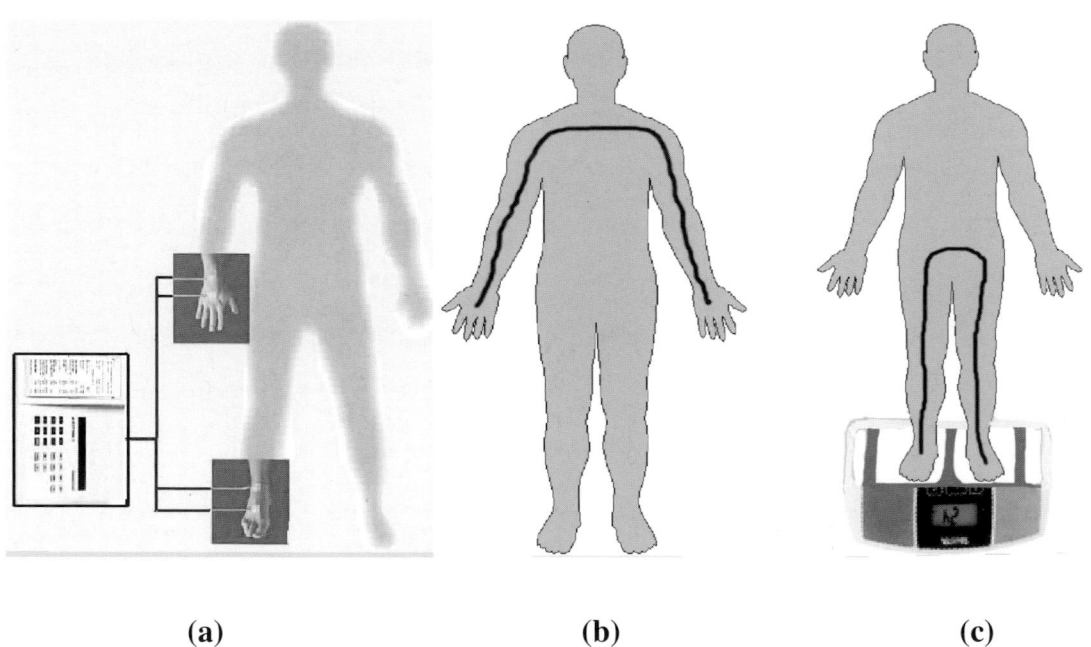

(a)   **(b)**   **(c)**

Figure I.14. Configuration of Electrodes and Path of the Electrical Current for Bioelectrical Impedance Analysis: Total Body (a), Upper Body Region (b), and Lower Body Region (c). (Source: Picture composed by the author).

Fat-Free Mass and Percent Body Fat

The estimates of percent body fat of the participants of NHANES III reported here were obtained using whole bioelectrical impedance (**Figure I.14a** and **Figure I.15**). The technique measures the impedance of a weak electrical current (800 μA; 50 KHz) passed between the right ankle and the right wrist of an individual. The measurements of bioelectric impedance (R) were obtained with a whole bioelectrical impedance analyzer (Valhalla 1990 Body Composition Analyzer, Valhalla Scientific, San Diego, CA).

Procedure. Subjects assumed a supine position with arms and feet spread apart and shoes and socks removed. The measurements of bioelectric impedance were performed by placing electrodes on the dorsal aspect of the right wrist midway between the radial and lunar processes, and the anterior aspect of the right foot (**see Figure I.15**). **Note:** the electrodes on the hand or foot should be no more than 2 inches apart. The measurement of BIA is based on the premise that when an electrical current is passed through the body, the voltage drop between two electrodes is proportional to the body's fluid volume in that region of the body. The voltage drop was measured and the resistance (R) calculated, while the current was kept constant. In these measurements it is assumed that the whole body acts like a cylindrical conductor and the conductor's length is proportional to the subject's height.

Therefore, the impedance index (Ht^2/R) is assumed to be proportional to the volume of the body.

Equations to Predict Body Composition from Bioelectric Impedance. Predictive equations for assessing body composition given in various instruments have been developed, using total body water measured by isotope dilution and underwater weighing as the reference methods (14,15). However, because these equations were based upon small, non-representative samples, they have limited applicability. To correct this problem, several equations for the prediction of body composition from measurement of bioelectric impedance based on large heterogeneous samples are being developed. Some equations estimate directly the lean body mass, while others first estimate total body water (TBW) and then compute the lean body mass (LBM). Generally, in adults and older children, the water content of the lean body mass (LBM) or fat-free mass (FFM) is constant at 0.732 L per kg (16). Under field conditions, total body water can be estimated using bioelectrical impedance analysis (14). Sun et al. (17), based on a statistically representative sample of 1474 whites and 355 blacks, ranging in age from 12 to 94 years, developed equations for estimating body water (TBW) and fat-free mass (FFM) from measurements of bioelectric resistance:

Males: FFM (kg) =

-10.678 + (0.262 x weight) + (0.652 x stature^2/resistance) + (0.02 x resistance)

Females: FFM (kg) =

-9.529 + (0.168 x weight) + (0.696 x stature^2/resistance) + (0.02 x resistance)

Estimates for total body fat (TBF) and percent body fat (%BF) for each participant were derived from their corresponding estimated FFM using the equations:

TBF (kg) = weight - FFM

%BF (%) = (TBF/weight) x 100

Fat-Free Mass and Fat Mass Indices

The fat-free mass index (FFMI) and fat mass index (FMI) have been proposed as indicators of nutritional status (18–22) and were derived by the following computations:

FFMI (kg/m^2) = FFM, kg/height, m^2

FMI (kg/m^2) = FM, kg/height, m^2

Advantages and Limitations. Bioelectrical impedance is safe and convenient, and the equipment is portable and relatively inexpensive. However, variability in hydration resulting from over-activity or physiological status can influence the measurements of resistance. In over-hydration, for example, resistance measurements will be higher, but lower in dehydration. For another example, vigorous exercise and consumption of excessive alcohol or excessive sweating can substantially alter the reading of impedance. Nevertheless, measurements of bioelectrical impedance do provide valuable information for assessing nutritional status and age-associated changes in body composition.

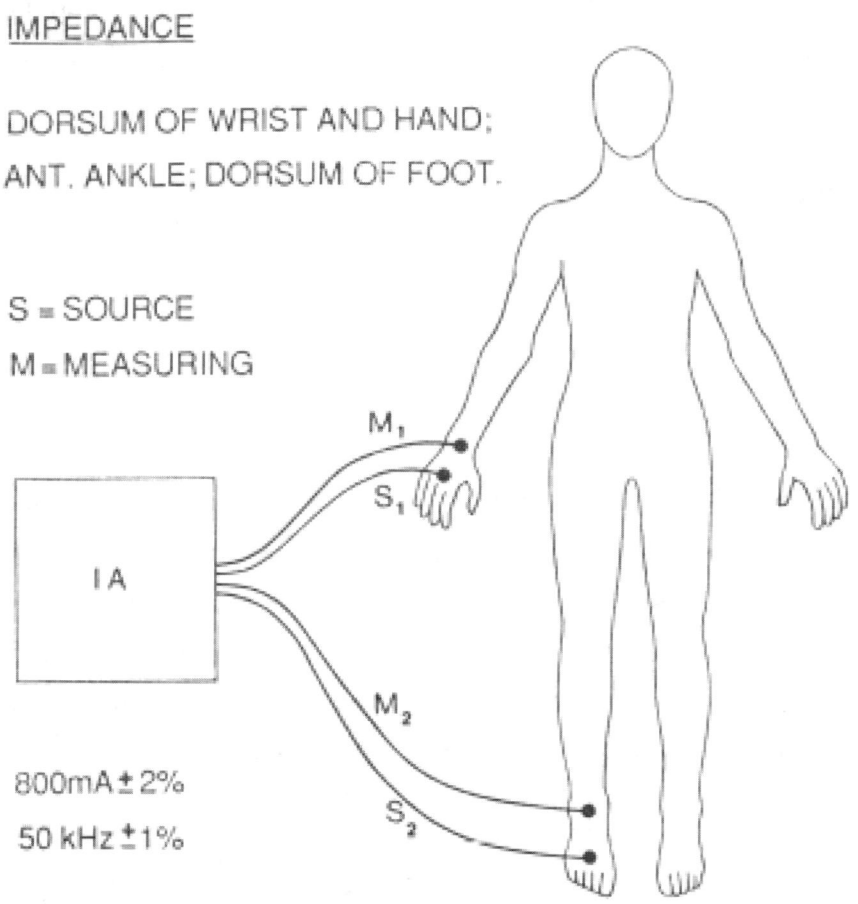

IMPEDANCE

DORSUM OF WRIST AND HAND;
ANT. ANKLE; DORSUM OF FOOT.

S = SOURCE
M = MEASURING

Figure I.15. Placement of Electrodes for the Measurements of Bioelectrical Impedance (R). **Note:** The electrodes on the hand or foot should be no more than 2 inches apart.

RELIABILITY OF ANTHROPOMETRIC MEASUREMENTS

Anthropometric evaluation, like other techniques, is subject to error in both data collection and interpretation. Therefore, researchers need to assess whether the degree of reliability of a given measurement is large or small. There are several statistical approaches for determining the reliability of obtaining information about anthropometric dimensions (23–26). A widely employed measure of replicability is the technical error of measurement. The technical error of measurement (**TEM**) is defined as the squared root of the sum of the squared differences (Σd^2) of replicates (the same measurements are taken on the same subject), divided by twice the number of pairs (2N). The mathematical expression is as follows:

$$\textbf{TEM} = [\sqrt{\Sigma} \ d^2/2N]$$

To adequately evaluate the validity of a given measurement, one needs to know both the inter- and intra-examiner technical measurement error. One way of assessing the accuracy of a given measurement is to compare the values of **TEM** with values obtained by well-trained anthropometrists (**Table I.3**). If the examiner's **TEM** comes close to the reference value (**Table I.2**) in a series of repeated measurements, and if there are no biases in measurement, then the measurements can be considered accurate. Reliability of a measurement can also be evaluated with reference to a coefficient calculated as:

$$\textbf{R} = 1 - (\textbf{TEM}^2/\textbf{s}^2)$$

where **R** is the coefficient of reliability that ranges from 0 to 1, **TEM**^{2} is the square of the technical error of measurement, and **s**^{2} is the square of the inter-subject variance. The coefficient indicates the degree to which a given measurement is error free. For example, a measurement reliability **R** = 0.80 indicates that the measurement is 80% free of error (23,24). With both the **TEM** and the **R** value the investigator can determine the permissible limits of accepting and interpreting inter- and intra-population differences in a given anthropometric dimension. Of course, such interpretation depends not only on the **TEM** but also on the scale of a given measurement. For example, when measuring upper arm tissues, it is best to evaluate them in terms of areas rather than actual circumferences. This point can be illustrated by the study of Hill et al. (26), which reports that the difference in measurements of upper arm circumference of patients before major surgery, and patients still in the hospital one week after, equaled only 1.1 cm (before = 23.3 cm and after = 22.2 cm). However, when the same values are expressed as areas, there is a difference of nearly 4 cm^2 (before = 43.19 cm^2 and after = 39.21 cm^2). For a comprehensive evaluation of inter-observer error in measurements of upper arm areas, the procedure of Hall et al. (27) should be used.

Table I.3. Reliability of Anthropometric Dimensions Given by Mean Intra- and Inter-Examiner Technical Error of Measurement*

Measurement	Technical Error of Measurement	
	Intra-Examiner	**Inter-Examiner**
	Mean	Mean
Height, Cervical (cm)	0.692	0.953
Sitting Height (cm)	0.535	0.705
Biacromial Breadth (cm)	0.544	0.915
Bitrochanteric Breadth (cm)	0.523	0.836
Elbow Breadth (cm)	0.117	0.154
Wrist Breadth (cm)	0.115	0.139
Upper Arm Circumference (cm)	0.347	0.425
Triceps Skinfold Thickness (mm)	0.800	1.890
Subscapular Skinfold Thickness (mm)	1.830	1.530
Midaxillary Skinfold Thickness (mm)	2.080	1.470

*Adapted from refer. #23: Malina et al. (1973), and refer. #24: Johnston et al. (1972).

As measuring techniques are usually learned via instruction of an expert or supervisor, there is a need to determine when a trainee or anthropometrist is ready to perform the measurement accurately. With this purpose in mind, Zerfas (28) has developed a versatile method that monitors the measuring ability of trainees as well as other sources of error. A basic principle of this method is to compare the measurements obtained by the trainee to the measurements obtained by the expert or supervisor. Based on more than 50 tests during large-scale nutrition tests on young children in developing countries and from various sources in the literature, four categories have been established for stature (or length), arm circumference, weight, and triceps skinfold thickness. These categories are given in **Table I.4**. From these data, it is evident that a difference of more than 20 mm (2 cm) between the expert's and the trainee's measurements indicates a gross error related to reading or recording imprecision. An error in the range of 10 to 19 mm indicates that the trainee is not yet ready to take accurate measurements. A difference in the expert's and trainee's measurements of 0 to 5 mm indicates that the trainee has reached an acceptable level of proficiency in measuring.

Table I.4. Evaluation of Measurement Error Among Trainees*

| Measurement | Difference Between Trainee and Supervisor | | | |
	Good	Fair	Poor	Gross Error
Height (mm)	0.0 to 5.0	6.0 to 9.0	10.0 to 19.0	20.0 or >
Arm Circumference (mm)	0.0 to 5.0	6.0 to 9.0	10.0 to 19.0	20.0 or >
Weight (kg)	0.0 to 0.1	>0.2	0.3 to 0.4	0.5 or >
Skinfold (mm)	0.0 to 0.9	1.0 to 1.9	2.0 to 4.9	5.0 or >

*Adapted from refer. #28: Zerfas (1985).

LITERATURE CITED

1. Frisancho, A.R. 1990. Anthropometric Standards for the Assessment of Growth and Nutritional Status. Ann Arbor, MI: University of Michigan Press.

2. National Center for Health Statistics. 1996. NHANES III reference manuals and reports. Hyattsville, MD: National Center for Health Statistics (CD-ROM).

3. Lohman, T.G., Roche, A.F., Martorell, R. (Eds.). 1988. In: Anthropometric Standardization Reference Manual. Champaign, IL: Human Kinetics Books.

4. Evidence Report of Clinical Guidelines on the Identification, Evaluation, and Treatment of Overweight and Obesity in Adults. 1998. NIH/National Heart, Lung, and Blood Institute (NHLBI).

5. Seidell, J.C. 2001. Waist and hip circumferences have independent and opposite effects on cardiovascular disease risk factors: the Quebec Family Study. Am. J. Clin. Nutr. 74:315–21.

6. Hsieh, S.D., Yoshinaga, H., Muto, T. 2003. Waist-to-height ratio, a simple and practical index for assessing central fat distribution and metabolic risk in Japanese men and women. Intern. J. Obesity 27:610–16.

7. Baker, P.T., Hunt, E.E. Jr., Sen, T. 1958. The growth and interrelations of skinfolds and brachial tissues in man. Am. J. Phys. Anthropol. 16:39–58.

8. Gurney, T.M., Jelliffe, D.B. 1973. Arm muscle circumference and cross-sectional muscle and fat areas. Am. J. Clin. Nutr. 26:912–15.

9. Heymsfield, S.B., McManus, C., Smith, J., Stevens, V., Nixon, D.W. 1982. Anthropometric measurement of muscle mass: revised equations for calculating bone-free arm muscle area. Am. J. Clin. Nutr. 36:680–90.

10. Forbes, G.B., Brown, M.R., Griffiths, H.J.L. 1988. Arm muscle plus bone area: anthropometry and CAT scan compared. Am. J. Clin. Nutr. 47:929–31.

11. Boye, K.R., Dimitriou, T., Manz, F., Schoenau, E., Neu, Ch., Wudy, S., Remer, T. 2002. Anthropometric assessment of muscularity during growth: estimating fat-free mass with 2 skinfold-thickness measurements is superior to measuring mid-upper arm muscle area in healthy prepubertal children. Am. J. Clin. Nutr. 76:628–32.

12. Himes, J.H., Frisancho, A.R. 1988. Estimating frame size. In: Lohman, T.G., Roche, A.F., Martorell, R., eds. Anthropometric Standardization Reference Manual. Champaign, IL: Human Kinetics Books. 121–24.

13. Chumlea, W.C, Wisemandle, W., Guo, S.S., Siervogel, R.M. 2002. Relations between frame size and body composition and bone mineral status. Am. J. Clin. Nutr. 75:1012–6.

14. Kushner, R.F., Schoeller, D.A., Fjeld, C.R., Danford, L. 1992. Is the impedance index (Ht^2/R) significant in predicting total body water? Am. J. Clin. Nutr. 56:835–39.

15. Ellis, K.J. 2001. Selected body composition methods can be used in field studies. J. Nutr. [Suppl] 131:1589–95.

16. Wang, Z.M., Deurenberg, P., Wang, W., Pietrobelli, A., Baumgartner, R.N., Heymsfield, S.B. 1999. Hydration of fat-free mass: review and critique of a classic body composition constant. Am. J. Clin. Nutr. 69:833–41.

17. Sun, S.S., Chumlea, W.C., Heymsfield, S.B., Lukaski, H.C., Schoeller, D., Friedl, K., Kuczmarski, R.J., Flegal, K.M., Johnson, C.L., Hubbard, V.S. 2003. Development of bioelectrical impedance analysis prediction equations for body composition with the use of a multicomponent model for use in epidemiologic surveys. Am. J. Clin. Nutr. 77:331–40.

18. VanItallie, T.B., Yang, M.U., Heymsfield, S.B., Funk, R.C., Boileau, R.A. 1990. Height-normalized indices of the body's fat-free mass and fat mass: potentially useful indicators of nutritional status. Am. J. Clin. Nutr. 52:953–59.

19. Bartlett, H.L., Puhl, S.M., Hodgson, J.L., Buskirk, E.R. 1991. Fat-free mass in relation to stature: ratios of fat-free mass to height in children, adults, and elderly subjects. Am. J. Clin. Nutr. 53:1112–16.

20. Hattori, K., Tatsumi, N., Tanaka, S. 1997. Assessment of body composition by using a new chart method. Am. J. Hum. Biol. 9:573–78.

21. Schutz, Y., Kyle, U.U.G., Pichard, C. 2002. Fat-free mass index and fat Caucasians aged 18–98 years. International Journal of Obesity 26:953–60.

22. Freedman, D.S., Wang, J., Maynard, L.M., Thornton, J.C., Meil, Z., Pierson, R.N. Jr., Dietz, W.H., Horlick, M. 2005. Relation of BMI to fat and fat-free mass among children and adolescents. International Journal of Obesity 29:1–8.

23. Malina, R.M., Hamill, P.V.V., Lemeshow, S. 1973. Selected body measurements of children 6–11 years. U.S. Vital & Health Statistics, Series 11, No. 123, USDHHS, Washington D.C.

24. Johnston, F.E., Hamill, P.V.V., Lemeshow, S. 1972. Skinfold thicknesses of children 6–11 years. U.S. Vital & Health Statistics, Series 11, No. 120, USDHHS, Washington D.C.

25. Mueller, W.H., Martorell, R. 1988. Reliability and accuracy of measurement. In: Lohman, T.G., Roche, A.F., Martorell, R., eds., Anthropometric Standardization Reference Manual. Champaign, IL: Human Kinetics Books.

26. Hill, G.L., Blackett, R.L., Pickford, I., Burkinshaw, L., Young, G.A., Warren, J.V., Schorah, C.J., Morgan, D.B. 1977. Malnutrition in surgical patients. Lancet 1:689.

27. Hall, J.C., O'Quigley, J., Giles, G.R., Appleton, N., Stocks, H. 1980. Upper limb anthropometry: the value of measurement variance studies. Am. J. Clin. Nutr. 33:1846–51.

28. Zerfas, A.J. 1985. Checking continuous measures: manual for anthropometry. Division of Epidemiology, School of Public Health, University of California, Los Angeles, CA 90024.

CHAPTER II
ANTHROPOMETRIC REFERENCES OF PREGNANCY WEIGHT GAIN AND PRENATAL GROWTH

REFERENCE OF PREGNANCY WEIGHT GAIN
Recommended Weight Gains During Pregnancy
Early Pattern of Weight Gain and Birth Weight

REFERENCE OF PRENATAL GROWTH AND BIRTH WEIGHT
Birth Weight Percentiles
Classification of Newborns by Gestational Length
Classification of Newborns by Birth Weight
Classification of Newborns by Both Gestational Age and Birth Weight
Evaluation of Prenatal Growth Status of African-American Black Newborns
Reference of Rohrer Index

SUMMARY

LITERATURE CITED

CHAPTER II
ANTHROPOMETRIC REFERENCES OF PREGNANCY
WEIGHT GAIN AND PRENATAL GROWTH

Pregnancy is associated with an increase in the nutritional requirements. On the average the energy cost of pregnancy is about 68,000 kcal. Thus, an extra 250 kcal/day must be ingested to support the increased nutritional requirements of pregnancy. The increased cost is associated with growth of new maternal and fetal tissues. The cumulative effect of the new tissue growth is reflected in the increased weight and fat gain of pregnancy. This chapter focuses on the anthropometric references to evaluate weight gain during pregnancy, prenatal growth, and nutritional status during pregnancy.

REFERENCE OF PREGNANCY WEIGHT GAIN
Recommended Weight Gains During Pregnancy

On the average the energy cost of pregnancy is about 68,000 kcal (1,2). Thus, an extra 250 kcal/day must be ingested to support the increased nutritional requirements of pregnancy. The increased cost is associated with the growth of new maternal and fetal tissues, which is reflected in the pregnancy weight gain. The weight gain during pregnancy is quite variable and no single maternal weight gain target meets the needs of all categories of pregnant women, but in general the recommended weight gain is different for adults and non-adults.

Adults. Individualized patterns of weight gain must be adjusted for height and pre-pregnancy weight. Since the body mass index (BMI) is a relative measure of weight per unit of height, it provides a good reference for determining targets of weight gain. Several studies have consistently found that prenatal weight gain within the suggested range for each pre-gravid BMI category is associated with more favorable outcomes than is weight gain above or below the suggested range (3,4). These outcomes include a reduction in the prevalence of low-birth-weight infants (<2500 g), small-for-gestational age infants, large-for-gestational age infants, high-birth-weight infants (>4500 g), cesarean deliveries (3,4), and preterm deliveries, as well as an increase in mean birth weight.

Accordingly, the Subcommittee on Nutritional Status and Weight Gain during Pregnancy of the U.S. National Academy of Sciences (5) recommends that weight gain during pregnancy should be done with reference to body mass index (BMI) **(Table II.1)**. Thus, the recommended weight gain for a woman with a low pre-pregnancy BMI is 12.5 to 18 kilograms (28 to 48 pounds), for a woman with an average pre-pregnancy BMI is 11.5 to 16 kilograms (25 to 35 pounds), and for a woman with a high pre-pregnancy BMI is 7.0 to 11.5 kilograms (15 to 25 pounds). These recommendations are related to the fact that greater weight gains are most effective in increasing birth weight among women of low pre-pregnancy weight, but are less effective in overweight women. The recommended target weight gain range for women carrying twins is 16 to 20.5 kilograms (35 to 45 pounds).

Table II.1. Recommended Amount of Pregnancy Weight Gain by Category of Weight and Body Mass Index*

Category	BMI[1] (kg/cm^2)	Weight Gain	
		(kg)	(lb.)
Underweight	<19.8	12.7-18.2	28-40
Average weight	19.8-26.0	11.4-16.0	25-35
Overweight	>26.0-29.0	6.8-11.4	15-25

*Adapted from refer. #5: Subcommittee on Nutritional Status and Weight Gain During Pregnancy, Nutritional Status and Weight Gain During Pregnancy of the Food and Nutrition Board, Institute of (1990).
[1]BMI in metric = (Weight, kg/Height, m^2; or BMI in English = [(Weight, lb./Height, in./Height, in.) x 703].

Non-adults. Previous studies indicate that for still-growing, non-adults under the age of 15 years, about 1 kilogram of the pregnancy weight gain represents the normal growth (6-10). Therefore, the recommended target weight gain range for still-growing non-adults under the age of 15 years should be increased by 1.0 kilograms (2.20 pounds).

Early Pattern of Weight Gain and Birth Weight

Various studies indicate that in both black and white women, increasing weight gain during pregnancy is associated with higher birth weight. These studies indicate a linear rate of about 0.66 pounds per week from 8 through 20 weeks of gestation and a linear rate of 1.06 pounds per week after week 20 (11). However, from a functional and evolutionary point of view, weight gain during the first trimester of pregnancy is an opportunistic adaptation whereby energy is stored early, when the growth needs of the fetus are low, to be used during the second and third trimester, when the energy needs for growth of the fetus are high. In this context, the pattern of early pregnancy weight gain would be even more advantageous under conditions of maternal undernutrition. In the developing nations chronically undernourished women are able to reproduce even though the cost of pregnancy (68,000 Kcalories or 250 kcal/day) exceeds their resources. Then, it is quite possible that women in such conditions gaining weight during the first trimester would be able to store energy that can be used to feed the growth needs of the fetus during the last trimester. This pattern of weight gain represents an opportunistic adaptation that enables women to reproduce even under the most limited nutritional conditions. Furthermore, a pattern of weight gain during the first or second trimester, rather than the third trimester, would also have adaptive significance for well-nourished women, since women who gain weight excessively after mid-pregnancy retained more weight after pregnancy. Therefore, gaining weight early in pregnancy may also be of benefit for promoting postpartum weight loss. Recent studies of 389 women from Minnesota (**Figure II.1**) indicate that maternal weight gain occurring primarily in the first and second trimesters of pregnancy is associated with higher birth weight than weight gain occurring in the third trimester (12).

In summary, it is recommended that evaluation of nutritional status during pregnancy be done through measurements of pregnancy weight gain with reference to body mass index, rather than height and weight only. These recommendations should done taking into account that a weight gain during the first trimester is more conducive to higher birth weight than is a uniform weight gain throughout pregnancy. Although women who gain excess weight account for a growing proportion of cesarean deliveries, extensive studies indicate that excess weight gain and macrosomia are not the primary factors that contribute to the recent increase in cesarean delivery (13,14).

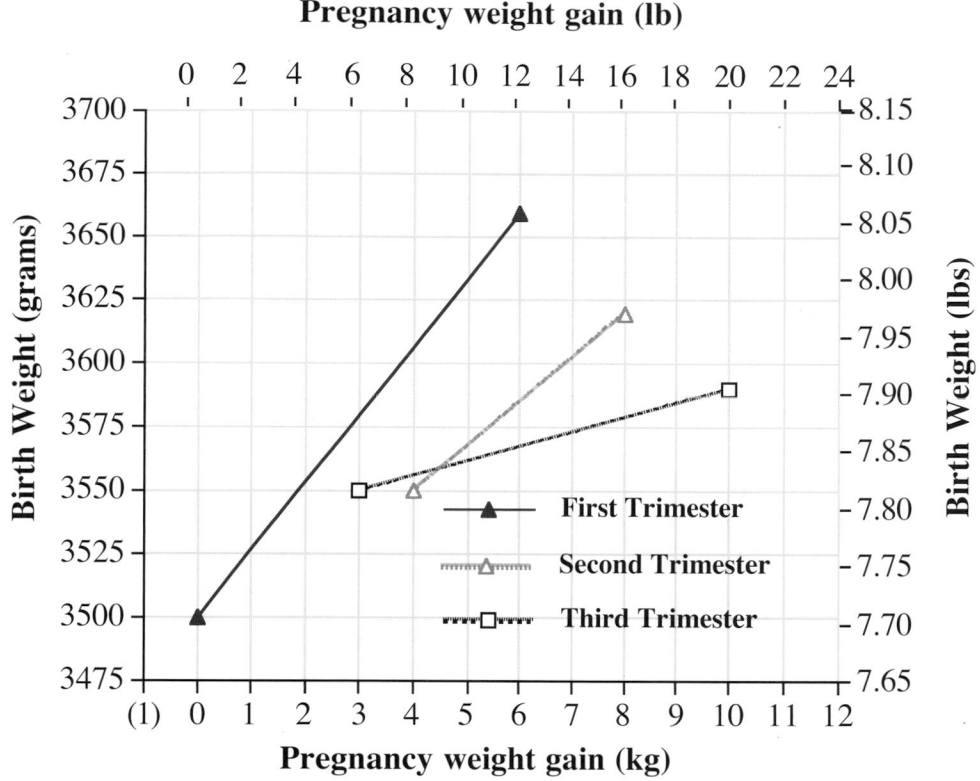

Figure II.1. Early Pregnancy Weight Gain and Birth Weight. Data from refer. #12: Brown et al. (2002).

REFERENCE OF PRENATAL GROWTH AND BIRTH WEIGHT

Birth Weight Percentiles

There are several references of birth weight percentiles that have been used by clinicians and researchers to assess fetal growth in individual infants and in populations (15,16). Recently, new references using the 2001-2002 nationwide United States Natality Datasets have been published (17,18). For the present series the references of birth weight for whites and black derived from population samples from the USA (17,18). In addition, the references of white newborns from Canada (19) have been selected. The rationale for the selection of these references is that they were (a) based on large representative samples, (b) excluded still-births, multiple pregnancies, malformations, and birth defects, and (c) the gestational ages, determined using ultrasound assessment and/or date of last menstrual period, are based on completed weeks. The World Health Organization (WHO) recommends basing gestational age on the number of completed weeks. The birth weight percentiles of the Canadians were based on a sample that included 347,570 singleton males and 329,035 singleton females, with recorded gestational ages of 22 to 43 weeks (19). The USA birth weight percentiles were based upon information derived from 6,690,717 singleton infants with recorded birth weight and sex born to United States resident mothers in 1999 and 2000, published by Oken (17) and originally derived from the US Natality Datasets published in 2002 (18). Given the recent and large size of the sample these percentiles are more appropriate than those given in previous references (15,16).

Classification of Newborns by Gestational Length

The average gestation length for full term infants is 37 weeks. Based on gestational age at delivery, newborns are classified into three categories. (a) Pre-term or premature. Infants born with gestational age of less than 37 weeks (less than 259 days). (b) Term or full term. Infants born with gestational age of more than 37 weeks (>259 to 293 days) but less than 42 completed weeks. (c) Post-term. Infants born with gestational age of more than 42 completed weeks (>294 days). Thus, the term *premature* is used for infants born before 37 weeks of gestation.

Classification of Newborns by Birth Weight

Birth weight is the final common pathway for the expression of pregnancy and pre-natal growth. The frequency of birth weight follows a normal (or bell-shaped) distribution (**Figure II. 2**). In general, at the individual and population level, birth weights that are between 5.5 and 4.5 kilograms (6 to 11 pounds), or are within the average for the population, have lower postnatal negative health risk factors than birth weights below 2.5 kilograms (<5.5 pounds) or above 5.5 kilograms (>12 pounds). Therefore, evaluation of birth weight provides retrospective information about the maturity and nutritional status of the newborn.

Classification of Newborns by Both Gestational Age and Birth Weight

Using as a reference the data presented in **Tables II.2, II.3,** and **II.4** and **Figures II.3** to **II.6**, newborns can be classified into three groups: small-for-gestational age (SGA), appropriate-for-gestational age (AGA), and large-for-gestational age (LGA).

Small-for-Gestational Age or Intra-Uterine Retarded. Small-for-gestational age (SGA) infant refers to weight status at birth, while the term intrauterine growth retardation (IUGR) is sometimes applied to SGA infants. Intrauterine growth retardation refers to fetal growth that has been limited by an inadequate prenatal environment. Infants that are born after at least 37 weeks of gestation and weigh less than 2500 grams (<5.5 pounds) at birth are considered intra-uterine growth retarded. Due to the difficulties of determining accurately the gestational age, low birth weight (<2500 grams) is often used as a proxy for IUGR.

Appropriate-for-Gestational Age. A newborn whose weight corresponds to gestational age, or is between the 10th and 90th percentiles for gestational age, is considered appropriate-for-gestational age (AGA).

Large-for-Gestational Age. A newborn that weighs above the 90th percentile for gestational age is considered large-for-gestational age (LGA).

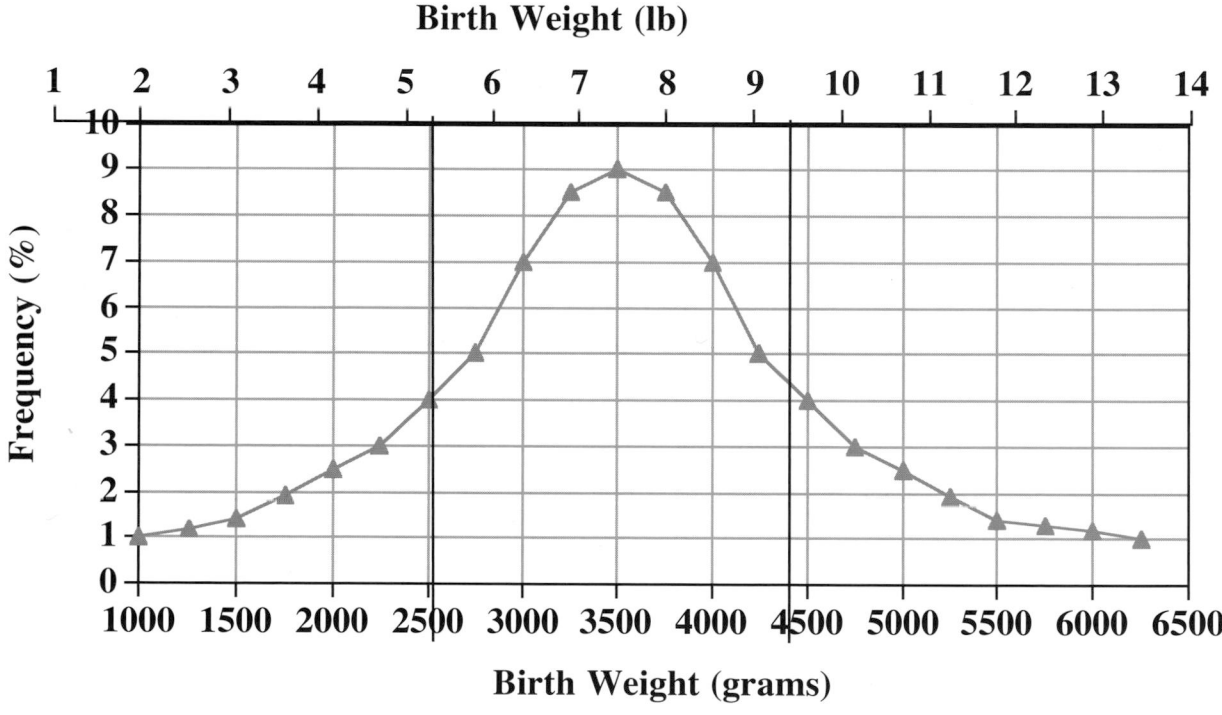

Figure II.2. Distribution of Birth Weights. In most populations birth weights fall in a normal or bell-shaped distribution. Data from refer. #20: Frisancho (2000).

Table II.2. Birth Weight Percentiles by Completed Gestational Ages and Sex*

Gestational Age (weeks)	Percentile: Males					Percentile: Females				
	10th	25th	50th	75th	90th	10th	25th	50th	75th	90th
22	394	454	520	606	755	364	424	482	568	725
23	454	531	597	686	814	419	482	564	645	781
24	502	595	680	784	917	473	551	626	732	872
25	558	675	771	889	1040	507	618	712	822	969
26	599	758	898	1047	1234	562	705	835	972	1186
27	680	856	1023	1187	1426	628	780	947	1112	1397
28	775	974	1170	1387	1762	699	891	1087	1306	1736
29	914	1134	1360	1616	2160	852	1054	1286	1593	2274
30	1052	1315	1577	1977	2601	976	1230	1500	1978	2642
31	1254	1535	1834	2401	2933	1188	1457	1777	2489	2965
32	1486	1764	2115	2726	3164	1401	1693	2061	2771	3185
33	1724	2027	2410	2984	3362	1651	1951	2371	2968	3334
34	1968	2278	2658	3140	3505	1883	2194	2597	3085	3449
35	2204	2505	2849	3255	3625	2110	2416	2771	3185	3544
36	2422	2704	3013	3353	3691	2310	2590	2904	3244	3584
37	2620	2895	3193	3504	3814	2507	2774	3068	3377	3674
38	2819	3077	3366	3669	3957	2705	2955	3232	3520	3815
39	2956	3203	3489	3788	4071	2842	3080	3354	3646	3925
40	3037	3288	3580	3880	4156	2928	3170	3441	3732	4013
41	3073	3334	3636	3944	4241	2959	3212	3494	3790	4071
42	2990	3271	3583	3903	4212	2903	3158	3451	3760	4042
43	2960	3236	3537	3857	4156	2857	3118	3408	3715	3992
44	2965	3244	3545	3858	4156	2873	3130	3411	3718	4014

*Percentiles calculated from refer. #17: Oken et al. 2003. A nearly continuous measure of birth weight for gestational age using a United States national reference. BMC Pediatr 8:3-6. http://www.biomedcentral.com/1471-2431/3/6.

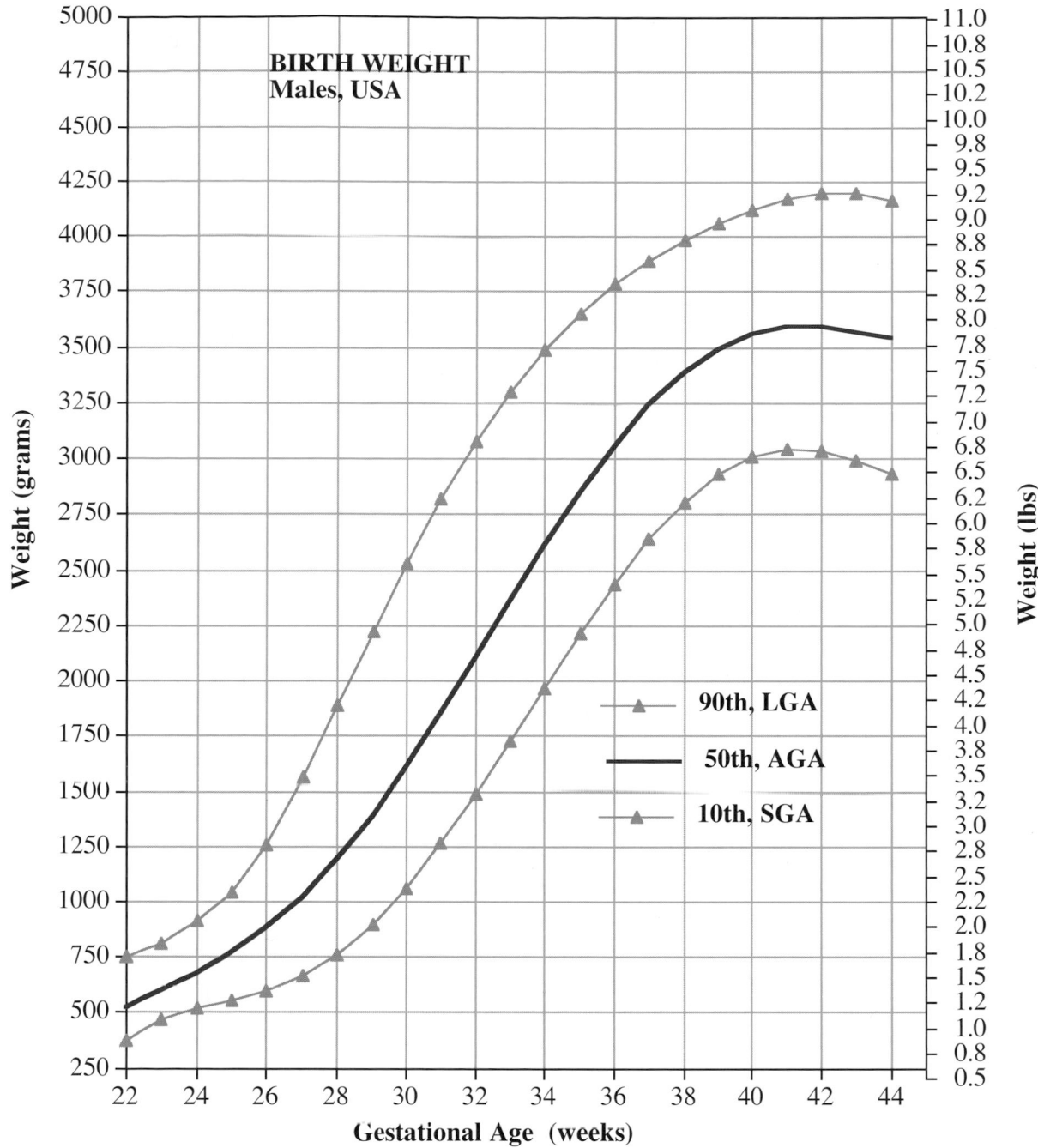

Figure II.3. Percentiles of Birth Weight (grams) for Determining Prenatal Growth Status for White Male Infants. SGA = a newborn that weighs below the 10th percentiles for gestational age, AGA = a newborn whose weight is between the 10th and 90th percentiles for gestational age, LGA = a newborn that weighs above the 90th percentiles for gestational age. (*Percentiles calculated from refer. #17: Oken et al. 2003. A nearly continuous measure of birth weight for gestational age using a United States national reference. BMC Pediatr 8:3-6. http://www.biomedcentral.com/1471-2431/3/6.)

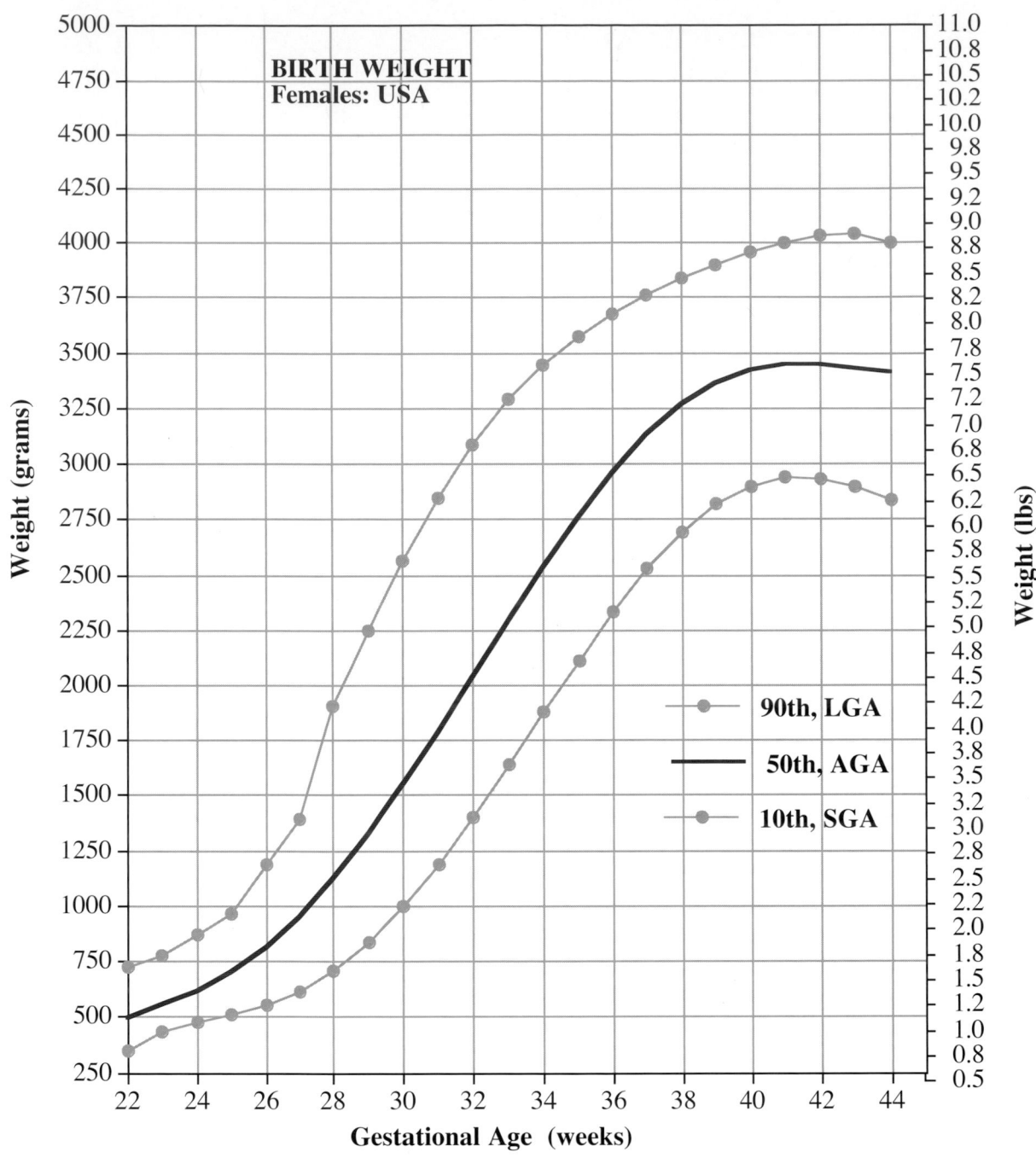

Figure II.4. Percentiles of Birth Weight (grams) for Determining Prenatal Growth Status for White Female Infants. SGA = a newborn that weighs below the 10th percentiles for gestational age, AGA = a newborn whose weight is between the 10th and 90th percentiles for gestational age, LGA = a newborn that weighs above the 90th percentiles for gestational age. (Percentiles calculated from refer. #17: Oken et al. 2003. A nearly continuous measure of birth weight for gestational age using a United States national reference. BMC Pediatr 8:3-6. http://www.biomedcentral.com/1471-2431/3/6.)

Table II.3. Birth Weight (g) for Gestational Age (weeks) for White Canadian Singleton Males*

Gestational Age (weeks)	N	3rd	5th	10th	Percentile 50th	90th	95th	97th	Mean	SD
22	82	338	368	401	490	587	627	659	501	111
23	114	406	434	475	589	714	762	797	598	114
24	156	468	498	547	690	844	902	940	697	125
25	202	521	557	617	795	981	1048	1092	800	147
26	234	571	614	686	908	1125	1200	1251	909	178
27	254	627	677	763	1033	1278	1358	1416	1026	209
28	330	694	752	853	1173	1445	1532	1598	1159	241
29	392	780	845	964	1332	1629	1729	1809	1312	273
30	467	885	959	1099	1507	1837	1955	2053	1487	306
31	584	1012	1098	1259	1698	2069	2209	2327	1682	339
32	997	1164	1266	1444	1906	2319	2478	2614	1896	369
33	1368	1344	1460	1648	2127	2580	2750	2897	2123	391
34	2553	1552	1677	1866	2360	2851	3029	3184	2361	410
35	4314	1783	1907	2091	2600	3132	3318	3475	2607	428
36	9648	2024	2144	2321	2845	3411	3604	3759	2855	443
37	19,965	2270	2384	2552	3080	3665	3857	4003	3091	449
38	51,947	2498	2605	2766	3290	3877	4065	4202	3306	448
39	77,623	2684	2786	2942	3465	4049	4232	4361	3489	445
40	112,737	2829	2927	3079	3613	4200	4382	4501	3638	447
41	54,139	2926	3025	3179	3733	4328	4512	4631	3745	459
42	8791	2960	3070	3233	3815	4433	4631	4773	3800	485
43	276	2954	3081	3249	3864	4528	4747	4941	3793	527

*Source: Refer. #19: Kramer, M.S., Platt, R.W., Wen, S.W., Joseph, K.S., Allen, A., Abrahamowicz, M., Blondel, B., Breart, G. Fetal/Infant Health Study Group of the Canadian Perinatal Surveillance System. 2001. A new and improved population-based Canadian reference for birth weight for gestational age. Pediatrics 108(2):E35.

Table II.4. Birth Weight (g) for Completed Gestational Age (weeks) for White Canadian Singleton Females*

Gestational Age (weeks)	N	3rd	5th	10th	Percentile 50th	90th	95th	97th	Mean	SD
22	80	332	347	385	466	552	576	576	472	72
23	106	379	403	450	557	669	706	726	564	95
24	148	424	456	513	651	790	839	887	656	121
25	184	469	508	578	751	918	982	1060	754	152
26	191	516	562	645	858	1060	1139	1247	860	186
27	188	569	624	717	976	1218	1313	1446	976	222
28	287	634	697	802	1109	1390	1499	1657	1107	254
29	299	716	787	903	1259	1578	1701	1885	1256	286
30	390	814	894	1022	1427	1783	1918	2121	1422	319
31	461	938	1026	1168	1613	2004	2150	2347	1604	345
32	795	1089	1184	1346	1817	2242	2399	2578	1808	368
33	1055	1264	1369	1548	2035	2494	2664	2825	2029	389
34	2018	1467	1581	1768	2266	2761	2948	3097	2266	409
35	3391	1695	1813	1998	2506	3037	3242	3384	2512	426
36	8203	1935	2052	2227	2744	3307	3523	3660	2754	439
37	17,308	2177	2286	2452	2968	3543	3752	3886	2981	443
38	47,516	2406	2502	2658	3169	3738	3931	4061	3181	439
39	75,068	2589	2680	2825	3334	3895	4076	4202	3350	434
40	110,738	2722	2814	2955	3470	4034	4212	4331	3486	434
41	52,063	2809	2906	3051	3576	4154	4330	4444	3588	439
42	7970	2849	2954	3114	3655	4251	4423	4554	3656	448
43	277	2862	2975	3159	3717	4333	4495	4685	3693	459

*Source: Refer. #19: Kramer, M.S., Platt, R.W., Wen, S.W., Joseph, K.S., Allen, A., Abrahamowicz, M., Blondel, B., Breart, G. Fetal/Infant Health Study Group of the Canadian Perinatal Surveillance System. 2001. A new and improved population-based Canadian reference for birth weight for gestational age. Pediatrics 108(2):E35.

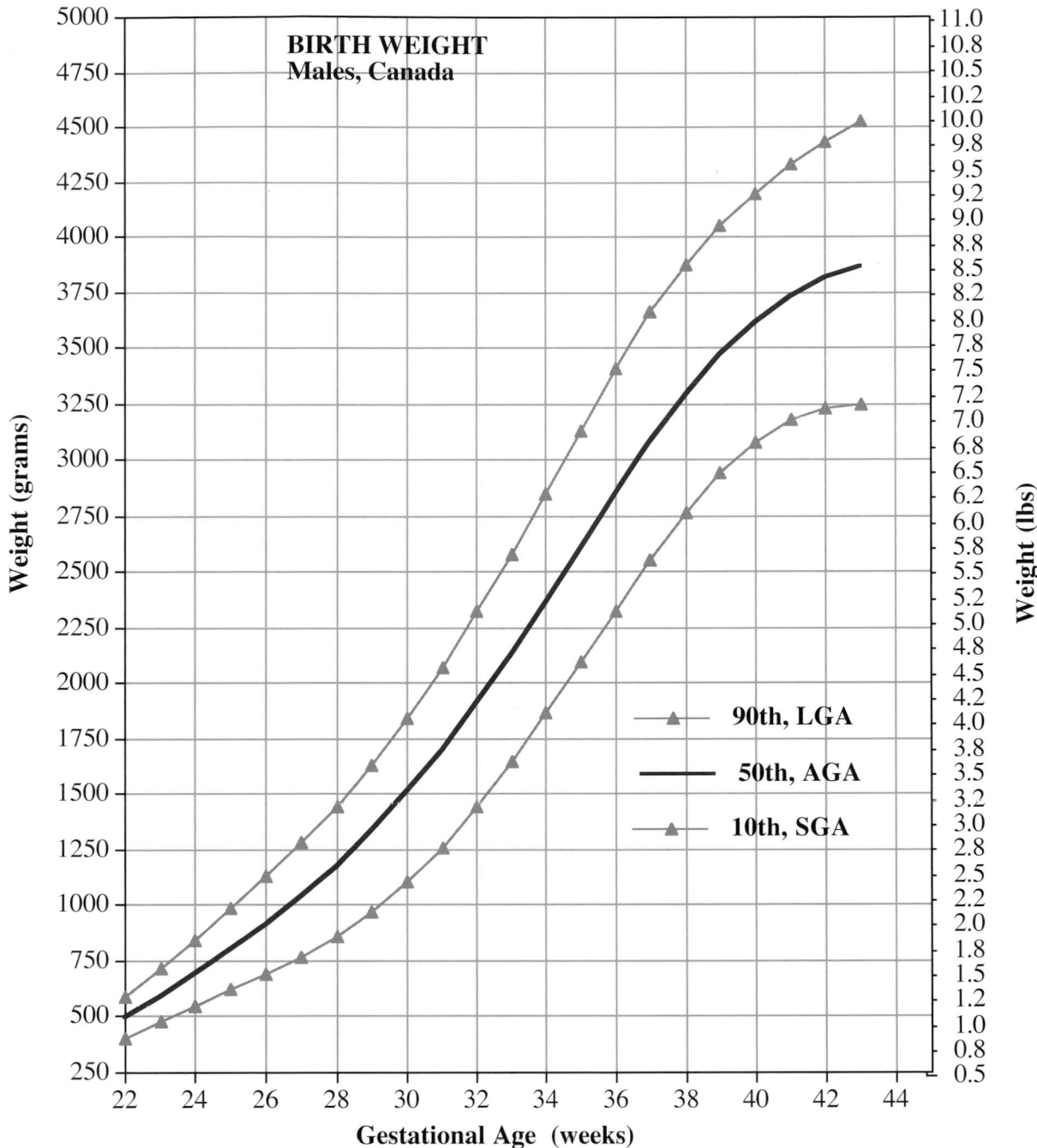

Figure II.5. Percentiles of Birth Weight (grams) for Determining Prenatal Growth Status for White Male Infants. SGA = a newborn that weighs below the 10th percentiles for gestational age, AGA = a newborn whose weight is between the 10th and 90th percentiles for gestational age, LGA = a newborn that weighs above the 90th percentiles for gestational age. (*Derived from the data given in refer. #19: Kramer et al. 2001. A new and improved population-based Canadian reference for birth weight and gestational age. Pediatrics 108:1-7.)

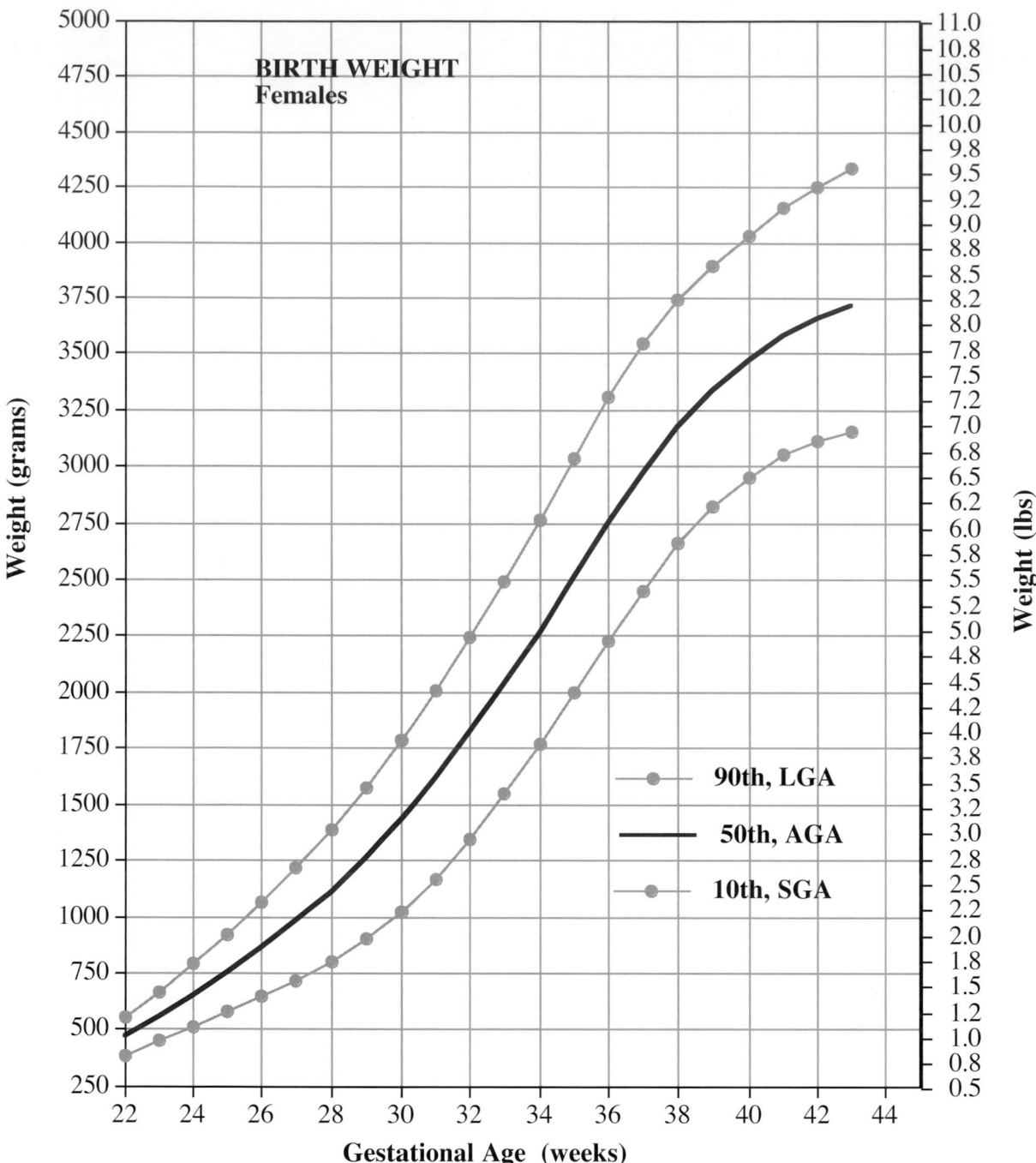

Figure II.6. Percentiles of Birth Weight (grams) for Determining Prenatal Growth Status for White Female Infants. SGA = a newborn that weighs below the 10th percentiles for gestational age, AGA = a newborn whose weight is between the 10th and 90th percentiles for gestational age, LGA = a newborn that weighs above the 90th percentiles for gestational age. (*Derived from the data given in refer. #19: Kramer et al. 2001. A new and improved population-based Canadian reference for birth weight and gestational age. Pediatrics 108:1-7.)

Evaluation of Prenatal Growth Status of African-American Black Newborns

Epidemiological studies conducted in the 1960's (21,22) have shown that the birth weight for full-term black infants (3100 ± 450 grams, or 6.82 lbs.) is significantly lower than the birth weight of white infants (3450 ± 450 grams).   The difference in birth weight persisted independently of numerous social and economic risk factors. In the 1967 National Collaborative Perinatal Project, only 1% of the total variance in birth weight among 18,000 infants was accounted for by socioeconomic variables (21). Epidemiological studies (22) indicate that the incidence of low birth weight (birth weight less than 2500 grams) varied between about 4 to 5% for infants born to white mothers, 5.27% for infants born to Native American mothers, and 5.31% for those born to Hispanic mothers. However, the incidence among infants born to black mothers was much higher (11.32%). Likewise, comparative studies of infants born to "mixed-race" parents in the United States in the year 1983 (23) found that the percentage of LBW when the mother was black and the father was white was higher than when the mother was white and the father was black. That is, the mother's ethnicity is a stronger predictor of low birth weight than is the ethnicity of the father. Recent analyses confirm that full-term newborns born to black mothers weigh on the average about 250 grams less than infants born to white mothers (17,18).

For the above reasons, birth weight percentiles for USA infants born to black mothers should be done with reference to the birth weight percentiles, as shown in **Table II.5** and **Figure II.7**. These percentiles were based upon information derived from birth weight percentiles for 954,021 non-Hispanic black infants born at 22-44 completed weeks of gestation published by Oken (17) and originally derived from the US Natality Datasets published in 2002 (18).

Table II.5. Birth Weight Percentiles in Grams by Gestational Age (weeks) for Infants Born to African-American Black Mothers*

Gestational Age (weeks)	Percentiles				
	10th	25th	50th	75th	90th
22	383	440	509	593	758
23	435	501	571	674	827
24	479	566	652	762	908
25	531	639	737	853	1001
26	567	709	857	1006	1234
27	646	820	977	1152	1453
28	716	925	1120	1345	1790
29	861	1073	1304	1612	2243
30	988	1248	1525	2024	2635
31	1199	1464	1804	2476	2937
32	1429	1692	2084	2760	3144
33	1628	1939	2358	2940	3303
34	1861	2166	2571	3050	3419
35	2082	2378	2733	3141	3504
36	2259	2549	2870	3207	3535
37	2450	2720	3014	3320	3623
38	2640	2882	3158	3456	3753
39	2759	3000	3277	3566	3843
40	2823	3072	3356	3653	3928
41	2847	3114	3399	3704	3985
42	2789	3049	3346	3658	3957
43	2778	3035	3316	3618	3915
44	2787	3044	3328	3631	3929

*Percentiles calculated from refer. #17: Oken et al. 2003. A nearly continuous measure of birth weight for gestational age using a United States national reference. BMC Pediatr 8:3-6. http://www.biomedcentral.com/1471-2431/3/6.

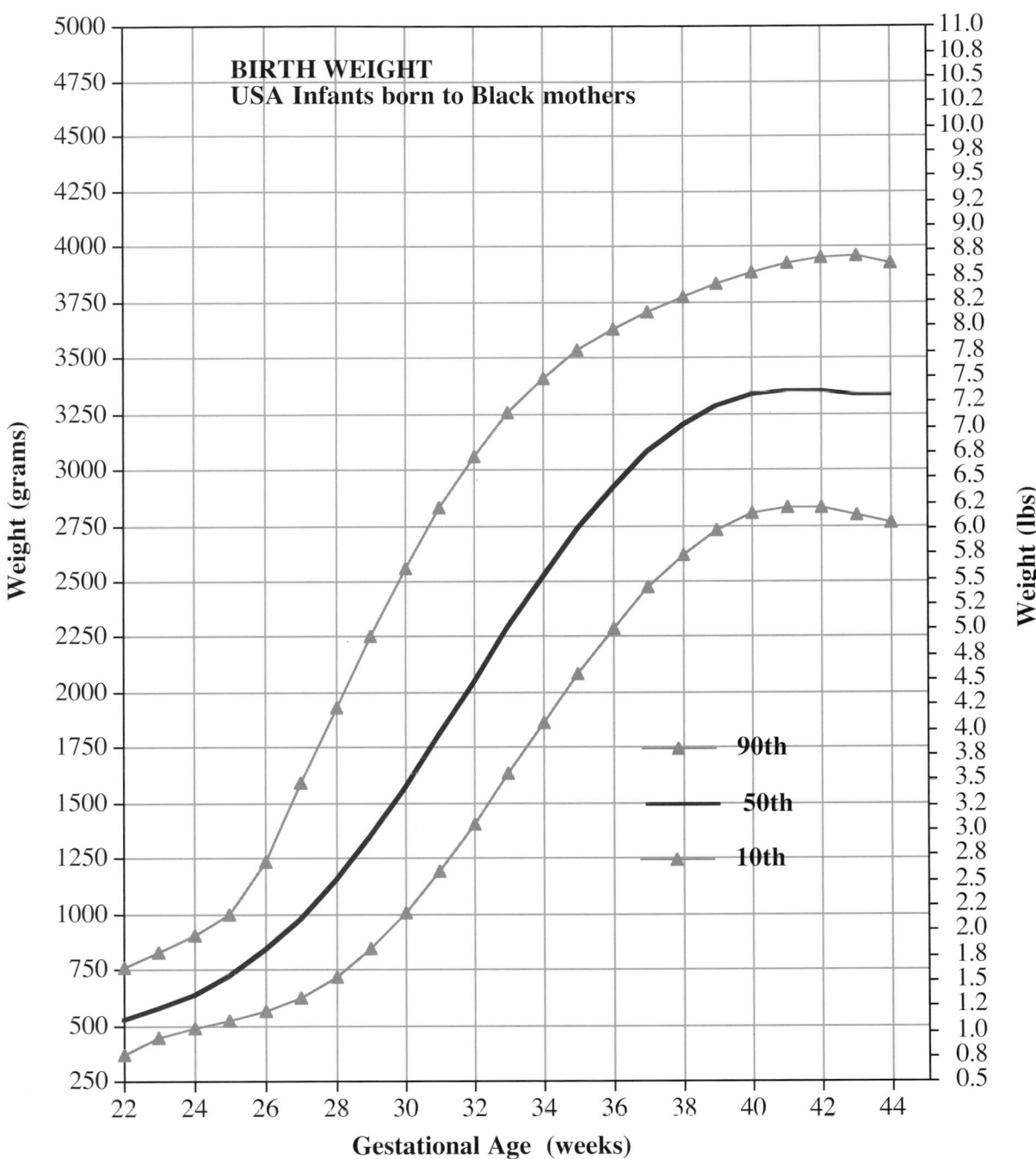

Figure II.7. Percentiles of Birth Weight (grams) for Determining Prenatal Growth Status of Infants Born to African-American Black Mothers. SGA = a newborn that weighs below the 10th percentiles for gestational age, AGA = a newborn whose weight is between the 10th and 90th percentiles for gestational age, LGA = a newborn that weighs above the 90th percentiles for gestational age. (*Percentiles calculated from refer. #17: Oken et al. 2003. A nearly continuous measure of birth weight for gestational age using a United States national reference. BMC Pediatr 8:3-6. http://www.biomedcentral.com/1471-2431/3/6.)

51

Reference of Rohrer Index

Although evaluation of birth weight with reference to population-based birth weight percentiles by age provides important information on the pre-natal growth influence of under- or over-nutrition, it does not reveal the effects on body proportions. There is evidence that the negative long-term post-natal effects of pre-natal under-nutrition are greater when they influence body proportions than when they reduce birth weight alone. The Rohrer index, also known as the ponderal index, has been shown to identify proportionality of growth. **Table II.6** presents the percentiles of Rohrer index by sex and age developed by Lehingue et al. (24). These references are based upon a sample of 88,581 French infants that excluded stillbirths, multiple pregnancies, malformations, and birth defects. The gestational ages were determined using ultrasound assessment, date of last menstrual period, and pediatric maturity assessments.

SUMMARY

The prenatal nutritional status is one of the most important stages in human development. Variability in nutrient and dietary intake can have profound influences on postnatal growth and during adulthood. Events occurring prenatally have long-term effects on future health and behavior. Deficient nutrition that leads to a reduction in birth weight is associated with postnatal growth delay and an increased risk of cardio-vascular diseases during adulthood. Studies of preterm infants and infants born small for gestational age have shown increased risk of cardio-vascular diseases associated with the metabolic syndrome of adulthood. Likewise, excessive weight at birth is associated with increased probabilities of obesity during childhood and adulthood. Conversely, low and high weight during pregnancy is conducive to postpartum health problems. Hence, it is recommended that evaluation of nutritional status during pregnancy be done through measurements of pregnancy weight gain, with reference to body mass index, rather than height and weight only. These recommendations should be considered while taking into account that a weight gain during the first trimester is more conducive to higher birth weight than is a uniform weight gain throughout pregnancy. As such, monitoring the nutritional status at all stages of pregnancy is essential for all concerned.

Table II.6. Percentiles of Rohrer Index (grams/cm^3) for Gestational Age and Sex*

Gestational Age (weeks)	Percentiles								
	5th	**10th**	**15th**	**25th**	**50th**	**75th**	**85th**	**90th**	**95th**
Males									
32	1.76	1.87	1.94	2.05	2.27	2.51	2.65	2.74	2.89
33	1.88	1.97	2.04	2.15	2.35	2.57	2.70	2.78	2.92
34	1.99	2.08	2.14	2.24	2.43	2.63	2.75	2.83	2.95
35	2.09	2.18	2.24	2.33	2.51	2.70	2.81	2.88	3.00
36	2.19	2.27	2.33	2.41	2.58	2.76	2.86	2.93	3.03
37	2.25	2.33	2.39	2.47	2.63	2.80	2.89	2.96	3.06
38	2.31	2.38	2.44	2.52	2.67	2.83	2.92	2.99	3.08
39	2.34	2.41	2.46	2.54	2.69	2.85	2.94	3.00	3.09
40	2.34	2.42	2.47	2.55	2.70	2.86	2.95	3.01	3.10
41	2.35	2.42	2.48	2.56	2.71	2.87	2.96	3.02	3.12
42	2.34	2.42	2.48	2.56	2.72	2.89	2.98	3.05	3.15
Females									
32	1.84	1.93	2.00	2.10	2.31	2.53	2.66	2.75	2.89
33	1.91	2.00	2.06	2.16	2.35	2.56	2.68	2.76	2.89
34	2.00	2.09	2.15	2.25	2.43	2.63	2.74	2.82	2.94
35	2.10	2.19	2.25	2.34	2.51	2.70	2.80	2.88	2.99
36	2.19	2.27	2.33	2.41	2.58	2.76	2.86	2.93	3.04
37	2.26	2.34	2.39	2.48	2.64	2.81	2.91	2.98	3.08
38	2.31	2.39	2.44	2.52	2.68	2.85	2.94	3.01	3.10
39	2.34	2.41	2.47	2.55	2.70	2.86	2.95	3.02	3.11
40	2.35	2.43	2.48	2.56	2.71	2.87	2.96	3.02	3.12
41	2.36	2.43	2.49	2.57	2.72	2.88	2.98	3.04	3.14
42	2.36	2.44	2.50	2.58	2.74	2.91	.3.003	3.07	3.17

*Derived from the data given in refer. #24: Lehingue, Y., Remontet, L., Munoz, F., Mamelle, N. 1998. Birth Ponderal Index and Body Mass Index Reference Curves in a Large Population. Am. J. Hum. Biol. 10:327-4.

LITERATURE CITED

1.   Hytten, F.E., Leitch, I. 1971. The physiology of human pregnancy, 2nd ed. Oxford: Blackwell Scientific Publications.

2.   Durnin, J.V.G.A. 1987. Energy requirements of pregnancy, an integration of the longitudinal data from the five-country study. Lancet 2:1131-33.

3.   Abrams, B., Selvin, S. 1995. Maternal weight gain pattern and birth weight. Obstet. Gynecol. 86:163-69.

4.   To, W.W., Cheung, W. 1998. The relationship between weight gain in pregnancy, birth-weight and postpartum weight retention. Aust. N. Z. J. Obstet. Gynecol. 38:176-79.

5.   Subcommittee on Nutritional Status and Weight Gain during Pregnancy, Nutritional Status and Weight Gain during Pregnancy of the Food and Nutrition Board, Institute of Medicine. Part 1. 1990. Washington D.C.: National Academy Press.

6.   Frisancho, A.R., Matos, J., Bollettino, L.A. 1984. Influence of growth status and placental function on birth weight of infants born to young still-growing teenagers. Am. J. Clin. Nutr. 40:801-7.

7.   Frisancho, A.R., Matos, J., Leonard, W.R., Yaroch, L.A. 1985. Developmental and nutritional determinants of pregnancy outcome among teenagers. Am. J. Phys. Anthropol. 66:247-61.

8.   Scholl, T.O., Hediger, M.L., Ances, I.G. 1990. Maternal growth during pregnancy and decreased infant birth weight. Am. J. Clin. Nutr. 51:790-93.

9.   Scholl, T.O., Hediger, M.L., Schall, J.I., Khoo, C.S., Fischer, R.L. 1994. Maternal growth during pregnancy and the competition for nutrients. Am. J. Clin. Nutr. 60:183-88.

10.   Scholl, T.O., Stein, P.T., Smith, W.K. 2000. Leptin and maternal growth during adolescent pregnancy. Am. J. Clin. Nutr. 72:1542-47.

11.   Petitti, D.B., Croughan-Minihane, M.S., Hiatt, R.A. 1991. Weight gain by gestational age in both black and white women delivered of normal-birth-weight and low-birth-weight infants. Am. J. Obstet. Gynecol. 164:801-5.

12.   Brown, J.E., Murtaugh, M.A., Jacobs, D.R. Jr., Margellos, H.C. 2002. Variation in newborn size according to pregnancy weight change by trimester. Am. J. Clin. Nutr. 76:205-20.

13.   Rhodes, J.C., Schoendorf, K.C., Parker, J.D. 2003. Contribution of excess weight gain

during pregnancy and macrosomia to the cesarean delivery rate, 1990-2000. Pediatrics 111:1181-85.

14. Giuliani, A., Tamussino, K., Basver, A., Haas, J., Petru, E. 2002. The impact of body mass index and weight gain during pregnancy on puerperal complications after spontaneous vaginal delivery. Wien. Klin. Wochenschr. 114:383-86.

15. Williams, R.L., Creasy, R.K., Cunningham, G.X., Hawes, W.E., Norris, F.D. 1982. Fetal growth and perinatal viability in California. Obstet. Gynecol. 59:624-32.

16. Amini, S.B., Catalano, P.M., Hirsch, V., Mann, L.I. 1994. An analysis of birth weight by gestational age using a computerized perinatal data base, 1975-1992. Obstet. Gynecol. 83:342-52.

17. Oken, E., Kleinman, K.P., Rich-Edwards, J., Gillman, M.W. 2003. A nearly continuous measure of birth weight for gestational age using a United States national reference. BMC Pediatr. 3:6.

18. National Vital Statistics System Birth Data. 2002. [http://www.cdc.gov/nchs/births.htm].

19. Kramer, M.S., Platt, R.W., Wen, S.W., Joseph, K.S., Allen, A., Abrahamowicz, M., Blondel, B., Breart, G. 2001. Fetal/Infant Health Study Group of the Canadian Perinatal Surveillance System: A new and improved population-based Canadian reference for birth weight for gestational age. Pediatrics 108(2):E35.

20. Frisancho, A.R. 2000. Prenatal compared with parental origins of adolescent fatness. Am. J. Clin. Nutr. 72:1186-90.

21. Naylor, A.F., Myrianthopoulos, N.C. 1967. The relation of ethnic and selected socio-economic factors to human birth-weight. Ann. Hum. Genet. 31:71-83.

22. Emanuel, I., Leisenring, W., Williams, M.A., Kimpo, C., Estee, S., O'Brien, W., Hale, C.B. 1999. The Washington State intergenerational study of birth outcomes: methodology and some comparisons of maternal birth weight and infant birthweight in four ethnic groups. Pediatr. & Perinat. Epidemiol. 13:352-69.

23. Migone, A., Emanuel, I., Mueller, B., Daling, J., Little, R.E. 1991. Gestational duration and birthweight in white, black and mixed-race babies. Pediatr. & Perinat. Epidemiol. 5:378-91.

24. Lehingue, Y., Remontet, L., Muñoz, F., Mamelle, N. 1998. Birth ponderal index and body mass index reference curves in a large population. Am. J. Hum. Biol. 10:327-40.

CHAPTER III
NON-SMOOTHED ANTHROPOMETRIC REFERENCE
BASED ON THE THIRD NATIONAL HEALTH AND
NUTRITION EXAMINATION SURVEY (NHANES III)

SAMPLE

STATISTICAL ANALYSIS

AGE GROUPS

THE NON-SMOOTHED NHANES III ANTHROPOMETRIC
REFERENCE DATA

LIST OF TABLES: NON-SMOOTHED NHANES III
ANTHROPOMETRIC REFERENCE DATA: ALL ETHNIC GROUPS
COMBINED

LIST OF TABLES: NON-SMOOTHED NHANES III
ANTHROPOMETRIC REFERENCE DATA: NON-HISPANIC WHITES

LIST OF TABLES: NON-SMOOTHED NHANES III
ANTHROPOMETRIC REFERENCE DATA: NON-HISPANIC BLACKS

LIST OF TABLES: NON-SMOOTHED NHANES III
ANTHROPOMETRIC REFERENCE DATA: MEXICAN-AMERICANS

LITERATURE CITED

CHAPTER III

NON-SMOOTHED ANTHROPOMETRIC REFERENCE BASED ON THE THIRD NATIONAL HEALTH AND NUTRITION EXAMINATION SURVEY (NHANES III)

This chapter describes the data source and the statistical analysis used to derive the measures of dispersion of the anthropometric variables. The results are presented as means, standard errors of the mean, and standard deviations, and each anthropometric variable is presented by age, gender, and ethnicity.

SAMPLE

The third National Health Examination Survey (NHANES III) was a nationally representative, two-phase, six-year cross-sectional survey conducted from 1988 until 1994 by the National Center for Health Statistics (NCHS) of the Centers for Disease Control (CDC) (1,2). The sampling plan used a complex stratified, multistage, probability cluster design. The total NHANES III sample consisted of 31,311 persons, aged 2 months to 94 years, who completed a standardized, detailed physical examination, of which 11,652 were non-Hispanic whites, 9074 non-Hispanic blacks, 9138 Mexican-Americans, and 1447 non-Mexican-American Hispanics and other. Recently, however, the NCHS has posted the Anthropometric Reference Data, United States, 1988-1994, based on 30,703 participants (2).

STATISTICAL ANALYSIS

Descriptive statistics including means, standard deviations, and standard errors for estimates of all the anthropometric variables were calculated for age, sex, and ethnic groups. These means, standard errors of the mean, and standard deviations for all anthropometric dimensions were estimated using SAS (3) and WesVarPC (4,5). These statistical programs, recommended by the National Center for Health Statistics (NCHS), incorporate the sample weights and complex sample design for calculating variance estimates. Sample weighting in NHANES III was used to a) compensate for differential probabilities of selection among subgroups (i.e., age-sex-race-ethnicity sub-domains, where persons living in different geographic strata were sampled at different rates); b) reduce biases arising from the fact that non respondents may be different from those who participate; c) bring sample data up to the dimensions of the target population totals; d) compensate, to the extent possible, for inadequacies in the sampling frame; and e) to reduce variances in the estimation procedure by using auxiliary information that is known with a high degree of accuracy. The sample weighting was carried out in three stages. The first stage involved the computation of weights to compensate for unequal probabilities of selection (Objective a above). The second stage adjusted for non-response (Objective b). The third stage used post-stratification of the sample weights to Census Bureau estimates of the U.S. population to simultaneously accomplish the third, fourth, and fifth objectives.

AGE GROUPS

Following the age classification given by the NCHS (1) children ranging in age from 2 to 48 months were stratified into seven specific age month groups (i.e., 2.0-2.9; 3.0-5.9; 6.0-8.9; 9.0-11.9; 12.0-23.9; 24.0-35.9; 36.0-47.9). Participants ranging in age from 2 to 19 years were classified by 1-year intervals (i.e., 2.0-2.9; 3.0-3.9;…19.0-19.9), and participants aged 20 to 90 years were defined at 10-year intervals (i.e. 20.0-29.9; 30.0-39.9;…80.0-90.9).

THE NON-SMOOTHED NHANES III ANTHROPOMETRIC REFERENCE DATA

The means, standard errors of the mean, and standard deviations for infants, children, and adults for all the anthropometric variables collected in the third National Health and Nutrition Examination Survey (2) are presented in **Tables III.1** to **III.11** for all ethnic groups combined (non-Hispanic white, non-Hispanic Black, Mexican-Americans, and other). The corresponding values for non-Hispanic whites are presented in **Tables III.12** to **III.22**, values for non-Hispanic Blacks are presented in **Tables III.23** to **III.33**, and values for Mexican-Americans are presented in **Tables III.34** to **III.44**. This information complements the "Anthropometric Reference Data" published by the

National Center for Health Statistics (2) and those published elsewhere (6-12). From this data it is evident that the measurements of weight, body mass index, and skinfold thickness are skewed to the right. For example, the coefficient of variance (SD/Mean) for adolescents and adults averages about 30 to 50% for body weight, body mass index, and skinfold thickness, which exceed the recommended values for anthropometric references (13-15). Obviously, the wide range of variability and excessive skewness will fail to identify those who are either excessively heavy or underweight. Therefore, these references **per se are not** appropriate anthropometric references for determining an individual's or a population's nutritional status. Hence, to construct an anthropometric reference based upon the NHANES III, anthropometric data sets must be normalized and the range of variance must be reduced within the acceptable limits. This topic is addressed in the next chapter.

LIST OF TABLES

NON-SMOOTHED NHANES III ANTHROPOMETRIC REFERENCE DATA: ALL ETHNIC GROUPS COMBINED

Table III.9. Mean (M), standard error of the mean (SE), and standard deviation (SD) of biacromial (cm) breadth and bi-iliac breadth (cm) by age for males and females for all ethnic groups combined of 2 to 90 years: NHANES III, 1988-1994.

Table III.10. Mean (M), standard error of the mean (SE), and standard deviation (SD) of knee height (cm) for males and females for all ethnic groups combined of 60 to 90 years: NHANES III, 1988-1994.

Table III.11. Mean (M), standard error of the mean (SE), and standard deviation (SD) of fat-free mass (kg), total body fat (kg), and percent body fat (%) for males and females for all ethnic groups combined of 12 to 90 years: NHANES III, 1988-1994.

Table III.1.
Mean (M), standard error of the mean (SE), and standard deviation (SD) of weight (kg), recumbent length (cm),
Rohrer index (100 g/cm^3), and head circumference (cm) by age of all ethnic groups combined of males
and females 2 months to 7 years: NHANES III, 1988-1994

Age Group (months)	Mean Age (months)	Males				Mean Age (months)	Females			
		N	M	SE	SD		N	M	SE	SD
Weight (kg)										
2.0-2.9	2.12	108	6.58	0.093	0.97	2.0	134	6.02	0.08	0.88
3.0-5.9	3.96	290	7.40	0.10	1.70	4.04	308	6.80	0.09	1.58
6.0-8.9	6.91	320	8.80	0.11	1.97	7.04	264	8.20	0.13	2.11
9.0-11.9	9.95	277	9.60	0.11	1.83	9.99	315	9.00	0.10	1.77
12.0-23.9	17.53	663	11.60	0.10	2.57	17.755	647	10.90	0.09	2.29
24.0-35.9	29.54	645	13.60	0.11	2.79	29.38	624	13.20	0.12	3.00
36.0-47.9	41.40	516	15.80	0.20	4.54	41.49	587	15.40	0.16	3.88
Recumbent Length (cm)										
2.0-2.9	2.12	108	61.42	0.318	3.31	2.0	134	59.95	0.31	3.61
3.0-5.9	3.96	291	64.40	0.29	4.95	4.04	309	62.40	0.24	4.22
6.0-8.9	6.91	321	70.00	0.26	4.66	7.04	264	68.10	0.23	3.74
9.0-11.9	9.95	277	73.80	0.29	4.83	9.99	316	72.00	0.23	4.09
12.0-23.9	17.53	657	82.20	0.28	7.18	17.75	636	80.70	0.22	5.55
24.0-35.9	29.54	616	91.70	0.23	5.71	29.38	598	90.60	0.22	5.38
36.0-47.9	41.40	508	100.00	0.27	6.09	41.49	585	99.40	0.23	5.56
Rohrer Index (100 g/cm^3)										
2.0-2.9	2.12	108	2.84	0.03	0.35	2.0	133	2.78	0.03	0.31
3.0-5.9	3.96	292	2.71	0.02	0.32	4.04	309	2.75	0.04	0.64
6.0-8.9	6.91	311	2.53	0.01	0.27	7.04	264	2.55	0.02	0.33
9.0-11.9	9.95	291	2.36	0.01	0.23	9.99	316	2.40	0.01	0.25
12.0-23.9	17.53	613	2.09	0.01	0.25	17.75	636	2.05	0.01	0.26
24.0-35.9	29.54	614	1.75	0.01	0.17	29.38	598	1.75	0.01	0.19
36.0-47.9	41.40	506	1.58	0.01	0.17	41.49	585	1.58	0.01	0.17
Head Circumference (cm)										
2.0-2.9	2.12	108	41.04	0.14	1.48	2.0	133	40.02	0.1	1.66
3.0-5.9	3.96	291	42.40	0.14	2.39	4.04	307	41.20	0.12	2.10
6.0-8.9	6.91	317	44.80	0.14	2.49	7.04	263	43.50	0.12	1.95
9.0-11.9	9.95	275	46.00	0.13	2.16	9.99	315	44.90	0.09	1.60
12.0-23.9	17.53	656	47.90	0.10	2.56	17.75	631	46.70	0.08	2.01
24.0-35.9	29.54	599	49.50	0.10	2.45	29.38	582	48.40	0.08	1.93
36.0-47.9	41.40	495	50.30	0.10	2.22	41.49	574	49.50	0.07	1.68
48.0-59.9	53.59	549	50.80	0.10	2.34	53.22	528	49.90	0.08	1.84
60.0-71.9	65.18	491	51.50	0.10	2.22	65.58	553	50.70	0.08	1.88
72.0-83.9	77.43	265	52.50	0.16	2.65	77.69	269	51.00	0.11	1.80

Table III.2.

Mean (M), standard error of the mean (SE), and standard deviation of weight (kg), stature (cm), and body mass index (w/s^2) by age of all ethnic groups combined of males and females of 2 to 90 years: NHANES III, 1988-1994

Age Group (years)	Mean Age (years)	Weight (kg)				Stature (cm)				Body Mass Index (kg/m^2)			
		N	M	SE	SD	N	M	SE	SD	N	M	SE	SD
Males													
2.0-2.9	2.46	645	13.60	0.11	2.79	589	90.90	0.27	6.55	588	16.50	0.09	2.18
3.0-3.9	3.45	516	15.80	0.20	4.54	513	98.80	0.32	7.25	512	16.10	0.16	3.62
4.0-4.9	4.47	549	17.70	0.18	4.22	551	105.20	0.33	7.75	547	15.90	0.10	2.34
5.0-5.9	5.43	497	20.10	0.25	5.57	497	112.30	0.38	8.47	495	15.90	0.13	2.89
6.0-6.9	6.45	283	23.30	0.57	9.59	283	118.90	0.65	10.93	282	16.30	0.26	4.37
7.0-7.9	7.47	269	26.30	0.56	9.18	270	125.90	0.68	11.17	269	16.50	0.24	3.94
8.0-8.9	8.46	266	30.20	0.83	13.54	269	131.30	0.60	9.84	266	17.30	0.34	5.55
9.0-9.9	9.50	281	34.40	0.87	14.58	280	137.70	0.65	10.88	279	18.00	0.33	5.51
10.0-10.9	10.45	297	37.30	0.87	14.99	297	142.00	0.83	14.30	297	18.40	0.30	5.17
11.0-11.9	11.44	281	42.50	1.18	19.78	285	147.40	0.76	12.83	280	19.40	0.40	6.69
12.0-12.9	12.47	203	49.10	1.43	20.37	207	155.50	0.89	12.80	203	20.10	0.44	6.27
13.0-13.9	13.47	187	54.00	1.72	23.52	190	161.60	1.06	14.61	187	20.50	0.49	6.70
14.0-14.9	14.49	188	64.10	2.73	37.43	191	169.00	0.91	12.58	188	22.30	0.84	11.52
15.0-15.9	15.45	187	66.90	2.03	27.76	188	172.80	0.99	13.57	187	22.30	0.56	7.66
16.0-16.9	16.45	194	68.80	2.23	31.06	197	175.00	0.92	12.91	194	22.30	0.56	7.80
17.0-17.9	17.45	196	72.90	1.75	24.50	196	176.50	1.03	14.42	196	23.40	0.53	7.42
18.0-18.9	18.46	176	71.30	2.09	27.73	176	177.30	0.99	13.13	176	22.60	0.56	7.43
19.0-19.9	19.43	168	73.00	1.82	23.59	169	175.50	0.69	8.97	168	23.70	0.53	6.87
20.0-29.9	24.96	1630	78.30	0.62	25.03	1631	176.10	0.27	10.90	1630	25.20	0.17	6.86
30.0-39.9	34.72	1481	83.00	0.68	26.17	1481	176.70	0.28	10.78	1481	26.50	0.18	6.93
40.0-49.9	44.35	1226	85.10	0.76	26.61	1226	176.30	0.30	10.50	1226	27.30	0.22	7.70
50.0-59.9	54.89	855	86.00	0.80	23.39	855	175.70	0.34	9.94	855	27.80	0.23	6.73
60.0-69.9	64.83	1175	83.10	0.65	22.28	1176	174.10	0.30	10.29	1175	27.30	0.18	6.17
70.0-79.9	74.16	875	79.00	0.71	21.00	875	171.90	0.33	9.76	875	26.70	0.21	6.21
80.0-90.9	84.09	700	71.80	0.74	19.58	699	169.40	0.40	10.58	699	25.00	0.22	5.82
Females													
2.0-2.9	2.45	624	13.20	0.12	3.00	564	89.70	0.33	7.84	562	16.40	0.13	3.08
3.0-3.9	3.46	587	15.40	0.16	3.88	590	98.20	0.33	8.02	582	15.90	0.14	3.38
4.0-4.9	4.44	537	17.90	0.27	6.26	535	105.10	0.36	8.33	533	16.00	0.21	4.85
5.0-5.9	5.47	554	20.20	0.27	6.36	557	112.20	0.41	9.68	554	15.90	0.17	4.00
6.0-6.9	6.47	272	22.60	0.55	9.07	274	117.90	0.61	10.10	272	16.10	0.32	5.28
7.0-7.9	7.44	274	26.40	0.69	11.42	275	124.30	0.67	11.11	274	16.90	0.35	5.79
8.0-8.9	8.47	248	29.90	0.80	12.60	247	131.100	0.70	11.00	247	17.30	0.42	6.60
9.0-9.9	9.43	280	34.40	1.03	17.24	282	136.60	0.70	11.75	280	18.20	0.47	7.86
10.0-10.9	10.43	258	37.90	1.05	16.87	262	142.70	0.74	11.98	258	18.40	0.46	7.39
11.0-11.9	11.46	275	44.20	1.08	17.91	275	150.20	0.75	12.44	275	19.40	0.45	7.46
12.0-12.9	12.46	236	49.00	1.30	19.97	239	155.50	0.88	13.60	236	20.20	0.57	8.76
13.0-13.9	13.45	220	55.80	1.53	22.69	225	159.90	0.83	12.45	220	21.80	0.63	9.34
14.0-14.9	14.47	218	58.50	1.45	21.41	226	161.20	0.83	12.48	218	22.40	0.59	8.71
15.0-15.9	15.47	191	58.10	1.25	17.28	201	162.80	0.70	9.92	191	21.90	0.53	7.32
16.0-16.9	16.47	208	61.30	1.79	25.82	221	163.10	0.74	11.00	208	23.00	0.72	10.38
17.0-17.9	17.45	201	62.40	1.55	21.98	217	163.40	0.78	11.49	201	23.30	0.66	9.36
18.0-18.9	18.43	175	61.20	1.88	24.87	193	163.20	0.88	12.23	175	22.90	0.74	9.79
19.0-19.9	19.48	177	63.20	1.96	26.08	194	163.80	0.81	11.28	177	23.70	0.89	11.84
20.0-29.9	24.91	1665	64.50	0.57	23.26	1867	162.70	0.26	11.23	1665	24.30	0.20	8.16
30.0-39.9	34.86	1775	70.10	0.66	27.81	1863	163.40	0.26	11.22	1775	26.30	0.24	10.11
40.0-49.9	44.28	1368	71.60	0.72	26.63	1371	162.80	0.28	10.37	1367	27.00	0.27	9.98
50.0-59.9	54.83	1006	74.40	0.84	26.64	1009	161.80	0.32	10.16	1006	28.40	0.31	9.83
60.0-69.9	64.82	1172	70.90	0.71	24.31	1177	160.20	0.30	10.29	1172	27.60	0.27	9.24
70.0-79.9	74.46	988	67.40	0.75	23.57	988	158.00	0.34	10.69	985	26.90	0.28	8.79
80.0-90.9	84.45	790	60.50	0.68	19.11	792	154.90	0.39	10.98	788	25.20	0.26	7.30

Table III.3.
Mean (M), standard error of the mean (SE), and standard deviation (SD) of sitting height (cm), upper arm length (cm),
and upper leg length (cm) by age of all ethnic groups combined of males and females of 2 to 90 years: NHANES III, 1988-1994

Age Group (years)	Mean Age (years)	Sitting Height (cm)				Upper Arm Length (cm)				Upper Leg Length (cm)			
		N	M	SE	SD	N	M	SE	SD	N	M	SE	SD
Males													
2.0-2.9	2.46	581	52.1	0.19	4.58	571	17.9	0.08	1.91	530	18.5	0.14	3.22
3.0-3.9	3.45	508	54.7	0.2	4.51	484	19.4	0.1	2.20	490	21.2	0.17	3.76
4.0-4.9	4.47	551	57.4	0.2	4.69	541	20.9	0.1	2.33	541	23.2	0.16	3.72
5.0-5.9	5.43	497	60.6	0.23	5.13	494	22.4	0.11	2.44	488	25.2	0.19	4.20
6.0-6.9	6.45	282	63.3	0.37	6.21	279	23.8	0.18	3.01	279	27.5	0.29	4.84
7.0-7.9	7.47	270	66	0.38	6.24	268	25.4	0.18	2.95	268	29.5	0.31	5.07
8.0-8.9	8.46	269	68.7	0.36	5.90	263	26.6	0.18	2.92	262	31.1	0.3	4.86
9.0-9.9	9.50	277	71.1	0.36	5.99	276	28.3	0.2	3.32	275	33	0.32	5.31
10.0-10.9	10.45	294	73.1	0.38	6.52	294	29.1	0.25	4.29	293	34.4	0.38	6.50
11.0-11.9	11.44	282	75.5	0.38	6.38	282	30.3	0.2	3.36	279	35.9	0.34	5.68
12.0-12.9	12.47	203	79.1	0.51	7.27	202	32.3	0.28	3.98	202	38.6	0.43	6.11
13.0-13.9	13.47	186	82.4	0.64	8.73	181	33.6	0.31	4.17	182	39.8	0.42	5.67
14.0-14.9	14.49	189	86.9	0.57	7.84	185	35.3	0.31	4.22	186	42	0.41	5.59
15.0-15.9	15.45	187	88.8	0.55	7.52	183	36.2	0.31	4.19	181	43.5	0.45	6.05
16.0-16.9	16.45	194	90.4	0.58	8.08	192	36.8	0.28	3.88	192	43.6	0.41	5.68
17.0-17.9	17.45	192	91.7	0.54	7.48	193	37.1	0.24	3.33	191	44.7	0.38	5.25
18.0-18.9	18.46	173	91.9	0.5	6.58	169	37.2	0.27	3.51	168	44.5	0.46	5.96
19.0-19.9	19.43	165	91.8	0.45	5.78	162	37.1	0.27	3.44	162	43.5	0.38	4.84
20.0-29.9	24.96	1611	92.2	0.15	6.02	1585	37.4	0.08	3.18	1579	43.2	0.15	5.96
30.0-39.9	34.72	1463	92.7	0.17	6.50	1435	37.8	0.08	3.03	1434	43.1	0.16	6.06
40.0-49.9	44.35	1200	92.5	0.18	6.24	1176	38	0.09	3.09	1170	42.2	0.17	5.81
50.0-59.9	54.89	831	92.2	0.2	5.77	820	38.1	0.11	3.15	816	41.7	0.2	5.71
60.0-69.9	64.83	1125	90.8	0.17	5.70	1112	38.1	0.09	3.00	1101	41	0.19	6.30
70.0-79.9	74.16	804	89.3	0.21	5.95	788	37.7	0.11	3.09	774	40.6	0.22	6.12
80.0-90.9	84.09	569	87.3	0.26	6.20	551	37.6	0.13	3.05	531	40.1	0.26	5.99
Females													
2.0-2.9	2.45	548	51.3	0.2	4.68	556	17.5	0.1	2.36	518	18.8	0.18	4.10
3.0-3.9	3.46	584	54.4	0.19	4.59	562	19.2	0.09	2.13	567	21.5	0.17	4.05
4.0-4.9	4.44	530	57.3	0.22	5.06	527	20.8	0.11	2.53	528	23.4	0.18	4.14
5.0-5.9	5.47	556	60.2	0.24	5.66	556	22.4	0.11	2.59	556	25.6	0.19	4.48
6.0-6.9	6.47	272	62.6	0.33	5.44	274	23.7	0.18	2.98	274	27.4	0.29	4.80
7.0-7.9	7.44	275	65.6	0.34	5.64	270	24.9	0.2	3.29	270	28.9	0.33	5.42
8.0-8.9	8.47	245	68.3	0.38	5.95	245	26.5	0.19	2.97	245	31.4	0.38	5.95
9.0-9.9	9.43	278	70.7	0.39	6.50	271	28.1	0.22	3.62	273	32.8	0.32	5.29
10.0-10.9	10.43	261	73.6	0.42	6.79	255	29.1	0.21	3.35	255	34.9	0.35	5.59
11.0-11.9	11.46	275	77.4	0.43	7.13	268	31	0.23	3.77	267	36.7	0.36	5.88
12.0-12.9	12.46	237	80.4	0.51	7.85	233	32.1	0.25	3.82	233	38.5	0.48	7.33
13.0-13.9	13.45	219	83.1	0.52	7.70	218	33.1	0.27	3.99	217	39.8	0.43	6.33
14.0-14.9	14.47	218	84.3	0.45	6.64	220	33.8	0.24	3.56	219	39.9	0.44	6.51
15.0-15.9	15.47	196	85.5	0.47	6.58	195	33.9	0.26	3.63	193	40.1	0.44	6.11
16.0-16.9	16.47	217	85.7	0.39	5.75	211	34.1	0.26	3.78	208	40.2	0.42	6.06
17.0-17.9	17.45	215	86	0.41	6.01	210	34.2	0.23	3.33	209	40.5	0.39	5.64
18.0-18.9	18.43	190	85.6	0.52	7.17	186	34	0.29	3.96	185	40.1	0.49	6.66
19.0-19.9	19.48	192	86.6	0.44	6.10	185	34	0.26	3.54	185	40.4	0.54	7.34
20.0-29.9	24.91	1837	86.1	0.13	5.57	1807	34.3	0.07	2.98	1802	39.6	0.14	5.94
30.0-39.9	34.86	1837	86.7	0.13	5.57	1791	34.6	0.06	2.54	1783	39.4	0.13	5.49
40.0-49.9	44.28	1338	86.5	0.15	5.49	1302	34.6	0.07	2.53	1295	38.8	0.17	6.12
50.0-59.9	54.83	981	85.5	0.17	5.32	964	34.8	0.09	2.79	958	38	0.2	6.19
60.0-69.9	64.82	1107	84	0.15	4.99	1089	34.6	0.09	2.97	1078	37.3	0.19	6.24
70.0-79.9	74.46	894	82.4	0.2	5.98	864	34.5	0.1	2.94	857	36.8	0.22	6.44
80.0-90.9	84.45	604	79.6	0.24	5.90	576	34.4	0.11	2.64	564	36.9	0.27	6.41

Table III.4.

Mean (M), standard error of the mean (SE), and standard deviation (SD) of triceps (mm) and subscapular (mm) by age of all ethnic groups combined of males and females of 2 to 90 years: NHANES III, 1988-1994

Age Group (years)	Mean Age (years)	Triceps (mm)				Subscapular (mm)			
		N	M	SE	SD	N	M	SE	SD
Males									
2.0-2.9	2.46	555	9.10	0.13	3.06	549	6.40	0.11	2.58
3.0-3.9	3.45	479	8.90	0.20	4.38	479	6.20	0.22	4.81
4.0-4.9	4.47	538	9.00	0.18	4.18	537	6.00	0.15	3.48
5.0-5.9	5.43	493	8.70	0.20	4.44	491	5.80	0.18	3.99
6.0-6.9	6.45	278	9.80	0.46	7.67	278	6.90	0.45	7.50
7.0-7.9	7.47	268	9.70	0.45	7.37	267	6.70	0.52	8.50
8.0-8.9	8.46	262	10.80	0.59	9.55	261	7.60	0.50	8.08
9.0-9.9	9.50	276	12.40	0.69	11.46	271	8.60	0.58	9.55
10.0-10.9	10.45	293	12.50	0.63	10.78	292	9.10	0.53	9.06
11.0-11.9	11.44	282	13.60	0.70	11.75	280	10.50	0.75	12.55
12.0-12.9	12.47	200	13.50	0.77	10.89	199	10.80	0.82	11.57
13.0-13.9	13.47	182	12.40	0.89	12.01	180	10.20	0.90	12.07
14.0-14.9	14.49	183	11.00	0.82	11.09	182	11.00	1.04	14.03
15.0-15.9	15.45	182	12.10	1.00	13.49	181	11.70	0.97	13.05
16.0-16.9	16.45	191	11.10	0.86	11.89	187	10.90	0.82	11.21
17.0-17.9	17.45	191	11.30	0.82	11.33	190	12.70	0.93	12.82
18.0-18.9	18.46	168	10.90	0.90	11.67	168	12.30	0.87	11.28
19.0-19.9	19.43	160	12.10	1.05	13.28	159	13.90	0.98	12.36
20.0-29.9	24.96	1556	12.00	0.22	8.68	1541	16.20	0.28	10.99
30.0-39.9	34.72	1419	13.00	0.23	8.66	1377	19.00	0.29	10.76
40.0-49.9	44.35	1164	13.50	0.25	8.53	1103	20.10	0.33	10.96
50.0-59.9	54.89	813	13.70	0.29	8.27	770	20.80	0.40	11.10
60.0-69.9	64.83	1122	14.20	0.25	8.37	1059	21.20	0.34	11.06
70.0-79.9	74.16	825	13.40	0.28	8.04	761	19.50	0.37	10.21
80.0-90.9	84.09	641	12.00	0.28	7.09	537	16.70	0.38	8.81
Females									
2.0-2.9	2.45	545	9.50	0.17	3.97	541	6.90	0.17	3.95
3.0-3.9	3.46	554	9.70	0.21	4.94	553	6.90	0.23	5.41
4.0-4.9	4.44	529	10.30	0.29	6.67	526	7.30	0.35	8.03
5.0-5.9	5.47	554	10.30	0.27	6.36	555	7.40	0.36	8.48
6.0-6.9	6.47	273	10.30	0.48	7.93	273	7.60	0.61	10.08
7.0-7.9	7.44	269	11.90	0.59	9.68	265	9.10	0.81	13.19
8.0-8.9	8.47	244	12.40	0.64	10.00	243	9.00	0.75	11.69
9.0-9.9	9.43	270	14.40	0.84	13.80	269	11.00	1.00	16.40
10.0-10.9	10.43	255	15.00	0.81	12.93	253	11.50	0.99	15.75
11.0-11.9	11.46	268	15.10	0.78	12.77	263	11.90	0.98	15.89
12.0-12.9	12.46	233	15.20	0.90	13.74	231	12.60	1.05	15.96
13.0-13.9	13.45	218	17.50	0.89	13.14	215	13.90	1.10	16.13
14.0-14.9	14.47	216	18.70	0.90	13.23	214	15.30	1.15	16.82
15.0-15.9	15.47	188	17.80	0.98	13.44	183	14.90	1.17	15.83
16.0-16.9	16.47	202	18.60	0.89	12.65	199	16.00	1.10	15.52
17.0-17.9	17.45	191	20.00	0.98	13.54	184	17.80	1.14	15.46
18.0-18.9	18.43	165	19.40	1.07	13.74	160	16.40	1.20	15.18
19.0-19.9	19.48	167	19.60	1.18	15.25	162	16.30	1.30	16.55
20.0-29.9	24.91	1579	20.90	0.33	13.11	1509	18.50	0.36	13.98
30.0-39.9	34.86	1623	23.60	0.35	14.10	1544	21.30	0.39	15.32
40.0-49.9	44.28	1237	25.30	0.35	12.31	1164	23.10	0.41	13.99
50.0-59.9	54.83	929	26.70	0.40	12.19	876	24.50	0.47	13.91
60.0-69.9	64.82	1090	24.20	0.37	12.22	1029	22.50	0.42	13.47
70.0-79.9	74.46	902	22.30	0.39	11.71	836	19.80	0.44	12.72
80.0-90.9	84.45	705	18.60	0.42	11.15	562	16.30	0.48	11.38

Table III.5.
Mean (M), standard error of the mean (SE), and standard deviation (SD) of suprailiac (mm) and thigh (mm)
by age of all ethnic groups combined of males and females of 2 to 90 years: NHANES III, 1988-1994

Age Group (years)	Mean Age (years)	Suprailiac (mm)				Thigh (mm)			
		N	M	SE	SD	N	M	SE	SD
Males									
2.0-2.9	2.46	500	5.30	0.11	2.46	505	12.20	0.22	4.94
3.0-3.9	3.45	478	5.30	0.19	4.15	478	11.20	0.22	4.81
4.0-4.9	4.47	537	5.40	0.19	4.40	536	11.50	0.26	6.02
5.0-5.9	5.43	488	5.40	0.23	5.08	485	11.30	0.29	6.39
6.0-6.9	6.45	277	6.90	0.60	9.99	278	12.80	0.72	12.00
7.0-7.9	7.47	266	7.60	0.69	11.25	264	12.30	0.55	8.94
8.0-8.9	8.46	257	8.50	0.72	11.54	254	13.60	0.73	11.63
9.0-9.9	9.50	271	10.80	0.97	15.97	263	15.10	0.89	14.43
10.0-10.9	10.45	289	11.70	0.90	15.30	281	16.50	0.87	14.58
11.0-11.9	11.44	275	13.20	1.03	17.08	259	15.90	0.75	12.07
12.0-12.9	12.47	199	15.20	1.24	17.49	192	16.20	0.89	12.33
13.0-13.9	13.47	181	13.50	1.28	17.22	171	14.40	0.98	12.82
14.0-14.9	14.49	178	11.90	1.04	13.88	171	13.20	0.98	12.82
15.0-15.9	15.45	178	14.50	1.38	18.41	170	12.40	0.95	12.39
16.0-16.9	16.45	186	12.90	1.22	16.64	181	11.70	0.70	9.42
17.0-17.9	17.45	185	15.30	1.34	18.23	181	11.60	0.74	9.96
18.0-18.9	18.46	164	13.60	1.25	16.01	162	11.50	0.78	9.93
19.0-19.9	19.43	159	16.40	1.55	19.54	149	13.40	1.15	14.04
20.0-29.9	24.96	1538	20.30	0.42	16.47	1493	13.60	0.29	11.21
30.0-39.9	34.72	1385	23.50	0.41	15.26	1375	14.70	0.32	11.87
40.0-49.9	44.35	1144	24.40	0.44	14.88	1128	15.10	0.36	12.09
50.0-59.9	54.89	794	23.60	0.50	14.09	796	15.50	0.42	11.85
60.0-69.9	64.83	1087	21.90	0.40	13.19	1079	15.00	0.37	12.15
70.0-79.9	74.16	770	18.50	0.46	12.76	752	14.60	0.44	12.07
80.0-90.9	84.09	540	15.40	0.46	10.69	522	14.30	0.49	11.20
Females									
2.0-2.9	2.45	492	5.90	0.20	4.44	494	14.20	0.29	6.45
3.0-3.9	3.46	553	6.40	0.29	6.82	555	13.80	0.31	7.30
4.0-4.9	4.44	526	6.70	0.39	8.94	525	14.20	0.34	7.79
5.0-5.9	5.47	552	6.90	0.35	8.22	554	14.60	0.40	9.41
6.0-6.9	6.47	273	7.60	0.73	12.06	269	14.40	0.57	9.35
7.0-7.9	7.44	266	9.80	0.99	16.15	262	16.50	0.76	12.30
8.0-8.9	8.47	242	9.70	0.93	14.47	233	16.80	0.71	10.84
9.0-9.9	9.43	270	12.70	1.18	19.39	165	19.10	0.77	9.89
10.0-10.9	10.43	254	13.50	1.20	19.12	238	18.40	0.84	12.96
11.0-11.9	11.46	267	14.30	1.15	18.79	243	19.30	0.80	12.47
12.0-12.9	12.46	227	14.90	1.29	19.44	200	18.90	0.95	13.44
13.0-13.9	13.45	215	16.30	1.34	19.65	190	21.60	0.98	13.51
14.0-14.9	14.47	210	18.20	1.32	19.13	190	23.90	0.99	13.65
15.0-15.9	15.47	184	16.80	1.38	18.72	164	23.40	1.10	14.09
16.0-16.9	16.47	197	17.00	1.26	17.68	179	25.20	1.03	13.78
17.0-17.9	17.45	183	18.70	1.31	17.72	152	25.80	1.08	13.32
18.0-18.9	18.43	163	17.40	1.37	17.49	147	25.30	1.12	13.58
19.0-19.9	19.48	163	17.00	1.43	18.26	139	25.10	1.28	15.09
20.0-29.9	24.91	1552	17.70	0.38	14.97	1336	26.70	0.34	12.43
30.0-39.9	34.86	1580	19.80	0.41	16.30	1261	29.00	0.36	12.78
40.0-49.9	44.28	1205	22.00	0.46	15.97	955	31.60	0.40	12.36
50.0-59.9	54.83	890	24.00	0.50	14.92	701	31.30	0.47	12.44
60.0-69.9	64.82	1005	21.10	0.44	13.95	906	30.20	0.44	13.24
70.0-79.9	74.46	816	18.70	0.48	13.71	740	29.10	0.47	12.79
80.0-90.9	84.45	554	15.70	0.48	11.30	513	27.30	0.54	12.23

Table III.6.
Mean (M), standard error of the mean (SE), and standard deviation (SD) of mid-upper arm circumference (cm)
and thigh circumference (cm) by age of all ethnic groups combined of males and females
of 2 to 90 years: NHANES III, 1988-1994

Age Group (years)	Mean Age (years)	Mid-Upper Arm Circumference (cm)				Thigh Circumference (cm)			
		N	M	SE	SD	N	M	SE	SD
Males									
2.0-2.9	2.46	574	16.50	0.08	1.92	522	28.10	0.15	3.43
3.0-3.9	3.45	483	16.90	0.13	2.86	482	29.20	0.21	4.61
4.0-4.9	4.47	542	17.30	0.11	2.56	539	30.20	0.18	4.18
5.0-5.9	5.43	495	17.90	0.13	2.89	489	31.60	0.22	4.86
6.0-6.9	6.45	279	18.90	0.28	4.68	279	33.70	0.44	7.35
7.0-7.9	7.47	268	19.30	0.24	3.93	268	34.90	0.40	6.55
8.0-8.9	8.46	261	20.40	0.31	5.01	260	36.70	0.48	7.74
9.0-9.9	9.50	276	21.70	0.34	5.65	273	39.40	0.53	8.76
10.0-10.9	10.45	294	22.60	0.34	5.83	293	40.50	0.47	8.05
11.0-11.9	11.44	281	23.60	0.38	6.37	279	42.90	0.61	10.19
12.0-12.9	12.47	202	25.20	0.45	6.40	201	44.90	0.65	9.22
13.0-13.9	13.47	181	25.70	0.49	6.59	181	45.90	0.72	9.69
14.0-14.9	14.49	185	28.10	0.78	10.61	185	49.50	1.05	14.28
15.0-15.9	15.45	183	28.50	0.51	6.90	180	50.70	0.74	9.93
16.0-16.9	16.45	191	29.20	0.50	6.91	191	50.50	0.76	10.50
17.0-17.9	17.45	193	30.70	0.51	7.09	191	51.70	0.62	8.57
18.0-18.9	18.46	168	30.10	0.55	7.13	169	50.70	0.79	10.27
19.0-19.9	19.43	161	31.50	0.52	6.60	161	51.70	0.66	8.37
20.0-29.9	24.96	1585	32.40	0.14	5.57	1574	52.40	0.18	7.14
30.0-39.9	34.72	1435	33.40	0.15	5.68	1430	53.00	0.19	7.18
40.0-49.9	44.35	1178	33.70	0.15	5.15	1170	52.30	0.20	6.84
50.0-59.9	54.89	824	33.70	0.18	5.17	815	51.60	0.22	6.28
60.0-69.9	64.83	1126	32.80	0.15	5.03	1091	49.80	0.18	5.95
70.0-79.9	74.16	832	31.50	0.17	4.90	764	48.10	0.24	6.63
80.0-90.9	84.09	642	29.50	0.19	4.81	525	46.10	0.25	5.73
Females									
2.0-2.9	2.45	556	16.30	0.09	2.12	508	28.40	0.17	3.83
3.0-3.9	3.46	561	17.00	0.11	2.61	560	29.50	0.19	4.50
4.0-4.9	4.44	527	17.60	0.17	3.90	527	31.10	0.28	6.43
5.0-5.9	5.47	555	18.10	0.15	3.53	556	32.10	0.25	5.89
6.0-6.9	6.47	273	18.70	0.28	4.63	274	33.40	0.45	7.45
7.0-7.9	7.44	270	19.90	0.34	5.59	268	35.30	0.50	8.19
8.0-8.9	8.47	245	20.60	0.35	5.48	245	37.40	0.51	7.98
9.0-9.9	9.43	272	22.10	0.47	7.75	271	39.40	0.64	10.54
10.0-10.9	10.43	255	22.60	0.42	6.71	255	40.60	0.61	9.74
11.0-11.9	11.46	268	23.70	0.40	6.55	268	43.10	0.57	9.33
12.0-12.9	12.46	233	24.50	0.48	7.33	231	44.80	0.70	10.64
13.0-13.9	13.45	217	26.30	0.53	7.81	218	47.90	0.71	10.48
14.0-14.9	14.47	218	26.90	0.49	7.23	217	48.80	0.71	10.46
15.0-15.9	15.47	189	26.70	0.49	6.74	187	48.70	0.64	8.75
16.0-16.9	16.47	204	27.30	0.47	6.71	202	49.50	0.65	9.24
17.0-17.9	17.45	195	27.70	0.50	6.98	192	49.90	0.73	10.12
18.0-18.9	18.43	170	27.40	0.59	7.69	169	49.60	0.88	11.44
19.0-19.9	19.48	168	28.20	0.63	8.17	168	51.00	0.92	11.92
20.0-29.9	24.91	1623	28.90	0.17	6.85	1615	50.70	0.23	9.24
30.0-39.9	34.86	1707	30.70	0.19	7.85	1690	52.40	0.26	10.69
40.0-49.9	44.28	1300	31.40	0.20	7.21	1289	52.10	0.29	10.41
50.0-59.9	54.83	970	32.50	0.25	7.79	957	52.00	0.34	10.52
60.0-69.9	64.82	1122	31.70	0.21	7.03	1071	49.80	0.30	9.82
70.0-79.9	74.46	914	30.50	0.23	6.95	848	48.60	0.33	9.61
80.0-90.9	84.45	712	28.50	0.25	6.67	552	46.80	0.37	8.69

Table III.7.

Mean (M), standard error of the mean (SE), and standard deviation (SD) of waist circumference (cm) and buttocks (hip) circumference (cm) by age of all ethnic groups combined of males and females of 2 to 90 years: NHANES III, 1988-1994

Age Group (years)	Mean Age (years)	Waist Circumference (cm)				Buttocks (hip) Circumference (cm)			
		N	M	SE	SD	N	M	SE	SD
Males									
2.0-2.9	2.46	524	47.90	0.20	4.58	524	51.00	0.23	5.26
3.0-3.9	3.45	485	49.80	0.31	6.83	484	52.40	0.32	7.04
4.0-4.9	4.47	542	51.40	0.25	5.82	540	54.60	0.27	6.27
5.0-5.9	5.43	492	53.00	0.31	6.88	491	57.30	0.33	7.31
6.0-6.9	6.45	279	55.70	0.64	10.69	278	61.00	0.68	11.34
7.0-7.9	7.47	268	57.40	0.63	10.31	268	64.10	0.64	10.48
8.0-8.9	8.46	262	60.00	0.72	11.65	260	67.80	0.76	12.25
9.0-9.9	9.50	273	63.30	0.91	15.04	273	72.30	0.82	13.55
10.0-10.9	10.45	293	65.10	0.83	14.21	293	74.50	0.75	12.84
11.0-11.9	11.44	281	68.70	1.02	17.10	280	78.20	0.94	15.73
12.0-12.9	12.47	202	72.20	1.20	17.06	202	82.60	1.03	14.64
13.0-13.9	13.47	181	73.00	1.35	18.16	181	85.30	1.15	15.47
14.0-14.9	14.49	185	77.40	1.91	25.98	185	90.80	1.74	23.67
15.0-15.9	15.45	182	78.70	1.54	20.78	181	92.50	1.21	16.28
16.0-16.9	16.45	191	78.30	1.25	17.28	191	93.20	1.06	14.65
17.0-17.9	17.45	190	81.00	1.26	17.37	191	95.00	0.96	13.27
18.0-18.9	18.46	169	80.20	1.35	17.55	169	94.70	1.18	15.34
19.0-19.9	19.43	162	82.10	1.33	16.93	161	96.00	1.20	15.23
20.0-29.9	24.96	1579	87.60	0.43	17.09	1578	97.40	0.32	12.71
30.0-39.9	34.72	1428	93.60	0.46	17.38	1428	99.60	0.34	12.85
40.0-49.9	44.35	1173	97.70	0.54	18.49	1174	100.70	0.43	14.73
50.0-59.9	54.89	816	100.50	0.58	16.57	817	101.10	0.40	11.43
60.0-69.9	64.83	1101	101.60	0.49	16.26	1103	100.60	0.36	11.96
70.0-79.9	74.16	773	100.10	0.57	15.85	772	99.60	0.43	11.95
80.0-90.9	84.09	540	97.60	0.67	15.57	539	97.50	0.46	10.68
Females									
2.0-2.9	2.45	507	48.00	0.28	6.30	508	50.80	0.28	6.31
3.0-3.9	3.46	562	49.80	0.35	8.30	560	52.70	0.28	6.63
4.0-4.9	4.44	527	52.10	0.46	10.56	525	55.80	0.40	9.17
5.0-5.9	5.47	554	53.30	0.41	9.65	556	58.40	0.39	9.20
6.0-6.9	6.47	273	54.60	0.78	12.89	273	60.90	0.67	11.07
7.0-7.9	7.44	268	57.60	0.92	15.06	268	65.20	0.79	12.93
8.0-8.9	8.47	244	59.40	0.94	14.68	244	69.40	0.85	13.28
9.0-9.9	9.43	273	62.90	1.14	18.84	272	72.80	0.97	16.00
10.0-10.9	10.43	254	64.70	1.22	19.44	255	75.80	0.92	14.69
11.0-11.9	11.46	266	67.40	1.05	17.12	267	81.20	0.90	14.71
12.0-12.9	12.46	233	69.90	1.36	20.76	233	85.50	1.11	16.94
13.0-13.9	13.45	216	74.00	1.49	21.90	218	91.00	1.13	16.68
14.0-14.9	14.47	217	76.40	1.40	20.62	217	93.90	1.12	16.50
15.0-15.9	15.47	188	74.10	1.43	19.61	188	93.40	1.14	15.63
16.0-16.9	16.47	204	76.50	1.69	24.14	204	95.60	1.27	18.14
17.0-17.9	17.45	191	78.50	1.50	20.73	193	97.60	1.25	17.37
18.0-18.9	18.43	169	76.50	1.72	22.36	169	95.80	1.35	17.55
19.0-19.9	19.48	170	78.60	1.88	24.51	170	97.60	1.48	19.30
20.0-29.9	24.91	1616	80.50	0.51	20.50	1616	98.20	0.41	16.48
30.0-39.9	34.86	1702	86.40	0.59	24.34	1699	102.70	0.47	19.37
40.0-49.9	44.28	1295	89.70	0.66	23.75	1299	104.00	0.53	19.10
50.0-59.9	54.83	962	94.40	0.75	23.26	962	105.40	0.63	19.54
60.0-69.9	64.82	1074	94.50	0.67	21.96	1076	103.10	0.56	18.37
70.0-79.9	74.46	852	93.60	0.73	21.31	854	101.40	0.58	16.95
80.0-90.9	84.45	560	91.70	0.73	17.27	562	99.40	0.62	14.70

Table III.8.
Mean (M), standard error of the mean (SE), and standard deviation (SD) of wrist breadth (cm) and elbow breadth (cm)
of all ethnic groups combined of males and females of 2 to 90 years: NHANES III, 1988-1994

Age Group (years)	Mean Age (years)	Wrist Breadth (cm)				Elbow Breadth (cm)			
		N	M	SE	SD	N	M	SE	SD
Males									
2.0-2.9	2.46	528	3.60	0.02	0.46	529	4.40	0.02	0.46
3.0-3.9	3.45	487	3.80	0.02	0.44	486	4.60	0.02	0.44
4.0-4.9	4.47	544	3.90	0.02	0.47	544	4.70	0.02	0.47
5.0-5.9	5.43	495	4.10	0.02	0.44	496	4.90	0.02	0.45
6.0-6.9	6.45	279	4.20	0.03	0.50	280	5.10	0.04	0.67
7.0-7.9	7.47	269	4.40	0.03	0.49	269	5.30	0.04	0.66
8.0-8.9	8.46	261	4.50	0.04	0.65	262	5.60	0.05	0.81
9.0-9.9	9.50	276	4.70	0.03	0.50	276	5.80	0.04	0.66
10.0-10.9	10.45	294	4.80	0.03	0.51	294	5.90	0.04	0.69
11.0-11.9	11.44	282	5.00	0.04	0.67	282	6.20	0.05	0.84
12.0-12.9	12.47	202	5.30	0.05	0.71	202	6.60	0.05	0.71
13.0-13.9	13.47	182	5.50	0.06	0.81	182	6.80	0.06	0.81
14.0-14.9	14.49	187	5.70	0.04	0.55	187	7.00	0.07	0.96
15.0-15.9	15.45	185	5.70	0.04	0.54	185	7.20	0.06	0.82
16.0-16.9	16.45	192	5.70	0.04	0.55	192	7.20	0.05	0.69
17.0-17.9	17.45	193	5.80	0.04	0.56	193	7.30	0.05	0.69
18.0-18.9	18.46	169	5.80	0.05	0.65	170	7.20	0.06	0.78
19.0-19.9	19.43	164	5.80	0.03	0.38	164	7.10	0.05	0.64
20.0-29.9	24.96	1588	5.80	0.01	0.40	1586	7.20	0.02	0.80
30.0-39.9	34.72	1435	5.90	0.01	0.38	1437	7.30	0.02	0.76
40.0-49.9	44.35	1180	5.90	0.02	0.69	1181	7.40	0.02	0.69
50.0-59.9	54.89	819	6.00	0.02	0.57	820	7.50	0.03	0.86
60.0-69.9	64.83	1117	6.10	0.02	0.67	1116	7.50	0.02	0.67
70.0-79.9	74.16	799	6.10	0.02	0.57	797	7.50	0.03	0.85
80.0-90.9	84.09	563	6.10	0.03	0.71	560	7.50	0.03	0.71
Females									
2.0-2.9	2.45	508	3.50	0.02	0.45	508	4.20	0.02	0.45
3.0-3.9	3.46	567	3.60	0.02	0.48	566	4.40	0.02	0.48
4.0-4.9	4.44	528	3.80	0.02	0.46	526	4.60	0.03	0.69
5.0-5.9	5.47	555	3.90	0.02	0.47	555	4.80	0.03	0.71
6.0-6.9	6.47	274	4.10	0.03	0.50	274	4.90	0.04	0.66
7.0-7.9	7.44	269	4.20	0.04	0.66	271	5.10	0.04	0.66
8.0-8.9	8.47	245	4.40	0.03	0.47	245	5.30	0.04	0.63
9.0-9.9	9.43	271	4.60	0.03	0.49	272	5.60	0.05	0.82
10.0-10.9	10.43	257	4.70	0.04	0.64	257	5.70	0.05	0.80
11.0-11.9	11.46	270	4.90	0.04	0.66	270	5.90	0.04	0.66
12.0-12.9	12.46	233	5.00	0.04	0.61	233	6.10	0.05	0.76
13.0-13.9	13.45	218	5.00	0.04	0.59	218	6.20	0.05	0.74
14.0-14.9	14.47	217	5.00	0.04	0.59	220	6.20	0.05	0.74
15.0-15.9	15.47	189	5.00	0.04	0.55	196	6.20	0.06	0.84
16.0-16.9	16.47	203	5.10	0.04	0.57	210	6.20	0.05	0.72
17.0-17.9	17.45	197	5.00	0.04	0.56	212	6.20	0.05	0.73
18.0-18.9	18.43	170	5.00	0.04	0.52	188	6.10	0.06	0.82
19.0-19.9	19.48	171	5.00	0.04	0.52	187	6.30	0.06	0.82
20.0-29.9	24.91	1619	5.00	0.01	0.40	1805	6.20	0.02	0.85
30.0-39.9	34.86	1713	5.10	0.01	0.41	1798	6.40	0.02	0.85
40.0-49.9	44.28	1305	5.20	0.01	0.36	1312	6.50	0.02	0.72
50.0-59.9	54.83	965	5.30	0.02	0.62	986	6.70	0.03	0.94
60.0-69.9	64.82	1091	5.30	0.02	0.66	1092	6.60	0.02	0.66
70.0-79.9	74.46	873	5.30	0.02	0.59	873	6.60	0.03	0.89
80.0-90.9	84.45	596	5.40	0.02	0.49	595	6.50	0.03	0.73

Table III.9.
Mean (M), standard error of the mean (SE), and standard deviation (SD) of biacromial breadth (cm) and bi-iliac breadth (cm)
of all ethnic groups combined of males and females of 2 to 90 years: NHANES III, 1988-1994

Age Group (years)	Mean Age (years)	Biacromial Breadth (cm)				Bi-liac Breadth (cm)			
		N	M	SE	SD	N	M	SE	SD
Males									
2.0-2.9	2.46					532	15.3	0.1	2.31
3.0-3.9	3.45	452	22.40	0.12	2.55	487	16.2	0.09	1.99
4.0-4.9	4.47	542	23.70	0.12	2.79	543	16.8	0.09	2.10
5.0-5.9	5.43	492	25.00	0.14	3.11	491	17.7	0.11	2.44
6.0-6.9	6.45	279	26.30	0.21	3.51	277	18.4	0.19	3.16
7.0-7.9	7.47	268	27.60	0.19	3.11	268	19.6	0.19	3.11
8.0-8.9	8.46	262	29.00	0.25	4.05	261	20	0.21	3.39
9.0-9.9	9.50	274	30.50	0.23	3.81	272	21.3	0.25	4.12
10.0-10.9	10.45	292	31.20	0.21	3.59	292	21.7	0.23	3.93
11.0-11.9	11.44	281	32.60	0.21	3.52	281	22.8	0.25	4.19
12.0-12.9	12.47	202	34.40	0.3	4.26	202	24.3	0.33	4.69
13.0-13.9	13.47	181	35.90	0.36	4.84	181	25.3	0.37	4.98
14.0-14.9	14.49	187	37.70	0.34	4.65	185	26.6	0.53	7.21
15.0-15.9	15.45	183	38.80	0.31	4.19	183	27	0.38	5.14
16.0-16.9	16.45	193	39.90	0.34	4.72	192	27.4	0.41	5.68
17.0-17.9	17.45	193	40.80	0.3	4.17	192	27.7	0.43	5.96
18.0-18.9	18.46	169	41.00	0.3	3.90	169	27.6	0.37	4.81
19.0-19.9	19.43	162	40.80	0.37	4.71	161	27.9	0.4	5.08
20.0-29.9	24.96	1587	41.50	0.1	3.98	1583	28.5	0.12	4.77
30.0-39.9	34.72	1434	41.50	0.1	3.79	1434	29.1	0.13	4.92
40.0-49.9	44.35	1177	41.30	0.11	3.77	1174	29.9	0.14	4.80
50.0-59.9	54.89	817	41.00	0.14	4.00	816	30.5	0.15	4.28
60.0-69.9	64.83	1114	40.50	0.13	4.34	1100	30.8	0.13	4.31
70.0-79.9	74.16	793	39.70	0.15	4.22	780	30.7	0.15	4.19
80.0-90.9	84.09	554	39.00	0.16	3.77	542	30.6	0.17	3.96
Females									
2.0-2.9	2.45					511	15.10	0.11	2.49
3.0-3.9	3.46	529	22.20	0.12	2.76	564	16.00	0.11	2.61
4.0-4.9	4.44	526	23.80	0.18	4.13	528	17.10	0.13	2.99
5.0-5.9	5.47	556	24.90	0.14	3.30	555	17.70	0.12	2.83
6.0-6.9	6.47	274	26.10	0.19	3.15	273	18.40	0.19	3.14
7.0-7.9	7.44	271	27.20	0.24	3.95	269	19.40	0.27	4.43
8.0-8.9	8.47	245	28.80	0.25	3.91	243	20.40	0.27	4.21
9.0-9.9	9.43	274	30.20	0.24	3.97	274	21.40	0.30	4.97
10.0-10.9	10.43	255	31.10	0.21	3.35	255	22.40	0.28	4.47
11.0-11.9	11.46	269	33.00	0.26	4.26	267	23.50	0.29	4.74
12.0-12.9	12.46	233	34.10	0.26	3.97	233	24.40	0.37	5.65
13.0-13.9	13.45	218	35.50	0.31	4.58	217	26.10	0.35	5.16
14.0-14.9	14.47	219	36.00	0.26	3.85	219	26.50	0.34	5.03
15.0-15.9	15.47	195	36.30	0.30	4.19	195	26.80	0.41	5.73
16.0-16.9	16.47	211	36.70	0.24	3.49	211	27.10	0.41	5.96
17.0-17.9	17.45	212	36.70	0.24	3.49	211	27.20	0.36	5.23
18.0-18.9	18.43	185	36.60	0.28	3.81	186	26.80	0.39	5.32
19.0-19.9	19.48	186	36.40	0.26	3.55	187	28.00	0.49	6.70
20.0-29.9	24.91	1805	36.90	0.09	3.82	1806	27.70	0.12	5.10
30.0-39.9	34.86	1795	37.00	0.09	3.81	1786	28.80	0.14	5.92
40.0-49.9	44.28	1305	36.90	0.11	3.97	1302	29.40	0.15	5.41
50.0-59.9	54.83	966	36.90	0.13	4.04	964	30.10	0.18	5.59
60.0-69.9	64.82	1091	36.40	0.12	3.96	1077	30.10	0.16	5.25
70.0-79.9	74.46	866	35.70	0.13	3.83	854	30.00	0.17	4.97
80.0-90.9	84.45	583	34.80	0.15	3.62	567	29.90	0.19	4.52

Table III.10.
Mean (M), standard error of the mean (SE), and standard deviation (SD) of knee height (cm)
by age of all ethnic groups combined of males and females of 60 to 90 years:
NHANES III, 1988-1994

Age Group (years)	Mean Age (years)	N	M	SE	SD
			Males		
60.0-69.9	64.83	1096	54.40	0.11	3.64
70.0-79.9	74.16	781	53.80	0.13	3.63
80.0-90.9	84.09	542	53.50	0.14	3.26
			Females		
60.0-69.9	64.82	1081	49.70	0.12	3.94
70.0-79.9	74.46	863	49.40	0.13	3.82
80.0-90.9	84.45	575	49.20	0.16	3.84

Table III.11.
Mean (M), standard error of the mean (SE), and standard deviation (SD) of fat-free mass (kg),
total body fat (kg), and percent body fat (%) by age of all ethnic groups combined of males and females of
12 to 90 years: NHANES III, 1988-1994

Age Group (years)	Mean (years)	N	Fat-Free Mass (kg) M	SE	SD	Body Fat Weight (kg) M	SE	SD	Body Fat (%) M	SE	SD
					Males						
12-13.9	13.00	355	41.1	0.47	8.9	11.9	0.43	**8.1**	20.9	0.43	8.2
14-15.9	15.00	334	51.0	0.50	9.1	12.90	0.49	8.9	18.9	0.40	7.4
16-17.9	17.00	361	54.7	0.45	8.6	14.20	0.39	7.4	19.7	0.34	6.5
18-19.9	18.90	318	56.9	0.50	8.9	16.40	0.45	7.9	21.5	0.35	6.3
20-29.9	25.00	1550	58.1	0.25	9.9	19.30	0.23	9.2	24.1	0.16	6.3
30-39.9	34.70	1387	60.6	0.28	10.3	21.10	0.23	8.7	25.1	0.16	6.0
40-49.9	44.30	1155	61.4	0.30	10.1	22.30	0.25	8.5	26.0	0.17	5.8
50-59.9	54.90	792	61.6	0.35	9.8	22.60	0.30	8.3	26.3	0.20	5.7
60-69.9	64.80	1053	59.4	0.29	9.3	22.30	0.24	7.6	26.8	0.17	5.6
70-79.9	74.00	723	57.0	0.33	9.0	20.50	0.26	7.0	25.9	0.21	5.6
80-90.9	83.30	473	54.0	0.36	7.9	18.60	0.30	6.6	25.1	0.28	6.1
					Females						
12-13.9	13.00	412	38.2	0.28	5.7	16.6	0.42	8.6	28.6	0.41	8.4
14-15.9	14.90	358	39.6	0.29	5.5	19.2	0.42	8.0	31.5	0.36	6.9
16-17.9	16.90	369	40.9	0.30	5.7	21.9	0.57	10.9	33.2	0.40	7.6
18-19.9	19.00	305	41.1	0.36	6.3	22.0	0.64	11.1	33.2	0.45	7.9
20-29.9	25.00	1511	42.1	0.16	6.2	24.0	0.28	10.7	34.9	0.20	7.6
30-39.9	35.00	1634	44.5	0.18	7.3	28.5	0.32	13.1	37.3	0.20	7.9
40-49.9	44.20	1249	44.8	0.20	7.1	29.7	0.33	11.6	38.7	0.19	6.7
50-59.9	54.80	908	44.8	0.23	7	30.6	0.39	11.9	39.3	0.23	6.8
60-69.9	64.80	1030	42.9	0.20	6.4	28.8	0.32	10.3	39.1	0.20	6.5
70-79.9	74.40	817	41.9	0.22	6.3	26.3	0.33	9.6	37.6	0.23	6.7
80-90.9	83.50	476	39.2	0.24	5.2	22.7	0.35	7.7	35.8	0.31	6.7

LIST OF TABLES

NON-SMOOTHED NHANES III ANTHROPOMETRIC REFERENCE DATA: NON-HISPANIC WHITES

Table III.21. Mean (M), standard error of the mean (SE), and standard deviation (SD) of knee height (cm) for males and females for non-Hispanic whites of 60 to 90 years: NHANES III, 1988-1994.

Table III.22. Mean (M), standard error of the mean (SE), and standard deviation (SD) of fat-free mass (kg), total body fat (kg) and percent body fat (%) for males and females for non-Hispanic whites of 12 to 90 years: NHANES III, 1988-1994.

Non-Smoothed NHANES III Anthropometric Reference Data: Non-Hispanic Whites

Table III.12.
Mean (M), standard error of the mean (SE), and standard deviation of weight (kg), recumbent length (cm), Rohrer's index (100 g/cm³), and head circumference (cm) by age for non-Hispanic white boys and girls of 2 months to 7 years: NHANES III, 1988-1994

Age Group (months)	Mean (months)	Boys N	M	SE	SD	Mean (months)	Girls N	M	SE	SD
				Weight (kg)						
2.0-2.9		52	6.8	0.1	0.8	2.00	77	6.0	0.1	0.9
3.0-5.9	4.02	167	7.8	0.1	1.0	4.10	164	7.1	0.1	0.9
6.0-8.9	6.85	190	8.8	0.1	1.1	7.10	165	8.4	0.1	1.3
9.0-11.9	9.95	167	9.9	0.1	1.1	9.94	160	9.3	0.1	1.1
12.0-23.9	17.51	203	11.7	0.1	1.4	17.63	212	10.9	0.1	1.3
24.0-35.9	29.38	208	13.6	0.1	1.5	29.41	212	13.4	0.1	1.8
36.0-47.9	41.86	136	15.6	0.2	2.1	41.50	153	15.4	0.2	2.1
				Recumbent Length (cm)						
2.0-2.9	2.00	52	61.8	0.5	3.2	2.00	78	60.0	0.4	3.5
3.0-5.9	4.02	168	66.2	0.3	3.6	4.10	164	64.3	0.3	3.7
6.0-8.9	6.85	190	70.5	0.2	3.2	7.10	165	69.4	0.2	2.9
9.0-11.9	9.95	166	74.6	0.2	3.0	9.94	160	73.0	0.3	4.0
12.0-23.9	17.51	201	83.0	0.4	5.2	17.63	209	81.6	0.3	4.3
24.0-35.9	29.38	197	91.9	0.3	4.2	29.41	206	91.5	0.3	5.0
36.0-47.9	41.86	134	100.3	0.4	4.3	41.50	148	99.7	0.4	5.0
				Rohrer's Index (100 g/cm³)						
2.0-2.9	2.00	52	2.88	0.06	0.42	2.00	77	2.74	0.03	0.23
3.0-5.9	4.02	167	2.71	0.03	0.33	4.10	164	2.69	0.03	0.33
6.0-8.9	6.85	190	2.51	0.02	0.25	7.10	165	2.53	0.03	0.37
9.0-11.9	9.95	166	2.38	0.02	0.21	9.94	160	2.40	0.02	0.26
12.0-23.9	17.51	201	2.06	0.02	0.27	17.63	209	2.01	0.01	0.21
24.0-35.9	29.38	197	1.75	0.01	0.16	29.41	206	1.75	0.01	0.20
36.0-47.9	41.86	134	1.54	0.01	0.15	41.50	148	1.55	0.01	0.16
				Head Circumference (cm)						
2.0-2.9	2.00	52	41.3	0.2	1.2	2.00	77	40.0	0.2	1.7
3.0-5.9	4.02	168	43.2	0.1	1.5	4.10	163	42.0	0.1	1.5
6.0-8.9	6.85	188	45.1	0.1	1.4	7.10	166	44.1	0.1	1.4
9.0-11.9	9.95	165	46.4	0.1	1.6	9.94	159	45.2	0.1	1.2
12.0-23.9	17.51	198	48.1	0.1	1.4	17.63	209	46.9	0.1	1.5
24.0-35.9	29.38	193	49.7	0.1	1.5	29.41	199	48.6	0.1	1.4
36.0-47.9	41.86	131	50.3	0.1	1.2	41.50	146	49.5	0.1	1.4
48.0-59.9	53.64	142	51.1	0.1	1.5	52.89	131	50.0	0.1	1.3
60.0-71.9	65.25	136	51.6	0.1	1.3	65.73	149	50.8	0.1	1.3
72.0-83.9	77.65	65	52.2	0.2	1.7	78.06	65	51.0	0.2	1.4

Table III.13.

Mean (M), standard error of the mean (SE), and standard deviation (SD) of weight (kg), stature (cm), and body mass index (w/s²) by age for non-Hispanic white males and females of 2 to 90 years: NHANES III, 1988-1994

Age Group (years)	Mean (years)	Weight				Stature				Body Mass Index			
		N	M	SE	SD	N	M	SE	SD	N	M	SE	SD
Males													
2.0-2.9	2.4	208	13.6	0.1	1.5	203	90.7	0.3	3.9	203	16.4	0.1	1.2
3.0-3.9	3.5	136	15.5	0.2	2.1	134	99.4	0.4	4.5	134	15.7	0.1	1.4
4.0-4.9	4.5	144	17.4	0.2	2.1	144	105.4	0.4	4.6	143	15.7	0.1	1.2
5.0-5.9	5.4	138	19.8	0.2	2.8	137	112.3	0.4	4.9	137	15.7	0.1	1.5
6.0-6.9	6.5	69	23.1	0.7	5.5	69	119.2	0.9	7.3	69	16.1	0.3	2.5
7.0-7.9	7.4	74	25.7	0.6	5.3	74	125.9	0.8	6.9	74	16.0	0.3	2.2
8.0-8.9	8.4	79	28.9	0.8	7.1	79	131.4	0.7	5.9	79	16.6	0.3	3.0
9.0-9.9	9.5	75	34.2	1.0	8.7	75	138.2	0.8	6.5	75	17.9	0.4	3.4
10.0-10.9	10.5	74	36.8	0.9	7.9	74	142.8	0.9	7.7	74	18.1	0.3	2.8
11.0-11.9	11.4	68	40.1	1.2	9.7	68	147.3	0.9	7.8	68	18.3	0.4	3.3
12.0-12.9	12.4	48	48.0	1.4	9.9	50	155.0	1.0	6.8	48	19.4	0.4	3.1
13.0-13.9	13.5	48	53.6	2.0	14.2	48	162.9	1.2	8.4	48	19.9	0.6	4.1
14.0-14.9	14.5	47	63.0	2.5	16.9	48	169.8	1.1	7.5	47	21.5	0.8	5.4
15.0-15.9	15.5	37	66.6	2.5	15.2	37	174.4	1.3	7.9	37	22.0	0.7	4.3
16.0-16.9	16.5	50	68.1	2.7	19.4	50	177.3	1.1	7.4	50	21.6	0.7	4.9
17.0-17.9	17.4	51	71.6	2.1	14.7	51	177.0	1.1	8.0	51	22.6	0.6	4.4
18.0-18.9	18.5	44	72.1	2.5	16.7	44	178.3	1.2	7.8	44	22.3	0.7	4.5
19.0-19.9	19.4	35	72.3	2.0	11.9	35	175.4	0.7	4.4	35	23.1	0.6	3.6
20.0-29.9	25.3	393	79.0	0.9	17.8	393	177.4	0.3	6.7	393	25.0	0.3	5.4
30.0-39.9	34.9	454	84.4	0.9	19.0	454	177.9	0.3	7.0	454	26.6	0.3	5.3
40.0-49.9	44.5	428	86.2	0.9	19.2	428	177.2	0.3	7.0	428	27.4	0.3	5.8
50.0-59.9	54.9	418	87.1	0.8	16.8	418	176.7	0.3	6.3	418	27.9	0.3	5.1
60.0-69.9	65.0	510	84.3	0.7	16.0	510	175.0	0.3	6.5	510	27.5	0.2	4.7
70.0-79.9	74.3	524	79.6	0.7	15.1	524	172.2	0.3	6.6	524	26.8	0.2	4.6
80.0-90.9	84.0	560	72.3	0.6	14.0	559	169.8	0.3	7.1	559	25.0	0.2	4.3
Females													
2.0-2.9	2.5	212	13.3	0.1	1.8	212	90.0	0.3	4.6	211	16.3	0.1	1.5
3.0-3.9	3.5	153	15.3	0.2	2.1	152	98.4	0.4	4.8	152	15.8	0.1	1.5
4.0-4.9	4.4	135	17.2	0.2	2.1	134	105.0	0.4	4.3	134	15.6	0.1	1.2
5.0-5.9	5.5	150	20.1	0.3	3.7	150	112.4	0.4	5.3	150	15.8	0.2	2.1
6.0-6.9	6.5	67	21.5	0.5	4.5	67	118.1	0.7	5.6	67	15.3	0.3	2.3
7.0-7.9	7.5	73	25.0	0.7	5.6	73	123.8	0.7	6.0	73	16.1	0.3	2.5
8.0-8.9	8.4	66	28.7	1.1	8.6	65	131.0	0.8	6.3	65	16.5	0.5	3.9
9.0-9.9	9.4	83	32.1	1.0	9.0	83	135.4	0.7	6.4	83	17.6	0.4	3.5
10.0-10.9	10.4	67	36.4	1.1	9.4	67	142.2	0.9	7.1	67	17.6	0.4	3.6
11.0-11.9	11.5	71	43.5	1.1	9.4	71	151.2	0.8	6.8	71	18.9	0.4	3.2
12.0-12.9	12.4	45	48.8	1.9	12.8	47	156.3	1.3	8.6	45	20.4	0.8	5.0
13.0-13.9	13.5	60	55.5	1.8	13.6	62	160.6	0.9	7.2	60	21.5	0.6	4.6
14.0-14.9	14.4	64	55.8	1.4	10.9	64	162.4	0.8	6.2	64	21.1	0.5	3.9
15.0-15.9	15.5	62	57.1	1.2	9.4	62	163.3	0.7	5.2	62	21.5	0.4	3.3
16.0-16.9	16.6	56	60.7	2.2	16.7	57	164.1	0.8	6.1	56	22.3	0.8	5.7
17.0-17.9	17.4	56	59.9	1.7	12.4	56	164.7	0.9	6.6	56	22.0	0.6	4.2
18.0-18.9	18.5	55	59.2	1.6	12.2	55	164.7	0.9	6.6	55	21.6	0.6	4.3
19.0-19.9	19.4	58	62.4	2.0	15.6	58	165.4	0.8	6.3	58	23.0	0.8	5.7
20.0-29.9	25.2	452	63.7	0.9	18.5	499	163.6	0.4	8.9	452	23.8	0.3	6.4
30.0-39.9	35.0	579	68.9	0.9	22.6	600	164.5	0.4	8.6	579	25.5	0.3	7.9
40.0-49.9	44.5	477	70.5	1.0	21.0	478	163.5	0.4	8.1	477	26.4	0.4	7.9
50.0-59.9	54.9	484	74.3	1.0	21.8	485	162.4	0.4	7.9	484	28.2	0.4	7.9
60.0-69.9	64.8	501	70.7	0.9	19.5	501	160.7	0.4	8.1	501	27.3	0.3	7.2
70.0-79.9	74.5	644	66.8	0.7	18.8	644	158.1	0.4	8.9	643	26.7	0.3	7.1
80.0-90.9	84.5	621	60.4	0.6	15.7	624	155.0	0.4	9.0	621	25.1	0.2	6.0

Non-Smoothed NHANES III Anthropometric Reference Data: Non-Hispanic Whites

Table III.14.

Mean (M), standard error of the mean (SE), and standard deviation (SD) of sitting height (cm), upper arm length (cm), and upper leg length (cm) by age for non-Hispanic white males and females of 2 to 90 years: NHANES III, 1988-1994

Age Group (years)	Mean (years)	Sitting Height				Upper Arm Length				Upper Leg Length			
		N	M	SE	SD	N	M	SE	SD	N	M	SE	SD
Males													
2.0-2.9	2.45	198	52.4	0.17	2.4	185	17.8	0.09	1.2	180	18.4	0.17	1.7
3.0-3.9	3.49	134	55.0	0.22	2.5	129	19.4	0.10	1.1	131	21.3	0.22	2.0
4.0-4.9	4.47	143	57.8	0.22	2.7	140	20.9	0.12	1.4	140	23.0	0.22	2.0
5.0-5.9	5.44	137	60.7	0.25	2.9	135	22.3	0.12	1.4	132	25.3	0.25	2.1
6.0-6.9	6.47	69	63.8	0.47	3.9	68	23.9	0.23	1.9	68	27.3	0.47	2.6
7.0-7.9	7.44	74	66.2	0.39	3.4	72	25.5	0.21	1.8	72	29.8	0.39	2.5
8.0-8.9	8.44	79	69.0	0.38	3.4	75	26.5	0.20	1.8	74	30.9	0.38	2.7
9.0-9.9	9.49	74	71.7	0.37	3.1	73	28.4	0.23	2.0	73	33.3	0.37	2.6
10.0-10.9	10.47	74	73.8	0.45	3.9	74	29.2	0.27	2.3	74	34.9	0.45	3.3
11.0-11.9	11.44	67	76.0	0.45	3.7	67	30.1	0.23	1.9	65	36.0	0.45	2.7
12.0-12.9	12.39	48	79.7	0.53	3.7	47	32.3	0.31	2.1	47	38.7	0.53	3.1
13.0-13.9	13.49	48	82.8	0.68	4.7	47	33.9	0.38	2.6	47	39.6	0.68	3.2
14.0-14.9	14.50	48	87.3	0.68	4.7	47	35.4	0.32	2.2	48	42.4	0.68	2.9
15.0-15.9	15.49	37	90.0	0.71	4.3	37	36.6	0.37	2.3	36	43.9	0.71	3.0
16.0-16.9	16.47	50	92.1	0.56	4.0	50	37.4	0.33	2.3	50	44.2	0.56	2.7
17.0-17.9	17.45	50	92.4	0.53	3.8	51	37.0	0.23	1.7	49	44.5	0.53	2.7
18.0-18.9	18.47	42	92.9	0.57	3.7	41	37.3	0.32	2.1	40	45.1	0.57	3.0
19.0-19.9	19.44	34	92.5	0.42	2.5	33	37.4	0.37	2.1	33	43.4	0.42	2.3
20.0-29.9	25.27	389	93.1	0.21	4.1	386	37.60	0.11	2.16	385	43.4	0.22	4.3
30.0-39.9	34.86	453	93.6	0.21	4.5	446	38.00	0.10	2.11	446	43.3	0.20	4.2
40.0-49.9	44.53	421	93.3	0.20	4.1	416	38.10	0.11	2.24	413	42.3	0.21	4.3
50.0-59.9	54.88	409	92.9	0.19	3.8	402	38.30	0.10	2.00	401	42.0	0.21	4.2
60.0-69.9	65.05	487	91.4	0.17	3.8	482	38.20	0.09	1.98	479	41.0	0.21	4.6
70.0-79.9	74.30	483	89.7	0.19	4.2	474	37.80	0.10	2.18	471	40.6	0.21	4.6
80.0-90.9	84.03	452	87.7	0.21	4.5	438	37.70	0.10	2.09	421	40.2	0.22	4.5
Females													
2.0-2.9	2.45	206	51.7	0.20	2.9	188	17.9	0.10	1.4	191	19.0	0.20	2.0
3.0-3.9	3.46	148	54.7	0.22	2.7	141	19.1	0.11	1.3	142	21.5	0.22	1.9
4.0-4.9	4.41	134	57.4	0.22	2.6	130	20.7	0.11	1.3	132	23.4	0.22	1.9
5.0-5.9	5.48	150	60.7	0.25	3.1	150	22.4	0.11	1.4	150	25.5	0.25	2.1
6.0-6.9	6.51	66	62.8	0.39	3.2	67	23.8	0.18	1.5	67	27.4	0.39	1.9
7.0-7.9	7.49	73	65.9	0.36	3.1	72	24.8	0.22	1.9	71	28.9	0.36	2.2
8.0-8.9	8.44	65	68.4	0.45	3.6	65	26.5	0.23	1.9	65	31.1	0.45	2.4
9.0-9.9	9.41	82	70.2	0.38	3.4	81	27.9	0.21	1.9	81	32.8	0.38	2.4
10.0-10.9	10.39	67	74.1	0.47	3.9	66	28.8	0.23	1.8	66	34.6	0.47	2.4
11.0-11.9	11.51	71	78.0	0.51	4.3	70	31.0	0.24	2.0	69	36.8	0.51	2.6
12.0-12.9	12.44	47	81.0	0.68	4.7	47	32.4	0.33	2.2	47	38.1	0.68	3.1
13.0-13.9	13.48	60	84.0	0.56	4.3	60	33.1	0.30	2.3	60	39.6	0.56	3.0
14.0-14.9	14.45	63	85.9	0.42	3.3	64	34.1	0.24	1.9	63	39.8	0.42	2.7
15.0-15.9	15.55	62	86.3	0.46	3.6	61	33.9	0.27	2.1	60	39.7	0.46	2.8
16.0-16.9	16.55	56	86.7	0.41	3.1	54	33.9	0.32	2.3	53	40.3	0.41	2.8
17.0-17.9	17.43	55	86.9	0.48	3.6	54	34.2	0.28	2.1	54	40.7	0.48	2.6
18.0-18.9	18.49	55	87.0	0.49	3.6	55	34.1	0.28	2.1	55	40.0	0.49	2.6
19.0-19.9	19.44	58	87.5	0.43	3.3	57	34.1	0.24	1.8	58	40.8	0.43	3.4
20.0-29.9	25.20	489	86.9	0.19	4.2	485	34.30	0.11	2.42	484	39.7	0.20	4.4
30.0-39.9	34.97	595	87.5	0.17	4.1	580	34.70	0.09	2.17	576	39.6	0.17	4.1
40.0-49.9	44.49	467	87.1	0.18	3.9	459	34.60	0.09	1.93	458	38.9	0.21	4.5
50.0-59.9	54.88	476	86.1	0.19	4.1	470	34.80	0.10	2.17	470	38.0	0.20	4.3
60.0-69.9	64.83	472	84.5	0.17	3.7	469	34.60	0.10	2.17	464	37.4	0.21	4.5
70.0-79.9	74.51	584	82.6	0.20	4.8	571	34.50	0.09	2.15	565	36.9	0.20	4.8
80.0-90.9	84.48	475	79.9	0.22	4.8	452	34.30	0.10	2.13	443	36.8	0.22	4.6

Table III.15.
Mean (M), standard error of the mean (SE), and standard deviation (SD) of triceps skinfold thickness (mm) and subscapular skinfold thickness (mm) by age for non-Hispanic white males and females of 2 to 90 years: NHANES III, 1988-1994

Age Group (years)	Mean (years)	Triceps Skinfold				Subscapular Skinfold			
		N	M	SE	SD	N	M	SE	SD
Males									
2.0-2.9	2.45	181	9.1	0.1	1.7	178	6.3	0.1	1.4
3.0-3.9	3.49	129	8.7	0.2	1.8	130	5.8	0.1	1.4
4.0-4.9	4.47	140	8.8	0.2	2.1	139	5.7	0.1	1.6
5.0-5.9	5.44	134	8.5	0.2	2.2	133	5.5	0.2	1.8
6.0-6.9	6.47	68	9.5	0.5	4.1	68	6.6	0.5	4.2
7.0-7.9	7.44	72	9.0	0.4	3.7	72	6.0	0.5	4.3
8.0-8.9	8.44	75	9.9	0.6	4.8	74	6.5	0.5	4.2
9.0-9.9	9.49	73	11.6	0.7	6.2	72	7.7	0.6	5.2
10.0-10.9	10.47	74	11.6	0.7	5.6	74	7.9	0.6	4.8
11.0-11.9	11.44	67	12.5	0.7	6.0	67	8.4	0.7	5.6
12.0-12.9	12.39	47	13.4	0.8	5.6	47	9.1	0.8	5.2
13.0-13.9	13.49	47	11.4	1.0	6.8	47	8.8	0.9	6.2
14.0-14.9	14.50	46	10.5	0.9	5.9	47	9.4	0.9	6.3
15.0-15.9	15.49	37	11.4	1.2	7.4	37	10.6	1.2	7.3
16.0-16.9	16.47	49	10.6	1.0	7.0	48	9.6	0.9	6.2
17.0-17.9	17.45	50	10.1	0.9	6.2	48	12.0	1.0	7.2
18.0-18.9	18.47	41	11.2	1.1	7.2	41	11.6	1.1	6.7
19.0-19.9	19.44	33	11.4	1.3	7.3	33	13.7	1.2	7.1
20.0-29.9	25.27	382	12.3	12.3	6.8	381	15.9	0.4	8.6
30.0-39.9	34.86	440	13.3	13.3	7.1	440	18.9	0.4	8.2
40.0-49.9	44.53	410	13.8	13.8	6.7	400	20.2	0.4	8.2
50.0-59.9	54.88	402	13.8	13.8	6.6	382	20.5	0.4	8.6
60.0-69.9	65.05	486	14.6	14.6	6.8	461	21.3	0.4	8.6
70.0-79.9	74.30	500	13.5	13.5	6.5	462	19.4	0.4	7.7
80.0-90.9	84.03	515	12.0	12.0	5.7	429	16.7	0.3	6.8
Females									
2.0-2.9	2.45	185	9.6	0.2	2.1	184	6.9	0.1	1.6
3.0-3.9	3.46	139	9.6	0.2	2.7	139	6.5	0.2	2.4
4.0-4.9	4.41	130	9.7	0.2	1.8	129	6.3	0.1	1.6
5.0-5.9	5.48	150	10.2	0.3	3.1	150	7.0	0.3	3.6
6.0-6.9	6.51	66	9.5	0.5	3.9	65	6.5	0.5	4.0
7.0-7.9	7.49	72	11.0	0.6	4.7	71	7.0	0.5	4.2
8.0-8.9	8.44	65	11.5	0.7	5.6	64	7.5	0.7	5.5
9.0-9.9	9.41	80	13.1	0.7	6.2	80	9.0	0.7	6.2
10.0-10.9	10.39	66	13.8	0.8	6.3	66	9.7	0.8	6.6
11.0-11.9	11.51	70	13.7	0.7	6.0	69	9.9	0.8	6.6
12.0-12.9	12.44	47	15.6	1.1	7.8	47	12.2	1.1	7.3
13.0-13.9	13.48	60	17.7	0.8	6.6	60	13.1	0.9	6.9
14.0-14.9	14.45	63	17.4	0.8	6.6	64	13.8	0.9	7.4
15.0-15.9	15.55	61	17.4	0.8	6.4	60	13.2	0.8	6.6
16.0-16.9	16.55	53	18.3	1.0	7.1	53	14.7	1.0	6.9
17.0-17.9	17.43	54	19.3	1.0	7.2	53	16.8	1.1	7.9
18.0-18.9	18.49	55	17.0	0.9	6.9	54	13.5	0.9	6.4
19.0-19.9	19.44	56	19.6	1.0	7.8	56	14.8	0.9	7.0
20.0-29.9	25.20	438	20.6	0.5	10.5	424	17.4	0.5	10.7
30.0-39.9	34.97	549	22.9	0.5	11.2	533	20.0	0.5	11.8
40.0-49.9	44.49	445	25.1	0.5	9.7	428	21.9	0.5	10.8
50.0-59.9	54.88	460	26.7	0.4	9.4	450	24.1	0.5	11.0
60.0-69.9	64.83	473	24.3	0.4	9.6	464	22.1	0.5	10.6
70.0-79.9	74.51	601	22.2	0.4	9.3	558	19.3	0.4	9.4
80.0-90.9	84.48	561	18.7	0.4	8.8	445	16.1	0.4	8.4

Table III.16.
Mean (M), standard error of the mean (SE), and standard deviation (SD) of supra-iliac skinfold thickness (mm) and thigh skinfold thickness (mm) by age for non-Hispanic white males and females of 2 to 90 years: NHANES III, 1988-1994

Age Group (years)	Mean (years)	Supra-iliac Skinfold Thickness				Thigh Skinfold Thickness			
		N	M	SE	SD	N	M	SE	SD
Males									
2.0-2.9	2.45	175	5.1	0.10	1.4	175	12.5	0.21	2.8
3.0-3.9	3.49	130	4.9	0.10	1.1	131	11.2	0.22	2.6
4.0-4.9	4.47	139	5.1	0.21	2.5	140	10.9	0.27	3.2
5.0-5.9	5.44	132	5.1	0.22	2.5	130	11.4	0.33	3.8
6.0-6.9	6.47	68	6.4	0.65	5.4	68	12.5	0.86	7.1
7.0-7.9	7.44	72	6.3	0.64	5.5	71	11.4	0.55	4.7
8.0-8.9	8.44	72	6.6	0.58	4.9	71	12.6	0.75	6.3
9.0-9.9	9.49	73	8.8	0.91	7.8	68	14.6	1.03	8.5
10.0-10.9	10.47	72	9.9	0.90	7.7	73	15.6	0.95	8.1
11.0-11.9	11.44	66	10.6	0.98	8.0	63	16.3	0.92	7.3
12.0-12.9	12.39	47	14.0	1.31	9.0	47	16.5	1.01	6.9
13.0-13.9	13.49	47	11.1	1.24	8.5	45	13.4	1.17	7.8
14.0-14.9	14.50	44	11.0	1.09	7.2	45	12.7	1.11	7.4
15.0-15.9	15.49	35	13.5	1.62	9.6	33	12.1	1.18	6.8
16.0-16.9	16.47	47	11.3	1.19	8.2	45	11.1	0.87	5.8
17.0-17.9	17.45	47	13.1	1.34	9.2	46	11.0	0.84	5.7
18.0-18.9	18.47	39	14.6	1.48	9.3	38	10.8	0.95	5.8
19.0-19.9	19.44	33	16.4	1.78	10.2	33	12.9	1.39	8.0
20.0-29.9	25.27	378	20.60	0.68	13.22	371	14.20	0.45	8.67
30.0-39.9	34.86	439	24.00	0.57	11.94	430	15.40	0.44	9.12
40.0-49.9	44.53	403	24.90	0.57	11.44	395	15.80	0.47	9.34
50.0-59.9	54.88	396	23.40	0.56	11.14	390	16.00	0.47	9.28
60.0-69.9	65.05	476	22.00	0.47	10.25	470	15.50	0.43	9.32
70.0-79.9	74.30	469	18.50	0.46	9.96	461	14.70	0.42	9.02
80.0-90.9	84.03	430	15.30	0.40	8.29	416	14.40	0.42	8.57
Females									
2.0-2.9	2.45	184	5.8	0.12	1.6	184	14.4	0.26	3.6
3.0-3.9	3.46	139	5.9	0.23	2.7	139	13.8	0.36	4.2
4.0-4.9	4.41	129	5.9	0.17	2.0	131	14.3	0.28	3.2
5.0-5.9	5.48	148	6.5	0.29	3.5	150	14.7	0.44	5.4
6.0-6.9	6.51	64	6.0	0.54	4.3	65	13.5	0.66	5.3
7.0-7.9	7.49	71	7.7	0.64	5.4	70	15.4	0.71	6.0
8.0-8.9	8.44	64	7.9	0.80	6.4	62	16.0	0.77	6.0
9.0-9.9	9.41	80	10.5	0.86	7.7	78	19.4	0.85	7.5
10.0-10.9	10.39	66	11.5	1.02	8.3	61	18.0	0.93	7.3
11.0-11.9	11.51	70	12.2	0.93	7.8	67	18.8	0.84	6.9
12.0-12.9	12.44	46	15.2	1.27	8.6	40	18.8	1.21	7.6
13.0-13.9	13.48	58	15.8	1.16	8.9	49	22.9	1.13	7.9
14.0-14.9	14.45	62	17.3	1.08	8.5	56	22.7	1.10	8.2
15.0-15.9	15.55	60	15.2	0.98	7.6	55	24.3	1.04	7.7
16.0-16.9	16.55	53	16.1	1.16	8.5	51	25.9	1.17	8.3
17.0-17.9	17.43	51	16.8	1.14	8.1	45	26.3	1.15	7.7
18.0-18.9	18.49	55	14.9	1.01	7.5	49	23.8	1.12	7.8
19.0-19.9	19.44	55	15.2	1.05	7.8	48	25.5	1.2	8.5
20.0-29.9	25.20	431	16.7	0.6	11.6	387	27.1	0.5	10.2
30.0-39.9	34.97	530	18.3	0.6	12.7	435	29.2	0.5	10.6
40.0-49.9	44.49	443	20.7	0.6	12.2	355	32.4	0.5	10.0
50.0-59.9	54.88	442	23.5	0.6	11.8	350	31.8	0.5	10.1
60.0-69.9	64.83	446	20.5	0.5	11.0	393	30.8	0.5	10.7
70.0-79.9	74.51	548	18.3	0.5	10.5	493	29.5	0.5	10.4
80.0-90.9	84.48	440	15.5	0.4	8.6	407	27.8	0.5	10.1

Table III.17.
Mean (M), standard error of the mean (SE), and standard deviation (SD) of upper arm circumference (cm) and thigh circumference (cm) by age for non-Hispanic white males and females of 2 to 90 years: NHANES III, 1988-1994

Age Group (years)	Mean (years)	Upper Arm Circumference				Thigh Circumference			
		N	M	SE	SD	N	M	SE	SD
Males									
2.0-2.9	2.45	187	16.4	0.08	1.1	180	27.8	0.08	2.0
3.0-3.9	3.49	129	16.8	0.11	1.2	131	28.7	0.11	2.1
4.0-4.9	4.47	140	17.2	0.11	1.3	140	29.9	0.11	2.2
5.0-5.9	5.44	135	17.8	0.13	1.6	132	31.1	0.13	2.7
6.0-6.9	6.47	68	18.8	0.32	2.7	68	33.7	0.32	4.4
7.0-7.9	7.44	72	19.1	0.24	2.1	72	34.2	0.24	3.7
8.0-8.9	8.44	75	19.9	0.31	2.6	74	35.9	0.31	4.5
9.0-9.9	9.49	73	21.5	0.39	3.3	73	39.2	0.39	5.5
10.0-10.9	10.47	74	22.4	0.37	3.2	74	40.5	0.37	4.6
11.0-11.9	11.44	67	22.9	0.42	3.4	65	41.3	0.42	5.5
12.0-12.9	12.39	47	24.7	0.47	3.2	47	44.2	0.47	4.6
13.0-13.9	13.49	47	25.1	0.55	3.8	47	45.0	0.55	5.9
14.0-14.9	14.50	47	27.7	0.70	4.8	47	49.2	0.70	6.9
15.0-15.9	15.49	37	28.7	0.60	3.6	35	50.5	0.60	5.8
16.0-16.9	16.47	49	29.0	0.59	4.1	49	49.7	0.59	6.6
17.0-17.9	17.45	51	30.3	0.57	4.0	49	51.2	0.57	5.6
18.0-18.9	18.47	41	30.6	0.70	4.5	41	50.6	0.70	6.3
19.0-19.9	19.44	33	31.6	0.63	3.6	33	51.2	0.63	4.7
20.0-29.9	25.27	386	32.5	0.2	3.9	384	52.2	0.3	5.3
30.0-39.9	34.86	444	33.6	0.2	4.0	444	53.2	0.3	5.5
40.0-49.9	44.53	417	33.9	0.2	3.9	413	52.4	0.3	5.1
50.0-59.9	54.88	406	33.7	0.2	3.8	401	51.7	0.2	4.6
60.0-69.9	65.05	487	32.9	0.2	3.5	476	49.9	0.2	4.6
70.0-79.9	74.30	502	31.6	0.2	3.6	468	48.1	0.2	5.0
80.0-90.9	84.03	517	29.5	0.2	3.6	418	46.1	0.2	4.3
Females									
2.0-2.9	2.45	188	16.4	0.09	1.2	187	28.4	0.09	2.2
3.0-3.9	3.46	142	16.9	0.10	1.2	141	29.3	0.10	2.4
4.0-4.9	4.41	129	17.3	0.11	1.2	130	30.4	0.11	2.3
5.0-5.9	5.48	150	18.2	0.16	1.9	150	31.8	0.16	3.5
6.0-6.9	6.51	67	18.1	0.27	2.2	66	32.5	0.27	3.6
7.0-7.9	7.49	72	19.6	0.31	2.7	71	34.6	0.31	4.0
8.0-8.9	8.44	65	20.0	0.40	3.2	65	36.4	0.40	4.8
9.0-9.9	9.41	81	21.5	0.42	3.8	81	38.4	0.42	5.3
10.0-10.9	10.39	66	22.1	0.42	3.4	66	39.9	0.42	5.3
11.0-11.9	11.51	70	23.6	0.38	3.1	70	43.0	0.38	4.9
12.0-12.9	12.44	47	24.7	0.65	4.4	47	44.8	0.65	6.6
13.0-13.9	13.48	60	26.5	0.53	4.1	60	47.8	0.53	5.8
14.0-14.9	14.45	64	26.2	0.48	3.8	63	47.6	0.48	5.2
15.0-15.9	15.55	61	26.5	0.40	3.1	60	48.4	0.40	4.4
16.0-16.9	16.55	54	27.3	0.50	3.7	52	48.9	0.50	6.4
17.0-17.9	17.43	54	27.0	0.49	3.6	53	48.8	0.49	4.7
18.0-18.9	18.49	55	26.5	0.50	3.7	55	48.5	0.50	6.1
19.0-19.9	19.44	57	27.5	0.56	4.2	57	49.7	0.56	6.8
20.0-29.9	25.20	442	28.6	0.3	5.3	440	50.2	0.3	7.1
30.0-39.9	34.97	561	30.2	0.3	6.4	553	51.7	0.4	8.5
40.0-49.9	44.49	459	31.0	0.3	5.8	456	51.8	0.4	8.1
50.0-59.9	54.88	472	32.4	0.3	6.1	469	51.8	0.4	8.4
60.0-69.9	64.83	485	31.5	0.3	5.7	463	49.6	0.4	7.5
70.0-79.9	74.51	608	30.4	0.2	5.4	559	48.4	0.3	7.6
80.0-90.9	84.48	568	28.5	0.2	5.5	435	46.7	0.3	6.9

Table III.18.
Mean (M), standard error of the mean (SE), and standard deviation (SD) of waist circumference (cm) and buttocks circumference (cm) by age for non-Hispanic white males and females of 2 to 90 years: NHANES III, 1988-1994

Age Group (years)	Mean (years)	Waist Circumference				Hip-Buttocks Circumference			
		N	M	SE	SD	N	M	SE	SD
Males									
2.0-2.9	2.45	184	47.8	0.21	2.9	182	50.9	0.22	3.0
3.0-3.9	3.49	130	49.4	0.25	2.9	131	51.9	0.26	2.9
4.0-4.9	4.47	140	51.5	0.29	3.4	140	54.5	0.29	3.5
5.0-5.9	5.44	134	53.0	0.34	4.0	134	57.0	0.36	4.2
6.0-6.9	6.47	68	55.7	0.80	6.6	68	61.1	0.82	6.7
7.0-7.9	7.44	72	56.6	0.77	6.5	72	63.3	0.75	6.4
8.0-8.9	8.44	74	58.4	0.80	6.8	74	66.4	0.77	6.7
9.0-9.9	9.49	73	62.3	1.24	10.6	73	72.5	0.99	8.5
10.0-10.9	10.47	74	64.8	1.10	9.5	74	74.4	0.87	7.5
11.0-11.9	11.44	66	65.5	1.14	9.2	65	76.2	1.03	8.3
12.0-12.9	12.39	47	71.0	1.38	9.5	47	81.9	1.10	7.6
13.0-13.9	13.49	47	71.8	1.74	11.9	47	85.1	1.41	9.7
14.0-14.9	14.50	47	76.5	2.03	13.9	47	89.9	1.72	11.8
15.0-15.9	15.49	37	78.2	2.12	12.9	36	92.4	1.57	9.4
16.0-16.9	16.47	49	77.2	1.57	11.0	49	92.5	1.25	8.7
17.0-17.9	17.45	49	79.7	1.65	11.5	49	94.1	1.21	8.5
18.0-18.9	18.47	41	80.9	1.91	12.2	41	95.0	1.50	9.6
19.0-19.9	19.44	33	82.3	1.76	10.1	33	95.7	1.41	8.1
20.0-29.9	25.27	383	88.10	0.63	12.33	385	97.70	0.45	8.83
30.0-39.9	34.86	445	94.60	0.61	12.87	442	100.10	0.43	9.04
40.0-49.9	44.53	416	98.40	0.66	13.46	415	101.30	0.53	10.80
50.0-59.9	54.88	402	100.90	0.61	12.23	402	101.50	0.40	8.02
60.0-69.9	65.05	479	102.30	0.55	12.04	480	101.30	0.39	8.54
70.0-79.9	74.30	469	100.70	0.52	11.26	468	99.90	0.39	8.44
80.0-90.9	84.03	430	98.20	0.55	11.41	428	97.80	0.37	7.65
Females									
2.0-2.9	2.45	188	48.2	0.23	3.2	189	51.0	0.26	3.6
3.0-3.9	3.46	140	49.7	0.33	3.9	141	52.7	0.31	3.7
4.0-4.9	4.41	129	51.3	0.29	3.3	128	55.1	0.29	3.3
5.0-5.9	5.48	149	53.4	0.44	5.4	150	58.3	0.47	5.7
6.0-6.9	6.51	65	53.1	0.77	6.2	65	59.9	0.71	5.8
7.0-7.9	7.49	72	56.1	0.81	6.9	72	63.7	0.77	6.5
8.0-8.9	8.44	64	57.9	1.06	8.5	64	67.7	1.02	8.1
9.0-9.9	9.41	81	61.4	1.05	9.4	80	71.9	0.98	8.8
10.0-10.9	10.39	66	63.0	1.22	9.9	66	74.6	1.02	8.3
11.0-11.9	11.51	70	66.7	1.00	8.4	70	80.3	0.92	7.7
12.0-12.9	12.44	47	70.4	1.80	12.3	47	86.3	1.65	11.3
13.0-13.9	13.48	60	73.2	1.53	11.9	60	91.0	1.27	9.9
14.0-14.9	14.45	63	74.1	1.18	9.3	63	92.4	1.05	8.3
15.0-15.9	15.55	60	73.0	1.10	8.5	60	92.8	0.90	7.0
16.0-16.9	16.55	54	75.1	1.91	14.1	54	94.9	1.59	11.6
17.0-17.9	17.43	53	77.0	1.43	10.4	54	95.1	1.32	9.7
18.0-18.9	18.49	55	75.8	1.38	10.2	55	95.2	1.25	9.3
19.0-19.9	19.44	58	76.6	1.81	13.8	58	96.8	1.53	11.6
20.0-29.9	25.20	440	79.40	0.76	15.94	440	97.70	0.63	13.21
30.0-39.9	34.97	558	84.80	0.79	18.66	556	101.90	0.67	15.80
40.0-49.9	44.49	457	88.40	0.85	18.17	458	103.50	0.71	15.19
50.0-59.9	54.88	469	94.00	0.86	18.62	469	105.40	0.73	15.81
60.0-69.9	64.83	466	94.00	0.79	17.05	464	102.90	0.68	14.65
70.0-79.9	74.51	564	93.30	0.70	16.62	564	101.10	0.58	13.77
80.0-90.9	84.48	441	91.80	0.63	13.23	443	99.40	0.57	12.00

Table III.19.

Mean (M), standard error of the mean (SE), and standard deviation (SD) of elbow breadth (mm) and wrist breadth (mm) by age for non-Hispanic white males and females of 2 to 90 years: NHANES III, 1988-1994

Age Group (years)	Mean (years)	Elbow Breadth				Wrist Breadth			
		N	M	SE	SD	N	M	SE	SD
Males									
2.0-2.9	2.45	186	43.8	0.19	2.6	185	35.9	0.15	2.0
3.0-3.9	3.49	131	45.2	0.23	2.7	131	37.2	0.20	2.3
4.0-4.9	4.47	140	47.1	0.24	2.9	140	38.9	0.19	2.3
5.0-5.9	5.44	135	49.6	0.25	2.9	135	40.8	0.24	2.8
6.0-6.9	6.47	68	51.6	0.48	4.0	68	42.5	0.40	3.3
7.0-7.9	7.44	73	53.7	0.47	4.0	73	43.3	0.34	2.9
8.0-8.9	8.44	74	55.1	0.50	4.3	74	44.7	0.35	3.0
9.0-9.9	9.49	73	58.3	0.49	4.2	73	47.7	0.37	3.2
10.0-10.9	10.47	74	59.7	0.45	3.9	74	48.7	0.40	3.5
11.0-11.9	11.44	67	60.6	0.50	4.1	67	49.9	0.41	3.4
12.0-12.9	12.39	47	65.5	0.60	4.1	47	52.4	0.54	3.7
13.0-13.9	13.49	47	67.9	0.70	4.8	47	55.7	0.66	4.6
14.0-14.9	14.50	48	70.5	0.64	4.4	48	56.9	0.47	3.3
15.0-15.9	15.49	37	72.3	0.67	4.1	37	57.0	0.44	2.7
16.0-16.9	16.47	49	72.2	0.66	4.6	49	58.0	0.37	2.6
17.0-17.9	17.45	51	73.0	0.61	4.4	51	58.2	0.44	3.1
18.0-18.9	18.47	41	72.9	0.75	4.8	40	58.4	0.64	4.0
19.0-19.9	19.44	33	71.2	0.61	3.5	33	57.3	0.42	2.4
20.0-29.9	25.27	386	5.80	0.02	0.39	385	7.30	0.02	0.39
30.0-39.9	34.86	445	5.90	0.02	0.42	447	7.40	0.03	0.63
40.0-49.9	44.53	418	5.90	0.02	0.41	418	7.40	0.03	0.61
50.0-59.9	54.88	403	6.00	0.02	0.40	403	7.60	0.03	0.60
60.0-69.9	65.05	483	6.10	0.02	0.44	484	7.60	0.02	0.44
70.0-79.9	74.30	477	6.10	0.02	0.44	477	7.50	0.03	0.66
80.0-90.9	84.03	446	6.10	0.02	0.42	445	7.50	0.03	0.63
Females									
2.0-2.9	2.45	189	42.2	0.21	2.9	190	34.9	0.16	2.2
3.0-3.9	3.46	144	44.0	0.22	2.6	144	36.1	0.18	2.2
4.0-4.9	4.41	129	45.2	0.23	2.6	131	37.9	0.21	2.4
5.0-5.9	5.48	150	48.1	0.29	3.6	150	39.8	0.22	2.7
6.0-6.9	6.51	67	48.4	0.42	3.4	67	40.7	0.33	2.7
7.0-7.9	7.49	72	51.3	0.42	3.5	71	42.0	0.36	3.1
8.0-8.9	8.44	65	52.7	0.54	4.4	65	43.3	0.38	3.1
9.0-9.9	9.41	80	55.3	0.47	4.2	80	45.3	0.35	3.1
10.0-10.9	10.39	66	57.1	0.50	4.1	66	46.2	0.40	3.3
11.0-11.9	11.51	70	59.8	0.46	3.8	70	49.1	0.39	3.2
12.0-12.9	12.44	47	60.9	0.60	4.1	47	49.9	0.45	3.1
13.0-13.9	13.48	60	62.0	0.51	4.0	60	50.2	0.39	3.1
14.0-14.9	14.45	64	62.9	0.50	4.0	64	50.8	0.36	2.8
15.0-15.9	15.55	62	62.2	0.51	4.0	62	50.2	0.38	3.0
16.0-16.9	16.55	54	62.6	0.57	4.2	54	50.9	0.41	3.0
17.0-17.9	17.43	55	61.5	0.54	4.0	55	50.0	0.39	2.9
18.0-18.9	18.49	55	62.0	0.47	3.5	55	50.2	0.33	2.4
19.0-19.9	19.44	58	62.8	0.58	4.4	58	50.1	0.36	2.8
20.0-29.9	25.20	440	5.00	0.02	0.42	485	6.30	0.02	0.44
30.0-39.9	34.97	559	5.10	0.01	0.24	581	6.40	0.03	0.72
40.0-49.9	44.49	461	5.20	0.02	0.43	462	6.50	0.03	0.64
50.0-59.9	54.88	470	5.30	0.02	0.43	472	6.70	0.03	0.65
60.0-69.9	64.83	468	5.30	0.02	0.43	469	6.60	0.03	0.65
70.0-79.9	74.51	571	5.30	0.02	0.48	571	6.60	0.03	0.72
80.0-90.9	84.48	463	5.30	0.02	0.43	462	6.50	0.03	0.64

Non-Smoothed NHANES III Anthropometric Reference Data: Non-Hispanic Whites

Table III.20.

Mean (M), standard error of the mean (SE), and standard deviation (SD) of biacromial breadth (cm) and bi-iliac breadth (cm) by age for non-Hispanic white males and females of 2 to 90 years: NHANES III, 1988-1994

Age Group (years)	Mean (years)	Biacromial Breadth				Bi-iliac Breadth			
		N	M	SE	SD	N	M	SE	SD
Males									
2.0-2.9	2.45	no data available				185	15.3	0.08	1.1
3.0-3.9	3.49	130	22.1	0.14	1.5	131	16.2	0.09	1.0
4.0-4.9	4.47	139	23.6	0.12	1.4	140	16.9	0.09	1.1
5.0-5.9	5.44	134	24.8	0.12	1.4	133	17.9	0.10	1.1
6.0-6.9	6.47	68	26.7	0.24	1.9	68	18.6	0.20	1.7
7.0-7.9	7.44	72	27.4	0.22	1.9	72	19.6	0.19	1.6
8.0-8.9	8.44	74	28.9	0.22	1.9	74	20.0	0.20	1.8
9.0-9.9	9.49	72	30.4	0.22	1.9	72	21.6	0.26	2.2
10.0-10.9	10.47	74	31.3	0.19	1.6	74	22.0	0.22	1.9
11.0-11.9	11.44	66	32.4	0.23	1.9	66	22.6	0.24	2.0
12.0-12.9	12.39	47	34.1	0.31	2.1	47	24.4	0.30	2.0
13.0-13.9	13.49	47	35.9	0.39	2.7	47	25.4	0.41	2.8
14.0-14.9	14.50	48	37.6	0.35	2.4	47	26.6	0.43	2.9
15.0-15.9	15.49	37	38.8	0.38	2.3	37	27.2	0.45	2.7
16.0-16.9	16.47	50	72.2	0.36	2.6	50	27.5	0.45	3.2
17.0-17.9	17.45	51	40.6	0.30	2.2	50	28.0	0.50	3.6
18.0-18.9	18.47	41	41.5	0.35	2.2	41	28.5	0.36	2.3
19.0-19.9	19.44	33	41.1	0.41	2.4	32	28.2	0.45	2.5
20.0-29.9	25.27	385	41.60	0.15	2.94	385	28.80	0.16	3.14
30.0-39.9	34.86	444	41.50	0.14	2.95	447	29.50	0.16	3.38
40.0-49.9	44.53	418	41.40	0.14	2.86	415	30.10	0.17	3.46
50.0-59.9	54.88	401	41.10	0.15	3.00	401	30.80	0.15	3.00
60.0-69.9	65.05	482	40.60	0.14	3.07	479	31.10	0.14	3.06
70.0-79.9	74.30	476	39.70	0.14	3.05	472	30.90	0.13	2.82
80.0-90.9	84.03	441	38.90	0.13	2.73	430	30.80	0.13	2.70
Females									
2.0-2.9	2.50	no data available				190	15.2	0.10	1.4
3.0-3.9	3.46	142	22.1	0.11	1.3	142	16.3	0.10	1.2
4.0-4.9	4.41	130	23.5	0.18	2.1	131	17.0	0.10	1.1
5.0-5.9	5.48	150	25.0	0.14	1.7	150	17.9	0.13	1.5
6.0-6.9	6.51	67	26.0	0.16	1.3	67	18.3	0.19	1.5
7.0-7.9	7.49	72	26.9	0.21	1.8	71	19.6	0.24	2.0
8.0-8.9	8.44	65	28.5	0.25	2.0	65	20.4	0.30	2.4
9.0-9.9	9.41	81	29.9	0.20	1.8	81	21.4	0.26	2.4
10.0-10.9	10.39	66	30.7	0.20	1.6	66	22.4	0.27	2.2
11.0-11.9	11.51	70	32.8	0.25	2.1	70	23.6	0.27	2.3
12.0-12.9	12.44	47	34.3	0.33	2.3	47	24.8	0.47	3.2
13.0-13.9	13.48	60	35.8	0.30	2.4	60	26.5	0.33	2.5
14.0-14.9	14.45	64	35.9	0.22	1.8	63	27.0	0.31	2.5
15.0-15.9	15.55	61	36.4	0.27	2.1	61	26.7	0.31	2.4
16.0-16.9	16.55	54	36.7	0.23	1.7	54	27.5	0.45	3.3
17.0-17.9	17.43	55	36.5	0.26	1.9	54	27.5	0.38	2.8
18.0-18.9	18.49	55	36.4	0.23	1.7	55	26.8	0.33	2.5
19.0-19.9	19.44	57	36.4	0.24	1.8	58	28.2	0.46	3.5
20.0-29.9	25.20	484	36.80	0.10	2.20	484	27.80	0.19	4.18
30.0-39.9	34.97	581	36.90	0.10	2.41	578	28.90	0.19	4.57
40.0-49.9	44.49	458	36.80	0.11	2.35	459	29.40	0.19	4.07
50.0-59.9	54.88	471	36.90	0.11	2.39	470	30.30	0.20	4.34
60.0-69.9	64.83	468	36.30	0.11	2.38	465	30.30	0.19	4.10
70.0-79.9	74.51	570	35.60	0.09	2.15	563	30.00	0.16	3.80
80.0-90.9	84.48	457	34.70	0.10	2.14	447	30.00	0.17	3.59

Table III.21.
Mean (M), standard error of the mean (SE), and standard deviation (SD)
of knee height (cm) by age for non-Hispanic white males and
females of 60 to 90 years: NHANES III, 1988-1994

Age Group (yrs)	Mean Age (yrs)	Knee Height			
		N	M	SE	SD
Males					
60.0-69.9	65.05	476	54.60	0.13	2.84
70.0-79.9	74.30	473	53.80	0.13	2.83
80.0-90.9	84.03	429	53.60	0.13	2.69
Females					
60.0-69.9	64.83	462	49.70	0.15	3.22
70.0-79.9	74.51	569	49.30	0.14	3.34
80.0-90.9	84.48	449	49.10	0.16	3.39

Table III.22.
Mean (M), standard error of the mean (SE), and standard deviation (SD) of fat-free mass (kg), total body fat weight (kg),
and percent body fat (%) for non-Hispanic white males and females of 12 to 90 years: NHANES III, 1988-1994

Age Group (years)	M (years)	Fat-Free Mass (kg)				Total Body Fat Weight (kg)			Body Fat (%)		
		N	M	SE	SD	M	SE	SD	M	SE	SD
Males											
12-13.9	12.94	88	41.8	1.00	8.2	10.00	0.70	6.0	18.4	1.00	7.3
14-15.9	14.93	82	54.3	1.20	9.6	14.00	1.60	12.2	18.4	1.20	8.3
16-17.9	16.98	96	57.8	1.00	8.4	13.10	0.90	7.5	17.7	0.90	6.8
18-19.9	18.91	76	58.0	1.10	8.0	15.10	1.10	8.5	19.6	1.00	6.9
20-29.9	25.32	384	61.3	0.60	9.5	17.90	0.50	8.7	21.8	0.40	6.2
30-39.9	34.90	436	63.6	0.60	10.5	20.40	0.50	8.5	23.6	0.40	5.8
40-49.9	44.47	410	64.6	0.60	10.6	21.30	0.50	8.5	24.2	0.40	5.7
50-59.9	54.88	396	64.6	0.50	8.8	22.30	0.50	8.3	25.1	0.40	6.0
60-69.9	65.00	465	62.3	0.50	8.9	22.70	0.40	7.7	26.2	0.30	5.5
70-79.9	74.15	447	59.1	0.50	8.6	20.30	0.40	6.8	25.1	0.30	5.5
80-90.9	83.23	372	54.6	0.39	7.4	18.82	0.35	6.7	25.1	0.32	6.2
Females											
12-13.9	13.05	101	38.1	0.7	5.6	14	1	8.7	24.8	1.20	9.7
14-15.9	14.99	120	40.4	0.6	4.8	17.4	0.8	6.9	29.1	0.80	6.5
16-17.9	16.99	104	41.6	0.7	5.5	19.5	1.2	10.1	30.7	0.90	6.9
18-19.9	18.98	90	43.1	0.8	5.6	20.6	1.3	10.3	30.8	1.00	7.9
20-29.9	25.26	426	42.8	0.4	5.9	20.5	0.6	9.6	31.0	0.50	7.5
30-39.9	35.14	543	45	0.4	6.9	24.1	0.6	12.3	33.0	0.50	8.5
40-49.9	44.48	454	44.8	0.4	6.9	25.9	0.6	10.9	35.4	0.40	6.9
50-59.9	54.85	454	45.4	0.4	6.7	28.6	0.7	11.6	37.3	0.40	7.1
60-69.9	64.76	447	43.6	0.4	6.3	26.7	0.6	9.9	36.9	0.40	6.9
70-79.9	74.41	538	42.3	0.4	6.5	24.8	0.5	9.3	35.9	0.40	6.9
80-90.9	83.56	379	39.5	0.26	5.0	22.6	0.38	7.5	35.5	0.34	6.6

LIST OF TABLES

NON-SMOOTHED NHANES III ANTHROPOMETRIC REFERENCE DATA: NON-HISPANIC BLACKS

Table III.32. Mean (M), standard error of the mean (SE), and standard deviation (SD) of knee height (cm) for non-Hispanic black males and females of 60 to 90 years: NHANES III, 1988-1994.

Table III.33. Mean (M), standard error of the mean (SE), and standard deviation (SD) of fat-free mass (kg), total body fat (kg), and percent body fat (%) for non-Hispanic black males and females of 12 to 90 years: NHANES III, 1988-1994.

Table III.23.
Mean (M), standard error of the mean (SE), and standard deviation (SD) of weight (kg), recumbent length (cm),
Rohrer's index (100 g/cm^3), and head circumference (cm) by age for non-Hispanic black boys and girls of 2 months to 7 years:
NHANES III, 1988-1994

Age Group	Mean	Boys				Mean	Girls			
(months)	(months)	N	M	SE	SD	(months)	N	M	SE	SD
					Weight (kg)					
2.0-2.9	2.00	24	6.3	0.25	1.2	2.00	20	6.0	0.22	1.0
3.0-5.9	4.02	48	7.7	0.18	1.2	3.93	43	7.2	0.20	1.3
6.0-8.9	7.04	54	9.0	0.15	1.1	6.83	41	8.2	0.20	1.3
9.0-11.9	9.70	37	9.5	0.17	1.0	9.92	49	9.1	0.17	1.2
12.0-23.9	17.34	170	11.5	0.12	1.6	17.85	202	11.1	0.11	1.6
24.0-35.9	29.42	202	13.7	0.12	1.6	29.54	157	13.1	0.16	2.0
36.0-47.9	41.50	171	16.0	0.16	2.1	41.76	200	15.6	0.19	2.7
					Recumbent Length (cm)					
2.0-2.9	2.00	24	60.9	0.76	3.7	2.00	20	59.6	1.05	4.7
3.0-5.9	4.02	48	65.3	0.47	3.3	3.93	44	63.6	0.62	4.1
6.0-8.9	7.04	54	71.1	0.57	4.2	6.83	41	68.2	0.48	3.1
9.0-11.9	9.70	37	73.9	0.56	3.4	9.92	49	72.3	0.44	3.1
12.0-23.9	17.34	169	82.1	0.35	4.5	17.85	199	81.7	0.38	5.3
24.0-35.9	29.42	195	92.2	0.30	4.1	29.54	147	91.5	0.36	4.4
36.0-47.9	41.50	167	101.0	0.35	4.5	41.76	200	100.2	0.37	5.2
					Rohrer's Index (100 g/cm^3)					
2.0-2.9	2.00	24	2.75	0.05	0.27	2.00	20	2.85	0.13	0.57
3.0-5.9	4.02	48	2.75	0.04	0.28	3.93	43	2.79	0.06	0.39
6.0-8.9	7.04	54	2.52	0.04	0.30	6.83	41	2.59	0.04	0.23
9.0-11.9	9.70	37	2.36	0.04	0.27	9.92	49	2.39	0.04	0.26
12.0-23.9	17.34	169	2.09	0.02	0.26	17.85	199	2.05	0.02	0.26
24.0-35.9	29.42	195	1.75	0.01	0.17	29.54	147	1.71	0.01	0.16
36.0-47.9	41.50	167	1.56	0.01	0.14	41.76	199	1.54	0.01	0.18
					Head Circumference (cm)					
2.0-2.9	2.00	24	40.9	0.39	1.9	2.00	20	40.1	0.45	2.0
3.0-5.9	4.02	48	43.0	0.25	1.7	3.93	44	41.6	0.27	1.8
6.0-8.9	7.04	53	45.2	0.21	1.5	6.83	40	43.6	0.28	1.7
9.0-11.9	9.70	37	45.9	0.22	1.4	9.92	48	45.3	0.20	1.4
12.0-23.9	17.34	169	47.8	0.13	1.6	17.85	192	47.0	0.11	1.5
24.0-35.9	29.42	193	49.3	0.10	1.4	29.54	145	48.2	0.13	1.6
36.0-47.9	41.50	164	50.1	0.11	1.4	41.76	194	49.4	0.10	1.4
48.0-59.9	53.37	178	50.7	0.10	1.3	53.19	163	50.1	0.14	1.8
60.0-71.9	65.22	160	51.5	0.12	1.5	65.54	174	50.8	0.12	1.6
72.0-83.9	77.33	84	51.5	0.23	2.1	77.65	91	51.4	0.20	1.9

Non-Smoothed NHANES III Anthropometric Reference Data: Non-Hispanic Blacks

Table III.24.

Mean (M), standard error of the mean (SE), and standard deviation (SD) of weight (kg), stature (cm),
and body mass index (w/s^2) by age for non-Hispanic black males and females of 2 to 90 years: NHANES III, 1988-1994

Age Group (years)	Mean (years)	Weight				Stature				Body Mass Index			
		N	M	SE	SD	N	M	SE	SD	N	M	SE	SD
Males													
2.0-2.9	2.45	202	13.6	0.11	1.6	198	91.5	0.31	4.3	198	16.3	0.10	1.5
3.0-3.9	3.46	171	16.0	0.16	2.1	170	100.1	0.34	4.5	170	16.0	0.10	1.3
4.0-4.9	4.45	178	18.1	0.19	2.6	178	107.5	0.35	4.7	178	15.8	0.11	1.5
5.0-5.9	5.44	163	20.9	0.30	3.9	162	114.7	0.41	5.2	162	15.8	0.15	2.0
6.0-6.9	6.44	87	23.0	0.54	5.0	87	120.4	0.63	5.9	86	15.8	0.24	2.2
7.0-7.9	7.46	94	26.3	0.61	5.9	95	127.6	0.60	5.9	94	16.2	0.27	2.6
8.0-8.9	8.49	86	30.0	0.71	6.6	86	132.2	0.60	5.6	86	16.7	0.34	3.1
9.0-9.9	9.50	106	33.1	0.86	8.8	105	138.6	0.68	6.9	105	17.1	0.35	3.6
10.0-10.9	10.44	106	37.3	1.07	11.0	106	143.8	0.80	8.2	106	17.9	0.37	3.8
11.0-11.9	11.43	95	43.8	1.32	12.9	95	149.8	0.86	8.4	95	19.4	0.43	4.2
12.0-12.9	12.51	79	48.2	1.82	16.2	80	154.5	1.04	9.3	79	19.9	0.58	5.1
13.0-13.9	13.48	57	54.7	2.30	17.3	57	163.5	1.32	10.0	57	20.4	0.68	5.2
14.0-14.9	14.49	72	62.0	2.17	18.4	73	169.8	0.92	7.8	72	21.4	0.67	5.7
15.0-15.9	15.43	69	65.3	2.07	17.2	69	172.2	0.85	7.1	69	21.9	0.67	5.5
16.0-16.9	16.43	71	66.5	1.89	16.0	71	172.9	0.91	7.6	71	22.2	0.50	4.2
17.0-17.9	17.46	65	69.2	1.80	14.5	65	174.3	0.95	7.7	65	22.4	0.58	4.7
18.0-18.9	18.42	59	75.2	2.50	19.2	59	176.9	0.86	6.6	59	23.6	0.66	5.1
19.0-19.9	19.41	67	72.4	1.93	15.8	67	175.3	0.92	7.6	67	23.6	0.62	5.0
20.0-29.9	25.02	488	82.60	0.97	21.43	488	177.00	0.35	7.73	488	26.20	0.28	6.19
30.0-39.9	34.90	497	82.90	0.91	20.29	497	177.20	0.32	7.13	497	26.40	0.27	6.02
40.0-49.9	44.02	370	84.30	0.96	18.47	370	176.70	0.40	7.69	370	26.90	0.27	5.19
50.0-59.9	55.13	217	84.60	1.41	20.77	217	175.40	0.48	7.07	217	27.40	0.42	6.19
60.0-69.9	64.81	295	80.40	1.02	17.52	295	173.50	0.42	7.21	295	26.70	0.31	5.32
70.0-79.9	74.01	187	77.20	1.19	16.27	187	172.40	0.54	7.38	187	25.90	0.38	5.20
80.0-90.9	84.55	59	70.70	2.04	15.67	59	168.80	1.22	9.37	59	24.90	0.78	5.99
Females													
2.0-2.9	2.46	157	13.0	0.16	2.0	152	90.5	0.38	4.6	152	15.9	0.12	1.4
3.0-3.9	3.48	200	15.4	0.19	2.7	200	99.2	0.34	4.9	199	15.6	0.13	1.8
4.0-4.9	4.43	165	17.9	0.22	2.9	165	106.4	0.35	4.5	165	15.6	0.14	1.8
5.0-5.9	5.46	175	20.6	0.27	3.6	176	114.3	0.42	5.6	175	15.6	0.15	2.0
6.0-6.9	6.47	92	24.0	0.70	6.7	92	121.1	0.64	6.2	92	16.2	0.35	3.4
7.0-7.9	7.43	88	27.4	0.80	7.5	88	127.1	0.69	6.5	88	16.7	0.38	3.5
8.0-8.9	8.51	81	31.4	0.90	8.1	81	134.2	0.77	6.9	81	17.4	0.38	3.4
9.0-9.9	9.45	94	34.6	0.93	9.0	95	139.2	0.76	7.4	94	17.7	0.40	3.9
10.0-10.9	10.48	93	40.1	1.12	10.8	93	145.7	0.74	7.2	93	18.5	0.43	4.1
11.0-11.9	11.44	91	46.7	1.34	12.8	91	152.9	0.83	7.9	91	19.8	0.46	4.4
12.0-12.9	12.47	90	52.8	1.50	14.2	90	158.3	0.77	7.3	90	21.1	0.53	5.0
13.0-13.9	13.46	82	59.6	1.60	14.5	84	160.7	0.67	6.1	82	22.7	0.55	5.0
14.0-14.9	14.51	65	61.2	2.29	18.5	69	161.9	0.81	6.8	65	23.4	0.80	6.5
15.0-15.9	15.45	61	62.9	1.86	14.5	62	163.8	0.73	5.8	61	23.3	0.64	5.0
16.0-16.9	16.43	88	62.5	1.66	15.6	92	163.3	0.75	7.2	88	23.1	0.59	5.6
17.0-17.9	17.47	71	63.9	2.02	17.0	71	162.9	0.93	7.8	71	24.0	0.73	6.2
18.0-18.9	18.37	73	66.8	2.54	21.7	73	163.3	0.79	6.7	73	24.8	0.89	7.6
19.0-19.9	19.44	60	64.3	2.03	15.8	60	165.1	0.77	5.9	60	23.8	0.76	5.9
20.0-29.9	24.87	563	70.80	0.83	19.69	624	163.70	0.29	8.13	563	26.30	0.30	7.12
30.0-39.9	34.82	626	76.80	0.92	23.02	654	163.60	0.31	7.24	626	28.70	0.34	8.51
40.0-49.9	44.06	456	81.90	1.15	24.56	457	164.10	0.33	7.93	456	30.40	0.42	8.97
50.0-59.9	54.94	275	80.80	1.34	22.22	275	162.80	0.42	7.05	275	30.50	0.50	8.29
60.0-69.9	64.91	300	78.80	1.29	22.34	301	161.30	0.42	6.96	300	30.30	0.49	8.49
70.0-79.9	74.74	182	75.50	1.57	21.18	182	159.80	0.51	7.29	181	29.40	0.59	7.94
80.0-90.9	84.65	93	63.10	1.66	16.01	92	156.10	0.77	6.88	92	25.90	0.66	6.33

Non-Smoothed NHANES III Anthropometric Reference Data: Non-Hispanic Blacks

Table III.25.

Mean (M), standard error of the mean (SE), and standard deviation (SD) of sitting height (cm), upper arm length (cm), and upper leg length (cm) by age for non-Hispanic black males and females of 2 to 90 years: NHANES III, 1988-1994

Age Group (years)	Mean (years)	Sitting Height				Upper Arm Length				Upper Leg Length			
		N	M	SE	SD	N	M	SE	SD	N	M	SE	SD
Males													
2.0-2.9	2.45	196	51.4	0.2	2.5	187	18.1	0.1	1.3	184	19.2	0.2	1.8
3.0-3.9	3.46	166	54.4	0.2	2.7	162	20.0	0.1	1.6	163	21.8	0.2	1.7
4.0-4.9	4.45	178	57.4	0.2	2.6	177	21.5	0.1	1.3	178	24.1	0.2	1.9
5.0-5.9	5.44	162	60.2	0.2	3.0	162	23.2	0.1	1.6	162	26.6	0.2	2.3
6.0-6.9	6.44	86	62.8	0.3	3.2	85	24.0	0.2	1.9	85	27.9	0.3	2.6
7.0-7.9	7.46	95	65.7	0.3	3.3	95	26.0	0.2	1.6	95	30.3	0.3	2.3
8.0-8.9	8.49	86	68.0	0.3	3.0	85	27.0	0.2	1.6	85	31.6	0.3	2.3
9.0-9.9	9.50	103	70.1	0.3	3.2	105	28.3	0.2	2.2	105	33.7	0.3	2.9
10.0-10.9	10.44	103	71.6	0.4	4.1	104	29.8	0.2	2.4	103	36.1	0.4	2.9
11.0-11.9	11.43	95	74.7	0.4	4.3	95	31.3	0.2	2.4	94	37.3	0.4	3.6
12.0-12.9	12.51	79	76.6	0.5	4.3	80	32.3	0.3	2.6	80	38.7	0.5	3.1
13.0-13.9	13.48	56	81.7	0.7	5.2	53	34.4	0.4	2.7	53	41.4	0.7	3.0
14.0-14.9	14.49	73	84.8	0.5	4.4	69	35.9	0.3	2.7	69	42.4	0.5	3.1
15.0-15.9	15.43	69	86.7	0.4	3.5	68	36.6	0.3	2.3	67	44.5	0.4	2.9
16.0-16.9	16.43	71	87.3	0.4	3.8	71	36.9	0.3	2.4	71	43.7	0.4	3.3
17.0-17.9	17.46	63	88.5	0.5	3.7	63	36.7	0.3	2.1	63	44.7	0.5	3.2
18.0-18.9	18.42	59	89.8	0.5	3.6	58	37.8	0.2	1.9	58	44.8	0.5	2.9
19.0-19.9	19.41	65	89.7	0.5	3.7	63	37.6	0.3	2.2	63	44.5	0.5	3.1
20.0-29.9	25.02	482	90.2	0.2	4.2	473	38.3	0.1	2.6	470	45.0	0.2	3.7
30.0-39.9	34.90	491	90.1	0.2	4.0	479	38.2	0.1	2.2	478	44.5	0.2	3.5
40.0-49.9	44.02	357	90.1	0.2	4.2	343	38.6	0.1	2.6	341	43.6	0.2	3.5
50.0-59.9	55.13	212	89.0	0.3	3.9	207	38.4	0.2	2.3	204	43.0	0.2	3.4
60.0-69.9	64.81	281	88.0	0.2	4.0	277	38.5	0.2	2.5	270	42.6	0.2	3.6
70.0-79.9	74.01	175	86.6	0.3	4.5	165	38.0	0.2	2.4	158	42.3	0.3	3.5
80.0-90.9	84.55	50	85.2	0.6	4.2	46	38.3	0.4	2.4	44	41.2	0.5	3.3
Females													
2.0-2.9	2.46	146	50.3	0.2	2.3	137.0	18.0	0.1	1.3	141.0	19.3	0.2	1.8
3.0-3.9	3.48	199	53.7	0.2	2.5	191.0	19.6	0.1	1.5	194.0	22.1	0.2	2.0
4.0-4.9	4.43	160	56.9	0.2	2.7	162.0	21.3	0.1	1.3	162.0	24.2	0.2	2.0
5.0-5.9	5.46	176	59.8	0.2	3.0	175.0	23.0	0.1	1.5	175.0	27.0	0.2	2.3
6.0-6.9	6.47	92	62.9	0.4	3.6	92.0	24.4	0.2	1.7	92.0	28.8	0.4	2.5
7.0-7.9	7.43	88	65.4	0.4	3.3	87.0	26.0	0.2	2.0	87.0	30.9	0.4	3.0
8.0-8.9	8.51	81	68.1	0.4	3.8	81.0	27.4	0.2	1.8	81.0	33.0	0.4	2.6
9.0-9.9	9.45	94	70.5	0.4	3.6	91.0	28.7	0.2	2.1	92.0	34.4	0.4	3.0
10.0-10.9	10.48	92	73.6	0.4	4.0	88.0	30.4	0.2	2.3	88.0	36.5	0.4	3.0
11.0-11.9	11.44	91	77.6	0.5	4.5	89.0	31.8	0.2	2.3	89.0	38.3	0.5	3.2
12.0-12.9	12.47	89	80.0	0.4	4.0	86.0	33.4	0.2	2.2	86.0	40.0	0.4	3.2
13.0-13.9	13.46	83	82.0	0.4	3.3	81.0	34.1	0.2	1.9	81.0	40.6	0.4	2.5
14.0-14.9	14.51	65	82.4	0.4	3.3	66.0	34.4	0.3	2.4	66.0	42.1	0.4	3.3
15.0-15.9	15.45	61	83.6	0.4	3.5	61.0	35.0	0.3	2.1	60.0	41.5	0.4	2.8
16.0-16.9	16.43	90	83.8	0.4	3.4	88.0	34.6	0.2	2.3	87.0	41.0	0.4	3.0
17.0-17.9	17.47	70	84.0	0.5	4.0	68.0	34.5	0.2	1.8	67.0	41.4	0.5	2.9
18.0-18.9	18.37	71	84.0	0.4	3.6	68.0	34.6	0.3	2.4	67.0	41.3	0.4	3.4
19.0-19.9	19.44	59	85.2	0.4	3.2	56.0	35.2	0.3	2.0	55.0	42.4	0.4	2.7
20.0-29.9	24.87	615	84.3	0.2	3.7	603.0	35.3	0.1	2.5	602.0	41.7	0.2	3.9
30.0-39.9	34.82	644	84.8	0.2	3.8	622.0	35.6	0.1	2.7	620.0	40.7	0.2	4.0
40.0-49.9	44.06	446	84.9	0.2	3.4	426.0	35.9	0.1	2.5	422.0	40.2	0.2	4.3
50.0-59.9	54.94	263	83.9	0.2	3.6	257.0	36.0	0.2	2.7	253.0	39.3	0.3	4.6
60.0-69.9	64.91	280	82.6	0.2	3.7	270.0	36.1	0.2	3.0	265.0	38.5	0.3	4.6
70.0-79.9	74.74	165	80.9	0.3	3.5	153.0	35.7	0.2	2.7	152.0	38.5	0.3	4.1
80.0-90.9	84.65	67	78.1	0.5	3.8	67.0	35.5	0.3	2.2	64.0	38.3	0.6	5.0

Table III.26.
Mean (M), standard error of the mean (SE), and standard deviation (SD) of triceps skinfold thickness (mm)
and subscapular skinfold thickness (mm) by age for non-Hispanic black males and females of 2 to 90 years: NHANES III, 1988-1994

Age Group (years)	Mean (years)	Triceps Skinfold				Subscapular Skinfold			
		N	M	SE	SD	N	M	SE	SD
Males									
2.0-2.9	2.45	173	8.4	0.14	1.9	171	6.2	0.11	1.4
3.0-3.9	3.46	160	8.2	0.17	2.2	160	6.0	0.15	1.9
4.0-4.9	4.45	177	7.9	0.17	2.2	177	5.6	0.12	1.5
5.0-5.9	5.44	161	7.8	0.25	3.1	161	5.8	0.22	2.9
6.0-6.9	6.44	84	7.8	0.38	3.5	84	5.7	0.31	2.8
7.0-7.9	7.46	95	8.4	0.48	4.7	95	6.3	0.37	3.6
8.0-8.9	8.49	84	8.7	0.57	5.3	84	6.8	0.53	4.9
9.0-9.9	9.50	105	9.2	0.52	5.4	104	6.8	0.41	4.2
10.0-10.9	10.44	103	10.4	0.63	6.4	103	7.8	0.50	5.1
11.0-11.9	11.43	94	11.7	0.71	6.9	94	9.2	0.73	7.1
12.0-12.9	12.51	78	11.1	0.84	7.4	78	9.3	0.83	7.4
13.0-13.9	13.48	53	9.7	0.87	6.4	53	9.5	1.07	7.8
14.0-14.9	14.49	68	9.1	0.83	6.9	66	9.0	0.67	5.4
15.0-15.9	15.43	66	8.8	0.68	5.5	66	9.6	0.67	5.5
16.0-16.9	16.43	70	8.4	0.64	5.3	70	10.3	0.67	5.6
17.0-17.9	17.46	63	8.3	0.75	5.9	62	10.3	0.74	5.8
18.0-18.9	18.42	56	8.8	0.64	4.8	57	11.3	0.69	5.2
19.0-19.9	19.41	62	8.1	0.67	5.3	61	11.6	0.82	6.4
20.0-29.9	25.02	456	11.8	11.8	7.5	450	17.2	0.4	8.3
30.0-39.9	34.90	471	11.8	11.8	6.7	443	18.2	0.4	8.8
40.0-49.9	44.02	341	12.5	12.5	7.2	320	20.1	0.5	8.6
50.0-59.9	55.13	200	12.5	12.5	6.8	187	20.8	0.6	8.6
60.0-69.9	64.81	279	12.6	12.6	7.3	257	20.8	0.6	9.0
70.0-79.9	74.01	168	12.5	12.5	7.0	154	20.5	0.7	8.2
80.0-90.9	84.55	50	11.6	11.6	6.2	44	17.6	1.0	6.8
Females									
2.0-2.9	2.46	133	8.8	0.22	2.5	132	6.6	0.16	1.8
3.0-3.9	3.48	186	8.7	0.19	2.6	186	6.5	0.19	2.6
4.0-4.9	4.43	163	9.2	0.24	3.0	161	6.6	0.22	2.8
5.0-5.9	5.46	174	9.0	0.25	3.2	174	6.7	0.27	3.6
6.0-6.9	6.47	91	10.3	0.52	4.9	91	7.5	0.54	5.2
7.0-7.9	7.43	87	10.8	0.63	5.9	85	8.2	0.62	5.7
8.0-8.9	8.51	80	11.8	0.61	5.5	81	9.2	0.62	5.6
9.0-9.9	9.45	91	11.9	0.68	6.5	90	9.7	0.65	6.2
10.0-10.9	10.48	88	13.0	0.77	7.3	86	9.9	0.65	6.0
11.0-11.9	11.44	89	14.1	0.80	7.5	87	10.8	0.70	6.6
12.0-12.9	12.47	86	15.5	0.88	8.2	84	13.4	0.91	8.3
13.0-13.9	13.46	81	16.7	0.91	8.2	79	14.8	0.95	8.4
14.0-14.9	14.51	65	17.6	1.07	8.6	63	16.2	1.07	8.5
15.0-15.9	15.45	60	18.8	1.05	8.1	58	15.7	0.98	7.4
16.0-16.9	16.43	87	17.3	0.89	8.3	84	16.2	0.96	8.8
17.0-17.9	17.47	66	18.0	1.07	8.7	65	16.9	0.98	7.9
18.0-18.9	18.37	65	18.2	1.14	9.2	61	17.7	1.10	8.6
19.0-19.9	19.44	55	18.4	1.15	8.6	51	16.2	1.09	7.8
20.0-29.9	24.87	517	21.9	0.5	10.5	493	21.6	0.5	10.4
30.0-39.9	34.82	546	25.4	0.5	11.2	505	25.0	0.5	11.5
40.0-49.9	44.06	389	27.3	0.5	10.5	350	27.6	0.6	10.3
50.0-59.9	54.94	240	27.5	0.7	10.4	212	27.6	0.7	10.8
60.0-69.9	64.91	268	26.0	0.6	10.0	239	26.7	0.6	9.9
70.0-79.9	74.74	154	23.9	0.8	9.9	143	24.3	0.9	10.4
80.0-90.9	84.65	77	17.1	1.0	8.6	62	18.9	1.3	10.1

Table III.27.

Mean (M), standard error of the mean (SE), and standard deviation (SD) of supra-iliac skinfold thickness (mm) and thigh skinfold thickness (mm) by age for non-Hispanic black males and females of 2 to 90 years: NHANES III, 1988-1994

Age Group (years)	Mean (years)	Supra-iliac Skinfold Thickness				Thigh Skinfold Thickness			
		N	M	SE	SD	N	M	SE	SD
Males									
2.0-2.9	2.45	168	4.9	0.10	1.3	172	10.7	0.19	2.5
3.0-3.9	3.46	158	4.8	0.16	2.0	160	9.9	0.24	3.1
4.0-4.9	4.45	177	4.6	0.12	1.6	176	9.4	0.25	3.3
5.0-5.9	5.44	161	4.9	0.26	3.3	160	9.3	0.36	4.6
6.0-6.9	6.44	83	4.9	0.41	3.7	84	8.6	0.41	3.8
7.0-7.9	7.46	95	5.6	0.47	4.6	94	9.9	0.63	6.1
8.0-8.9	8.49	83	6.3	0.61	5.5	82	10.5	0.68	6.1
9.0-9.9	9.50	102	6.4	0.57	5.8	101	10.5	0.64	6.4
10.0-10.9	10.44	102	8.4	0.74	7.5	97	11.9	0.78	7.6
11.0-11.9	11.43	92	9.7	0.87	8.4	87	12.6	0.82	7.6
12.0-12.9	12.51	78	10.1	1.01	9.0	72	11.7	0.93	7.9
13.0-13.9	13.48	52	9.1	1.15	8.3	48	10.8	1.17	8.1
14.0-14.9	14.49	66	9.4	1.00	8.1	64	9.2	0.72	5.8
15.0-15.9	15.43	67	9.3	0.96	7.9	61	8.9	0.61	4.7
16.0-16.9	16.43	68	8.8	0.81	6.7	68	8.2	0.42	3.5
17.0-17.9	17.46	62	9.2	0.98	7.7	60	8.1	0.64	4.9
18.0-18.9	18.42	56	10.6	1.02	7.6	57	9.1	0.68	5.1
19.0-19.9	19.41	61	9.8	0.95	7.4	54	8.0	0.76	5.6
20.0-29.9	25.02	451	18.3	0.6	12.1	438	11.6	0.3	7.1
30.0-39.9	34.90	452	19.6	0.6	11.9	453	12.3	0.3	7.0
40.0-49.9	44.02	336	21.9	0.7	11.9	327	12.6	0.4	7.4
50.0-59.9	55.13	192	21.4	0.8	10.5	197	12.5	0.6	7.7
60.0-69.9	64.81	262	20.2	0.7	10.8	262	12.3	0.5	7.4
70.0-79.9	74.01	160	18.8	0.8	10.2	150	13.4	0.7	8.3
80.0-90.9	84.55	45	16.2	1.2	7.8	42	13.4	1.2	7.5
Females									
2.0-2.9	2.46	131	5.3	0.16	1.8	132	12.1	0.34	3.9
3.0-3.9	3.48	184	5.4	0.18	2.4	187	11.7	0.32	4.4
4.0-4.9	4.43	161	5.5	0.20	2.5	162	12.0	0.36	4.6
5.0-5.9	5.46	173	5.7	0.26	3.4	174	12.3	0.39	5.1
6.0-6.9	6.47	92	7.2	0.68	6.6	88	13.4	0.66	6.1
7.0-7.9	7.43	86	7.9	0.71	6.6	85	14.5	0.84	7.8
8.0-8.9	8.51	79	8.7	0.70	6.2	75	15.3	0.81	7.0
9.0-9.9	9.45	92	10.0	0.79	7.6	89	15.9	0.81	7.7
10.0-10.9	10.48	87	10.6	0.82	7.6	85	15.8	0.83	7.7
11.0-11.9	11.44	89	12.4	0.84	8.0	75	17.2	0.95	8.3
12.0-12.9	12.47	82	14.6	1.02	9.2	70	17.8	0.93	7.8
13.0-13.9	13.46	81	16.7	1.10	9.9	69	19.9	1.05	8.7
14.0-14.9	14.51	62	15.7	1.19	9.3	57	22.2	1.29	9.7
15.0-15.9	15.45	57	16.6	1.24	9.4	50	23.2	1.39	9.8
16.0-16.9	16.43	84	16.1	0.99	9.1	70	23.0	0.97	8.1
17.0-17.9	17.47	64	16.3	1.16	9.3	51	22.1	1.15	8.2
18.0-18.9	18.37	62	17.5	1.33	10.5	55	22.6	1.18	8.8
19.0-19.9	19.44	52	14.9	1.30	9.4	45	22.7	1.18	7.9
20.0-29.9	24.87	516	19.9	0.5	12.0	425	26.2	0.5	10.3
30.0-39.9	34.82	531	22.8	0.5	12.4	401	28.8	0.6	11.0
40.0-49.9	44.06	372	26.4	0.6	11.4	276	30.7	0.6	10.5
50.0-59.9	54.94	225	26.3	0.8	11.7	170	29.4	0.9	11.5
60.0-69.9	64.91	238	24.7	0.7	10.5	200	29.8	0.8	11.0
70.0-79.9	74.74	139	22.3	0.9	11.0	121	28.4	0.9	10.1
80.0-90.9	84.65	62	17.0	1.4	10.7	55	25.8	1.4	10.3

Table III.28.
Mean (M), standard error of the mean (SE), and standard deviation (SD) of mid-upper arm circumference (cm) and thigh circumference (cm) by age for non-Hispanic black males and females of 2 to 90 years: NHANES III, 1988-1994

Age Group (years)	Mean (years)	Mid-Upper Arm Circumference				Thigh Circumference			
		N	M	SE	SD	N	M	SE	SD
Males									
2.0-2.9	2.45	187	16.3	0.1	1.2	182	28.5	0.08	2.2
3.0-3.9	3.46	162	17.0	0.1	1.3	161	29.9	0.10	2.4
4.0-4.9	4.45	178	17.3	0.1	1.5	178	31.1		2.7
5.0-5.9	5.44	162	18.0	0.2	1.9	162	32.7	0.15	3.5
6.0-6.9	6.44	85	18.4	0.2	2.3	85	33.4	0.25	4.2
7.0-7.9	7.46	95	19.3	0.3	2.6	95	35.6	0.27	4.4
8.0-8.9	8.49	84	20.2	0.3	2.9	85	37.2	0.32	5.0
9.0-9.9	9.50	105	20.8	0.3	3.0	103	38.5	0.29	5.3
10.0-10.9	10.44	104	22.3	0.4	3.8	103	41.0	0.37	6.2
11.0-11.9	11.43	95	23.6	0.4	4.1	95	44.0	0.42	7.0
12.0-12.9	12.51	80	24.6	0.5	4.6	80	45.2	0.52	7.5
13.0-13.9	13.48	53	26.0	0.6	4.7	53	48.0	0.64	7.9
14.0-14.9	14.49	69	27.4	0.6	5.1	69	48.6	0.62	8.1
15.0-15.9	15.43	68	28.3	0.5	4.5	67	50.7	0.55	7.1
16.0-16.9	16.43	71	29.0	0.5	4.5	71	51.4	0.53	6.2
17.0-17.9	17.46	63	29.9	0.5	3.7	63	52.5	0.47	5.8
18.0-18.9	18.42	58	31.2	0.6	4.5	58	53.5	0.59	7.4
19.0-19.9	19.41	63	30.4	0.5	3.9	62	52.3	0.49	6.1
20.0-29.9	25.02	473	33.7	0.2	5.0	470	55.4	0.3	7.2
30.0-39.9	34.90	480	33.9	0.2	4.6	477	54.3	0.3	6.6
40.0-49.9	44.02	344	33.9	0.2	4.3	342	53.3	0.3	5.9
50.0-59.9	55.13	207	33.9	0.4	5.0	203	51.9	0.4	6.3
60.0-69.9	64.81	282	32.9	0.3	4.7	265	50.7	0.4	6.2
70.0-79.9	74.01	172	31.9	0.3	4.3	156	49.1	0.5	6.0
80.0-90.9	84.55	50	30.0	0.7	4.6	43	48.2	0.7	4.3
Females									
2.0-2.9	2.46	137	16.1	0.1	1.4	137	28.2	0.12	2.5
3.0-3.9	3.48	190	16.6	0.1	1.6	191	29.8	0.12	3.2
4.0-4.9	4.43	163	17.4	0.1	1.6	163	31.5	0.13	2.9
5.0-5.9	5.46	174	17.9	0.2	2.0	175	33.1	0.15	3.4
6.0-6.9	6.47	92	19.1	0.3	3.2	92	35.5	0.34	5.8
7.0-7.9	7.43	87	19.9	0.4	3.5	87	36.7	0.37	5.5
8.0-8.9	8.51	81	20.9	0.4	3.3	81	39.1	0.37	5.2
9.0-9.9	9.45	92	21.7	0.4	3.5	91	40.5	0.37	5.9
10.0-10.9	10.48	88	22.7	0.4	4.0	88	42.1	0.43	6.2
11.0-11.9	11.44	89	24.1	0.4	4.2	89	45.2	0.45	6.6
12.0-12.9	12.47	86	25.8	0.5	4.6	85	47.4	0.50	7.0
13.0-13.9	13.46	81	26.6	0.5	4.8	81	50.5	0.54	7.0
14.0-14.9	14.51	66	27.2	0.6	5.2	66	51.3	0.64	8.7
15.0-15.9	15.45	61	28.0	0.7	5.3	60	51.3	0.68	7.8
16.0-16.9	16.43	88	27.9	0.5	4.7	88	51.4	0.50	6.9
17.0-17.9	17.47	68	28.0	0.6	5.2	67	52.1	0.63	7.1
18.0-18.9	18.37	69	28.2	0.7	6.1	67	52.1	0.73	9.0
19.0-19.9	19.44	56	27.9	0.6	4.6	55	51.9	0.62	7.3
20.0-29.9	24.87	548	30.3	0.2	5.6	546	54.4	0.4	8.2
30.0-39.9	34.82	593	32.4	0.3	6.3	589	55.8	0.4	9.0
40.0-49.9	44.06	426	34.0	0.3	6.8	421	56.3	0.4	9.0
50.0-59.9	54.94	261	34.1	0.4	6.6	253	55.0	0.5	8.6
60.0-69.9	64.91	280	34.0	0.4	6.5	260	54.4	0.6	9.2
70.0-79.9	74.74	161	32.8	0.5	6.5	151	52.6	0.7	8.7
80.0-90.9	84.65	78	28.9	0.6	5.6	61	49.4	0.9	7.3

Table III.29.
Mean (M), standard error of the mean (SE), and standard deviation (SD) of waist circumference (cm) and hip-buttocks circumference (cm) by age for non-Hispanic black males and females of 2 to 90 years: NHANES III, 1988-1994

Age Group (years)	Mean (years)	Waist Circumference				Hip-Buttocks Circumference			
		N	M	SE	SD	N	M	SE	SD
Males									
2.0-2.9	2.45	183	47.4		2.9	183	50.4	0.23	3.1
3.0-3.9	3.46	162	49.1	0.25	3.2	162	52.4	0.28	3.5
4.0-4.9	4.45	178	50.3	0.27	3.6	178	55.0	0.31	4.1
5.0-5.9	5.44	162	52.5	0.39	5.0	161	58.0	0.42	5.3
6.0-6.9	6.44	85	53.0	0.63	5.8	84	60.5	0.63	5.8
7.0-7.9	7.46	95	55.8	0.68	6.6	95	63.6	0.74	7.2
8.0-8.9	8.49	85	57.6	0.86	7.9	84	67.9	0.87	7.9
9.0-9.9	9.50	103	59.6	0.87	8.8	103	70.4	0.79	8.0
10.0-10.9	10.44	103	62.6	0.96	9.8	103	74.1	0.99	10.0
11.0-11.9	11.43	95	66.6	1.28	12.5	95	79.1	1.13	11.0
12.0-12.9	12.51	80	68.6	1.64	14.7	80	80.6	1.40	12.5
13.0-13.9	13.48	53	70.4	2.04	14.9	53	85.6	1.73	12.6
14.0-14.9	14.49	69	72.2	1.74	14.4	69	88.0	1.58	13.1
15.0-15.9	15.43	68	74.2	1.71	14.1	67	91.7	1.40	11.5
16.0-16.9	16.43	71	73.7	1.33	11.2	71	90.4	1.15	9.7
17.0-17.9	17.46	63	74.8	1.49	11.8	63	91.8	1.19	9.4
18.0-18.9	18.42	58	78.5	1.58	12.0	58	95.7	1.56	11.9
19.0-19.9	19.41	63	78.0	1.59	12.6	62	93.7	1.30	10.2
20.0-29.9	25.02	473	87.1	0.7	15.7	472	99.6	0.6	12.6
30.0-39.9	34.90	473	90.3	0.7	15.0	476	99.4	0.5	11.1
40.0-49.9	44.02	341	93.9	0.8	14.2	343	99.5	0.6	10.2
50.0-59.9	55.13	203	97.1	1.1	15.4	204	99.5	0.8	11.7
60.0-69.9	64.81	271	97.7	0.9	14.0	271	98.6	0.6	10.5
70.0-79.9	74.01	162	96.7	1.1	13.4	161	98.6	0.8	10.3
80.0-90.9	84.55	46	94.0	1.7	11.8	46	97.3	1.4	9.2
Females									
2.0-2.9	2.46	137	46.5	0.32	3.7	137	49.7	0.37	4.3
3.0-3.9	3.48	191	48.8	0.30	4.2	188	52.6	0.33	4.5
4.0-4.9	4.43	163	50.5	0.34	4.3	163	55.6	0.34	4.3
5.0-5.9	5.46	174	52.2	0.35	4.6	175	58.8	0.39	5.2
6.0-6.9	6.47	92	55.1	0.91	8.8	91	62.6	0.96	9.2
7.0-7.9	7.43	87	56.8	0.96	9.0	87	66.0	0.96	9.0
8.0-8.9	8.51	81	59.3	0.99	8.9	81	71.2	0.99	8.9
9.0-9.9	9.45	93	61.0	0.99	9.6	93	73.6	0.92	8.8
10.0-10.9	10.48	87	63.4	1.09	10.2	88	77.3	1.08	10.1
11.0-11.9	11.44	89	67.7	1.11	10.5	89	83.2	1.18	11.1
12.0-12.9	12.47	85	70.5	1.21	11.2	86	88.6	1.16	10.8
13.0-13.9	13.46	81	74.0	1.36	12.3	81	92.5	1.32	11.8
14.0-14.9	14.51	66	74.9	1.79	14.5	66	95.4	1.78	14.5
15.0-15.9	15.45	61	78.4	2.03	15.8	61	96.5	1.79	14.0
16.0-16.9	16.43	88	77.3	1.42	13.3	88	97.2	1.20	11.3
17.0-17.9	17.47	66	77.9	1.83	14.9	66	98.5	1.60	13.0
18.0-18.9	18.37	68	79.7	2.27	18.7	68	97.8	1.79	14.8
19.0-19.9	19.44	56	77.8	1.79	13.4	56	98.2	1.56	11.7
20.0-29.9	24.87	547	84.6	0.7	16.6	547	102.4	0.6	14.3
30.0-39.9	34.82	593	91.4	0.8	19.5	593	106.4	0.7	16.1
40.0-49.9	44.06	424	96.7	1.0	20.2	426	109.6	0.8	17.1
50.0-59.9	54.94	257	99.3	1.1	18.0	256	108.4	1.0	16.5
60.0-69.9	64.91	261	100.6	1.1	17.6	262	108.3	1.1	17.6
70.0-79.9	74.74	151	97.9	1.3	15.9	152	106.0	1.2	15.0
80.0-90.9	84.65	63	91.2	2.0	15.5	63	100.2	1.7	13.5

Table III.30.
Mean (M), standard error of the mean (SE), and standard deviation (SD) of elbow breadth (cm) and wrist breadth (cm)
by age for non-Hispanic black males and females of 2 to 90 years: NHANES III, 1988-1994

Age Group (years)	Mean (years)	Elbow Breadth				Wrist Breadth			
		N	M	SE	SD	N	M	SE	SD
Males									
2.0-2.9	2.45	180	4.41	0.02	0.26	179	3.61	0.03	0.23
3.0-3.9	3.46	163	4.61	0.02	0.28	163	3.81	0.03	0.25
4.0-4.9	4.45	178	4.81	0.02	0.31	178	3.97	0.03	0.25
5.0-5.9	5.44	163	5.00	0.03	0.33	162	4.10	0.02	0.30
6.0-6.9	6.44	86	5.17	0.05	0.44	86	4.28	0.04	0.35
7.0-7.9	7.46	95	5.49	0.05	0.44	95	4.49	0.04	0.35
8.0-8.9	8.49	85	5.61	0.04	0.40	85	4.60	0.04	0.31
9.0-9.9	9.50	105	5.82	0.05	0.48	105	4.70	0.03	0.35
10.0-10.9	10.44	104	5.96	0.05	0.52	104	4.88	0.03	0.41
11.0-11.9	11.43	95	6.39	0.06	0.54	95	5.09	0.04	0.40
12.0-12.9	12.51	80	6.54	0.06	0.51	80	5.24	0.04	0.40
13.0-13.9	13.48	54	6.84	0.06	0.45	54	5.56	0.05	0.38
14.0-14.9	14.49	72	6.99	0.07	0.55	72	5.63	0.04	0.39
15.0-15.9	15.43	68	7.11	0.04	0.37	68	5.72	0.05	0.27
16.0-16.9	16.43	71	7.13	0.05	0.44	71	5.77	0.04	0.35
17.0-17.9	17.46	63	7.13	0.06	0.50	63	5.78	0.00	0.35
18.0-18.9	18.42	59	7.30	0.07	0.53	59	5.79	0.03	0.40
19.0-19.9	19.41	65	7.21	0.05	0.38	65	5.73	0.03	0.30
20.0-29.9	25.02	476	7.30	0.02	0.44	476	5.80	0.02	0.44
30.0-39.9	34.90	480	7.40	0.02	0.44	479	5.90	0.02	0.44
40.0-49.9	44.02	346	7.40	0.03	0.56	346	6.00	0.02	0.37
50.0-59.9	55.13	207	7.60	0.03	0.43	206	6.00	0.03	0.43
60.0-69.9	64.81	279	7.50	0.03	0.50	281	6.10	0.03	0.50
70.0-79.9	74.01	170	7.60	0.04	0.52	171	6.20	0.04	0.52
80.0-90.9	84.55	49	7.50	0.06	0.42	50	6.20	0.05	0.35
Females									
2.0-2.9	2.46	137	4.20	0.02	0.28	137	3.42	0.03	0.23
3.0-3.9	3.48	190	4.40	0.02	0.33	191	3.62	0.02	0.25
4.0-4.9	4.43	162	4.63	0.02	0.31	162	3.82	0.02	0.26
5.0-5.9	5.46	174	4.81	0.03	0.34	174	3.98	0.02	0.28
6.0-6.9	6.47	92	5.06	0.05	0.44	92	4.18	0.03	0.29
7.0-7.9	7.43	88	5.28	0.05	0.45	87	4.31	0.03	0.34
8.0-8.9	8.51	81	5.43	0.05	0.42	81	4.50	0.04	0.30
9.0-9.9	9.45	93	5.63	0.04	0.39	93	4.62	0.03	0.34
10.0-10.9	10.48	90	5.87	0.04	0.41	90	4.78	0.03	0.30
11.0-11.9	11.44	90	6.10	0.05	0.48	90	4.92	0.03	0.35
12.0-12.9	12.47	86	6.16	0.05	0.44	86	5.10	0.03	0.30
13.0-13.9	13.46	81	6.30	0.05	0.46	81	5.04	0.04	0.29
14.0-14.9	14.51	66	6.26	0.06	0.53	65	5.03	0.05	0.32
15.0-15.9	15.45	61	6.33	0.08	0.61	60	5.11	0.05	0.31
16.0-16.9	16.43	88	6.29	0.05	0.47	87	5.10	0.04	0.33
17.0-17.9	17.47	69	6.27	0.05	0.42	69	5.01	0.00	0.30
18.0-18.9	18.37	70	6.34	0.06	0.53	70	5.11	0.00	0.35
19.0-19.9	19.44	57	6.35	0.05	0.40	57	5.13	0.00	0.28
20.0-29.9	24.87	603	6.40	0.02	0.49	548	5.10	0.02	0.47
30.0-39.9	34.82	628	6.50	0.03	0.75	601	5.20	0.02	0.49
40.0-49.9	44.06	432	6.80	0.04	0.83	430	5.30	0.02	0.41
50.0-59.9	54.94	259	6.90	0.05	0.80	258	5.40	0.03	0.48
60.0-69.9	64.91	273	6.90	0.05	0.83	273	5.50	0.03	0.50
70.0-79.9	74.74	160	6.80	0.06	0.76	160	5.50	0.04	0.51
80.0-90.9	84.65	72	6.70	0.07	0.59	72	5.50	0.06	0.51

Table III.31.

Mean (M), standard error of the mean (SE), and standard deviation (SD) of biacromial breadth (cm) and bi-iliac breadth (cm) by age for non-Hispanic black males and females of 2 to 90 years: NHANES III, 1988-1994

Age Group (years)	Mean (years)	Biacromial Breadth				Bi-iliac Breadth			
		N	M	SE	SD	N	M	SE	SD
Males									
2.0-2.9	2.50		no data available			186	14.95	0.11	1.45
3.0-3.9	3.46	163	22.87	0.10	1.28	161	15.74	0.08	1.07
4.0-4.9	4.45	178	24.27	0.10	1.35	178	16.44	0.08	1.08
5.0-5.9	5.44	161	25.68	0.13	1.70	161	17.25	0.10	1.26
6.0-6.9	6.44	85	26.61	0.21	1.94	84	17.73	0.16	1.45
7.0-7.9	7.46	95	28.27	0.21	2.00	95	18.76	0.19	1.82
8.0-8.9	8.49	85	29.57	0.20	1.81	84	19.31	0.20	1.80
9.0-9.9	9.50	105	30.92	0.21	2.14	103	20.28	0.19	1.91
10.0-10.9	10.44	102	31.77	0.25	2.52	102	20.97	0.25	2.49
11.0-11.9	11.43	95	33.45	0.23	2.27	95	22.36	0.27	2.61
12.0-12.9	12.51	80	34.91	0.31	2.77	80	23.06	0.36	3.26
13.0-13.9	13.48	53	36.59	0.44	3.19	53	24.14	0.48	3.50
14.0-14.9	14.49	70	38.29	0.31	2.61	69	24.80	0.38	3.15
15.0-15.9	15.43	68	39.46	0.26	2.18	68	25.85	0.34	2.81
16.0-16.9	16.43	71	40.02	0.28	2.40	71	25.63	0.30	2.57
17.0-17.9	17.46	63	40.65	0.33	2.61	63	25.65	0.33	2.60
18.0-18.9	18.42	58	41.26	0.29	2.19	58	26.07	0.41	3.10
19.0-19.9	19.41	63	41.41	0.31	2.44	63	25.65	0.34	2.67
20.0-29.9	25.02	475	42.00	0.13	2.83	474	27.50	0.17	3.70
30.0-39.9	34.90	480	42.20	0.13	2.85	477	27.90	0.16	3.49
40.0-49.9	44.02	342	41.80	0.13	2.40	343	28.30	0.17	3.15
50.0-59.9	55.13	205	41.60	0.19	2.72	204	29.00	0.26	3.71
60.0-69.9	64.81	279	41.10	0.18	3.01	270	29.20	0.19	3.12
70.0-79.9	74.01	167	40.30	0.21	2.71	164	29.30	0.24	3.07
80.0-90.9	84.55	46	39.90	0.34	2.31	46	29.50	0.35	2.37
Females									
2.0-2.9	2.50		no data available			138	14.60	0.13	1.49
3.0-3.9	3.48	192	22.51	0.11	1.49	190	15.34	0.09	1.30
4.0-4.9	4.43	162	24.18	0.11	1.36	162	16.43	0.09	1.19
5.0-5.9	5.46	175	25.53	0.12	1.58	174	17.22	0.10	1.27
6.0-6.9	6.47	92	26.97	0.21	2.02	91	18.15	0.24	2.25
7.0-7.9	7.43	87	28.19	0.22	2.09	87	18.98	0.23	2.11
8.0-8.9	8.51	81	29.59	0.25	2.25	81	19.78	0.22	1.96
9.0-9.9	9.45	93	30.51	0.22	2.14	93	20.78	0.28	2.70
10.0-10.9	10.48	88	32.09	0.25	2.35	88	21.67	0.27	2.52
11.0-11.9	11.44	89	33.67	0.29	2.69	88	23.12	0.30	2.78
12.0-12.9	12.47	86	35.06	0.25	2.32	86	24.23	0.30	2.79
13.0-13.9	13.46	81	36.41	0.24	2.19	81	25.38	0.35	3.17
14.0-14.9	14.51	65	36.57	0.29	2.30	66	25.30	0.47	3.85
15.0-15.9	15.45	61	37.04	0.30	2.33	61	26.28	0.49	3.86
16.0-16.9	16.43	88	36.98	0.24	2.23	88	25.66	0.34	3.18
17.0-17.9	17.47	69	37.24	0.27	2.20	69	26.05	0.40	3.29
18.0-18.9	18.37	67	37.14	0.34	2.79	68	26.65	0.52	4.32
19.0-19.9	19.44	57	37.52	0.26	1.98	57	26.49	0.34	2.58
20.0-29.9	24.87	604	37.40	0.11	2.70	603	27.40	0.16	3.93
30.0-39.9	34.82	625	37.80	0.12	3.00	622	28.40	0.18	4.49
40.0-49.9	44.06	429	38.20	0.14	2.90	425	29.60	0.23	4.74
50.0-59.9	54.94	258	38.10	0.18	2.89	257	29.90	0.26	4.17
60.0-69.9	64.91	272	37.80	0.20	3.30	265	29.90	0.27	4.40
70.0-79.9	74.74	155	37.10	0.23	2.86	152	29.80	0.32	3.95
80.0-90.9	84.65	68	35.90	0.29	2.39	65	28.90	0.49	3.95

95

Table III.32.
Mean (M), standard error of the mean (SE), and standard deviation (SD)
of knee height (cm) for non-Hispanic black males and females
of 60 to 90 years: NHANES III, 1988-1994

Age Group (years)	Mean (years)	Knee Height			
		N	M	SE	SD
Males					
60.0-69.9	64.81	271	55.60	0.21	3.46
70.0-79.9	74.01	161	55.40	0.27	3.43
80.0-90.9	84.55	46	54.70	0.44	2.98
Females					
60.0-69.9	64.91	269	51.50	0.20	3.28
70.0-79.9	74.74	154	51.30	0.26	3.23
80.0-90.9	84.65	67	50.80	0.35	2.86

Table III.33.
Mean (M), standard error of the mean (SE), and standard deviation (SD) of fat-free mass (kg), total body fat weight (kg),
and percent body fat (%) for non-Hispanic black males and females of 12 to 90 years: NHANES III, 1988-1994

Age Group (years)	Mean (years)	Fat-Free Mass (kg)				Total Body Fat Weight (kg)			Percent Body Fat (%)		
		N	M	SE	SD	M	SE	SD	M	SE	SD
Males											
12-13.9	12.93	124	40.9	0.9	9.3	11.2	0.7	9.1	19.5	1.1	8.9
14-15.9	14.95	131	52.2	0.9	9.0	12.2	1.6	8.4	17.8	9.0	7.5
16-17.9	16.91	126	55.3	0.9	8.9	13.4	0.9	7.3	18.6	0.8	6.4
18-19.9	18.94	118	59.2	1.0	10.2	15.5	1.1	7.9	19.9	0.8	6.0
20-29.9	25.02	462	62.2	0.6	11.1	20.7	0.5	11.4	23.7	0.4	7.0
30-39.9	34.90	454	62.6	0.5	10.5	20.3	0.5	9.5	23.6	0.4	6.7
40-49.9	44.02	339	62.2	0.6	10.3	21.4	0.5	8.7	24.9	0.5	6.1
50-59.9	55.20	191	61.9	0.9	11.5	21.8	0.5	9.7	25.1	0.7	6.7
60-69.9	64.70	258	60.1	0.7	10.3	20.7	0.4	8.3	24.9	0.6	6.6
70-79.9	73.92	145	58.0	0.9	10.0	19.3	0.4	7.7	24.3	0.7	6.3
80-90.9	83.27	40	56.0	1.5	9.2	17.2	1.0	6.4	23.1	1.0	6.2
Females											
12-13.9	12.95	156	39.3	0.5	5.5	15.8	0.8	8.7	26.9	0.8	8.8
14-15.9	14.96	102	41.8	0.9	7.0	20.2	1.1	10.1	30.9	0.9	8.0
16-17.9	16.88	126	42.0	0.6	5.6	22.0	1.1	11.4	32.6	0.9	8.5
18-19.9	18.88	110	42.6	0.8	7.1	23.2	1.3	12.6	33.3	1.0	8.7
20-29.9	24.96	510	44.3	0.4	6.5	26.0	0.6	11.3	35.5	0.4	7.5
30-39.9	34.92	569	46.4	0.4	7.8	30.4	0.6	13.5	38.0	0.4	7.7
40-49.9	44.00	395	48.2	0.5	7.9	33.3	0.8	14.1	39.4	0.4	7.0
50-59.9	55.00	231	47.3	0.6	7.6	33.4	1.0	12.9	40.0	0.6	7.5
60-69.9	64.76	258	45.7	0.6	7.3	31.9	0.8	12.1	39.8	0.5	6.9
70-79.9	74.80	149	44.7	0.7	6.8	29.3	1.0	10.8	38.5	0.6	6.7
80-90.9	83.53	49	40.8	0.73	5.1	24.5	1.3	9.1	36.4	1.05	7.4

96

LIST OF TABLES
NON-SMOOTHED NHANES III ANTHROPOMETRIC REFERENCE
DATA: MEXICAN-AMERICANS

Table III.43. Mean (M), standard error of the mean (SE), and standard deviation (SD) of knee height (cm) for Mexican-American males and females of 60 to 90 years: NHANES III, 1988-1994.

Table III.44. Mean (M), standard error of the mean (SE), and standard deviation (SD) of fat-free mass (kg), total body fat (kg), and percent body fat (%) for Mexican-American males and females of 12 to 90 years: NHANES III, 1988-1994.

Table III.34.
Mean (M), standard error of the mean (SE), and standard deviation (SD) of weight (kg), recumbent length (cm), Rohrer's index (100 g/cm³), and head circumference (cm) by age for Mexican-American males and females of 2 months to 7 years: NHANES III, 1988-1994

Age Group (months)	Mean (months)	Boys				Mean (months)	Girls			
		N	M	SE	SD		N	M	SE	SD
Weight (kg)										
2.0-2.9	2.00	23	6.5	0.2	1.1	2.00	25	6.2	0.2	0.7
3.0-5.9	3.80	51	7.8	0.1	1.0	3.93	44	7.4	0.2	1.2
6.0-8.9	6.96	47	9.3	0.1	0.9	7.08	49	8.4	0.1	0.9
9.0-11.9	10.05	61	10.2	0.1	1.0	10.24	51	9.4	0.1	1.0
12.0-23.9	17.71	206	11.9	0.1	1.7	17.91	200	11.3	0.1	1.8
24.0-35.9	29.80	199	13.8	0.1	1.8	29.40	209	13.4	0.1	2.1
36.0-47.9	40.84	180	16.1	0.2	2.3	41.28	214	15.5	0.2	2.3
Recumbent Length (cm)										
2.0-2.9	2.00	23	61.2	0.7	3.5	2.00	24	60.3	0.7	3.2
3.0-5.9	3.80	51	66.2	0.7	5.0	3.93	44	64.1	0.7	4.6
6.0-8.9	6.96	48	70.6	0.4	2.9	7.08	49	68.6	0.4	2.9
9.0-11.9	10.05	61	75.9	0.5	3.6	10.24	51	73.1	0.4	2.9
12.0-23.9	17.71	206	82.5	0.3	4.9	17.91	194	81.8	0.4	4.9
24.0-35.9	29.80	191	92.1	0.3	4.5	29.40	205	90.8	0.3	4.4
36.0-47.9	40.84	178	99.8	0.3	4.1	41.28	216	98.8	0.3	4.5
Rohrer's Index (100 g/cm³)										
2.0-2.9	2.00	23	2.83	0.1	0.29	2.00	24	2.81	0.1	0.26
3.0-5.9	3.80	51	2.71	0.1	0.36	3.93	44	2.96	0.2	1.39
6.0-8.9	6.96	47	2.64	0.0	0.30	7.08	49	2.61	0.0	0.31
9.0-11.9	10.05	61	2.35	0.0	0.23	10.24	51	2.41	0.0	0.25
12.0-23.9	17.71	202	2.13	0.0	0.23	17.91	193	2.07	0.0	0.30
24.0-35.9	29.80	190	1.76	0.0	0.19	29 40	203	1.78	0.0	0.21
36.0-47.9	40.84	177	1.62	0.0	0.17	41.28	210	1.61	0.0	0.16
Head Circumference (cm)										
2.0-2.9	2.00	23	40.7	0.3	1.6	2.00	24	40.2	0.3	1.4
3.0-5.9	3.80	50	42.6	0.3	1.8	3.93	43	41.9	0.2	1.2
6.0-8.9	6.96	48	45.0	0.2	1.4	7.08	49	43.8	0.2	1.3
9.0-11.9	10.05	61	46.4	0.2	1.2	10.24	51	45.1	0.2	1.1
12.0-23.9	17.71	206	47.6	0.1	1.5	17.91	195	46.6	0.1	1.6
24.0-35.9	29.80	179	49.1	0.1	1.3	29.40	199	47.9	0.1	1.3
36.0-47.9	40.84	173	50.0	0.1	1.4	41.28	214	48.9	0.1	1.3
48.0-59.9	53.86	203	50.7	0.1	1.6	53.34	202	49.6	0.1	1.3
60.0-71.9	65.03	171	51.0	0.1	1.2	65.40	190	50.0	0.1	1.5
72.0-83.9	77.55	86	51.2	0.1	1.1	77.57	105	50.3	0.1	1.5

Non-Smoothed NHANES III Anthropometric Reference Data: Mexican-Americans

Table III.35.

Mean (M), standard error of the mean (SE), and standard deviation (SD) of weight (kg), stature (cm),
and body mass index (w/s^2) by age for Mexican-American males and females of 2 to 90 years: NHANES III, 1988-1994

Age Group (years)	Mean Age (years)	Weight (kg)				Stature (cm)				Body Mass Index (w/s^2)			
		N	M	SE	SD	N	M	SE	SD	N	M	SE	SD
Males													
2.0-2.9	2.48	199	13.7	0.1	1.8	194	91.6	0.3	4.2	193	16.3	0.1	1.5
3.0-3.9	3.40	180	16.2	0.2	2.3	180	98.6	0.3	4.2	179	16.6	0.1	1.6
4.0-4.9	4.49	200	18.5	0.3	3.6	202	105.5	0.3	4.9	199	16.6	0.2	2.2
5.0-5.9	5.42	174	20.3	0.3	3.9	174	111.0	0.3	4.2	174	16.4	0.2	2.5
6.0-6.9	6.46	88	23.0	0.4	3.7	88	118.0	0.5	4.7	88	16.5	0.2	2.2
7.0-7.9	7.50	91	27.9	0.7	7.1	92	125.1	0.7	6.7	91	17.6	0.3	3.3
8.0-8.9	8.45	90	31.2	0.8	7.8	92	130.7	0.6	6.1	90	18.1	0.4	3.4
9.0-9.9	9.49	93	34.6	0.9	9.1	94	136.3	0.7	6.5	93	18.4	0.4	3.7
10.0-10.9	10.47	96	37.4	1.1	10.4	96	140.3	0.6	6.3	96	18.9	0.4	3.9
11.0-11.9	11.46	100	46.4	1.3	13.2	104	146.4	0.8	8.7	99	21.3	0.5	4.6
12.0-12.9	12.50	72	47.7	1.6	13.8	73	151.5	1.0	8.7	72	20.6	0.5	4.6
13.0-13.9	13.45	74	55.5	1.7	14.3	77	158.6	1.0	8.4	74	21.8	0.5	4.5
14.0-14.9	14.50	57	57.2	1.4	10.4	57	163.8	1.1	8.4	57	21.3	0.5	3.6
15.0-15.9	15.44	65	64.5	2.1	16.7	68	168.1	1.0	8.1	65	22.7	0.6	5.0
16.0-16.9	16.44	65	67.2	1.5	12.1	66	171.0	0.8	6.3	65	23.0	0.5	3.8
17.0-17.9	17.44	74	68.9	1.4	12.4	74	170.2	0.8	6.8	74	23.7	0.4	3.6
18.0-18.9	18.48	66	71.1	1.7	13.6	66	171.5	0.7	6.0	66	24.2	0.6	4.5
19.0-19.9	19.46	52	71.2	1.8	13.1	53	170.9	0.9	6.6	52	23.9	0.6	4.2
20.0-29.9	24.76	674	73.8	0.7	17.1	675	169.8	0.3	7.8	674	25.5	0.2	5.2
30.0-39.9	34.39	474	78.7	0.8	18.1	474	170.6	0.4	8.3	474	27.0	0.3	5.4
40.0-49.9	44.48	381	82.5	1.0	18.9	381	169.8	0.4	7.6	381	28.5	0.3	5.5
50.0-59.9	54.74	178	82.8	1.4	18.7	178	169.3	0.5	7.1	178	28.8	0.4	5.5
60.0-69.9	64.58	337	78.3	0.9	16.0	338	168.4	0.4	7.2	337	27.6	0.3	5.0
70.0-79.9	73.85	149	73.1	1.3	16.0	149	165.7	0.6	6.8	149	26.5	0.4	4.9
80.0-90.9	84.17	63	66.3	1.6	12.9	63	162.6	0.9	7.1	63	25.0	0.5	4.0
Females													
2.0-2.9	2.45	209	13.3	0.1	2.1	207	90.3	0.3	4.4	204	16.3	0.1	1.8
3.0-3.9	3.44	214	15.7	0.2	2.3	218	97.9	0.3	4.5	212	16.4	0.1	1.6
4.0-4.9	4.45	205	17.8	0.2	3.5	203	104.1	0.3	4.4	202	16.3	0.2	2.4
5.0-5.9	5.45	189	20.3	0.3	3.9	191	110.9	0.4	4.9	189	16.4	0.2	2.2
6.0-6.9	6.46	105	23.2	0.5	5.3	107	117.4	0.6	5.9	105	16.7	0.3	2.9
7.0-7.9	7.42	98	25.4	0.7	7.0	99	122.5	0.6	6.4	98	16.8	0.3	3.3
8.0-8.9	8.46	95	30.7	0.8	8.0	95	129.1	0.6	6.2	95	18.2	0.4	3.5
9.0-9.9	9.42	87	35.4	1.0	9.1	88	136.5	0.7	6.6	87	18.8	0.4	3.7
10.0-10.9	10.43	90	37.3	0.9	8.1	92	142.8	0.8	7.4	90	18.2	0.3	3.1
11.0-11.9	11.43	110	50.0	1.2	12.4	110	150.6	0.7	7.2	110	21.8	0.4	4.4
12.0-12.9	12.42	75	52.0	1.5	12.7	76	154.1	0.8	6.7	75	21.8	0.5	4.4
13.0-13.9	13.43	77	53.2	1.3	11.4	78	156.1	0.8	6.7	77	21.7	0.5	4.0
14.0-14.9	14.45	77	55.6	1.3	11.5	80	156.6	0.7	6.4	77	22.6	0.5	4.1
15.0-15.9	15.40	55	58.0	1.7	12.9	57	158.6	1.0	7.6	55	23.1	0.7	4.9
16.0-16.9	16.45	66	57.0	1.4	11.6	67	157.9	0.6	5.1	66	22.9	0.6	4.6
17.0-17.9	17.42	69	65.7	1.9	16.0	69	160.9	0.7	6.1	69	25.3	0.7	5.8
18.0-18.9	18.46	55	58.4	1.6	12.1	55	157.1	0.8	5.8	55	23.6	0.6	4.3
19.0-19.9	19.55	64	60.1	1.7	13.5	65	157.6	0.8	6.3	64	24.3	0.6	5.1
20.0-29.9	24.77	575	64.8	0.8	18.2	663	157.4	0.3	7.5	575	26.1	0.3	7.2
30.0-39.9	34.73	493	70.3	0.9	20.6	530	157.1	0.4	8.1	493	28.5	0.4	8.0
40.0-49.9	44.30	367	74.1	1.0	18.6	368	157.4	0.4	6.9	366	29.9	0.4	7.8
50.0-59.9	54.60	193	70.9	1.2	16.7	195	155.7	0.5	7.0	193	29.2	0.5	6.8
60.0-69.9	64.74	321	70.2	1.0	17.7	325	154.2	0.4	7.2	321	29.5	0.4	7.5
70.0-79.9	73.95	127	63.7	1.4	15.6	127	152.6	0.8	8.5	126	27.4	0.6	6.7
80.0-90.9	84.30	59	53.8	1.7	13.4	59	146.3	1.0	8.0	58	25.1	0.7	5.5

Table III.36.

Mean (M), standard error of the mean (SE), and standard deviation (SD) of sitting height (cm), upper arm length (cm), and upper leg length (cm) by age for Mexican-American males and females of 2 to 90 years: NHANES III, 1988-1994

Age Group (years)	Mean (years)	Sitting Height (cm)				Upper Arm Length (cm)				Upper Leg Length (cm)			
		N	M	SE	SD	N	M	SE	SD	N	M	SE	SD
Males													
2.0-2.9	2.48	193	52.1	0.2	2.3	165	17.9	0.1	1.2	171	18.6	0.2	1.6
3.0-3.9	3.40	179	54.9	0.2	2.4	168	19.4	0.1	1.2	171	21.0	0.2	1.8
4.0-4.9	4.49	203	57.6	0.2	2.9	200	21.0	0.1	1.4	198	23.2	0.2	2.0
5.0-5.9	5.42	174	60.3	0.2	2.6	173	22.4	0.1	1.2	170	25.4	0.2	2.2
6.0-6.9	6.46	88	63.1	0.3	2.8	87	23.9	0.2	1.6	87	27.0	0.3	2.0
7.0-7.9	7.50	92	66.3	0.4	3.9	92	25.4	0.2	1.9	92	29.0	0.4	2.4
8.0-8.9	8.45	92	67.9	0.4	3.4	90	26.3	0.2	1.8	90	31.2	0.4	2.4
9.0-9.9	9.49	93	71.1	0.3	3.2	92	28.1	0.2	2.1	92	32.2	0.3	2.6
10.0-10.9	10.47	96	72.9	0.4	3.6	96	29.0	0.2	2.0	96	33.7	0.4	2.6
11.0-11.9	11.46	102	74.3	0.5	4.8	101	30.3	0.2	2.3	101	35.4	0.5	3.2
12.0-12.9	12.50	72	77.8	0.6	4.7	71	31.5	0.3	2.3	72	36.5	0.6	3.5
13.0-13.9	13.45	74	82.8	0.6	4.8	74	33.3	0.3	2.3	74	39.7	0.6	3.0
14.0-14.9	14.50	56	84.3	0.6	4.4	56	34.1	0.3	1.9	56	40.6	0.6	3.0
15.0-15.9	15.44	65	87.6	0.6	4.7	63	35.2	0.3	2.2	63	42.2	0.6	3.3
16.0-16.9	16.44	65	88.8	0.4	3.4	64	36.0	0.2	1.8	64	42.5	0.4	2.8
17.0-17.9	17.44	73	89.0	0.4	3.6	72	36.3	0.3	2.3	72	42.3	0.4	3.3
18.0-18.9	18.48	66	89.9	0.4	3.0	65	36.0	0.3	2.3	65	41.8	0.4	2.8
19.0-19.9	19.46	52	90.1	0.5	3.6	51	36.6	0.3	1.9	51	42.4	0.5	2.3
20.0-29.9	24.76	665	89.5	0.2	4.6	654	36.3	0.1	2.3	653	41.3	0.1	3.6
30.0-39.9	34.39	463	90.3	0.2	4.7	456	36.6	0.1	2.3	456	40.9	0.2	3.8
40.0-49.9	44.48	375	89.9	0.2	4.5	371	36.8	0.1	2.3	370	40.0	0.2	3.7
50.0-59.9	54.74	168	89.4	0.3	4.0	169	36.7	0.2	2.3	169	39.5	0.3	3.8
60.0-69.9	64.58	324	88.5	0.2	4.1	321	36.6	0.1	2.5	321	39.2	0.2	4.1
70.0-79.9	73.85	134	86.5	0.4	4.4	136	36.2	0.2	1.9	132	38.2	0.3	3.7
80.0-90.9	84.17	51	84.1	0.6	4.3	51	36.4	0.3	2.0	50	37.0	0.5	3.8
Females													
2.0-2.9	2.45	203	51.2	0.2	2.2	194	17.5	0.1	1.3	195	18.5	0.2	1.7
3.0-3.9	3.44	217	54.1	0.2	2.8	210	19.1	0.1	1.3	211	20.9	0.2	1.7
4.0-4.9	4.45	203	56.9	0.2	2.7	203	20.6	0.1	1.3	202	23.4	0.2	2.1
5.0-5.9	5.45	190	59.5	0.2	3.1	191	22.0	0.1	1.4	191	25.2	0.2	2.1
6.0-6.9	6.46	106	62.1	0.3	3.3	107	23.5	0.2	1.6	107	27.1	0.3	2.2
7.0-7.9	7.42	99	64.7	0.3	3.3	96	24.7	0.2	1.8	97	29.0	0.3	2.0
8.0-8.9	8.46	93	67.6	0.4	3.4	92	26.3	0.2	1.7	92	30.4	0.4	2.6
9.0-9.9	9.42	87	70.4	0.4	3.9	86	27.4	0.2	1.9	87	32.3	0.4	2.0
10.0-10.9	10.43	92	73.0	0.4	4.1	91	28.9	0.2	1.9	91	34.1	0.4	2.8
11.0-11.9	11.43	109	77.5	0.4	4.2	107	31.2	0.2	2.0	107	36.8	0.4	2.9
12.0-12.9	12.42	75	80.6	0.5	4.4	73	32.0	0.2	1.9	73	37.8	0.5	2.4
13.0-13.9	13.43	76	82.0	0.4	3.8	76	32.4	0.2	2.0	75	37.9	0.4	2.9
14.0-14.9	14.45	76	83.1	0.4	3.7	78	33.0	0.2	1.8	78	38.4	0.4	2.6
15.0-15.9	15.40	54	84.0	0.7	5.0	54	33.3	0.3	1.9	53	38.9	0.7	2.5
16.0-16.9	16.45	66	83.9	0.3	2.4	65	32.8	0.2	1.4	65	38.5	0.3	2.5
17.0-17.9	17.42	69	84.9	0.3	2.9	68	33.4	0.2	1.8	68	38.9	0.3	2.8
18.0-18.9	18.46	53	82.9	0.4	3.2	51	33.0	0.3	1.8	51	37.9	0.4	2.6
19.0-19.9	19.55	64	84.0	0.4	3.2	62	33.1	0.3	2.0	62	38.5	0.4	2.5
20.0-29.9	24.77	654	83.9	0.2	4.1	640	33.5	0.1	2.3	637	37.6	0.2	4.0
30.0-39.9	34.73	520	84.0	0.2	4.3	515	33.6	0.1	2.3	513	37.2	0.2	4.3
40.0-49.9	44.30	357	84.1	0.2	3.8	350	33.9	0.1	2.2	348	36.6	0.2	4.3
50.0-59.9	54.60	189	82.9	0.3	3.7	185	33.8	0.2	2.2	183	35.7	0.3	4.2
60.0-69.9	64.74	307	81.6	0.2	4.0	302	33.7	0.1	2.3	301	34.3	0.3	5.0
70.0-79.9	73.95	117	79.7	0.5	4.9	112	33.6	0.2	2.3	111	34.2	0.5	5.0
80.0-90.9	84.30	49	74.2	0.7	4.7	45	32.3	0.3	1.9	45	32.4	0.6	4.3

Table III.37.
Mean (M), standard error of the mean (SE), and standard deviation (SD) of triceps skinfold thickness (mm) and subscapular skinfold thickness (mm) by age for Mexican-American males and females of 2 to 90 years: NHANES III, 1988-1994

Age Group (years)	Mean (years)	Triceps Skinfold (mm)				Subscapular Skinfold (mm)			
		N	M	SE	SD	N	M	SE	SD
Males									
2.0-2.9	2.48	167	8.9	0.2	2.1	166	6.4	0.1	1.6
3.0-3.9	3.40	167	9.0	0.2	2.5	167	6.3	0.2	2.3
4.0-4.9	4.49	199	9.4	0.2	3.0	198	6.3	0.2	3.1
5.0-5.9	5.42	174	8.9	0.2	3.1	173	6.1	0.2	2.9
6.0-6.9	6.46	87	8.9	0.4	3.5	87	6.2	0.3	2.9
7.0-7.9	7.50	92	10.0	0.6	5.3	91	7.2	0.6	5.8
8.0-8.9	8.45	90	10.5	0.5	4.9	90	7.4	0.6	5.3
9.0-9.9	9.49	92	11.6	0.6	5.3	89	8.2	0.6	5.3
10.0-10.9	10.47	96	11.9	0.6	6.3	96	8.7	0.6	6.1
11.0-11.9	11.46	102	13.1	0.7	7.1	100	9.7	0.6	6.1
12.0-12.9	12.50	71	12.9	0.8	6.5	70	10.3	0.8	6.8
13.0-13.9	13.45	75	13.1	0.9	7.5	73	10.4	0.8	7.0
14.0-14.9	14.50	56	10.1	0.7	5.1	56	9.5	0.7	5.1
15.0-15.9	15.44	64	10.4	0.7	5.8	63	10.3	0.7	5.7
16.0-16.9	16.44	64	11.5	0.7	5.5	62	11.0	0.7	5.7
17.0-17.9	17.44	72	11.3	0.7	5.6	73	12.9	0.7	5.6
18.0-18.9	18.48	65	12.3	0.8	6.4	65	14.3	0.8	6.5
19.0-19.9	19.46	51	10.6	0.7	4.9	50	13.5	0.9	6.2
20.0-29.9	24.76	646	11.7	0.3	6.6	639	17.5	0.3	8.6
30.0-39.9	34.39	455	12.8	0.4	7.5	442	20.2	0.4	8.8
40.0-49.9	44.48	368	12.5	0.4	6.7	342	21.5	0.5	8.7
50.0-59.9	54.74	169	13.6	0.6	7.9	159	22.6	0.7	8.3
60.0-69.9	64.58	325	12.2	0.3	6.1	313	21.9	0.5	9.0
70.0-79.9	73.85	143	10.7	0.4	4.8	133	18.5	0.6	7.3
80.0-90.9	84.17	58	11.2	0.6	4.4	49	16.7	0.9	6.0
Females									
2.0-2.9	2.45	192	9.4	0.2	2.4	191	7.0	0.2	2.4
3.0-3.9	3.44	209	9.8	0.2	2.3	209	7.0	0.2	2.6
4.0-4.9	4.45	204	10.2	0.3	3.8	204	7.4	0.3	3.9
5.0-5.9	5.45	190	10.3	0.3	3.8	191	7.3	0.3	4.1
6.0-6.9	6.46	107	10.2	0.4	4.1	107	7.0	0.4	4.2
7.0-7.9	7.42	96	11.2	0.4	4.3	96	7.9	0.5	4.5
8.0-8.9	8.46	92	12.7	0.6	5.4	91	9.9	0.6	5.7
9.0-9.9	9.42	86	13.4	0.7	6.1	86	10.7	0.7	6.5
10.0-10.9	10.43	91	13.3	0.6	5.5	91	10.8	0.7	6.4
11.0-11.9	11.43	107	15.3	0.6	6.7	105	12.6	0.7	6.8
12.0-12.9	12.42	73	17.6	0.8	6.4	73	15.0	0.8	7.2
13.0-13.9	13.43	76	16.4	0.7	6.3	75	13.4	0.8	6.7
14.0-14.9	14.45	78	17.8	0.8	6.9	77	15.8	0.9	7.5
15.0-15.9	15.40	54	21.4	1.1	8.0	51	17.9	1.1	8.2
16.0-16.9	16.45	65	19.3	0.8	6.8	64	17.0	0.9	7.5
17.0-17.9	17.42	65	20.7	1.0	8.2	61	18.6	1.1	8.2
18.0-18.9	18.46	51	18.4	0.9	6.5	51	18.7	1.2	8.5
19.0-19.9	19.55	62	20.8	1.0	8.1	61	20.4	1.1	8.6
20.0-29.9	24.77	553	22.8	0.4	9.9	522	22.2	0.5	10.3
30.0-39.9	34.73	460	25.5	0.5	10.5	442	25.2	0.5	10.7
40.0-49.9	44.30	338	27.5	0.5	8.6	321	27.3	0.5	8.4
50.0-59.9	54.60	179	26.1	0.7	9.0	173	25.9	0.7	8.9
60.0-69.9	64.74	301	24.8	0.5	8.5	282	25.1	0.6	9.6
70.0-79.9	73.95	117	21.0	0.9	9.4	108	20.5	0.9	9.4
80.0-90.9	84.30	52	16.1	1.0	7.4	44	15.2	1.2	7.7

Table III.38.
Mean (M), standard error of the mean (SE), and standard deviation (SD) of supra-iliac skinfold thickness (mm) and
thigh skinfold thickness (mm) by age for Mexican-American males and females of 2 to 90 years:
NHANES III, 1988-1994

Age Group (years)	Mean (years)	Supra-iliac Skinfold Thickness (mm)				Thigh Skinfold Thickness (mm)			
		N	M	SE	SD	N	M	SE	SD
Males									
2.0-2.9	2.48	165	5.4	0.1	1.5	163	11.6	0.2	2.9
3.0-3.9	3.40	167	5.5	0.2	2.4	166	11.2	0.3	4.0
4.0-4.9	4.49	198	6.0	0.3	3.7	197	11.4	0.3	4.6
5.0-5.9	5.42	171	6.0	0.3	4.3	171	10.8	0.3	4.5
6.0-6.9	6.46	87	6.3	0.5	4.5	87	10.8	0.6	5.5
7.0-7.9	7.50	89	7.3	0.7	6.3	89	11.7	0.6	5.8
8.0-8.9	8.45	90	8.6	0.7	7.0	88	13.0	0.7	6.7
9.0-9.9	9.49	91	10.1	0.8	7.7	88	13.8	0.7	6.2
10.0-10.9	10.47	93	10.6	0.8	8.0	91	13.8	0.7	6.8
11.0-11.9	11.46	100	12.9	1.0	9.7	92	13.7	0.7	6.8
12.0-12.9	12.50	70	13.8	1.2	9.9	68	14.5	0.9	7.3
13.0-13.9	13.45	74	14.6	1.2	10.0	70	14.0	0.9	7.8
14.0-14.9	14.50	56	12.7	1.1	8.2	53	10.8	0.8	6.1
15.0-15.9	15.44	62	12.7	1.1	8.9	61	11.5	0.9	7.2
16.0-16.9	16.44	63	15.5	1.1	9.0	61	11.8	0.8	6.4
17.0-17.9	17.44	69	17.1	1.1	9.2	69	11.0	0.5	4.2
18.0-18.9	18.48	64	18.5	1.2	9.5	62	11.7	0.7	5.7
19.0-19.9	19.46	50	17.3	1.3	9.5	47	11.0	0.8	5.8
20.0-29.9	24.76	638	21.8	0.6	14.4	617	12.2	0.3	7.0
30.0-39.9	34.39	443	24.9	0.7	14.1	443	12.8	0.3	6.9
40.0-49.9	44.48	361	24.5	0.7	12.5	362	12.0	0.4	6.7
50.0-59.9	54.74	164	24.1	0.9	11.9	168	12.8	0.6	7.6
60.0-69.9	64.58	317	22.6	0.7	12.8	318	11.9	0.4	6.8
70.0-79.9	73.85	128	18.2	1.0	11.1	128	10.8	0.5	5.5
80.0-90.9	84.17	49	16.5	1.2	8.3	48	11.7	1.0	6.7
Females									
2.0-2.9	2.45	188	6.3	0.2	2.6	188	13.5	0.3	4.2
3.0-3.9	3.44	210	6.4	0.2	2.6	209	13.4	0.3	3.7
4.0-4.9	4.45	204	6.8	0.3	4.3	201	13.7	0.4	5.6
5.0-5.9	5.45	191	6.8	0.3	4.8	190	13.4	0.3	4.8
6.0-6.9	6.46	107	7.2	0.5	5.2	105	14.0	0.6	6.0
7.0-7.9	7.42	96	8.2	0.6	6.1	95	15.0	0.7	6.4
8.0-8.9	8.46	92	11.2	0.8	7.3	87	16.4	0.8	7.1
9.0-9.9	9.42	85	12.3	0.9	8.3	85	17.7	0.8	7.2
10.0-10.9	10.43	91	12.8	0.8	7.8	83	16.6	0.7	6.4
11.0-11.9	11.43	106	17.0	0.9	9.6	99	18.3	0.8	8.0
12.0-12.9	12.42	72	19.7	1.1	9.5	66	19.3	0.9	7.1
13.0-13.9	13.43	75	16.3	1.0	8.8	71	19.9	0.8	6.8
14.0-14.9	14.45	76	17.5	0.9	8.1	68	21.3	0.8	6.7
15.0-15.9	15.40	54	21.0	1.3	9.7	45	24.4	1.2	7.8
16.0-16.9	16.45	63	18.0	1.0	7.8	60	22.9	0.9	7.2
17.0-17.9	17.42	62	20.7	1.2	9.6	54	23.5	1.0	7.3
18.0-18.9	18.46	51	18.9	1.1	8.2	46	22.8	1.1	7.5
19.0-19.9	19.55	61	20.7	1.2	9.2	52	23.4	1.1	7.8
20.0-29.9	24.77	536	21.8	0.5	12.5	458	25.7	0.5	10.1
30.0-39.9	34.73	451	24.4	0.6	13.4	373	27.6	0.5	9.8
40.0-49.9	44.30	326	27.8	0.6	11.2	276	29.7	0.6	10.1
50.0-59.9	54.60	176	27.3	0.9	11.7	146	28.2	0.8	9.8
60.0-69.9	64.74	275	26.2	0.7	11.9	270	27.3	0.7	10.7
70.0-79.9	73.95	104	21.7	1.2	12.0	103	24.0	1.0	9.6
80.0-90.9	84.30	42	16.5	1.6	10.6	43	18.7	1.5	9.9

Non-Smoothed NHANES III Anthropometric Reference Data: Mexican-Americans

Table III.39.

Mean (M), standard error of the mean (SE), and standard deviation (SD) of mid-upper arm circumference (cm)
and thigh circumference (cm) by age for Mexican-American males and females of 2 to 90 years: NHANES III, 1988-1994

Age Group (years)	Mean (years)	Mid-Upper Arm Circumference (cm)				Thigh Circumference (cm)			
		N	M	SE	SD	N	M	SE	SD
Males									
2.0-2.9	2.48	166	16.2	0.1	1.3	165	28.0	0.2	2.6
3.0-3.9	3.40	167	17.1	0.1	1.6	166	29.4	0.2	2.8
4.0-4.9	4.49	200	17.6	0.1	1.9	197	30.6	0.2	3.3
5.0-5.9	5.42	174	17.9	0.1	1.9	171	31.6	0.3	3.5
6.0-6.9	6.46	87	18.2	0.2	1.9	87	32.7	0.4	3.4
7.0-7.9	7.50	92	19.7	0.3	3.0	92	35.3	0.5	4.9
8.0-8.9	8.45	89	20.5	0.3	3.0	88	36.7	0.5	4.8
9.0-9.9	9.49	92	21.6	0.3	3.1	92	39.1	0.5	4.8
10.0-10.9	10.47	96	22.1	0.4	3.7	96	40.2	0.6	5.8
11.0-11.9	11.46	100	23.2	0.4	4.3	100	41.8	0.7	6.6
12.0-12.9	12.50	71	24.6	0.5	4.1	70	43.6	0.8	6.4
13.0-13.9	13.45	74	26.2	0.5	4.1	74	47.0	0.7	6.2
14.0-14.9	14.50	56	26.6	0.4	3.3	56	46.8	0.7	5.2
15.0-15.9	15.44	63	27.8	0.5	3.9	63	48.5	0.8	6.6
16.0-16.9	16.44	64	29.1	0.4	3.6	64	50.2	0.7	5.5
17.0-17.9	17.44	71	29.9	0.4	3.4	72	50.0	0.6	4.9
18.0-18.9	18.48	65	30.9	0.5	3.7	65	51.4	0.6	5.1
19.0-19.9	19.46	50	31.0	0.6	4.1	51	50.6	0.8	5.8
20.0-29.9	24.76	655	31.7	0.2	4.1	650	51.0	0.2	5.6
30.0-39.9	34.39	457	33.0	0.2	4.3	455	51.4	0.3	5.8
40.0-49.9	44.48	371	33.7	0.2	4.0	369	51.3	0.3	5.8
50.0-59.9	54.74	169	33.5	0.3	3.9	169	50.5	0.4	5.5
60.0-69.9	64.58	325	31.9	0.2	3.8	319	48.0	0.3	5.4
70.0-79.9	73.85	145	30.3	0.3	3.9	128	46.4	0.5	5.2
80.0-90.9	84.17	58	28.4	0.4	3.3	48	44.5	0.7	4.8
Females									
2.0-2.9	2.45	193	16.1	0.1	1.5	192	27.8	0.2	2.6
3.0-3.9	3.44	210	16.8	0.1	1.4	209	29.3	0.2	2.6
4.0-4.9	4.45	203	17.4	0.1	2.0	202	30.6	0.2	3.4
5.0-5.9	5.45	191	17.8	0.1	2.0	191	31.5	0.2	3.4
6.0-6.9	6.46	106	18.0	0.2	2.3	107	32.7	0.4	3.9
7.0-7.9	7.42	96	19.3	0.3	2.7	96	34.9	0.4	4.2
8.0-8.9	8.46	92	20.5	0.3	3.1	92	37.0	0.5	5.0
9.0-9.9	9.42	86	21.3	0.4	3.6	86	39.1	0.6	5.8
10.0-10.9	10.43	91	21.9	0.3	2.7	91	39.7	0.5	4.4
11.0-11.9	11.43	107	24.2	0.4	4.0	107	43.7	0.6	5.8
12.0-12.9	12.42	73	25.4	0.4	3.5	72	46.0	0.7	5.8
13.0-13.9	13.43	75	25.6	0.4	3.6	76	45.9	0.6	5.3
14.0-14.9	14.45	78	26.3	0.4	3.8	78	47.3	0.6	5.6
15.0-15.9	15.40	54	27.5	0.6	4.4	53	48.8	0.8	5.6
16.0-16.9	16.45	65	27.0	0.5	3.9	65	48.1	0.7	5.7
17.0-17.9	17.42	68	28.3	0.6	4.7	67	50.2	0.8	6.9
18.0-18.9	18.46	51	27.0	0.6	4.1	51	47.8	0.8	5.5
19.0-19.9	19.55	61	27.8	0.5	4.2	62	48.2	0.8	6.2
20.0-29.9	24.77	559	29.7	0.2	5.7	555	50.3	0.3	7.3
30.0-39.9	34.73	481	31.9	0.3	5.9	476	51.6	0.4	8.1
40.0-49.9	44.30	348	33.1	0.3	5.4	345	51.9	0.4	7.4
50.0-59.9	54.60	185	32.9	0.4	5.6	183	50.1	0.5	7.2
60.0-69.9	64.74	309	32.8	0.3	6.0	300	48.5	0.4	7.3
70.0-79.9	73.95	115	30.5	0.6	6.6	110	46.2	0.7	7.2
80.0-90.9	84.30	51	27.2	0.8	5.4	44	42.0	0.9	5.8

Table III.40.

Mean (M), standard error of the mean (SE), and standard deviation (SD) of waist circumference (cm) and buttocks circumference (cm) by age for Mexican-American males and females of 2 to 90 years: NHANES III, 1988-1994

Age Group (years)	Mean (years)	Waist Circumference (cm)				Hip Circumference (cm)			
		N	M	SE	SD	N	M	SE	SD
Males									
2.0-2.9	2.48	164	48.3	0.3	3.2	164	50.6	0.3	3.8
3.0-3.9	3.40	167	50.9	0.3	3.8	166	53.0	0.3	3.9
4.0-4.9	4.49	199	53.3	0.4	5.3	197	55.4	0.4	5.1
5.0-5.9	5.42	172	54.0	0.4	5.6	173	57.6	0.4	5.6
6.0-6.9	6.46	87	55.6	0.6	5.8	87	60.1	0.6	5.5
7.0-7.9	7.50	92	59.0	0.9	9.0	92	65.2	0.8	8.1
8.0-8.9	8.45	90	60.8	0.9	8.6	89	67.4	0.9	8.0
9.0-9.9	9.49	92	63.8	1.0	9.9	92	72.5	0.8	8.1
10.0-10.9	10.47	96	66.0	1.1	11.0	96	74.2	0.9	9.1
11.0-11.9	11.46	101	68.9	1.3	13.0	101	77.9	1.1	10.7
12.0-12.9	12.50	71	72.3	1.6	13.7	71	80.3	1.3	10.7
13.0-13.9	13.45	74	74.9	1.5	12.6	74	87.0	1.2	10.2
14.0-14.9	14.50	56	73.3	1.2	9.1	56	86.9	1.0	7.3
15.0-15.9	15.44	63	76.6	1.7	13.6	63	89.9	1.3	10.5
16.0-16.9	16.44	64	80.0	1.4	11.5	63	92.6	1.1	8.9
17.0-17.9	17.44	71	81.9	1.2	10.2	72	94.1	0.9	7.7
18.0-18.9	18.48	65	83.2	1.4	11.1	65	95.4	1.0	8.2
19.0-19.9	19.46	51	83.2	1.5	10.6	51	94.1	1.1	8.2
20.0-29.9	24.76	652	87.8	0.5	13.3	650	95.5	0.4	9.7
30.0-39.9	34.39	456	93.7	0.6	13.2	456	97.7	0.5	10.5
40.0-49.9	44.48	370	99.0	0.8	14.4	370	99.4	0.6	11.3
50.0-59.9	54.74	169	101.9	1.1	14.3	169	100.3	0.9	11.8
60.0-69.9	64.58	319	100.9	0.7	12.0	320	98.2	0.5	9.7
70.0-79.9	73.85	130	98.3	1.2	14.1	131	96.7	1.2	13.3
80.0-90.9	84.17	48	95.4	1.5	10.2	49	94.8	1.2	8.1
Females									
2.0-2.9	2.45	191	48.5	0.3	3.7	191	50.5	0.3	4.4
3.0-3.9	3.44	211	50.6	0.3	4.1	211	52.8	0.3	3.7
4.0-4.9	4.45	203	52.3	0.4	5.6	202	55.4	0.4	5.4
5.0-5.9	5.45	191	53.7	0.4	5.9	191	57.8	0.4	5.5
6.0-6.9	6.46	106	54.5	0.7	6.7	107	60.9	0.6	6.3
7.0-7.9	7.42	96	57.0	0.8	8.1	96	64.1	0.8	7.5
8.0-8.9	8.46	92	61.2	0.9	8.9	92	69.0	0.8	8.1
9.0-9.9	9.42	86	62.0	1.1	10.4	86	72.6	1.0	9.4
10.0-10.9	10.43	90	64.7	0.9	8.7	91	75.8	0.8	8.0
11.0-11.9	11.43	106	70.7	1.0	10.6	106	84.0	1.0	10.3
12.0-12.9	12.42	73	73.4	1.2	10.5	73	88.7	1.1	9.7
13.0-13.9	13.43	75	73.0	1.2	10.8	76	88.7	1.0	8.5
14.0-14.9	14.45	78	74.5	1.2	10.7	78	91.7	1.0	9.2
15.0-15.9	15.40	54	77.8	1.6	11.5	54	93.6	1.2	9.2
16.0-16.9	16.45	65	74.8	1.3	10.6	65	93.4	1.2	9.8
17.0-17.9	17.42	67	82.4	1.7	14.2	67	98.2	1.5	12.1
18.0-18.9	18.46	51	78.2	1.6	11.4	51	93.6	1.3	9.3
19.0-19.9	19.55	62	80.8	1.4	11.4	62	95.4	1.3	9.9
20.0-29.9	24.77	555	84.7	0.7	16.5	555	99.2	0.6	14.6
30.0-39.9	34.73	479	90.6	0.8	17.9	478	103.7	0.8	17.1
40.0-49.9	44.30	347	95.8	0.9	15.8	348	106.3	0.9	16.0
50.0-59.9	54.60	185	96.3	1.1	15.4	185	103.7	1.1	14.4
60.0-69.9	64.74	299	99.2	1.0	17.3	302	104.6	1.0	17.6
70.0-79.9	73.95	110	96.7	1.6	16.5	110	100.2	1.4	14.9
80.0-90.9	84.30	44	90.3	2.0	13.4	44	93.6	1.7	11.3

Table III.41.

Mean (M), standard error of the mean (SE), and standard deviation (SD) of elbow breadth (cm) and wrist breadth (cm) by age for Mexican-American males and females of 2 to 90 years: NHANES III, 1988-1994

Age Group (years)	Mean (years)	Elbow Breadth (cm)				Wrist Breadth (cm)			
		N	M	SE	SD	N	M	SE	SD
Males									
2.0-2.9	2.48	168	4.2	0.0	0.3	170	3.6	0.0	0.3
3.0-3.9	3.40	167	4.5	0.0	0.3	167	3.7	0.0	0.3
4.0-4.9	4.49	201	4.7	0.0	0.3	201	3.9	0.0	0.3
5.0-5.9	5.42	174	4.8	0.0	0.3	173	4.0	0.0	0.3
6.0-6.9	6.46	87	5.0	0.0	0.3	87	4.1	0.0	0.3
7.0-7.9	7.50	92	5.3	0.0	0.4	92	4.4	0.0	0.3
8.0-8.9	8.45	90	5.5	0.1	0.4	89	4.5	0.0	0.3
9.0-9.9	9.49	92	5.8	0.1	0.4	92	4.7	0.0	0.4
10.0-10.9	10.47	96	5.9	0.0	0.4	96	4.8	0.0	0.3
11.0-11.9	11.46	101	6.1	0.1	0.5	101	4.9	0.0	0.4
12.0-12.9	12.50	71	6.3	0.1	0.5	71	5.1	0.0	0.3
13.0-13.9	13.45	74	6.7	0.1	0.5	74	5.4	0.0	0.4
14.0-14.9	14.50	56	6.7	0.1	0.4	56	5.5	0.0	0.3
15.0-15.9	15.44	63	6.9	0.1	0.5	63	5.6	0.1	0.4
16.0-16.9	16.44	64	7.0	0.1	0.4	64	5.6	0.0	0.3
17.0-17.9	17.44	72	7.0	0.0	0.3	72	5.6	0.0	0.3
18.0-18.9	18.48	65	7.0	0.1	0.5	65	5.7	0.1	0.4
19.0-19.9	19.46	51	7.0	0.0	0.3	51	5.7	0.0	0.3
20.0-29.9	24.76	653	7.0	0.0	0.5	654	5.7	0.0	0.5
30.0-39.9	34.39	456	7.1	0.0	0.4	457	5.8	0.0	0.4
40.0-49.9	44.48	371	7.2	0.0	0.6	370	5.8	0.0	0.4
50.0-59.9	54.74	168	7.3	0.0	0.5	168	5.9	0.0	0.4
60.0-69.9	64.58	321	7.3	0.0	0.5	321	6.0	0.0	0.4
70.0-79.9	73.85	137	7.3	0.1	0.6	138	5.9	0.0	0.5
80.0-90.9	84.17	50	7.2	0.1	0.6	51	5.9	0.1	0.4
Females									
2.0-2.9	2.45	192	4.2	0.0	0.3	191	3.4	0.0	0.2
3.0-3.9	3.44	212	4.3	0.0	0.3	212	3.6	0.0	0.3
4.0-4.9	4.45	203	4.4	0.0	0.3	203	3.7	0.0	0.2
5.0-5.9	5.45	191	4.6	0.0	0.3	191	3.9	0.0	0.3
6.0-6.9	6.46	107	4.8	0.0	0.4	107	4.0	0.0	0.3
7.0-7.9	7.42	96	5.0	0.0	0.4	96	4.2	0.0	0.3
8.0-8.9	8.46	92	5.2	0.0	0.4	92	4.3	0.0	0.3
9.0-9.9	9.42	86	5.5	0.1	0.4	85	4.5	0.0	0.3
10.0-10.9	10.43	91	5.6	0.0	0.4	91	4.7	0.0	0.3
11.0-11.9	11.43	107	5.9	0.0	0.4	107	4.9	0.0	0.3
12.0-12.9	12.42	73	6.0	0.1	0.4	73	5.0	0.0	0.3
13.0-13.9	13.43	76	6.0	0.0	0.4	76	5.0	0.0	0.3
14.0-14.9	14.45	78	6.0	0.1	0.4	78	5.0	0.0	0.3
15.0-15.9	15.40	54	6.0	0.1	0.4	54	4.9	0.0	0.3
16.0-16.9	16.45	64	6.0	0.1	0.4	65	5.0	0.0	0.3
17.0-17.9	17.42	68	6.1	0.1	0.5	68	5.0	0.0	0.3
18.0-18.9	18.46	51	5.9	0.1	0.4	51	4.8	0.0	0.3
19.0-19.9	19.55	62	6.0	0.1	0.4	62	5.0	0.0	0.3
20.0-29.9	24.77	638	6.1	0.0	0.5	557	5.0	0.0	0.5
30.0-39.9	34.73	515	6.4	0.0	0.7	481	5.1	0.0	0.4
40.0-49.9	44.30	351	6.5	0.0	0.7	347	5.2	0.0	0.4
50.0-59.9	54.60	185	6.6	0.1	0.7	185	5.2	0.0	0.4
60.0-69.9	64.74	302	6.6	0.0	0.7	303	5.2	0.0	0.3
70.0-79.9	73.95	113	6.5	0.1	0.5	113	5.3	0.0	0.4
80.0-90.9	84.30	49	6.3	0.1	0.5	49	5.2	0.1	0.4

Table III.42.

Mean (M), standard error of the mean (SE), and standard deviation (SD) of biacromial breadth (cm) and bi-iliac breadth (cm) by age for Mexican-American males and females of 2 to 90 years: NHANES III, 1988-1994

Age Group (years)	Mean (years)	Biacromial Breadth (cm)				Bi-iliac Breadth (cm)			
		N	M	SE	SD	N	M	SE	SD
Males									
2.0-2.9	2.45	no data available				168	15.4	0.1	1.4
3.0-3.9	3.40	169	22.5	0.7	1.3	169	16.3	0.1	1.1
4.0-4.9	4.49	200	23.9	0.8	1.6	200	17.2	0.1	1.4
5.0-5.9	5.42	173	25.2	0.9	2.1	174	17.9	0.1	1.4
6.0-6.9	6.46	87	26.3	0.6	1.4	86	18.7	0.1	1.3
7.0-7.9	7.50	92	27.6	0.7	1.8	92	19.9	0.2	2.0
8.0-8.9	8.45	89	28.9	0.7	1.9	90	20.4	0.2	1.9
9.0-9.9	9.49	92	30.6	0.7	2.1	92	21.7	0.2	2.3
10.0-10.9	10.47	96	31.2	0.6	2.1	96	22.1	0.2	2.3
11.0-11.9	11.46	101	32.4	0.8	2.6	101	23.1	0.3	2.8
12.0-12.9	12.50	71	33.7	0.6	2.3	71	24.1	0.3	2.9
13.0-13.9	13.45	74	36.2	0.7	2.5	74	25.8	0.3	2.6
14.0-14.9	14.50	56	36.9	0.5	1.9	56	25.8	0.3	1.9
15.0-15.9	15.44	63	38.9	0.6	2.3	63	26.6	0.3	2.7
16.0-16.9	16.44	64	39.5	0.5	2.0	63	27.1	0.3	2.2
17.0-17.9	17.44	72	40.2	0.5	2.1	72	27.5	0.3	2.5
18.0-18.9	18.48	65	40.5	0.5	2.3	65	27.8	0.3	2.6
19.0-19.9	19.46	51	40.7	0.5	2.2	51	27.9	0.3	2.2
20.0-29.9	24.76	655	41.0	0.1	2.6	653	28.3	0.1	3.1
30.0-39.9	34.39	456	41.1	0.1	2.8	456	29.0	0.2	3.2
40.0-49.9	44.48	371	41.1	0.1	2.7	371	29.9	0.2	3.7
50.0-59.9	54.74	169	41.1	0.2	2.6	169	30.6	0.2	3.1
60.0-69.9	64.58	321	40.4	0.2	2.7	320	30.5	0.2	2.9
70.0-79.9	73.85	137	39.3	0.2	2.8	132	30.2	0.3	3.0
80.0-90.9	84.17	51	38.6	0.3	2.3	50	30.3	0.3	2.3
Females									
2.0-2.9	2.50	no data available				192	15.2	0.1	1.1
3.0-3.9	3.44	211	22.2	0.8	1.4	212	16.1	0.1	1.4
4.0-4.9	4.45	203	23.4	0.7	1.5	203	17.1	0.1	1.4
5.0-5.9	5.45	191	24.8	0.6	1.5	191	17.7	0.1	1.6
6.0-6.9	6.46	107	26.1	0.7	1.7	107	18.5	0.1	1.5
7.0-7.9	7.42	97	27.2	0.7	1.8	95	19.6	0.2	1.9
8.0-8.9	8.46	92	28.6	0.6	1.8	91	20.8	0.2	2.1
9.0-9.9	9.42	87	30.2	0.7	2.1	87	21.8	0.3	2.4
10.0-10.9	10.43	91	31.1	0.6	1.8	91	22.3	0.2	2.1
11.0-11.9	11.43	107	33.0	0.7	2.2	107	24.6	0.3	2.6
12.0-12.9	12.42	73	34.5	0.6	2.0	73	25.9	0.3	2.6
13.0-13.9	13.43	76	35.0	0.5	2.0	75	25.6	0.3	2.8
14.0 14.9	14.45	78	35.2	0.6	2.2	78	26.3	0.3	2.4
15.0-15.9	15.40	54	35.9	0.4	1.7	54	27.1	0.4	2.7
16.0-16.9	16.45	65	36.0	0.4	1.8	65	26.5	0.3	2.7
17.0-17.9	17.42	68	36.7	0.5	1.9	68	27.7	0.4	3.5
18.0-18.9	18.46	51	35.8	0.4	1.9	51	27.0	0.4	2.8
19.0-19.9	19.55	62	36.3	0.4	1.9	62	27.4	0.4	3.2
20.0-29.9	24.77	638	36.7	0.1	2.5	640	28.1	0.2	4.0
30.0-39.9	34.73	515	37.0	0.1	2.7	513	29.4	0.2	4.3
40.0-49.9	44.30	351	37.2	0.1	2.4	351	29.9	0.2	3.9
50.0-59.9	54.60	185	36.7	0.2	2.3	185	30.0	0.3	3.8
60.0-69.9	64.74	303	36.5	0.1	2.4	300	30.4	0.2	3.8
70.0-79.9	73.95	112	35.5	0.2	2.2	111	30.1	0.3	3.6
80.0-90.9	84.30	46	34.2	0.3	2.3	43	29.4	0.6	3.7

Table III.43.
Mean (M), standard error of the mean (SE), and standard deviation (SD)
of knee height (cm) by age for Mexican-American
males and females of 60 to 90 years: NHANES III, 1988-1994

Age Group (years)	Mean (years)	Knee Height (cm)			
		N	M	SE	SD
Males					
60.0-69.9	64.58	318	52.5	0.2	3.2
70.0-79.9	73.85	134	51.7	0.3	2.9
80.0-90.9	84.17	51	51.2	0.5	3.4
Females					
60.0-69.9	64.74	302	47.7	0.2	3.5
70.0-79.9	73.95	111	47.7	0.3	3.2
80.0-90.9	84.30	47	46.9	0.4	2.9

Table III.44.
Mean (M), standard error of the mean (SE), and standard deviation (SD) of fat-free body mass (kg), total body fat weight (kg),
and percent body fat (%) by age for Mexican-Americans of 12 to 90 years: NHANES III, 1988-1994

Age Group (years)	Mean (years)	N	Fat-Free Body Mass (kg)			Total Body Fat Weight (kg)			Percent Body Fat (%)		
			M	SE	SD	M	SE	SD	M	SE	SD
Males											
12-13.9	13.00	131	40.3	0.9	8.2	12.3	0.8	7.5	22.0	1.0	8.2
14-15.9	15.00	107	49.8	1.2	9.3	12.6	1.1	8.9	18.8	1.1	7.7
16-17.9	17.00	126	53.0	0.9	7.5	14.9	0.7	6.1	21.3	0.7	5.4
18-19.9	18.90	109	55.7	1.0	8.0	17.1	0.9	7.2	22.7	0.8	5.7
20-29.9	24.80	631	55.7	0.4	8.3	18.3	0.4	7.3	24.1	0.4	6.0
30-39.9	34.40	443	58.1	0.5	8.9	20.3	0.4	7.1	25.4	0.4	5.4
40-49.9	44.40	361	59.8	0.6	8.9	22.2	0.5	7.3	26.6	0.4	5.3
50-59.9	54.60	164	60.2	1.0	9.6	22.4	0.7	7.1	26.7	0.6	5.3
60-69.9	64.60	301	57.0	0.6	7.9	21.2	0.5	6.7	26.7	0.4	5.2
70-79.9	73.80	118	53.1	1.0	8.3	19.2	0.7	5.8	26.1	0.7	5.2
80-90.9	83.50	45	49.1	1.1	7.0	18.8	0.9	6.2	27.2	0.8	5.1
Females											
12-13.9	12.90	139	37.3	0.6	5.3	16.0	0.8	7.6	28.6	0.8	7.6
14-15.9	14.80	113	37.8	0.6	4.8	18.4	0.8	6.9	31.8	0.7	6.3
16-17.9	16.90	112	40.5	0.7	6.0	21.6	1.2	10.3	33.3	0.8	7.1
18-19.9	19.10	90	38.8	0.7	4.9	20.7	1.1	8.9	33.5	0.9	6.8
20-29.9	24.90	509	40.8	0.3	5.6	24.1	0.5	9.8	35.8	0.4	7.0
30-39.9	34.90	451	42.8	0.4	6.4	27.8	0.6	11.5	38.0	0.4	7.1
40-49.9	44.20	333	43.5	0.4	5.5	29.9	0.6	9.4	39.9	0.4	5.5
50-59.9	54.50	171	42.6	0.6	5.8	28.7	0.8	9.0	39.4	0.5	5.7
60-69.9	64.80	278	41.9	0.5	6.0	28.1	0.7	9.3	39.4	0.4	5.7
70-79.9	73.90	101	39.8	0.7	5.6	25.2	1.0	8.8	37.8	0.8	6.8
80-90.9	82.90	34	33.6	0.67	3.9	21.0	1.1	6.7	37.6	1.05	6.2

LITERATURE CITED

1. US Department of Health and Human Services. National Center for Health Statistics. 1996. The Third National Health and Nutrition Examination Survey (NHANES III, 1988-1994): Centers for Disease Control and Prevention: Washington D.C.

2. National Health and Nutrition Examination Survey. Anthropometric Reference Data, United States, 1988-1994. Available online at:
    http://www.cdc.gov/nchs/about/major/nhanes/Anthropometric%20Measures.htm.

3. SAS I. 1990. SAS Procedures Guide, Version 6, 3rd ed. SAS Institute Inc.: Cary, NC.

4. WesVarPC Manual. Westat, 1650 Research Boulevard, Rockville, MD 20850.

5. Shah, B.V., Barnwell, B.G., Bieler, G.S. 1995. SUDAAN User's manual, Release 6.40. Research Triangle Institute: Research Triangle Park, NC.

6. Ballew, C., Khan, L.K., Kaufmann, R., Mokdad, A., Miller, D.T., Gunter, E.W. 1999. Blood lead concentration and children's anthropometric dimensions in the Third National Health and Nutrition Examination Survey (NHANES III), 1988-1994. J. Pediatr. 134:623-30.

7. Ryan, A.S., Roche, A.F., Kuczmarski, R.J. 1999. Weight, stature, and body mass index data for Mexican Americans from the third national health and nutrition examination survey (NHANES III, 1988-1994). Am. J. Hum. Biol. 11:673-86.

8. Hediger, M.L., Overpeck, M.D., McGlynn, A., Kuczmarski, R.J., Maurer, K.R., Davis, W.W. 1999. Growth and fatness at three to six years of age of children born small- or large-for-gestational age. Pediatrics 104:e33.

9. Chumlea, W.C., Guo, S.S., Kuczmarski, R.J., Flegal, K.M., Johnson, C.L., Heymsfield, S.B., Lukaski, H.C., Friedl, K., Hubbard, V.S. 2002. Body composition estimates from NHANES III bioelectrical impedance data. Int. J. Obes. Relat. Metab. Disord. 26:1596-1609.

10. Fernandez, J.R., Redden, D.T., Pietrobelli, A., Allison, D.B. 2004. Waist circumference percentiles in nationally representative samples of African-American, European-American, and Mexican-American children and adolescents. J. Pediatr. 145:439-44.

11. Obisesan, T.O., Aliyu, M.H., Bond, V., Adams, R.G., Akomolafe, A., Rotimi, C.N. 2005. Ethnic and age-related fat free mass loss in older Americans: the Third National Health and Nutrition Examination Survey (NHANES III). BMC Public Health 5:41-49.

12. Kuczmarski, M.F., Kuczmarski, R.J., Najjar, M. 2000. Descriptive anthropometric reference data for older Americans. J. Am. Diet. Assoc. 100:59-66.

13. Frisancho, A.R. 1990. Anthropometric Standards for the Assessment of Growth and Nutritional Status. Ann Arbor, MI: University of Michigan Press.

14. Malina, R.M., Hamill, P.V.V., Lemeshow, S., 1973. Selected body measurements of children 6-11 years. US Vital & Health Statistics, Series 11, No. 123, USDHHS, Washington D.C.

15. Johnston F.E., Hamill, P.V.V., Lemeshow, S. 1972. Skinfold thicknesses of children 6-11 years. US Vital & Health Statistics, Series 11, No. 120, USDHHS, Washington D.C.

CHAPTER IV
POSTNATAL ANTHROPOMETRIC REFERENCE BASED ON NHANES III FOR CHILDREN AND ADULTS

DEVELOPMENT OF SMOOTHED NORMALIZED ANTHROPOMETRIC DISTANCE PERCENTILE CURVES
Skewness Factor
Curve Smoothing
Comparison of Smoothed and Non-Smoothed Anthropometric Variables

SMOOTHED ANTHROPOMETRIC REFERENCE FOR THE EVALUATIONS OF GROWTH AND NUTRITIONAL STATUS

LIST OF TABLES: SMOOTHED ANTHROPOMETRIC REFERENCE

LIST OF FIGURES: SMOOTHED ANTHROPOMETRIC REFERENCE

LITERATURE CITED

CHAPTER IV

POSTNATAL ANTHROPOMETRIC REFERENCE BASED ON NHANES III FOR CHILDREN AND ADULTS

This chapter focuses on the various statistical approaches and the methodology used in the development of the anthropometric reference. The resulting new anthropometric references for the evaluation of growth and nutritional status of children and adults from 2 months to 90 years of age are presented in tabular and graphic form. These references give the medians, generalized coefficients of variation, and percentiles by age and gender for each of the body measures collected in the third National Health and Nutrition Examination Survey. This chapter also includes the statistical rationale for using Z-scores and percentiles when evaluating anthropometric nutritional status of children and adults.

DEVELOPMENT OF SMOOTHED NORMALIZED ANTHROPOMETRIC DISTANCE PERCENTILE CURVES

Skewness Factor

The purpose of a dimensional reference or standard is to provide a uniform, normally distributed baseline. However, anthropometric variables, especially those that indicate body composition (e.g., weight, body mass index, fat, etc.), are not normally distributed (3) and are skewed with the right tail of the distribution longer than the left. Therefore, evaluation of nutritional status using as a reference non-normalized anthropometric data and employing conventional statistical methods that assume a normal distribution can lead to erroneous conclusions. For this reason, to construct a normally distributed anthropometric reference, the skewness factor was removed from the distribution of all the anthropometric variables. For this purpose we used the LMS method (1,2). The LMS method provides a way to obtain normalized percentile anthropometric measurements (e.g., height, weight, circumferences, or skinfolds). This method uses a power transformation referred to as L (for lambda), which stretches one tail of the distribution and shrinks the other, removing the skewness for each of a series of age groups. In addition, the LMS method calculates the median (Md) and the coefficient of variation (S) for

112

each of a series of age groups, and then causes them to change smoothly with age. The resulting L, Md, and S curves contain information to draw any percentile curve, and to convert measurements (even extreme values) into exact SD scores.

The skewness factor (L) and Z-score were derived using the following formula (2):

$$L = -LOG (Sa/Sh)/[2 \times LOG(Sa \times Sh/(Sg^2))]$$

where:

Sa = Standard deviation of the measurement/natural log of the geometric mean;

Sh = Reciprocal of the standard deviation x the natural log of the geometric mean;

Sg = Natural log of the coefficient of variation.

The Z-scores were derived using the following formula (1,2):

$$Z\text{-Score} = [(X/Md)^L - 1.0]/(L \times S)$$

where X is the physical measurement (e.g., birth weight, Rohrer index, etc.), L is the skewness variable (L), Md is the median or 50th percentile value for the measurement, and S is the coefficient of variation corresponding to the measurement. $(X/Md)^L$ means raising the quantity (X/Md) to the Lth power.

The normalization of the anthropometric data was developed in two stages. In the first stage, to obtain the LMS parameters, the anthropometric data of each individual was converted to the natural log and reciprocal values, from which the LMS values were calculated. In the second stage, the LMS were derived from the means of the anthropometric dimensions. For this purpose, the descriptive statistics (adjusted for sampling size), such as means, standard errors of the mean, standard deviations, medians, coefficients of variation, and geometric means, were calculated for age group and sex for all of the anthropometric variables. Then, the LMS parameters were calculated. The results of these estimates were averaged.

Curve Smoothing

The Md and S parameters were smoothed using several order polynomial regressions given in the software of StatView, version 5.0 (Abacus Concepts, Berkeley, CA, USA), and Cricket graph (4,5). Then, the L values were applied to calculate the percentiles. These estimations were done until the resulting distant curves approached a normal distribution. As a result of the several estimations, the L values, medians (Md), generalized coefficients (S), and percentiles differ from those derived by one single computation. Finally, the age-specific and sex-specific percentiles for each variable were determined by computation using the equation of the LMS method (1,2):

Percentile = Md $(1 + LSZ)^{(1/L)}$

where Md is the median or 50th percentile value for the measurement, L is the average skewness factor, S is the generalized coefficient of variation, Z is the Z-score that corresponds to the percentile, and 1/L means raising the quantity $(1 + L \times S \times Z)$ to the 1/Lth power. Therefore, the percentiles for each variable were obtained by computation:

5th percentile = Md x $(1 + L \times S \times -1.645)^{(1/L)}$

10th percentile = Md x $(1 + L \times S \times -1.282)^{(1/L)}$

15th percentile = Md x $(1 + L \times S \times -1.036)^{(1/L)}$

25th percentile = Md x $(1 + L \times S \times -0.674)^{(1/L)}$

50th percentile = Md x $(1 + L \times S \times 0.0)^{(1/L)}$

75th percentile = Md x $(1 + L \times S \times 0.674)^{(1/L)}$

85th percentile = Md x $(1 + L \times S \times 1.036)^{(1/L)}$

90th percentile = Md x $(1 + L \times S \times 1.282)^{(1/L)}$

95th percentile = Md x $(1 + L \times S \times 1.645)^{(1/L)}$

Comparison of Smoothed and Non-Smoothed Anthropometric Variables

Figures IV.1 to **IV.6** compare the smoothed (s90th and s75th) and non-smoothed and non-normalized raw percentiles (r90th and r75th) for height, body weight, body mass index, sitting height, leg lengths, upper arm length, skinfold thickness, and percent body fat. From this data it is evident that the smoothed and normalized percentiles across all ages and in both genders provide a more uniform reference than the non-smoothed and non-normalized percentiles. The transformation of the original anthropometric data, followed by the derivation of a robust median (Md) and a generalized coefficient of variation (S), reduces the extremes and provides normalized percentile curves, where the proportion of individuals above or below the mean are equally distributed. Therefore, the resulting anthropometric reference can be used to evaluate growth and nutritional status of individuals and populations using statistical methods that assume a normal distribution. Furthermore, as a result of the several estimates, the effects of sampling size "weigh" on the LMS values and the percentiles become negligible when compared to the raw means.

This reference is not divided by ethnicity. The reason for the exclusion of ethnic groups is based upon several factors. First, as pointed out in the previous chapter, the sample size by ethnicity for children in both males and females at each age group was quite small (N < 110). For example, among 6- to 19-year-old white males, the sample size ranges from 45 to 75, while in blacks the corresponding sample size ranges from 59 to 106, and for Mexican-Americans the sample size ranges from 52 to 88. In females, the sample size by age and ethnicity for non-adults was also small. In other words, despite the fact that the individuals included in the NHANES data sets represent a large sample size, and even when the data are adjusted with sampling weights, the sample size is too small for establishing reliable percentile references. Hence, a population-specific percentile for children would be unreliable due to an insufficient sample size and would not meet standards of reliability or precision that are necessary for establishing a valid point of reference.

In summary, although the anthropometric information has been derived from the data sets of NHANES III, due to the effect of statistical approaches used for smoothing the resulting means and standard deviations are lesser and the percentile ranges are narrower than those given in chapter III. Yet, because the anthropometric references were developed using a large sample size and statistical methods applicable to all populations they provide a uniform baseline useful for evaluating growth and nutritional status of individuals and populations, irrespective of ethnicity.

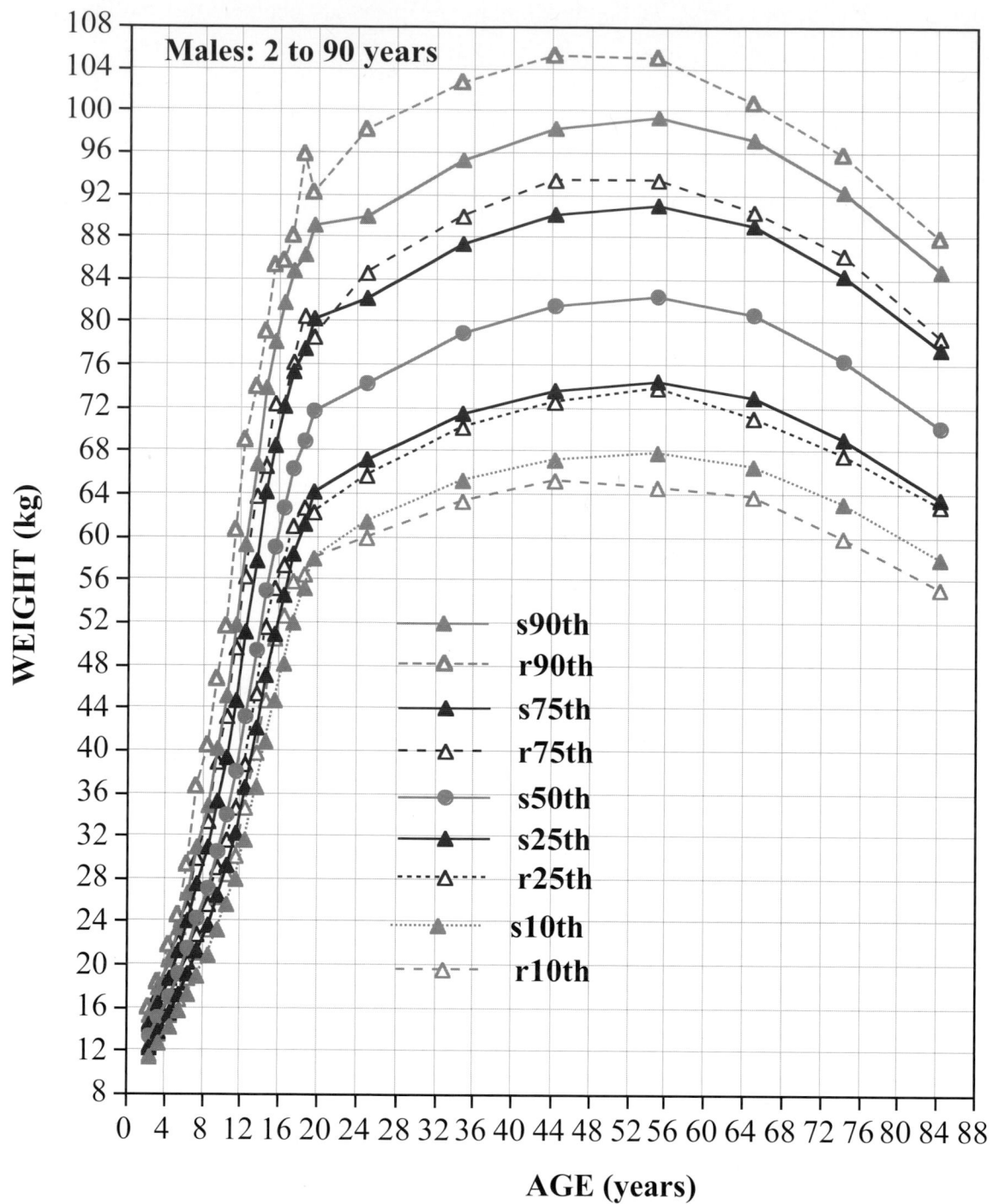

Figure IV.1. Comparison of the Smoothed Percentiles and Raw Percentiles of Weight for Males. Note that the smoothed and normalized percentiles across all ages provide a more uniform reference than the non-smoothed and non-normalized percentiles.

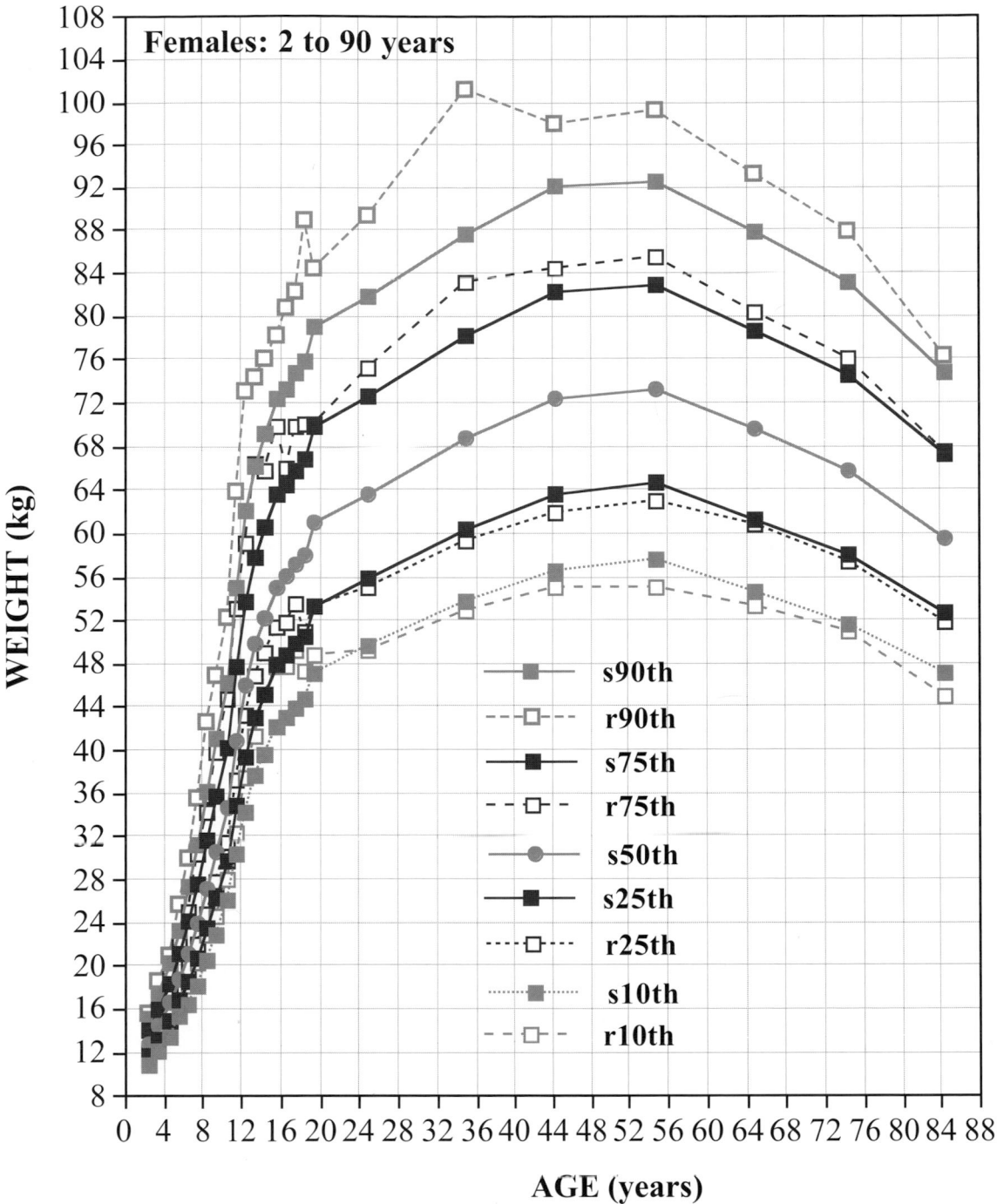

Figure IV.2. Comparison of the Smoothed Percentiles and Raw Percentiles of Weight for Females. Note that the smoothed and normalized percentiles across all ages provide a more uniform reference than the non-smoothed and non-normalized percentiles.

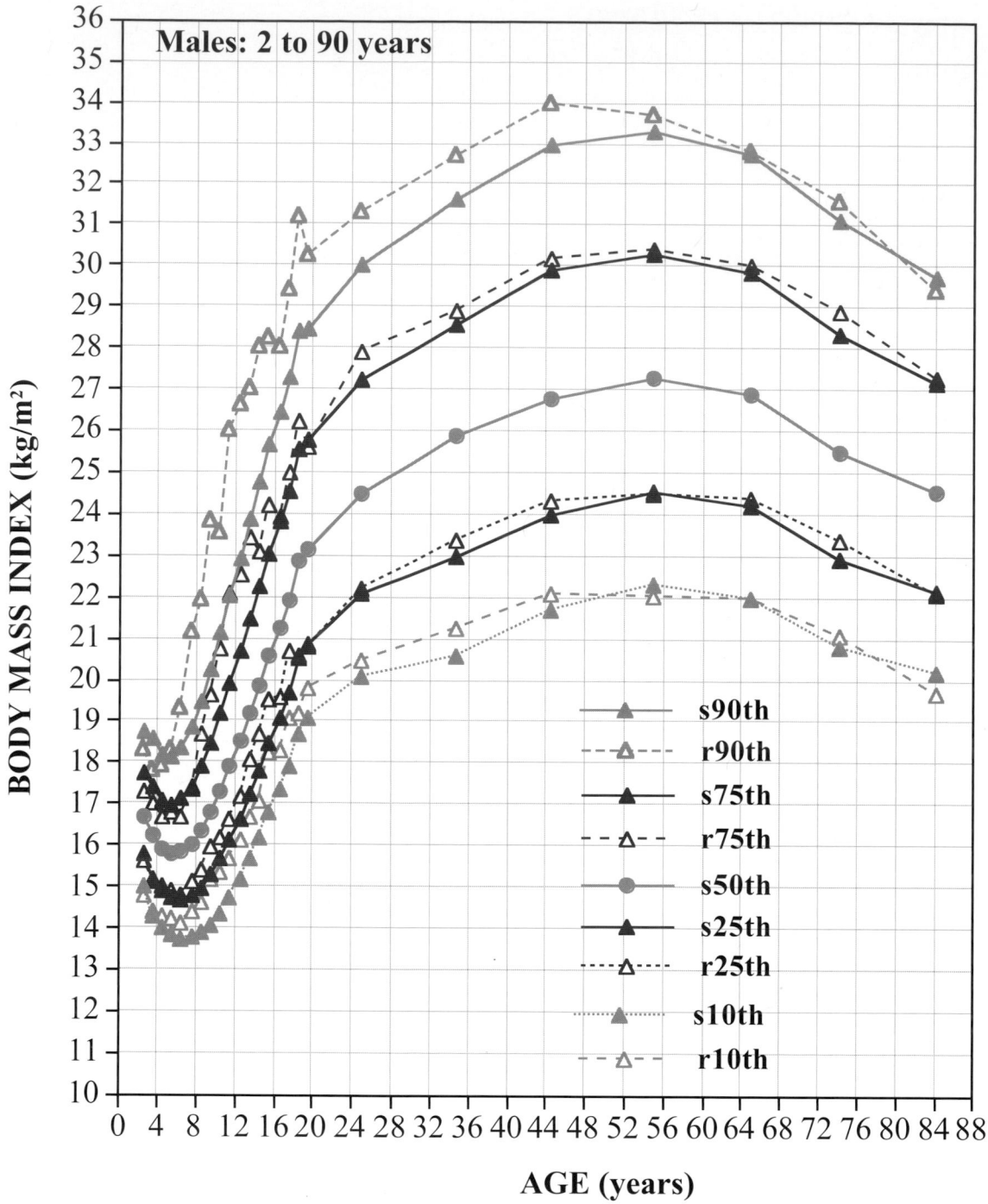

Figure IV.3. Comparison of the Smoothed Percentiles and Raw Percentiles of Body Mass Index (kg/m²) for Males. Note that the smoothed and normalized percentiles across all ages provide a more uniform reference than the non-smoothed and non-normalized percentiles.

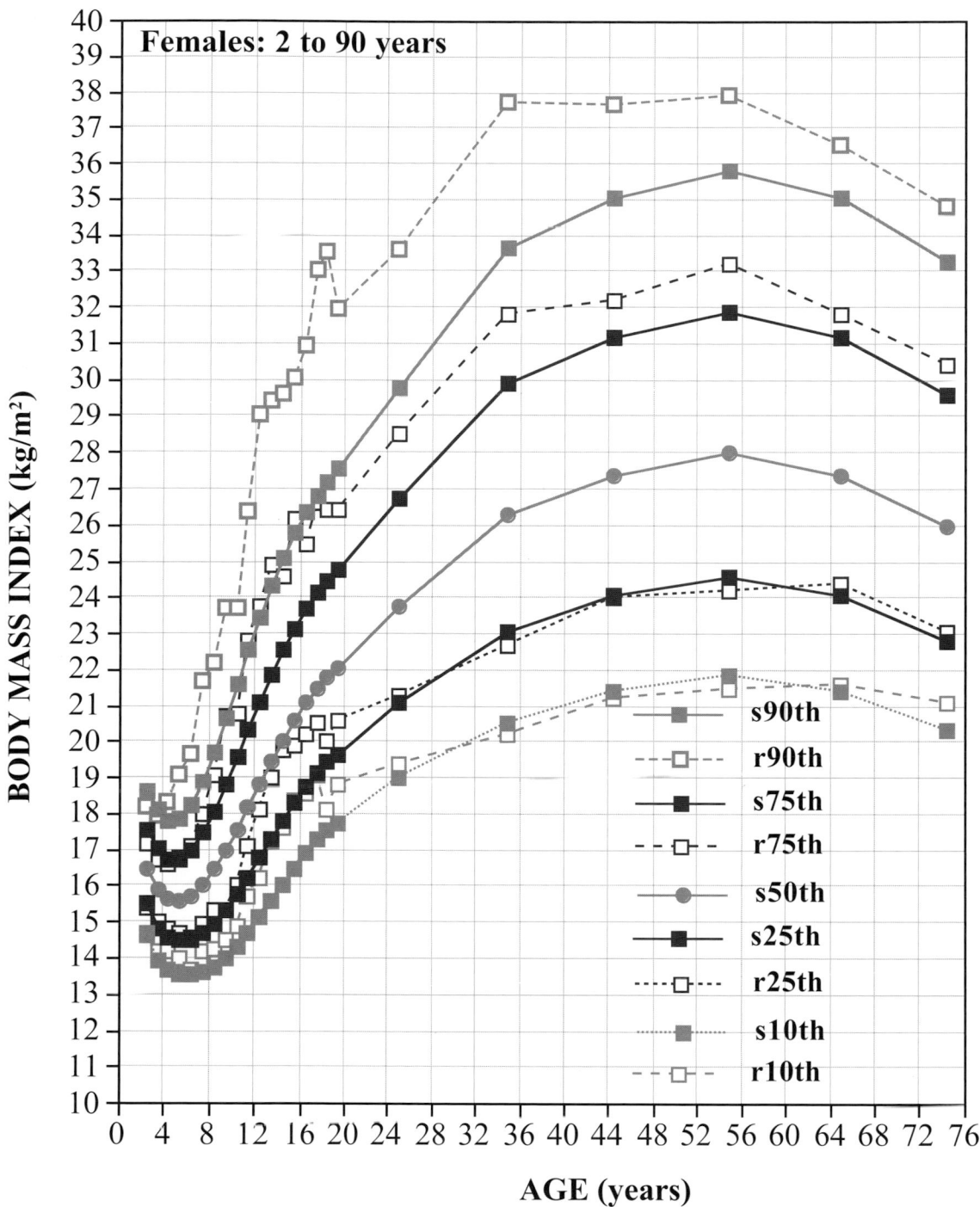

Figure IV.4. Comparison of the Smoothed Percentiles and Raw Percentiles of Body Mass Index (kg/m²) for Females. Note that the smoothed and normalized percentiles across all ages provide a more uniform reference than the non-smoothed and non-normalized percentiles.

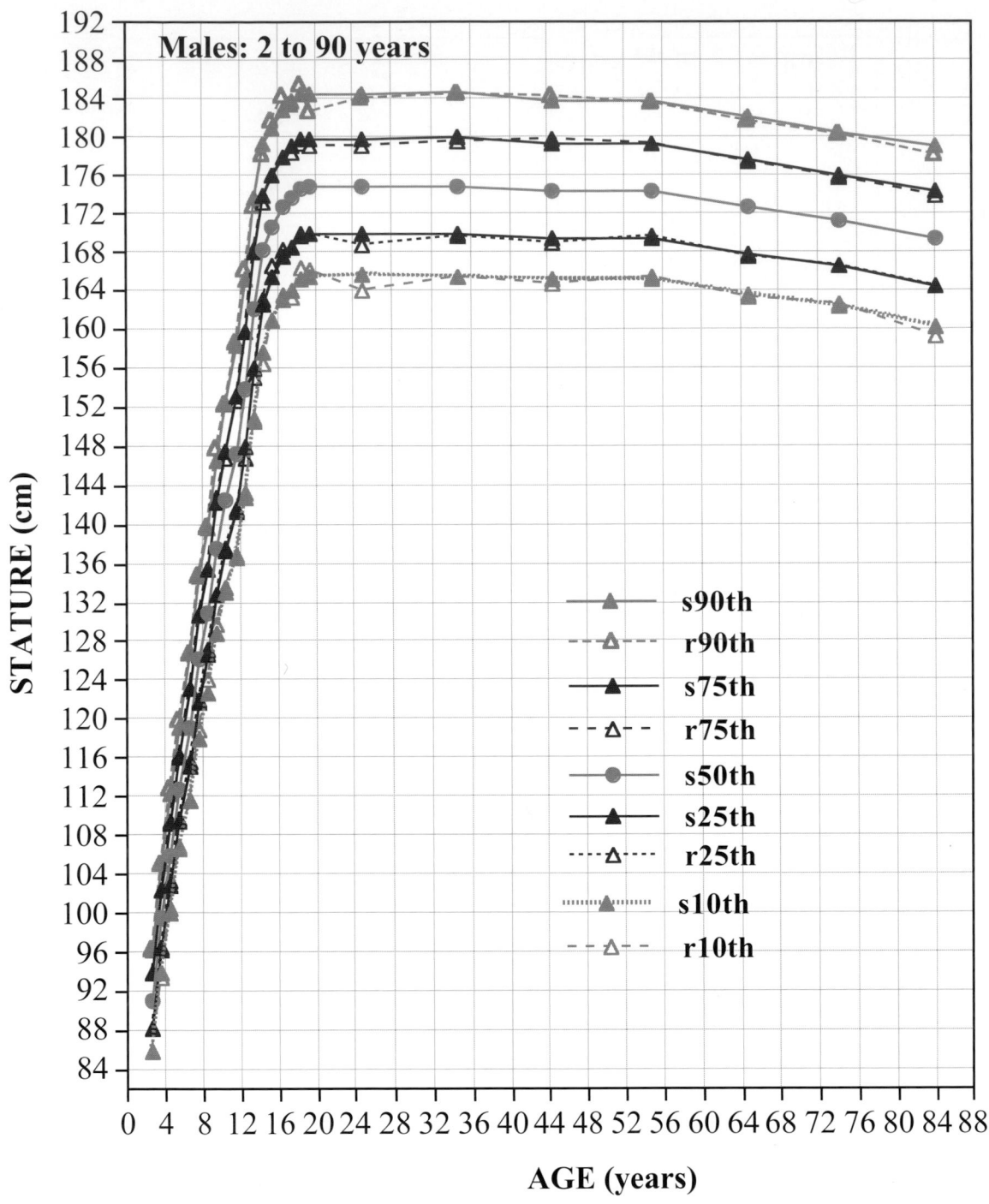

Figure IV.5. Comparison of the Smoothed Percentiles and Raw Percentiles of Height (cm) for Males. Note that the smoothed and normalized percentiles across all ages provide a more uniform reference than the non-smoothed and non-normalized percentiles.

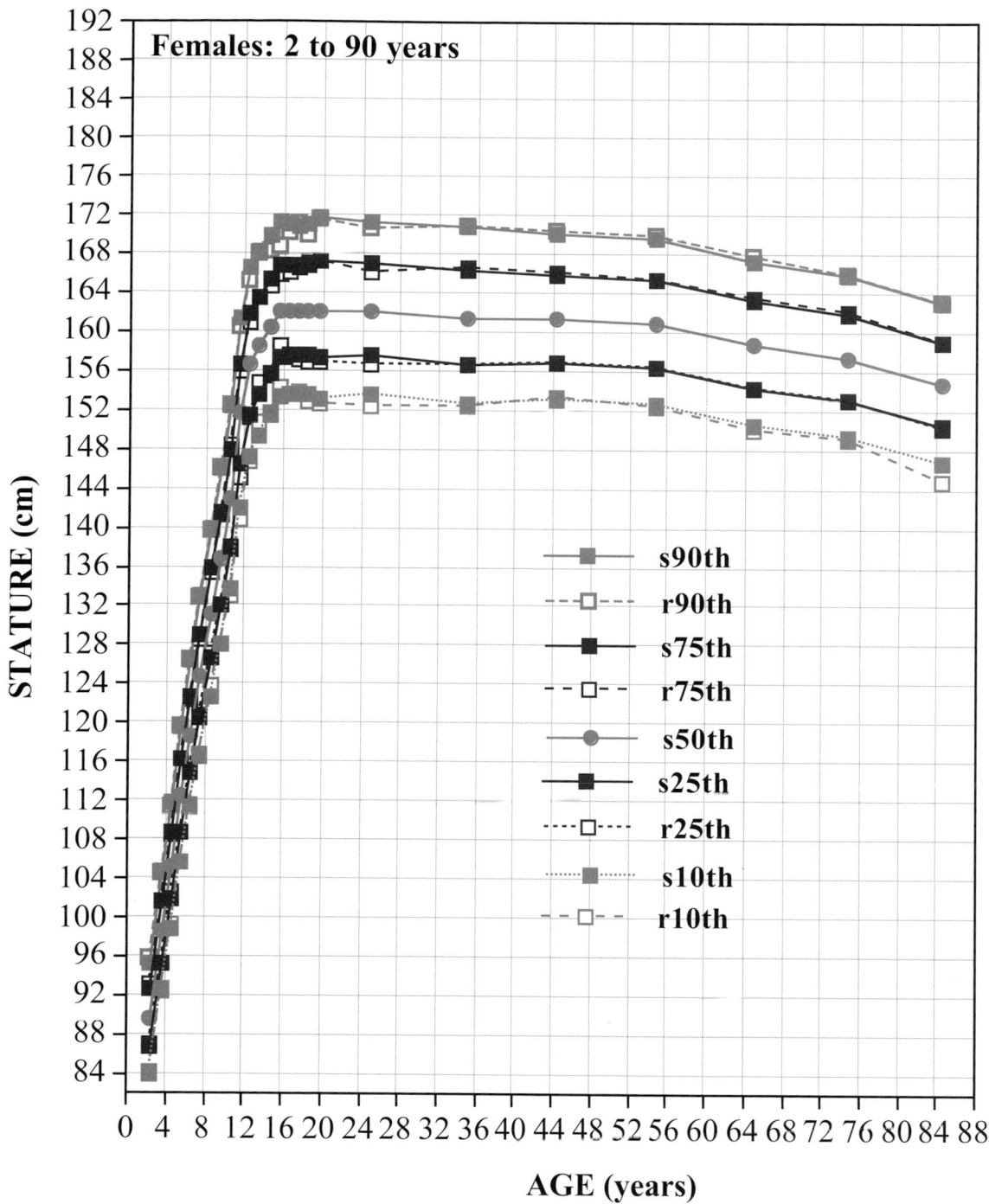

Figure IV.6. Comparison of the Smoothed Percentiles and Raw Percentiles of Height (cm) for Females. Note that the smoothed and normalized percentiles across all ages provide a more uniform reference than the non-smoothed and non-normalized percentiles.

SMOOTHED ANTHROPOMETRIC REFERENCE FOR THE EVALUATIONS OF GROWTH AND NUTRITIONAL STATUS

The means (M) and standard deviations (SD), along with the percentiles of the anthropometric variables, are presented in **Tables IV.1** to **IV.40**. This section also includes graphs (**Figures IV.7** to **IV.40**) of the age-associated changes in body size and body composition of children and adults traditionally used in the evaluation of growth and nutritional status.

LIST OF TABLES
SMOOTHED ANTHROPOMETRIC REFERENCE

Table IV.12. Mean (M), standard deviation (SD), and percentiles of lower leg length (cm) by age for males and females of 2 to 90 years.

Table IV.13. Mean (M), standard deviation (SD), and percentiles of lower leg length index (lower leg length/stature x 100) by age for males and females of 2 to 90 years.

Table IV.14. Mean (M), standard deviation (SD), and percentiles of total leg length (cm) by age for males and females of 2 to 90 years

Table IV.15. Mean (M), standard deviation (SD), and percentiles of total leg length index (total leg length/stature x 100) by age for males and females of 2 to 90 years.

Table IV.16. Mean (M), standard deviation (SD), and percentiles of upper arm length (cm) by age for males and females of 2 to 90 years.

Table IV.17. Mean (M), standard deviation (SD), and percentiles of biacromial breadth (cm) by age for males and females of 3 to 90 years.

Table IV.18. Mean (M), standard deviation (SD), and percentiles of bi-iliac breadth (cm) by age for males and females of 2 to 90 years.

Table IV.19. Mean (M), standard deviation (SD), and percentiles of elbow breadth (mm) by age for males and females of 2 to 90 years.

Table IV.20. Mean (M), standard deviation (SD), and percentiles of wrist breadth (mm) by age for males and females of 2 to 90 years.

Table IV.21. Mean (M), standard deviation (SD), and percentiles of waist circumference (cm) by age for males and females of 2 to 90 years.

Table IV.22. Mean (M), standard deviation (SD), and percentiles of buttock (hip) circumference (cm) by age for males and females of 2 to 90 years.

Table IV.23. Mean (M), standard deviation (SD), and percentiles of waist-buttock (hip) ratio by age for males and females of 2 to 90 years.

Table IV.24. Mean (M), standard deviation (SD), and percentiles of thigh circumference (cm) by age for males and females of 2 to 90 years.

Table IV.25. Mean (M), standard deviation (SD), and percentiles of triceps skinfold thickness (mm) by age for males and females of 2 to 90 years.

Table IV.26. Mean (M), standard deviation (SD), and percentiles of subscapular skinfold thickness (mm) by age for males and females of 2 to 90 years.

Table IV.27. Mean (M), standard deviation (SD), and percentiles of sum of two-site skinfold thickness (mm) (triceps and subscapular skinfold thickness) by age for males and females of 2 to 90 years.

Table IV.28. Mean (M), standard deviation (SD), and percentiles of suprailiac skinfold thickness (mm) by age for males and females of 2 to 90 years.

Table IV.29. Mean (M), standard deviation (SD), and percentiles of thigh skinfold thickness (mm) by age for males and females of 2 to 90 years.

Table IV.30. Mean (M), standard deviation (SD), and percentiles of the sum of four-site skinfold thickness (mm) (triceps, subscapular, suprailiac, and thigh) by age for males and females of 2 to 90 years.

Table IV.31. Mean (M), standard deviation (SD), and percentiles of mid-upper arm circumference (cm) by age for males and females of 2 to 90 years.

Table IV.32. Mean (M), standard deviation (SD), and percentiles of mid-upper arm area (cm^2) by age for males and females of 2 to 90 years.

Table IV.33. Mean (M), standard deviation (SD), and percentiles of mid-upper arm muscle area (cm^2) by age for males and females of 2 to 90 years.

Table IV.34. Mean (M), standard deviation (SD), and percentiles of mid-upper arm fat area (cm^2) by age for males and females of 2 to 90 years.

Table IV.35. Mean (M), standard deviation (SD), and percentiles of mid-upper arm fat index (arm fat area/total arm area x 100) by age for males and females of 2 to 90 years.

Table IV.36. Mean (M), standard deviation (SD), and percentiles of total fat-free mass (kg) by age for males and females of 12 to 90 years.

Table IV.37. Mean (M), standard deviation (SD), and percentiles of total fat-free mass index (kg/m^2) by age for males and females of 12 to 90 years.

Table IV.38. Mean (M), standard deviation (SD), and percentiles of total body fat mass (kg) by age for males and females of 12 to 90 years.

Table IV.39. Mean (M), standard deviation (SD), and percentiles of total body fat mass index ($kg\ fat/m^2$) by age for males and females of 12 to 90 years.

Table IV.40. Mean (M), standard deviation (SD), and percentiles of percent body fat (%) by age for males and females of 12 to 90 years.

Table IV.1.

Mean (M), standard deviation (SD), and percentiles of weight (kg) by age for males and females of 2 to 48 months

Age Group (months)	Mean Age (months)	N	M	SD	Percentiles								
					5th	10th	15th	25th	50th	75th	85th	90th	95th
Males													
2.0-2.9	2.00	108	6.9	1.0	5.4	5.6	5.8	6.1	6.7	7.4	7.9	8.2	8.7
3.0-5.9	3.96	292	7.7	1.0	6.3	6.5	6.7	7.0	7.7	8.4	8.9	9.2	9.7
6.0-8.9	6.91	311	8.8	1.1	7.2	7.5	7.7	8.0	8.7	9.5	9.9	10.2	10.7
9.0-11.9	9.95	292	9.7	1.2	8.0	8.3	8.6	8.9	9.7	10.5	11.0	11.3	11.9
12.0-17.9	14.49	310	11.0	1.3	9.0	9.4	9.6	10.0	10.9	11.8	12.4	12.8	13.4
18.0-23.9	20.55	311	12.4	1.5	10.1	10.5	10.8	11.3	12.3	13.3	14.0	14.4	15.1
24.0-29.9	26.60	315	13.5	1.6	11.0	11.5	11.8	12.3	13.4	14.5	15.2	15.7	16.4
30.0-35.9	32.32	330	14.4	1.8	11.8	12.3	12.6	13.2	14.3	15.6	16.3	16.8	17.6
36.0-41.9	38.54	268	15.4	1.9	12.4	13.0	13.4	14.0	15.2	16.6	17.4	17.9	18.8
42.0-47.9	44.53	247	16.5	2.4	12.8	13.4	13.9	14.7	16.1	17.8	18.7	19.4	20.4
Females													
2.0-2.9	2.00	134	6.2	0.9	4.8	5.0	5.2	5.5	6.0	6.7	7.1	7.3	7.8
3.0-5.9	4.04	273	7.1	1.0	5.6	5.9	6.1	6.4	7.0	7.7	8.2	8.5	9.0
6.0-8.9	7.04	282	8.2	1.1	6.5	6.8	7.1	7.4	8.1	8.9	9.4	9.7	10.3
9.0-11.9	9.99	298	9.2	1.2	7.4	7.7	8.0	8.3	9.1	9.9	10.4	10.8	11.4
12.0-17.9	14.66	304	10.5	1.3	8.5	8.8	9.1	9.5	10.3	11.3	11.8	12.2	12.8
18.0-23.9	20.61	326	11.8	1.5	9.4	9.9	10.2	10.7	11.6	12.7	13.3	13.8	14.5
24.0-29.9	26.53	318	12.9	1.8	10.1	10.6	11.0	11.6	12.7	13.9	14.7	15.2	16.0
30.0-35.9	32.42	294	13.9	2.0	10.8	11.3	11.7	12.4	13.6	15.1	15.9	16.5	17.5
36.0-41.9	38.35	284	15.0	2.3	11.4	12.0	12.5	13.2	14.6	16.2	17.1	17.8	18.9
42.0-47.9	44.46	305	16.2	2.7	11.9	12.7	13.2	14.0	15.7	17.6	18.7	19.5	20.7

Table IV.2.

Mean (M), standard deviation (SD), and percentiles of recumbent length (cm) by age for males and females of 2 to 48 months

Age Group (months)	Mean Age (months)	N	M	SD	Percentiles								
					5th	10th	15th	25th	50th	75th	85th	90th	95th
Males													
2.0-2.9	2.00	108	61.7	3.3	56.4	57.5	58.3	59.4	61.6	63.9	65.2	66.1	67.4
3.0-5.9	3.96	293	65.6	3.7	59.7	61.0	61.8	63.1	65.6	68.2	69.6	70.6	72.1
6.0-8.9	6.91	312	70.6	3.4	65.3	66.4	67.2	68.4	70.6	72.9	74.2	75.1	76.4
9.0-11.9	9.95	291	74.9	3.4	69.5	70.6	71.4	72.6	74.8	77.1	78.4	79.3	80.6
12.0-17.9	14.49	309	80.0	3.6	74.2	75.4	76.2	77.5	79.9	82.3	83.7	84.6	86.0
18.0-23.9	20.55	308	85.3	4.4	78.3	79.8	80.8	82.3	85.2	88.2	89.8	90.9	92.6
24.0-29.9	26.60	295	89.9	3.8	83.9	85.2	86.0	87.4	89.9	92.4	93.9	94.8	96.3
30.0-35.9	32.32	320	94.1	3.8	88.2	89.5	90.4	91.7	94.2	96.7	98.2	99.1	100.6
36.0-41.9	38.54	261	98.6	3.7	92.2	93.5	94.4	95.8	98.4	101.1	102.6	103.6	105.1
42.0-47.9	44.53	247	102.5	4.1	95.6	97.0	98.0	99.4	102.1	104.9	106.4	107.5	109.0
Females													
2.0-2.9	2.00	134	60.2	3.6	54.5	55.7	56.6	57.8	60.2	62.7	64.0	65.0	3.5
3.0-5.9	4.04	274	63.9	3.8	57.8	59.1	60.0	61.3	63.8	66.5	67.9	68.9	3.3
6.0-8.9	7.04	283	68.8	3.0	64.0	65.0	65.7	66.7	68.7	70.7	71.8	72.6	3.0
9.0-11.9	9.99	298	73.0	3.5	67.4	68.5	69.4	70.6	72.9	75.3	76.6	77.5	2.8
12.0-17.9	14.66	299	78.7	3.5	73.0	74.2	75.0	76.2	78.6	81.0	82.3	83.3	2.6
18.0-23.9	20.61	319	84.5	3.8	78.5	79.7	80.6	81.9	84.5	87.1	88.5	89.5	2.3
24.0-29.9	26.53	301	89.2	4.3	82.5	83.9	84.9	86.4	89.2	92.2	93.8	94.9	2.1
30.0-35.9	32.42	287	93.4	3.9	87.2	88.5	89.4	90.8	93.4	96.1	97.5	98.6	2.0
36.0-41.9	38.35	281	97.3	4.4	90.3	91.8	92.8	94.3	97.2	100.2	101.9	103.0	104.7
42.0-47.9	44.46	305	101.6	4.5	94.4	95.9	97.0	98.5	101.5	104.6	106.2	107.4	109.1

Table IV.3.
Mean (M), standard deviation (SD), and percentiles of Rohrer's index (gram/cm^3 x 100) by age for males and females of 2 to 48 months

Age Group (months)	Mean Age (months)	N	M	SD	Percentiles								
					5th	10th	15th	25th	50th	75th	85th	90th	95th
Males													
2.0-2.9	2.00	108	2.84	0.35	2.34	2.43	2.50	2.61	2.83	3.08	3.24	3.35	3.53
3.0-5.9	3.96	292	2.71	0.32	2.25	2.34	2.40	2.50	2.70	2.93	3.07	3.17	3.33
6.0-8.9	6.91	311	2.53	0.27	2.15	2.22	2.28	2.36	2.53	2.72	2.83	2.91	3.04
9.0-11.9	9.95	291	2.38	0.23	2.04	2.11	2.16	2.23	2.38	2.54	2.64	2.71	2.82
12.0-17.9	14.49	307	2.19	0.21	1.88	1.94	1.98	2.05	2.18	2.34	2.43	2.49	2.59
18.0-23.9	20.55	306	1.98	0.19	1.70	1.75	1.79	1.85	1.98	2.11	2.19	2.25	2.34
24.0-29.9	26.60	295	1.82	0.17	1.57	1.62	1.65	1.70	1.81	1.92	1.99	2.04	2.12
30.0-35.9	32.32	319	1.69	0.16	1.45	1.50	1.53	1.58	1.68	1.80	1.86	1.91	1.98
36.0-41.9	38.54	260	1.62	0.14	1.40	1.44	1.47	1.51	1.60	1.70	1.75	1.79	1.86
42.0-47.9	44.53	246	1.53	0.14	1.31	1.36	1.38	1.43	1.52	1.62	1.68	1.72	1.78
Females													
2.0-2.9	2.00	133	2.80	0.33	2.32	2.41	2.47	2.57	2.78	3.01	3.15	3.25	3.42
3.0-5.9	4.04	273	2.71	0.28	2.27	2.35	2.41	2.50	2.68	2.88	2.99	3.08	3.21
6.0-8.9	7.04	282	2.56	0.27	2.15	2.22	2.27	2.36	2.52	2.71	2.82	2.90	3.02
9.0-11.9	9.99	298	2.41	0.25	2.02	2.09	2.14	2.22	2.37	2.55	2.65	2.73	2.85
12.0-17.9	14.66	299	2.17	0.23	1.83	1.90	1.94	2.01	2.15	2.32	2.41	2.48	2.59
18.0-23.9	20.61	318	1.93	0.20	1.65	1.71	1.75	1.81	1.93	2.07	2.16	2.22	2.31
24.0-29.9	26.53	301	1.79	0.20	1.50	1.56	1.60	1.66	1.79	1.93	2.01	2.08	2.17
30.0-35.9	32.42	285	1.71	0.19	1.43	1.48	1.52	1.58	1.70	1.83	1.91	1.97	2.06
36.0-41.9	38.35	276	1.62	0.17	1.35	1.40	1.43	1.49	1.60	1.72	1.79	1.85	1.93
42.0-47.9	44.46	303	1.54	0.17	1.29	1.33	1.37	1.42	1.52	1.64	1.71	1.76	1.84

Table IV.4.

Mean (M), standard deviation (SD), and percentiles of head circumference (cm) by age for males and females of 2 to 84 months

Age Group (months)	Mean Age (months)	N	M	SD	Percentiles								
					5th	10th	15th	25th	50th	75th	85th	90th	95th
Males													
2.0-2.9	2.00	108	41.7	1.50	38.9	39.4	39.7	40.2	41.2	42.2	42.8	43.2	43.7
3.0-5.9	3.96	292	42.9	1.63	40.3	40.9	41.3	41.8	42.9	44.0	44.6	45.1	45.7
6.0-8.9	6.91	309	44.5	1.43	42.8	43.3	43.6	44.1	45.1	46.1	46.6	47.0	47.6
9.0-11.9	9.95	290	45.9	1.47	44.0	44.5	44.8	45.3	46.3	47.3	47.9	48.3	48.8
12.0-17.9	14.49	307	47.4	1.33	45.3	45.7	46.1	46.5	47.4	48.3	48.8	49.2	49.7
18.0-23.9	20.55	308	48.7	1.36	46.1	46.5	46.8	47.3	48.2	49.1	49.6	50.0	50.5
24.0-29.9	26.60	283	49.4	1.38	46.9	47.4	47.7	48.2	49.1	50.0	50.6	50.9	51.4
30.0-35.9	32.32	313	49.7	1.39	47.3	47.8	48.1	48.6	49.5	50.5	51.0	51.3	51.9
36.0-41.9	38.54	255	50.0	1.38	47.8	48.3	48.6	49.1	50.0	50.9	51.5	51.8	52.3
42.0-47.9	44.53	242	50.3	1.37	48.2	48.6	49.0	49.4	50.3	51.3	51.8	52.1	52.7
48.0-53.9	50.54	272	50.7	1.38	48.5	48.9	49.3	49.7	50.7	51.6	52.1	52.5	53.0
54.0-59.9	56.55	280	50.9	1.38	48.7	49.2	49.5	50.0	50.9	51.9	52.4	52.7	53.3
60.0-65.9	62.15	260	51.3	1.37	49.0	49.5	49.8	50.3	51.2	52.1	52.6	53.0	53.5
66.0-71.9	68.65	230	51.4	1.41	49.2	49.6	50.0	50.5	51.4	52.4	52.9	53.3	53.8
72.0-77.9	74.37	132	51.4	1.60	49.1	49.6	50.0	50.5	51.6	52.7	53.3	53.7	54.3
78.0-83.9	80.71	122	51.8	1.56	49.3	49.9	50.2	50.8	51.8	52.9	53.5	53.9	54.5
Females													
2.0-2.9	2.00	133	40.5	1.70	37.6	38.1	38.5	39.1	40.2	41.4	42.0	42.5	43.1
3.0-5.9	4.04	272	41.8	1.46	39.7	40.2	40.5	41.0	42.0	43.0	43.6	43.9	44.5
6.0-8.9	7.04	283	43.5	1.43	41.7	42.2	42.5	43.0	44.0	45.0	45.5	45.9	46.5
9.0-11.9	9.99	296	44.8	1.21	43.3	43.7	44.0	44.4	45.2	46.0	46.5	46.8	47.3
12.0-17.9	14.66	294	46.3	1.34	44.1	44.5	44.8	45.3	46.2	47.1	47.6	48.0	48.5
18.0-23.9	20.61	318	47.6	1.38	45.2	45.7	46.0	46.5	47.4	48.3	48.9	49.2	49.7
24.0-29.9	26.53	294	48.3	1.40	45.7	46.2	46.5	47.0	47.9	48.9	49.4	49.7	50.3
30.0-35.9	32.42	278	48.7	1.41	46.4	46.8	47.2	47.7	48.6	49.6	50.1	50.5	51.0
36.0-41.9	38.35	276	49.0	1.34	46.8	47.3	47.6	48.1	49.0	50.0	50.5	50.9	51.4
42.0-47.9	44.46	300	49.4	1.41	47.1	47.6	48.0	48.5	49.4	50.4	51.0	51.3	51.9
48.0-53.9	50.41	277	49.7	1.47	47.4	47.9	48.3	48.8	49.8	50.8	51.3	51.7	52.3
54.0-59.9	56.39	250	50.1	1.40	47.7	48.2	48.5	49.0	50.0	51.0	51.6	52.0	52.5
60.0-65.9	62.48	264	50.4	1.50	47.9	48.4	48.8	49.3	50.3	51.3	51.9	52.2	52.8
66.0-71.9	68.54	276	50.6	1.51	48.0	48.6	48.9	49.5	50.5	51.6	52.2	52.6	53.2
72.0-77.9	74.63	133	50.8	1.66	48.2	48.7	49.1	49.7	50.8	52.0	52.6	53.0	53.7
78.0-83.9	80.68	137	50.9	1.73	48.2	48.7	49.2	49.8	50.9	52.1	52.7	53.2	53.9

Table IV.5.

Mean (M), standard deviation (SD), and percentiles of weight (kg) by age for males and females of 2 to 90 years

Age Group (years)	Mean Age (years)	N	M	SD	Percentiles								
					5th	10th	15th	25th	50th	75th	85th	90th	95th
Males													
2.0-2.9	2.46	645	13.7	1.6	11.0	11.5	11.8	12.3	13.3	14.3	15.0	15.4	16.0
3.0-3.9	3.45	515	14.9	1.9	12.2	12.8	13.2	13.8	15.1	16.5	17.3	17.8	18.7
4.0-4.9	4.47	552	16.0	2.3	13.4	14.1	14.6	15.4	17.0	18.7	19.7	20.4	21.5
5.0-5.9	5.43	497	18.4	2.9	14.9	15.8	16.4	17.3	19.2	21.4	22.6	23.5	24.9
6.0-6.9	6.45	263	21.9	3.8	16.1	17.1	17.9	19.1	21.4	24.1	25.7	26.8	28.5
7.0-7.9	7.47	271	26.2	5.0	17.7	18.9	19.9	21.3	24.2	27.6	29.6	31.0	33.2
8.0-8.9	8.46	265	30.7	6.1	19.5	20.9	22.0	23.6	27.0	30.9	33.2	34.9	37.5
9.0-9.9	9.50	286	35.7	7.7	21.5	23.2	24.5	26.5	30.6	35.3	38.2	40.2	43.5
10.0-10.9	10.45	291	40.4	9.0	23.5	25.5	27.0	29.2	33.9	39.4	42.8	45.2	49.0
11.0-11.9	11.44	274	45.2	10.9	25.5	27.9	29.6	32.3	38.0	44.7	48.8	51.8	56.5
12.0-12.9	12.47	204	49.9	12.3	28.9	31.6	33.5	36.6	43.2	51.0	55.8	59.3	64.9
13.0-13.9	13.47	193	54.3	12.8	33.5	36.5	38.7	42.1	49.4	57.8	63.0	66.8	72.7
14.0-14.9	14.49	185	58.4	13.4	37.7	40.9	43.3	47.0	54.9	64.1	69.7	73.8	80.3
15.0-15.9	15.45	182	61.9	13.6	41.2	44.6	47.1	51.0	59.1	68.5	74.1	78.3	84.8
16.0-16.9	16.45	196	65.2	13.5	44.7	48.1	50.6	54.6	62.8	72.2	77.8	81.9	88.4
17.0-17.9	17.45	195	68.0	13.0	48.5	51.9	54.4	58.3	66.4	75.5	80.9	84.8	90.8
18.0-18.9	18.45	175	70.5	12.3	51.8	55.1	57.5	61.3	68.9	77.6	82.7	86.3	92.0
19.0-19.9	19.43	163	72.6	11.4	55.5	58.8	61.1	64.6	71.8	79.8	84.5	87.8	93.0
20.0-29.9	24.96	1639	74.3	11.0	58.3	61.5	63.8	67.3	74.4	82.2	86.8	90.0	95.0
30.0-39.9	34.72	1470	79.4	11.8	61.7	65.2	67.7	71.5	79.1	87.4	92.1	95.4	100.6
40.0-49.9	44.35	1222	80.9	12.0	63.6	67.3	69.8	73.8	81.6	90.1	95.0	98.4	103.7
50.0-59.9	54.89	858	82.0	12.2	64.2	67.9	70.5	74.5	82.4	91.0	95.9	99.4	104.7
60.0-69.9	64.83	1179	79.3	11.8	62.9	66.5	69.1	72.9	80.7	89.1	93.9	97.3	102.5
70.0-79.9	74.16	870	76.2	11.3	59.7	63.1	65.5	69.1	76.5	84.5	89.0	92.3	97.2
80.0-90.9	84.09	696	69.3	10.3	54.8	58.0	60.2	63.5	70.3	77.6	81.8	84.8	89.3
Females													
2.0-2.9	2.45	612	13.7	1.7	10.2	10.7	11.0	11.5	12.5	13.7	14.3	14.8	15.5
3.0-3.9	3.46	589	13.7	1.9	11.4	11.9	12.4	13.0	14.2	15.6	16.4	17.0	17.9
4.0-4.9	4.43	536	15.5	2.4	12.6	13.3	13.8	14.6	16.2	18.0	19.1	19.9	21.0
5.0-5.9	5.46	541	18.8	3.0	14.2	15.1	15.7	16.6	18.5	20.6	21.9	22.8	24.2
6.0-6.9	6.47	273	22.8	4.5	15.0	16.1	16.9	18.2	20.7	23.7	25.5	26.7	28.8
7.0-7.9	7.44	267	27.2	5.6	16.7	18.0	18.9	20.3	23.4	26.9	29.0	30.5	33.0
8.0-8.9	8.47	250	32.0	7.0	18.7	20.2	21.3	23.0	26.6	30.9	33.5	35.3	38.3
9.0-9.9	9.43	275	36.5	8.1	20.9	22.6	23.9	25.9	30.0	34.9	37.9	40.1	43.5
10.0-10.9	10.43	257	41.0	9.0	23.7	25.7	27.1	29.3	33.9	39.4	42.7	45.1	49.0
11.0-11.9	11.46	289	45.3	10.3	27.6	29.9	31.6	34.3	40.0	46.6	50.7	53.7	58.4
12.0-12.9	12.46	220	49.1	11.1	31.2	33.8	35.7	38.7	45.1	52.6	57.1	60.4	65.7
13.0-13.9	13.45	227	52.5	11.3	34.5	37.2	39.2	42.3	48.9	56.5	61.1	64.5	69.8
14.0-14.9	14.47	218	55.5	11.8	36.3	39.1	41.2	44.4	51.2	59.2	63.9	67.4	73.0
15.0-15.9	15.47	190	58.0	11.9	38.7	41.6	43.7	47.1	54.1	62.1	67.0	70.5	76.1
16.0-16.9	16.46	222	58.8	12.0	39.5	42.4	44.6	47.9	55.0	63.1	68.0	71.5	77.1
17.0-17.9	17.45	215	61.6	12.5	40.3	43.3	45.5	49.0	56.1	64.4	69.3	72.9	78.6
18.0-18.9	18.43	190	62.1	12.5	41.1	44.1	46.3	49.8	57.0	65.3	70.3	73.9	79.6
19.0-19.9	19.48	192	63.2	12.5	42.9	46.1	48.4	51.9	59.3	67.8	72.8	76.5	82.2
20.0-29.9	24.91	1868	64.7	12.6	46.0	49.4	51.8	55.6	63.4	72.4	77.6	81.5	87.4
30.0-39.9	34.85	1860	69.4	13.0	49.3	52.9	55.4	59.4	67.5	76.4	81.7	85.4	91.3
40.0-49.9	44.28	1363	72.3	13.5	51.9	55.7	58.4	62.6	71.1	80.5	86.0	89.9	95.9
50.0-59.9	54.83	1006	72.2	13.1	52.9	56.7	59.4	63.5	71.8	81.1	86.4	90.2	96.1
60.0-69.9	64.82	1174	69.4	12.6	50.2	53.8	56.4	60.3	68.2	77.0	82.1	85.7	91.3
70.0-79.9	74.46	988	65.6	11.9	47.5	50.9	53.3	57.0	64.5	72.8	77.7	81.1	86.4
80.0-90.9	84.45	783	58.7	10.3	43.4	46.4	48.5	51.8	58.4	65.7	69.9	72.9	77.5

Table IV.6.

Mean (M), standard deviation (SD), and percentiles of stature (cm) by age for males and females of 2 to 90 years

Age Group (years)	Mean Age (years)	N	M	SD	Percentiles								
					5th	10th	15th	25th	50th	75th	85th	90th	95th
Males													
2.0-2.9	2.46	628	91.1	4.1	84.5	85.9	86.8	88.3	91.0	93.8	95.3	96.4	97.9
3.0-3.9	3.45	513	99.4	4.4	92.5	94.0	95.0	96.6	99.5	102.5	104.1	105.2	106.9
4.0-4.9	4.47	554	106.3	4.8	98.4	100.0	101.1	102.8	106.0	109.3	111.0	112.3	114.1
5.0-5.9	5.43	496	113.0	5.0	104.8	106.5	107.7	109.4	112.8	116.1	118.0	119.3	121.1
6.0-6.9	6.45	263	119.3	6.0	109.6	111.7	113.1	115.1	119.1	123.2	125.4	126.9	129.2
7.0-7.9	7.47	273	126.3	6.6	115.7	118.0	119.5	121.8	126.2	130.7	133.1	134.8	137.3
8.0-8.9	8.46	267	131.5	6.6	120.5	122.7	124.3	126.6	131.0	135.5	138.0	139.7	142.2
9.0-9.9	9.50	285	138.0	6.9	126.5	128.9	130.5	132.9	137.5	142.2	144.8	146.5	149.2
10.0-10.9	10.45	291	142.4	7.5	130.4	133.0	134.7	137.4	142.4	147.6	150.4	152.3	155.2
11.0-11.9	11.44	278	147.3	8.6	133.6	136.5	138.5	141.5	147.2	153.0	156.2	158.4	161.7
12.0-12.9	12.47	208	154.0	8.8	139.8	142.8	144.9	147.9	153.8	159.7	163.0	165.3	168.7
13.0-13.9	13.47	196	161.7	8.9	147.8	150.9	153.0	156.1	162.0	168.1	171.4	173.7	177.1
14.0-14.9	14.49	188	167.7	8.4	154.8	157.7	159.7	162.6	168.2	173.9	177.1	179.2	182.5
15.0-15.9	15.45	185	171.2	7.9	158.1	160.9	162.7	165.5	170.7	176.1	179.0	181.0	184.0
16.0-16.9	16.45	197	173.3	7.8	160.3	162.9	164.8	167.5	172.7	178.0	180.9	182.9	185.8
17.0-17.9	17.45	195	173.2	7.8	161.2	163.9	165.7	168.5	173.7	179.0	181.9	183.9	186.9
18.0-18.9	18.45	175	175.2	7.5	162.6	165.2	167.0	169.6	174.6	179.7	182.5	184.4	187.3
19.0-19.9	19.43	164	174.2	7.5	162.8	165.4	167.1	169.8	174.8	179.9	182.7	184.6	187.5
20.0-29.9	24.96	1640	173.8	7.3	163.1	165.6	167.4	169.9	174.8	179.8	182.6	184.5	187.3
30.0-39.9	34.72	1470	174.9	7.5	162.9	165.4	167.2	169.8	174.8	179.9	182.8	184.7	187.6
40.0-49.9	44.35	1222	174.4	7.3	162.7	165.2	166.9	169.4	174.3	179.3	182.0	183.9	186.8
50.0-59.9	54.89	858	174.5	7.3	162.7	165.2	166.9	169.4	174.3	179.3	182.1	183.9	186.8
60.0-69.9	64.83	1180	172.4	7.2	161.2	163.6	165.3	167.9	172.7	177.7	180.4	182.2	185.0
70.0-79.9	74.16	870	171.3	7.0	160.0	162.4	164.1	166.5	171.2	176.0	178.6	180.4	183.1
80.0-90.9	84.09	695	169.1	7.3	157.8	160.3	162.0	164.6	169.4	174.4	177.1	179.0	181.8
Females													
2.0-2.9	2.45	601	90.0	4.4	82.7	84.2	85.3	86.8	89.7	92.7	94.3	95.4	97.0
3.0-3.9	3.46	592	98.5	4.7	90.9	92.6	93.7	95.4	98.5	101.7	103.5	104.6	106.4
4.0-4.9	4.43	533	105.4	5.1	97.2	98.9	100.1	101.9	105.3	108.7	110.6	111.9	113.8
5.0-5.9	5.46	544	112.6	5.5	103.7	105.6	106.9	108.8	112.5	116.2	118.3	119.7	121.7
6.0-6.9	6.47	275	118.9	5.9	109.2	111.3	112.7	114.8	118.7	122.7	124.9	126.4	128.7
7.0-7.9	7.44	268	124.9	6.3	114.6	116.8	118.3	120.5	124.7	129.0	131.3	132.9	135.3
8.0-8.9	8.47	249	131.5	6.7	120.4	122.8	124.4	126.7	131.2	135.8	138.3	140.0	142.5
9.0-9.9	9.43	277	136.9	7.0	125.6	128.0	129.7	132.1	136.8	141.6	144.2	146.0	148.6
10.0-10.9	10.43	261	143.0	7.3	131.2	133.8	135.5	138.1	142.9	147.8	150.5	152.4	155.1
11.0-11.9	11.46	289	150.8	7.5	139.5	142.1	143.9	146.6	151.6	156.7	159.5	161.5	164.3
12.0-12.9	12.46	223	156.2	7.6	144.5	147.1	148.9	151.6	156.6	161.8	164.6	166.6	169.5
13.0-13.9	13.45	232	159.0	7.4	146.8	149.3	151.0	153.6	158.5	163.6	166.4	168.3	171.2
14.0-14.9	14.47	225	160.1	7.2	149.2	151.6	153.3	155.8	160.5	165.4	168.1	170.0	172.8
15.0-15.9	15.47	193	162.0	6.9	151.1	153.4	155.0	157.5	162.1	166.8	169.4	171.2	174.0
16.0-16.9	16.46	228	161.7	6.7	151.4	153.7	155.3	157.6	162.1	166.7	169.2	171.0	173.6
17.0-17.9	17.45	215	162.2	6.7	151.5	153.8	155.3	157.7	162.1	166.7	169.2	170.9	173.5
18.0-18.9	18.43	190	161.7	6.8	151.3	153.6	155.2	157.6	162.1	166.8	169.3	171.1	173.8
19.0-19.9	19.48	193	162.2	6.9	151.2	153.6	155.2	157.6	162.2	166.9	169.5	171.3	173.9
20.0-29.9	24.91	1871	161.3	6.9	151.1	153.5	155.1	157.6	162.2	167.0	169.6	171.4	174.1
30.0-39.9	34.85	1863	161.6	7.1	150.1	152.5	154.2	156.7	161.4	166.3	168.9	170.7	173.5
40.0-49.9	44.28	1362	161.6	6.6	150.8	153.1	154.7	157.0	161.4	165.9	168.4	170.1	172.6
50.0-59.9	54.83	1008	161.0	6.6	150.4	152.6	154.2	156.5	160.9	165.4	167.9	169.6	172.1
60.0-69.9	64.82	1179	158.9	6.6	148.2	150.5	152.0	154.3	158.7	163.2	165.6	167.3	169.8
70.0-79.9	74.46	988	157.4	6.5	147.0	149.3	150.8	153.1	157.4	161.8	164.3	165.9	168.4
80.0-90.9	84.45	785	154.3	6.4	144.4	146.6	148.2	150.4	154.7	159.1	161.5	163.1	165.6

Table IV.7.

Mean (M), standard deviation (SD), and percentiles of body mass index (kg/m^2) by age for males and females of 2 to 90 years

Age Group (years)	Mean Age (years)	N	M	SD	Percentiles								
					5th	10th	15th	25th	50th	75th	85th	90th	95th
Males													
2.0-2.9	2.46	627	16.22	1.4	14.32	14.73	15.03	15.48	16.37	17.36	17.93	18.34	18.96
3.0-3.9	3.45	511	15.75	1.5	13.62	14.08	14.41	14.90	15.90	16.99	17.62	18.07	18.76
4.0-4.9	4.47	550	15.61	1.6	13.29	13.76	14.09	14.60	15.60	16.71	17.35	17.80	18.50
5.0-5.9	5.43	495	15.74	1.6	13.11	13.58	13.92	14.44	15.48	16.62	17.28	17.75	18.47
6.0-6.9	6.45	262	16.08	1.8	13.00	13.51	13.86	14.41	15.52	16.74	17.45	17.96	18.74
7.0-7.9	7.47	271	16.59	2.0	12.98	13.53	13.91	14.51	15.71	17.05	17.84	18.40	19.27
8.0-8.9	8.46	265	17.18	2.2	13.05	13.64	14.06	14.71	16.03	17.52	18.39	19.02	20.01
9.0-9.9	9.50	284	17.87	2.5	13.21	13.85	14.30	15.01	16.45	18.09	19.06	19.76	20.86
10.0-10.9	10.45	291	18.54	2.7	13.44	14.12	14.61	15.38	16.95	18.76	19.83	20.61	21.84
11.0-11.9	11.44	273	19.25	3.0	13.77	14.50	15.02	15.84	17.53	19.47	20.63	21.48	22.82
12.0-12.9	12.47	204	19.97	3.2	14.15	14.92	15.48	16.35	18.15	20.23	21.48	22.40	23.84
13.0-13.9	13.47	193	20.64	3.3	14.60	15.41	15.99	16.91	18.81	21.01	22.33	23.30	24.84
14.0-14.9	14.49	185	21.28	3.5	15.09	15.94	16.55	17.50	19.49	21.78	23.16	24.16	25.75
15.0-15.9	15.45	182	21.85	3.5	15.62	16.50	17.13	18.12	20.17	22.54	23.97	25.01	26.66
16.0-16.9	16.45	196	22.38	3.6	16.18	17.08	17.73	18.74	20.85	23.29	24.75	25.82	27.51
17.0-17.9	17.45	195	22.87	3.7	16.56	17.48	18.14	19.17	21.32	23.79	25.28	26.36	28.07
18.0-18.9	18.45	175	23.30	3.7	17.30	18.25	18.92	19.98	22.17	24.69	26.19	27.29	29.02
19.0-19.9	19.43	163	23.66	3.6	17.74	18.68	19.36	20.42	22.60	25.10	26.59	27.67	29.38
20.0-29.9	24.96	1639	25.01	3.8	18.73	19.78	20.53	21.68	24.02	26.64	28.18	29.27	30.98
30.0-39.9	34.72	1470	26.13	4.3	19.13	20.28	21.11	22.39	24.99	27.92	29.64	30.87	32.79
40.0-49.9	44.35	1222	27.09	4.3	20.16	21.38	22.25	23.58	26.26	29.23	30.96	32.18	34.07
50.0-59.9	54.89	858	27.15	4.2	20.74	21.95	22.81	24.12	26.75	29.64	31.31	32.49	34.31
60.0-69.9	64.83	1179	26.84	4.1	20.46	21.65	22.49	23.78	26.36	29.20	30.84	32.00	33.78
70.0-79.9	74.16	870	25.86	4.0	19.33	20.47	21.27	22.51	24.99	27.72	29.29	30.41	32.13
80.0-90.9	84.09	695	24.36	3.6	18.78	19.85	20.60	21.76	24.06	26.57	28.01	29.03	30.59
Females													
2.0-2.9	2.45	597	15.97	1.4	14.03	14.46	14.76	15.22	16.15	17.17	17.76	18.18	18.83
3.0-3.9	3.46	585	15.59	1.6	13.23	13.71	14.05	14.57	15.58	16.67	17.29	17.73	18.40
4.0-4.9	4.43	532	15.51	1.6	12.99	13.47	13.80	14.31	15.30	16.38	16.99	17.42	18.07
5.0-5.9	5.46	541	15.46	1.6	12.85	13.35	13.69	14.22	15.26	16.38	17.03	17.48	18.17
6.0-6.9	6.47	273	15.64	1.8	12.79	13.32	13.70	14.27	15.40	16.64	17.35	17.85	18.61
7.0-7.9	7.44	267	16.25	2.0	12.79	13.38	13.79	14.43	15.70	17.09	17.90	18.47	19.35
8.0-8.9	8.47	249	16.80	2.3	12.88	13.53	13.99	14.69	16.12	17.69	18.60	19.25	20.26
9.0-9.9	9.43	275	17.30	2.6	13.06	13.77	14.27	15.05	16.62	18.38	19.40	20.14	21.27
10.0-10.9	10.43	257	17.83	2.8	13.32	14.08	14.63	15.47	17.19	19.12	20.26	21.07	22.33
11.0-11.9	11.46	289	19.30	3.2	13.64	14.46	15.04	15.95	17.80	19.89	21.12	22.01	23.39
12.0-12.9	12.46	220	20.68	3.5	14.03	14.89	15.50	16.46	18.42	20.64	21.95	22.90	24.37
13.0-13.9	13.45	227	21.34	3.7	14.43	15.33	15.97	16.98	19.04	21.37	22.76	23.75	25.31
14.0-14.9	14.47	218	21.76	3.7	14.87	15.80	16.47	17.50	19.63	22.03	23.46	24.49	26.09
15.0-15.9	15.47	190	22.14	3.8	15.28	16.24	16.92	17.99	20.17	22.64	24.11	25.16	26.81
16.0-16.9	16.46	222	22.20	3.8	15.70	16.67	17.36	18.44	20.65	23.15	24.63	25.70	27.36
17.0-17.9	17.45	215	22.64	3.8	16.03	17.02	17.72	18.82	21.06	23.59	25.09	26.17	27.86
18.0-18.9	18.43	190	22.93	3.8	16.30	17.30	18.01	19.12	21.38	23.94	25.45	26.54	28.24
19.0-19.9	19.48	192	23.29	3.9	16.42	17.44	18.16	19.29	21.60	24.22	25.77	26.88	28.62
20.0-29.9	24.91	1868	24.40	4.2	17.60	18.71	19.50	20.73	23.27	26.14	27.84	29.07	30.98
30.0-39.9	34.85	1860	26.69	5.0	18.90	20.24	21.20	22.70	25.77	29.27	31.34	32.84	35.17
40.0-49.9	44.28	1362	27.67	5.2	19.70	21.09	22.09	23.65	26.85	30.49	32.65	34.20	36.62
50.0-59.9	54.83	1006	28.14	5.3	20.13	21.56	22.58	24.17	27.44	31.16	33.36	34.94	37.42
60.0-69.9	64.82	1174	27.56	5.2	19.71	21.10	22.10	23.65	26.85	30.49	32.64	34.19	36.61
70.0-79.9	74.46	985	26.48	5.0	18.70	20.02	20.97	22.45	25.48	28.93	30.97	32.44	34.73
80.0-90.9	84.45	781	24.62	4.6	17.72	18.94	19.82	21.20	24.01	27.20	29.09	30.44	32.56

Table IV.8.

Mean (M), standard deviation (SD), and percentiles of sitting height (cm) by age for males and females of 2 to 90 years

Age Group (years)	Mean Age (years)	N	M	SD	5th	10th	15th	25th	50th	75th	85th	90th	95th
								Males					
2.0-2.9	2.46	620	52.3	2.5	48.1	48.9	49.5	50.4	52.0	53.7	54.7	55.3	56.3
3.0-3.9	3.45	508	54.9	2.6	50.7	51.6	52.2	53.1	54.8	56.6	57.5	58.2	59.2
4.0-4.9	4.47	554	57.4	2.7	53.2	54.1	54.8	55.7	57.5	59.4	60.4	61.1	62.1
5.0-5.9	5.43	496	59.9	2.8	55.9	56.9	57.5	58.5	60.4	62.4	63.4	64.2	65.3
6.0-6.9	6.45	262	62.6	3.3	57.8	58.9	59.7	60.8	63.0	65.3	66.5	67.4	68.6
7.0-7.9	7.47	273	65.4	3.5	60.3	61.5	62.3	63.6	65.9	68.3	69.7	70.6	72.0
8.0-8.9	8.46	267	68.2	3.3	62.8	64.0	64.7	65.8	68.0	70.2	71.5	72.3	73.6
9.0-9.9	9.50	282	71.2	3.3	65.6	66.8	67.5	68.7	70.9	73.2	74.4	75.3	76.6
10.0-10.9	10.45	288	73.9	4.0	66.5	67.8	68.8	70.1	72.7	75.4	76.9	77.9	79.5
11.0-11.9	11.44	275	76.6	4.4	67.9	69.4	70.3	71.8	74.7	77.7	79.3	80.5	82.2
12.0-12.9	12.47	204	79.4	4.5	70.9	72.4	73.4	75.0	77.9	81.0	82.6	83.8	85.6
13.0-13.9	13.47	192	81.8	4.9	74.8	76.4	77.6	79.3	82.6	86.0	87.8	89.2	91.1
14.0-14.9	14.49	186	84.1	4.6	78.5	80.1	81.1	82.8	85.9	89.1	90.9	92.2	94.0
15.0-15.9	15.45	182	86.1	4.1	81.0	82.4	83.4	84.8	87.6	90.5	92.1	93.2	94.8
16.0-16.9	16.45	196	87.8	4.2	82.1	83.5	84.5	86.0	88.8	91.7	93.3	94.4	96.1
17.0-17.9	17.45	191	89.3	3.9	83.2	84.5	85.4	86.8	89.4	92.1	93.6	94.6	96.1
18.0-18.9	18.45	172	90.4	3.6	84.6	85.8	86.7	88.0	90.5	93.0	94.4	95.3	96.8
19.0-19.9	19.43	160	90.3	3.6	84.7	85.9	86.7	88.0	90.4	92.9	94.2	95.2	96.6
20.0-29.9	24.96	1620	90.4	3.6	84.7	85.9	86.7	88.0	90.4	92.9	94.2	95.2	96.6
30.0-39.9	34.72	1452	91.2	3.8	85.0	86.3	87.2	88.6	91.1	93.7	95.2	96.1	97.6
40.0-49.9	44.35	1195	91.1	3.8	85.0	86.3	87.2	88.6	91.1	93.7	95.2	96.1	97.6
50.0-59.9	54.89	835	91.0	3.8	84.8	86.1	87.0	88.4	90.9	93.5	94.9	95.9	97.4
60.0-69.9	64.83	1129	89.5	3.8	83.5	84.8	85.7	87.0	89.5	92.1	93.5	94.5	95.9
70.0-79.9	74.16	798	88.6	3.7	82.7	84.0	84.8	86.1	88.6	91.1	92.5	93.5	94.9
80.0-90.9	84.09	566	87.1	3.7	81.3	82.5	83.4	84.7	87.1	89.6	91.0	91.9	93.3
								Females					
2.0-2.9	2.45	585	52.0	2.6	47.2	48.0	48.6	49.5	51.2	53.0	53.9	54.6	55.6
3.0-3.9	3.46	586	53.7	2.7	49.8	50.8	51.4	52.3	54.1	56.0	57.0	57.7	58.8
4.0-4.9	4.43	528	56.1	2.7	52.7	53.6	54.2	55.2	57.0	58.9	59.9	60.6	61.7
5.0-5.9	5.46	543	59.2	3.1	55.0	56.0	56.8	57.8	59.9	62.0	63.2	64.0	65.3
6.0-6.9	6.47	273	62.4	3.4	57.2	58.3	59.1	60.3	62.5	64.8	66.1	67.0	68.3
7.0-7.9	7.44	268	65.6	3.2	60.1	61.2	62.0	63.1	65.3	67.5	68.7	69.6	70.9
8.0-8.9	8.47	247	68.9	3.6	62.2	63.4	64.3	65.5	67.9	70.4	71.7	72.7	74.1
9.0-9.9	9.43	273	71.9	3.7	64.3	65.5	66.3	67.6	70.0	72.5	73.9	74.8	76.3
10.0-10.9	10.43	260	74.7	4.0	67.1	68.5	69.4	70.8	73.5	76.3	77.8	78.9	80.5
11.0-11.9	11.46	288	77.2	4.3	71.1	72.6	73.5	75.0	77.9	80.8	82.4	83.5	85.2
12.0-12.9	12.46	221	79.3	4.2	73.7	75.1	76.1	77.6	80.4	83.3	84.9	86.1	87.7
13.0-13.9	13.45	227	81.1	3.9	76.4	77.8	78.7	80.1	82.7	85.4	86.9	88.0	89.5
14.0-14.9	14.47	216	82.6	3.8	77.3	78.6	79.5	80.8	83.4	86.0	87.4	88.4	89.9
15.0-15.9	15.47	189	83.8	3.4	79.1	80.3	81.1	82.3	84.6	87.0	88.2	89.1	90.4
16.0-16.9	16.46	224	84.6	3.6	78.8	80.1	80.9	82.2	84.6	87.1	88.5	89.4	90.8
17.0-17.9	17.45	213	85.2	3.7	79.2	80.4	81.3	82.6	85.0	87.5	88.9	89.8	91.2
18.0-18.9	18.43	186	85.6	3.8	79.1	80.4	81.2	82.5	85.0	87.6	89.0	90.0	91.4
19.0-19.9	19.48	191	85.8	3.6	79.5	80.8	81.6	82.8	85.2	87.7	89.0	89.9	91.3
20.0-29.9	24.91	1842	85.1	3.6	79.2	80.5	81.3	82.5	84.9	87.3	88.7	89.6	91.0
30.0-39.9	34.85	1837	85.2	3.6	79.6	80.8	81.7	82.9	85.3	87.8	89.1	90.0	91.4
40.0-49.9	44.28	1328	85.3	3.4	79.9	81.0	81.8	83.0	85.3	87.6	88.9	89.8	91.1
50.0-59.9	54.83	979	84.3	3.5	79.1	80.3	81.1	82.3	84.7	87.1	88.5	89.4	90.8
60.0-69.9	64.82	1110	83.3	3.5	77.6	78.8	79.6	80.8	83.1	85.5	86.8	87.7	89.1
70.0-79.9	74.46	893	81.8	3.5	76.4	77.6	78.4	79.7	82.0	84.4	85.7	86.6	88.0
80.0-90.9	84.45	599	79.2	3.4	73.9	75.0	75.8	77.0	79.3	81.6	82.9	83.8	85.1

Table IV.9.

Mean (M), standard deviation (SD), and percentiles of sitting height index (sitting height/stature x 100) by age for males and females of 2 to 90 years

Age Group (years)	Mean Age (years)	N	M	SD	Percentiles								
					5th	10th	15th	25th	50th	75th	85th	90th	95th
Males													
2.0-2.9	2.46	619	56.9	2.01	53.7	54.4	54.9	55.6	56.9	58.3	59.0	59.6	60.3
3.0-3.9	3.45	508	55.5	1.8	52.6	53.2	53.6	54.3	55.6	56.8	57.5	58.0	58.7
4.0-4.9	4.47	553	54.4	1.8	51.6	52.2	52.6	53.2	54.4	55.6	56.3	56.7	57.4
5.0-5.9	5.43	496	53.5	1.7	50.8	51.4	51.8	52.4	53.5	54.6	55.3	55.7	56.3
6.0-6.9	6.45	262	52.7	1.6	50.2	50.7	51.1	51.7	52.7	53.8	54.4	54.8	55.5
7.0-7.9	7.47	273	52.1	0.0	49.7	50.2	50.6	51.1	52.2	53.2	53.8	54.2	54.8
8.0-8.9	8.46	267	51.7	0.1	49.3	49.8	50.2	50.7	51.7	52.8	53.3	53.7	54.3
9.0-9.9	9.50	281	51.4	0.1	49.0	49.5	49.9	50.4	51.4	52.4	53.0	53.4	53.9
10.0-10.9	10.45	288	51.2	1.5	48.8	49.3	49.7	50.2	51.2	52.2	52.8	53.1	53.7
11.0-11.9	11.44	275	51.0	1.4	48.7	49.2	49.6	50.1	51.1	52.1	52.6	53.0	53.6
12.0-12.9	12.47	204	51.0	1.4	48.7	49.2	49.5	50.0	51.0	52.0	52.6	52.9	53.5
13.0-13.9	13.47	192	51.0	1.4	48.7	49.2	49.5	50.0	51.0	52.0	52.6	52.9	53.5
14.0-14.9	14.49	186	51.1	1.5	48.7	49.2	49.6	50.1	51.1	52.1	52.6	53.0	53.6
15.0-15.9	15.45	182	51.2	1.5	48.8	49.3	49.6	50.2	51.1	52.2	52.7	53.1	53.7
16.0-16.9	16.45	196	51.3	1.5	48.9	49.4	49.7	50.3	51.3	52.3	52.8	53.2	53.8
17.0-17.9	17.45	191	51.4	1.5	49.0	49.5	49.8	50.4	51.4	52.4	53.0	53.4	53.9
18.0-18.9	18.45	172	51.6	1.5	49.1	49.6	50.0	50.5	51.5	52.6	53.1	53.5	54.1
19.0-19.9	19.43	160	51.7	1.5	49.2	49.7	50.1	50.6	51.7	52.7	53.3	53.7	54.3
20.0-29.9	24.96	1620	52.3	1.5	49.8	50.3	50.7	51.2	52.2	53.3	53.8	54.2	54.8
30.0-39.9	34.72	1452	52.4	1.6	49.9	50.4	50.8	51.3	52.4	53.4	54.0	54.4	55.0
40.0-49.9	44.35	1195	52.2	1.5	49.9	50.4	50.8	51.3	52.3	53.4	53.9	54.3	54.9
50.0-59.9	54.89	835	52.1	1.5	49.8	50.3	50.7	51.2	52.2	53.3	53.8	54.2	54.8
60.0-69.9	64.83	1129	51.9	1.5	49.7	50.2	50.6	51.1	52.1	53.1	53.6	54.0	54.5
70.0-79.9	74.16	798	51.7	1.4	49.5	50.0	50.4	50.9	51.8	52.8	53.3	53.7	54.2
80.0-90.9	84.09	566	51.5	1.4	49.3	49.8	50.1	50.6	51.5	52.5	53.0	53.3	53.9
Females													
2.0-2.9	2.45	584	56.9	1.9	52.9	53.5	54.0	54.7	55.9	57.2	57.9	58.4	59.1
3.0-3.9	3.46	586	55.3	1.8	52.1	52.7	53.2	53.8	55.0	56.2	56.9	57.4	58.1
4.0-4.9	4.43	528	54.1	1.6	51.5	52.1	52.5	53.1	54.3	55.4	56.1	56.5	57.2
5.0-5.9	5.46	543	53.2	1.6	50.9	51.5	51.9	52.5	53.6	54.7	55.4	55.8	56.4
6.0-6.9	6.47	273	52.5	1.6	50.4	51.0	51.4	52.0	53.1	54.2	54.8	55.2	55.8
7.0-7.9	7.44	268	52.1	1.4	50.1	50.7	51.0	51.6	52.7	53.7	54.3	54.7	55.3
8.0-8.9	8.47	247	51.8	1.5	49.8	50.4	50.7	51.3	52.3	53.4	54.0	54.3	54.9
9.0-9.9	9.43	273	51.7	1.5	49.6	50.1	50.5	51.0	52.1	53.1	53.7	54.1	54.7
10.0-10.9	10.43	260	51.6	1.5	49.5	50.0	50.3	50.9	51.9	52.9	53.5	53.9	54.4
11.0-11.9	11.46	288	51.6	1.4	49.4	49.9	50.2	50.8	51.8	52.8	53.3	53.7	54.3
12.0-12.9	12.46	221	51.7	1.5	49.3	49.9	50.2	50.7	51.7	52.7	53.3	53.6	54.2
13.0-13.9	13.45	227	51.8	1.5	49.3	49.8	50.2	50.7	51.7	52.7	53.2	53.6	54.2
14.0-14.9	14.47	216	52.0	1.5	49.4	49.9	50.2	50.7	51.7	52.7	53.3	53.6	54.2
15.0-15.9	15.47	189	52.1	1.5	49.4	50.0	50.3	50.8	51.8	52.8	53.3	53.7	54.2
16.0-16.9	16.46	224	52.2	1.5	49.5	50.0	50.4	50.9	51.9	52.9	53.4	53.8	54.3
17.0-17.9	17.45	213	52.4	1.4	49.6	50.1	50.5	51.0	52.0	53.0	53.5	53.9	54.4
18.0-18.9	18.43	186	52.5	1.4	49.8	50.3	50.6	51.1	52.1	53.1	53.6	54.0	54.6
19.0-19.9	19.48	191	52.6	1.3	49.9	50.4	50.8	51.3	52.3	53.2	53.8	54.2	54.7
20.0-29.9	24.91	1842	52.9	1.5	50.2	50.8	51.1	51.7	52.7	53.8	54.3	54.7	55.3
30.0-39.9	34.85	1837	52.8	1.5	50.5	51.0	51.4	51.9	52.9	53.9	54.5	54.9	55.5
40.0-49.9	44.28	1328	52.8	1.5	50.5	51.1	51.4	51.9	52.9	53.9	54.5	54.9	55.4
50.0-59.9	54.83	979	52.8	1.5	50.4	50.9	51.3	51.8	52.8	53.8	54.3	54.7	55.2
60.0-69.9	64.82	1110	52.3	1.5	50.1	50.6	50.9	51.4	52.4	53.4	54.0	54.3	54.9
70.0-79.9	74.46	893	52.0	1.5	49.5	50.0	50.4	50.9	51.9	52.9	53.5	53.9	54.4
80.0-90.9	84.45	599	51.1	1.5	48.8	49.3	49.7	50.2	51.2	52.2	52.8	53.2	53.8

Table IV.10.

Mean (M), standard deviation (SD), and percentiles of upper leg length (cm) by age for males and females of 2 to 90 years

Age Group (years)	Mean Age (years)	N	M	SD	5th	10th	15th	25th	50th	75th	85th	90th	95th
Males													
2.0-2.9	2.46	565	19.4	1.7	16.0	16.5	16.9	17.5	18.6	19.8	20.5	20.9	21.7
3.0-3.9	3.45	494	21.0	1.8	18.5	19.1	19.5	20.1	21.3	22.6	23.3	23.8	24.6
4.0-4.9	4.47	544	23.0	2.0	20.4	21.1	21.6	22.2	23.6	25.0	25.8	26.4	27.2
5.0-5.9	5.43	487	25.0	2.2	22.1	22.8	23.3	24.0	25.5	27.1	27.9	28.6	29.5
6.0-6.9	6.45	259	27.3	2.4	23.8	24.6	25.1	25.9	27.5	29.2	30.1	30.7	31.7
7.0-7.9	7.47	271	29.5	2.5	25.7	26.5	27.0	27.9	29.5	31.2	32.1	32.8	33.8
8.0-8.9	8.46	259	31.6	2.5	27.4	28.2	28.8	29.6	31.3	33.1	34.1	34.7	35.8
9.0-9.9	9.50	281	33.7	2.8	28.8	29.7	30.3	31.2	33.0	34.9	36.0	36.8	37.9
10.0-10.9	10.45	287	35.5	3.0	30.0	30.9	31.6	32.6	34.6	36.6	37.8	38.6	39.9
11.0-11.9	11.44	271	37.2	3.3	31.2	32.3	33.0	34.1	36.2	38.5	39.7	40.6	42.0
12.0-12.9	12.47	204	38.7	3.4	33.0	34.0	34.8	35.9	38.1	40.4	41.7	42.6	44.0
13.0-13.9	13.47	188	40.0	3.1	35.0	36.0	36.8	37.9	40.0	42.3	43.5	44.4	45.8
14.0-14.9	14.49	182	41.1	3.1	37.0	38.0	38.7	39.8	41.8	43.9	45.1	46.0	47.2
15.0-15.9	15.45	177	42.0	3.0	38.3	39.3	40.0	41.0	43.0	45.1	46.3	47.1	48.3
16.0-16.9	16.45	194	42.7	3.1	38.6	39.7	40.4	41.5	43.6	45.8	47.0	47.8	49.1
17.0-17.9	17.45	189	43.2	3.1	38.7	39.7	40.4	41.5	43.6	45.8	47.0	47.8	49.1
18.0-18.9	18.45	168	43.7	3.2	38.6	39.6	40.3	41.4	43.5	45.7	46.9	47.8	49.1
19.0-19.9	19.43	156	43.9	2.9	38.2	39.3	40.1	41.2	43.4	45.8	47.1	48.0	49.4
20.0-29.9	24.96	1589	43.8	3.3	37.4	38.5	39.2	40.4	42.5	44.8	46.1	47.0	48.4
30.0-39.9	34.72	1423	42.3	3.3	37.3	38.4	39.2	40.3	42.4	44.7	46.0	46.9	48.3
40.0-49.9	44.35	1165	42.2	3.3	37.1	38.1	38.9	40.0	42.1	44.4	45.7	46.6	47.9
50.0-59.9	54.89	820	41.7	3.2	36.4	37.5	38.2	39.3	41.5	43.7	45.0	45.9	47.2
60.0-69.9	64.83	1105	40.8	3.4	35.8	36.9	37.6	38.8	41.0	43.4	44.7	45.6	47.0
70.0-79.9	74.16	768	40.6	3.4	35.5	36.6	37.3	38.5	40.7	43.0	44.3	45.2	46.6
80.0-90.9	84.09	528	40.0	3.2	35.0	36.1	36.8	37.9	40.0	42.2	43.5	44.4	45.7
Females													
2.0-2.9	2.45	555	19.2	1.9	16.1	16.7	17.1	17.7	18.9	20.2	20.9	21.4	22.2
3.0-3.9	3.46	568	21.2	1.9	18.6	19.2	19.7	20.3	21.6	22.9	23.7	24.2	25.0
4.0-4.9	4.43	527	23.3	2.0	20.4	21.1	21.5	22.2	23.5	24.9	25.7	26.3	27.1
5.0-5.9	5.46	543	25.6	2.3	22.3	23.0	23.5	24.3	25.7	27.3	28.1	28.7	29.7
6.0-6.9	6.47	275	27.9	2.4	24.0	24.8	25.3	26.1	27.7	29.4	30.3	31.0	32.0
7.0-7.9	7.44	263	29.9	2.6	25.5	26.3	26.9	27.7	29.4	31.2	32.2	32.9	34.0
8.0-8.9	8.47	246	32.0	2.8	27.1	27.9	28.5	29.4	31.2	33.1	34.1	34.9	36.0
9.0-9.9	9.43	269	33.7	2.7	28.8	29.7	30.3	31.2	33.0	34.9	36.0	36.8	37.9
10.0-10.9	10.43	254	35.3	2.9	30.7	31.6	32.2	33.2	35.1	37.0	38.2	38.9	40.1
11.0-11.9	11.46	280	36.7	2.9	32.5	33.4	34.1	35.1	37.0	39.1	40.2	41.0	42.2
12.0-12.9	12.46	216	37.8	3.0	33.8	34.8	35.4	36.5	38.5	40.6	41.8	42.6	43.9
13.0-13.9	13.45	224	38.7	3.0	34.5	35.5	36.2	37.3	39.4	41.5	42.7	43.6	44.9
14.0-14.9	14.47	219	39.4	3.1	34.9	35.9	36.6	37.7	39.7	41.9	43.1	43.9	45.2
15.0-15.9	15.47	185	39.9	2.9	35.2	36.2	36.9	37.9	39.9	41.9	43.1	43.9	45.1
16.0-16.9	16.46	216	40.3	2.9	35.6	36.5	37.1	38.1	40.0	42.0	43.1	43.9	45.1
17.0-17.9	17.45	207	40.4	2.9	35.5	36.5	37.1	38.1	40.0	42.1	43.2	44.0	45.2
18.0-18.9	18.43	180	40.5	3.2	34.7	35.7	36.5	37.5	39.6	41.8	43.1	43.9	45.2
19.0-19.9	19.48	185	40.5	3.2	35.0	36.0	36.8	37.8	39.9	42.1	43.3	44.2	45.5
20.0-29.9	24.91	1807	39.4	3.2	34.5	35.4	36.3	37.4	39.5	41.8	43.0	43.9	45.2
30.0-39.9	34.85	1783	38.7	3.2	33.9	35.0	35.7	36.8	38.9	41.1	42.3	43.2	44.5
40.0-49.9	44.28	1284	39.0	3.4	33.1	34.2	34.9	36.1	38.3	40.7	42.0	42.9	44.3
50.0-59.9	54.83	957	37.4	3.4	32.5	33.6	34.3	35.5	37.7	40.1	41.5	42.4	43.9
60.0-69.9	64.82	1080	37.1	3.4	32.0	33.1	33.9	35.0	37.3	39.7	41.0	42.0	43.4
70.0-79.9	74.46	857	36.6	3.4	31.6	32.7	33.5	34.6	36.9	39.3	40.7	41.6	43.1
80.0-90.9	84.45	559	36.8	3.4	31.3	32.4	33.2	34.3	36.6	39.0	40.3	41.3	42.7

134

Table IV.11.

Mean (M), standard deviation (SD), and percentiles of upper leg length index (upper leg length/stature x 100) by age for males and females of 2 to 90 years

Age Group (years)	Mean Age (years)	N	M	SD	Percentiles								
					5th	10th	15th	25th	50th	75th	85th	90th	95th
Males													
2.0-2.9	2.46	563	20.7	1.5	18.4	18.8	19.2	19.7	20.6	21.6	22.2	22.6	23.2
3.0-3.9	3.45	493	21.4	1.5	19.1	19.6	19.9	20.4	21.4	22.4	23.0	23.4	24.0
4.0-4.9	4.47	543	22.1	1.4	19.8	20.2	20.6	21.1	22.0	23.1	23.6	24.0	24.6
5.0-5.9	5.43	487	22.6	1.5	20.3	20.8	21.1	21.6	22.6	23.6	24.2	24.6	25.2
6.0-6.9	6.45	258	23.1	1.4	20.8	21.3	21.6	22.1	23.1	24.1	24.7	25.0	25.6
7.0-7.9	7.47	271	23.5	1.4	21.2	21.7	22.0	22.5	23.5	24.5	25.1	25.4	26.0
8.0-8.9	8.46	259	23.9	1.4	21.6	22.0	22.4	22.9	23.8	24.8	25.4	25.8	26.4
9.0-9.9	9.50	280	24.2	1.5	21.9	22.3	22.7	23.2	24.1	25.1	25.7	26.0	26.6
10.0-10.9	10.45	287	24.4	1.4	22.1	22.6	22.9	23.4	24.3	25.3	25.9	26.3	26.8
11.0-11.9	11.44	271	24.6	1.4	22.3	22.7	23.1	23.6	24.5	25.5	26.0	26.4	27.0
12.0-12.9	12.47	204	24.8	1.4	22.4	22.9	23.2	23.7	24.7	25.6	26.2	26.6	27.1
13.0-13.9	13.47	188	24.9	1.4	22.5	23.0	23.3	23.8	24.8	25.7	26.3	26.7	27.2
14.0-14.9	14.49	182	25.0	1.4	22.6	23.1	23.4	23.9	24.8	25.8	26.4	26.7	27.3
15.0-15.9	15.45	177	25.0	1.4	22.7	23.1	23.5	24.0	24.9	25.9	26.4	26.8	27.3
16.0-16.9	16.45	194	25.0	1.4	22.7	23.2	23.5	24.0	24.9	25.9	26.4	26.8	27.4
17.0-17.9	17.45	189	25.0	1.4	22.7	23.2	23.5	24.0	24.9	25.9	26.4	26.8	27.4
18.0-18.9	18.45	168	25.0	1.4	22.7	23.2	23.5	24.0	24.9	25.9	26.4	26.8	27.3
19.0-19.9	19.43	156	25.0	1.4	22.7	23.2	23.5	24.0	24.9	25.9	26.4	26.8	27.3
20.0-29.9	24.96	1589	24.8	1.4	22.5	23.0	23.3	23.8	24.7	25.7	26.2	26.6	27.2
30.0-39.9	34.72	1423	24.4	1.4	22.1	22.5	22.9	23.4	24.3	25.3	25.8	26.2	26.8
40.0-49.9	44.35	1165	24.1	1.4	21.8	22.3	22.6	23.1	24.0	25.0	25.6	26.0	26.6
50.0-59.9	54.89	820	23.8	1.5	21.5	22.0	22.3	22.8	23.8	24.8	25.3	25.7	26.3
60.0-69.9	64.83	1105	23.7	1.5	21.3	21.8	22.1	22.6	23.6	24.6	25.1	25.5	26.1
70.0-79.9	74.16	768	23.7	1.4	21.4	21.9	22.2	22.7	23.7	24.7	25.2	25.6	26.2
80.0-90.9	84.09	528	23.6	1.4	21.3	21.8	22.1	22.6	23.6	24.6	25.1	25.5	26.1
Females													
2.0-2.9	2.45	555	21.0	1.5	18.7	19.2	19.5	20.0	21.0	22.1	22.7	23.1	23.7
3.0-3.9	3.46	566	21.8	1.5	19.4	19.9	20.3	20.8	21.8	22.8	23.4	23.8	24.4
4.0-4.9	4.43	526	22.4	1.5	20.1	20.5	20.9	21.4	22.4	23.4	24.0	24.4	25.0
5.0-5.9	5.46	543	23.0	1.5	20.6	21.1	21.4	21.9	22.9	23.9	24.5	24.9	25.5
6.0-6.9	6.47	275	23.4	1.5	21.1	21.6	21.9	22.4	23.4	24.4	24.9	25.3	25.9
7.0-7.9	7.44	263	23.8	1.5	21.5	21.9	22.3	22.8	23.7	24.7	25.3	25.6	26.2
8.0-8.9	8.47	246	24.1	1.4	21.8	22.3	22.6	23.1	24.0	25.0	25.6	25.9	26.5
9.0-9.9	9.43	269	24.3	1.4	22.0	22.5	22.8	23.3	24.2	25.2	25.8	26.2	26.7
10.0-10.9	10.43	254	24.5	1.4	22.2	22.7	23.0	23.5	24.4	25.4	26.0	26.3	26.9
11.0-11.9	11.46	280	24.6	1.4	22.4	22.8	23.2	23.6	24.6	25.6	26.1	26.5	27.0
12.0-12.9	12.46	216	24.7	1.4	22.5	22.9	23.3	23.7	24.7	25.7	26.2	26.6	27.1
13.0-13.9	13.45	224	24.8	1.4	22.5	23.0	23.3	23.8	24.7	25.7	26.3	26.6	27.2
14.0-14.9	14.47	219	24.8	1.4	22.6	23.0	23.4	23.8	24.8	25.8	26.3	26.7	27.2
15.0-15.9	15.47	185	24.8	1.4	22.6	23.0	23.4	23.9	24.8	25.8	26.3	26.7	27.3
16.0-16.9	16.46	216	24.8	1.4	22.6	23.0	23.4	23.9	24.8	25.8	26.3	26.7	27.3
17.0-17.9	17.45	207	24.8	1.4	22.5	23.0	23.3	23.8	24.8	25.8	26.3	26.7	27.3
18.0-18.9	18.43	180	24.7	1.5	22.5	23.0	23.3	23.8	24.7	25.7	26.3	26.7	27.3
19.0-19.9	19.48	185	24.7	1.5	22.4	22.9	23.2	23.7	24.7	25.7	26.3	26.7	27.2
20.0-29.9	24.91	1807	24.4	1.5	22.0	22.5	22.9	23.4	24.4	25.5	26.0	26.4	27.0
30.0-39.9	34.85	1783	24.2	1.6	21.5	22.0	22.4	22.9	24.0	25.1	25.7	26.2	26.8
40.0-49.9	44.28	1284	23.9	1.7	21.2	21.8	22.1	22.7	23.8	25.0	25.6	26.1	26.7
50.0-59.9	54.83	957	23.4	1.7	20.9	21.5	21.9	22.5	23.6	24.8	25.4	25.9	26.6
60.0-69.9	64.82	1080	23.2	1.7	20.7	21.3	21.7	22.2	23.4	24.6	25.2	25.7	26.4
70.0-79.9	74.46	857	23.3	1.7	20.8	21.4	21.8	22.3	23.5	24.6	25.3	25.8	26.4
80.0-90.9	84.45	558	23.7	1.7	20.9	21.4	21.8	22.4	23.5	24.7	25.4	25.8	26.5

Table IV.12.

Mean (M), standard deviation (SD), and percentiles of lower leg length (cm) by age for males and females of 2 to 90 years

Age Group (years)	Mean Age (years)	N	M	SD	Percentiles								
					5th	10th	15th	25th	50th	75th	85th	90th	95th
Males													
2.0-2.9	2.46	561	20.9	2.5	16.6	17.4	17.9	18.7	20.3	22.0	23.0	23.7	24.8
3.0-3.9	3.45	492	22.7	2.5	19.3	20.0	20.6	21.4	23.0	24.7	25.7	26.4	27.5
4.0-4.9	4.47	542	24.7	2.4	21.4	22.2	22.7	23.5	25.1	26.9	27.9	28.5	29.6
5.0-5.9	5.43	487	26.6	2.6	22.9	23.7	24.3	25.2	26.9	28.7	29.7	30.4	31.5
6.0-6.9	6.45	258	28.7	2.8	24.5	25.3	25.9	26.9	28.7	30.6	31.7	32.5	33.7
7.0-7.9	7.47	271	30.6	2.9	26.1	27.0	27.6	28.6	30.5	32.5	33.7	34.5	35.7
8.0-8.9	8.46	259	32.4	3.1	27.5	28.5	29.1	30.2	32.1	34.2	35.4	36.3	37.5
9.0-9.9	9.50	278	34.1	3.2	28.9	29.9	30.5	31.6	33.6	35.8	37.0	37.9	39.2
10.0-10.9	10.45	286	35.4	3.3	29.9	31.0	31.7	32.8	34.9	37.1	38.4	39.3	40.7
11.0-11.9	11.44	271	36.7	3.5	31.0	32.1	32.8	34.0	36.2	38.6	40.0	40.9	42.4
12.0-12.9	12.47	203	37.8	3.6	32.3	33.4	34.2	35.4	37.8	40.3	41.7	42.7	44.2
13.0-13.9	13.47	187	38.7	3.7	33.6	34.8	35.6	36.8	39.3	41.9	43.3	44.4	45.9
14.0-14.9	14.49	181	39.4	3.6	34.8	36.0	36.8	38.0	40.4	43.0	44.5	45.5	47.0
15.0-15.9	15.45	177	40.0	3.5	35.3	36.5	37.3	38.5	40.8	43.3	44.7	45.7	47.2
16.0-16.9	16.45	194	40.4	3.5	35.5	36.6	37.4	38.5	40.8	43.3	44.6	45.6	47.0
17.0-17.9	17.45	188	40.7	3.4	35.4	36.6	37.3	38.5	40.8	43.3	44.6	45.6	47.0
18.0-18.9	18.45	168	40.9	3.6	35.4	36.5	37.3	38.5	40.8	43.3	44.7	45.7	47.1
19.0-19.9	19.43	155	40.9	3.5	35.4	36.5	37.3	38.5	40.8	43.3	44.7	45.7	47.1
20.0-29.9	24.96	1587	40.5	3.6	35.3	36.5	37.3	38.5	40.8	43.3	44.7	45.7	47.2
30.0-39.9	34.72	1421	40.5	3.6	35.2	36.4	37.2	38.4	40.8	43.4	44.8	45.8	47.3
40.0-49.9	44.35	1165	41.1	3.7	35.2	36.4	37.2	38.4	40.8	43.4	44.8	45.8	47.4
50.0-59.9	54.89	819	41.8	3.8	35.2	36.4	37.2	38.4	40.8	43.4	44.8	45.8	47.3
60.0-69.9	64.83	1105	42.1	3.7	35.3	36.5	37.3	38.5	40.8	43.3	44.7	45.7	47.2
70.0-79.9	74.16	759	42.1	3.6	35.5	36.6	37.4	38.5	40.8	43.2	44.6	45.5	47.0
80.0-90.9	84.09	524	42.1	3.4	35.7	36.8	37.5	38.7	40.8	43.1	44.4	45.3	46.7
Females													
2.0-2.9	2.45	549	20.0	2.5	16.5	17.3	17.8	18.6	20.2	22.0	23.0	23.7	24.8
3.0-3.9	3.46	566	22.4	2.5	18.5	19.3	19.8	20.7	22.3	24.1	25.1	25.8	26.9
4.0-4.9	4.43	523	24.5	2.4	20.7	21.4	22.0	22.8	24.3	26.0	27.0	27.6	28.7
5.0-5.9	5.46	542	26.7	2.6	22.6	23.4	24.0	24.8	26.5	28.2	29.2	29.9	31.0
6.0-6.9	6.47	273	28.7	2.8	24.2	25.1	25.7	26.6	28.4	30.4	31.5	32.2	33.4
7.0-7.9	7.44	263	30.4	2.8	25.7	26.6	27.3	28.3	30.2	32.3	33.5	34.3	35.6
8.0-8.9	8.47	246	32.0	2.9	27.2	28.2	28.9	29.9	31.9	34.1	35.3	36.2	37.5
9.0-9.9	9.43	269	33.3	3.1	28.6	29.6	30.3	31.3	33.3	35.5	36.7	37.6	38.9
10.0-10.9	10.43	254	34.4	3.1	29.8	30.8	31.5	32.5	34.6	36.7	38.0	38.8	40.1
11.0-11.9	11.46	280	35.4	3.0	30.7	31.7	32.4	33.5	35.6	37.8	39.1	39.9	41.3
12.0-12.9	12.46	216	36.1	3.3	31.3	32.3	33.1	34.2	36.3	38.7	40.0	40.9	42.3
13.0-13.9	13.45	223	36.6	3.4	31.7	32.8	33.5	34.7	36.9	39.2	40.5	41.5	42.9
14.0-14.9	14.47	215	37.0	3.2	32.0	33.0	33.8	34.9	37.2	39.5	40.9	41.8	43.2
15.0-15.9	15.47	184	37.2	3.4	32.0	33.1	33.9	35.0	37.3	39.6	41.0	41.9	43.3
16.0-16.9	16.46	216	37.4	3.4	32.0	33.1	33.8	35.0	37.2	39.6	40.9	41.9	43.3
17.0-17.9	17.45	207	37.4	3.4	31.9	32.9	33.7	34.8	37.1	39.4	40.8	41.7	43.1
18.0-18.9	18.43	180	37.3	3.4	31.7	32.7	33.5	34.6	36.8	39.2	40.5	41.4	42.8
19.0-19.9	19.48	185	37.2	3.4	31.5	32.5	33.3	34.4	36.6	38.9	40.2	41.2	42.6
20.0-29.9	24.91	1805	36.4	3.3	31.3	32.3	33.1	34.2	36.4	38.7	40.0	40.9	42.3
30.0-39.9	34.85	1780	36.8	3.4	31.5	32.6	33.4	34.5	36.7	39.0	40.3	41.3	42.7
40.0-49.9	44.28	1283	37.1	3.4	32.3	33.4	34.2	35.3	37.6	40.0	41.3	42.3	43.7
50.0-59.9	54.83	957	38.0	3.5	32.7	33.8	34.6	35.7	38.0	40.4	41.8	42.8	44.2
60.0-69.9	64.82	1078	38.4	3.5	33.5	34.7	35.5	36.7	39.0	41.5	42.9	43.9	45.4
70.0-79.9	74.46	855	38.7	3.6	33.5	34.6	35.4	36.6	39.0	41.4	42.8	43.8	45.3
80.0-90.9	84.45	554	39.0	3.6	33.5	34.7	35.5	36.7	39.0	41.5	42.9	43.9	45.4

Postnatal Anthropometric Reference

Table IV.13.

Mean (M), standard deviation (SD), and percentiles of lower leg length index (lower leg length/stature x 100) by age for males and females of 2 to 90 years

Age Group (years)	Mean Age (yrs)	N	M	SD	Percentiles								
					5th	10th	15th	25th	50th	75th	85th	90th	95th
Males													
2.0-2.9	2.46	561	22.5	2.1	19.3	19.9	20.4	21.1	22.4	23.9	24.7	25.3	26.1
3.0-3.9	3.45	492	23.1	2.0	20.0	20.6	21.1	21.7	23.1	24.5	25.3	25.8	26.6
4.0-4.9	4.47	542	23.6	2.0	20.5	21.2	21.6	22.3	23.5	24.9	25.7	26.2	27.0
5.0-5.9	5.43	487	23.9	1.9	20.9	21.6	22.0	22.6	23.9	25.2	26.0	26.5	27.3
6.0-6.9	6.45	258	24.2	1.9	21.3	21.9	22.3	22.9	24.2	25.5	26.2	26.7	27.5
7.0-7.9	7.47	271	24.4	1.8	21.5	22.1	22.5	23.1	24.3	25.6	26.3	26.8	27.5
8.0-8.9	8.46	259	24.4	1.8	21.7	22.2	22.6	23.2	24.4	25.7	26.4	26.8	27.6
9.0-9.9	9.50	278	24.5	1.8	21.7	22.3	22.7	23.3	24.5	25.7	26.4	26.8	27.6
10.0-10.9	10.45	286	24.4	1.7	21.8	22.3	22.7	23.3	24.4	25.7	26.3	26.8	27.5
11.0-11.9	11.44	271	24.4	1.7	21.7	22.3	22.7	23.3	24.4	25.6	26.3	26.7	27.4
12.0-12.9	12.47	203	24.3	1.7	21.7	22.2	22.6	23.2	24.3	25.5	26.2	26.6	27.3
13.0-13.9	13.47	187	24.1	1.7	21.6	22.1	22.5	23.1	24.2	25.4	26.0	26.5	27.2
14.0-14.9	14.49	181	24.0	1.7	21.5	22.0	22.4	23.0	24.1	25.3	25.9	26.4	27.0
15.0-15.9	15.45	177	23.8	1.7	21.4	21.9	22.3	22.9	24.0	25.1	25.8	26.2	26.9
16.0-16.9	16.45	194	23.7	1.7	21.3	21.8	22.2	22.7	23.8	25.0	25.6	26.1	26.8
17.0-17.9	17.45	188	23.6	1.7	21.1	21.7	22.0	22.6	23.7	24.9	25.5	26.0	26.6
18.0-18.9	18.45	168	23.4	1.7	21.0	21.6	21.9	22.5	23.6	24.7	25.4	25.8	26.5
19.0-19.9	19.43	155	23.3	1.7	20.9	21.4	21.8	22.4	23.5	24.6	25.3	25.7	26.4
20.0-29.9	24.96	1587	22.9	1.6	20.5	21.0	21.4	22.0	23.0	24.2	24.8	25.3	25.9
30.0-39.9	34.72	1421	23.3	1.7	20.6	21.2	21.5	22.1	23.2	24.3	24.9	25.4	26.1
40.0-49.9	44.35	1165	23.6	1.6	21.0	21.5	21.9	22.4	23.5	24.6	25.3	25.7	26.4
50.0-59.9	54.89	819	23.9	1.7	21.0	21.5	21.9	22.5	23.6	24.8	25.4	25.9	26.6
60.0-69.9	64.83	1105	24.3	1.8	20.9	21.5	21.9	22.5	23.6	24.8	25.5	25.9	26.7
70.0-79.9	74.16	759	24.5	1.7	21.0	21.6	21.9	22.5	23.6	24.8	25.4	25.9	26.5
80.0-90.9	84.09	524	24.8	1.7	21.1	21.7	22.0	22.6	23.6	24.7	25.3	25.8	26.4
Females													
2.0-2.9	2.45	549	22.2	2.2	19.0	19.7	20.2	20.9	22.4	24.0	24.9	25.5	26.4
3.0-3.9	3.46	566	23.0	2.1	19.7	20.4	20.8	21.6	22.9	24.4	25.3	25.9	26.8
4.0-4.9	4.43	523	23.5	2.1	20.2	20.9	21.3	22.0	23.3	24.8	25.6	26.1	27.0
5.0-5.9	5.46	542	23.9	2.0	20.6	21.3	21.7	22.4	23.6	25.0	25.8	26.3	27.1
6.0-6.9	6.47	273	24.1	1.9	20.9	21.5	22.0	22.6	23.8	25.1	25.8	26.4	27.1
7.0-7.9	7.44	263	24.1	1.8	21.1	21.7	22.1	22.7	23.9	25.2	25.9	26.4	27.1
8.0-8.9	8.47	246	24.1	1.8	21.2	21.8	22.2	22.8	23.9	25.2	25.8	26.3	27.0
9.0-9.9	9.43	269	24.0	1.7	21.3	21.8	22.2	22.8	23.9	25.1	25.8	26.2	26.9
10.0-10.9	10.43	254	23.9	1.7	21.2	21.8	22.2	22.7	23.9	25.0	25.7	26.1	26.8
11.0-11.9	11.46	280	23.8	1.7	21.2	21.7	22.1	22.7	23.8	24.9	25.5	26.0	26.7
12.0-12.9	12.46	216	23.6	1.6	21.1	21.6	22.0	22.6	23.6	24.8	25.4	25.8	26.5
13.0-13.9	13.45	223	23.4	1.6	21.0	21.5	21.9	22.4	23.5	24.6	25.2	25.7	26.3
14.0-14.9	14.47	215	23.3	1.6	20.8	21.4	21.7	22.3	23.3	24.5	25.1	25.5	26.2
15.0-15.9	15.47	184	23.1	1.6	20.7	21.2	21.6	22.1	23.2	24.3	24.9	25.4	26.0
16.0-16.9	16.46	216	23.0	1.6	20.5	21.1	21.4	22.0	23.0	24.2	24.8	25.2	25.9
17.0-17.9	17.45	207	22.9	1.6	20.4	20.9	21.3	21.8	22.9	24.0	24.6	25.1	25.7
18.0-18.9	18.43	180	22.8	1.6	20.2	20.8	21.1	21.7	22.8	23.9	24.5	25.0	25.6
19.0-19.9	19.48	185	22.8	1.6	20.1	20.6	21.0	21.6	22.6	23.8	24.4	24.8	25.5
20.0-29.9	24.91	1805	22.7	1.7	19.6	20.2	20.6	21.1	22.2	23.4	24.1	24.5	25.2
30.0-39.9	34.85	1780	23.0	1.8	19.8	20.4	20.8	21.4	22.6	23.8	24.5	25.0	25.7
40.0-49.9	44.28	1283	23.3	1.9	20.2	20.8	21.2	21.8	23.0	24.3	25.0	25.5	26.3
50.0-59.9	54.83	957	23.9	2.0	20.3	20.9	21.3	22.0	23.2	24.5	25.3	25.8	26.6
60.0-69.9	64.82	1078	24.5	2.0	20.3	21.0	21.4	22.0	23.3	24.7	25.4	26.0	26.8
70.0-79.9	74.46	855	24.8	2.0	20.7	21.3	21.7	22.4	23.6	24.9	25.6	26.1	26.9
80.0-90.9	84.45	554	25.1	2.1	20.7	21.4	21.8	22.5	23.7	25.1	25.9	26.4	27.2

Postnatal Anthropometric Reference

Table IV.14.

Mean (M), standard deviation (SD), and percentiles of total leg length (cm) by age for males and females of 2 to 90 years

Age Group (years)	Mean Age (years)	N	M	SD	5th	10th	15th	25th	50th	75th	85th	90th	95th
Males													
2.0-2.9	2.46	619	40.4	3.1	34.3	35.3	35.9	36.9	38.9	41.0	42.2	43.0	44.2
3.0-3.9	3.45	508	43.7	3.0	39.9	40.9	41.6	42.6	44.6	46.7	47.9	48.7	50.0
4.0-4.9	4.47	553	47.7	3.1	43.8	44.9	45.6	46.7	48.7	50.9	52.1	53.0	54.2
5.0-5.9	5.43	496	51.7	3.4	47.0	48.1	48.9	50.1	52.3	54.7	56.0	56.9	58.3
6.0-6.9	6.45	262	56.0	3.7	50.4	51.6	52.5	53.7	56.2	58.7	60.1	61.1	62.6
7.0-7.9	7.47	273	60.1	4.0	53.8	55.1	56.0	57.4	60.0	62.7	64.2	65.2	66.8
8.0-8.9	8.46	267	64.0	4.2	56.9	58.3	59.2	60.6	63.3	66.2	67.8	68.9	70.6
9.0-9.9	9.50	281	67.8	4.5	59.7	61.2	62.2	63.7	66.6	69.6	71.3	72.5	74.3
10.0-10.9	10.45	288	70.9	4.8	62.1	63.7	64.7	66.3	69.5	72.7	74.5	75.8	77.7
11.0-11.9	11.44	275	73.8	5.1	64.7	66.4	67.5	69.3	72.6	76.0	78.0	79.3	81.3
12.0-12.9	12.47	204	76.5	5.3	67.9	69.6	70.8	72.6	76.0	79.6	81.6	83.0	85.1
13.0-13.9	13.47	192	78.6	5.2	71.2	72.9	74.1	75.9	79.3	82.9	84.9	86.3	88.4
14.0-14.9	14.49	186	80.5	5.0	74.1	75.8	76.9	78.7	82.1	85.6	87.6	88.9	90.9
15.0-15.9	15.45	182	81.9	5.0	75.6	77.3	78.5	80.2	83.6	87.1	89.0	90.4	92.4
16.0-16.9	16.45	196	83.1	5.2	75.8	77.5	78.7	80.5	83.9	87.5	89.5	90.9	92.9
17.0-17.9	17.45	191	83.9	5.4	75.3	77.0	78.3	80.1	83.6	87.3	89.3	90.7	92.9
18.0-18.9	18.45	172	84.5	5.3	75.5	77.2	78.4	80.2	83.7	87.3	89.3	90.7	92.7
19.0-19.9	19.43	160	84.9	5.3	75.6	77.3	78.5	80.3	83.8	87.4	89.4	90.7	92.8
20.0-29.9	24.96	1620	84.4	5.4	75.1	76.8	78.0	79.8	83.3	87.0	89.0	90.4	92.5
30.0-39.9	34.72	1452	82.6	5.2	75.1	76.8	78.0	79.8	83.2	86.8	88.8	90.2	92.3
40.0-49.9	44.35	1195	83.5	5.1	75.3	77.0	78.2	79.9	83.3	86.8	88.8	90.1	92.2
50.0-59.9	54.89	835	83.4	5.0	75.4	77.1	78.2	79.9	83.2	86.6	88.5	89.9	91.8
60.0-69.9	64.83	1129	83.0	4.8	75.5	77.1	78.2	79.8	83.0	86.3	88.1	89.4	91.3
70.0-79.9	74.16	798	82.8	4.6	75.5	77.0	78.1	79.7	82.7	85.9	87.6	88.8	90.6
80.0-90.9	84.09	566	82.2	4.4	75.4	76.8	77.8	79.3	82.2	85.2	86.9	88.0	89.7
Females													
2.0-2.9	2.45	584	39.3	3.2	34.1	35.1	35.8	36.9	38.9	41.1	42.3	43.1	44.4
3.0-3.9	3.46	586	43.6	3.1	39.4	40.4	41.1	42.2	44.2	46.4	47.6	48.4	49.7
4.0-4.9	4.43	528	47.9	3.0	43.6	44.6	45.3	46.3	48.3	50.4	51.6	52.4	53.6
5.0-5.9	5.46	543	52.4	3.3	47.5	48.5	49.3	50.4	52.6	54.9	56.1	57.0	58.3
6.0-6.9	6.47	273	56.7	3.8	50.5	51.7	52.6	53.9	56.4	59.0	60.4	61.4	62.9
7.0-7.9	7.44	268	60.4	4.2	53.0	54.4	55.3	56.8	59.5	62.4	64.0	65.1	66.8
8.0-8.9	8.47	247	64.1	4.5	56.0	57.5	58.5	60.0	62.9	65.9	67.6	68.8	70.5
9.0-9.9	9.43	273	67.1	4.5	59.3	60.8	61.8	63.3	66.2	69.3	71.0	72.2	74.0
10.0-10.9	10.43	260	69.8	4.5	62.9	64.4	65.4	67.0	69.9	73.0	74.7	75.9	77.6
11.0-11.9	11.46	288	72.1	4.4	66.2	67.7	68.7	70.2	73.2	76.3	78.0	79.2	81.0
12.0-12.9	12.46	221	74.0	4.5	68.2	69.7	70.8	72.4	75.4	78.6	80.3	81.5	83.4
13.0-13.9	13.45	227	75.4	4.7	69.0	70.5	71.6	73.2	76.3	79.6	81.4	82.6	84.5
14.0-14.9	14.47	216	76.5	4.8	68.9	70.5	71.6	73.2	76.4	79.7	81.5	82.8	84.7
15.0-15.9	15.47	189	77.2	4.9	69.0	70.6	71.7	73.4	76.6	79.9	81.7	83.0	84.9
16.0-16.9	16.46	224	77.6	4.8	69.2	70.8	71.9	73.6	76.7	80.0	81.8	83.1	85.0
17.0-17.9	17.45	213	77.8	4.8	69.6	71.2	72.3	73.9	77.0	80.3	82.0	83.3	85.1
18.0-18.9	18.43	186	77.8	4.6	69.9	71.4	72.5	74.0	77.0	80.2	81.9	83.1	84.9
19.0-19.9	19.48	191	77.7	4.7	69.8	71.3	72.4	74.0	77.0	80.2	82.0	83.2	85.0
20.0-29.9	24.91	1842	75.8	4.8	68.7	70.3	71.4	73.1	76.3	79.6	81.4	82.7	84.6
30.0-39.9	34.85	1837	75.5	4.7	68.7	70.2	71.3	72.9	76.1	79.3	81.1	82.4	84.2
40.0-49.9	44.28	1328	76.1	4.7	68.7	70.2	71.3	72.9	75.9	79.1	80.9	82.1	84.0
50.0-59.9	54.83	979	75.5	4.5	68.7	70.2	71.3	72.8	75.8	78.9	80.6	81.8	83.6
60.0-69.9	64.82	1110	76.0	4.4	68.8	70.3	71.3	72.8	75.7	78.8	80.4	81.6	83.3
70.0-79.9	74.46	893	75.5	4.3	68.9	70.4	71.4	72.8	75.7	78.6	80.3	81.4	83.1
80.0-90.9	84.45	599	75.8	4.2	69.1	70.5	71.5	72.9	75.7	78.5	80.1	81.2	82.8

Table IV.15.

Mean (M), standard deviation (SD), and percentiles of total leg length index (total leg length/stature x 100) by age for males and females of 2 to 90 years

Age Group (years)	Mean Age (years)	N	M	SD	Percentiles								
					5th	10th	15th	25th	50th	75th	85th	90th	95th
Males													
2.0-2.9	2.46	619	43.1	1.8	40.1	40.7	41.1	41.7	42.9	44.1	44.7	45.2	45.9
3.0-3.9	3.45	508	44.5	1.8	41.9	42.5	43.0	43.6	44.8	46.0	46.7	47.2	47.9
4.0-4.9	4.47	553	45.6	1.7	43.1	43.7	44.1	44.7	45.8	46.9	47.6	48.0	48.6
5.0-5.9	5.43	496	46.5	1.6	43.8	44.4	44.8	45.4	46.4	47.6	48.2	48.6	49.2
6.0-6.9	6.45	262	47.3	1.6	44.5	45.0	45.4	46.0	47.0	48.1	48.7	49.1	49.8
7.0-7.9	7.47	273	47.9	1.6	45.1	45.6	46.0	46.5	47.6	48.7	49.2	49.6	50.2
8.0-8.9	8.46	267	48.3	1.5	45.7	46.2	46.6	47.1	48.1	49.1	49.7	50.1	50.7
9.0-9.9	9.50	281	48.6	1.5	46.2	46.8	47.1	47.6	48.6	49.6	50.1	50.5	51.1
10.0-10.9	10.45	288	48.8	1.4	46.6	47.1	47.5	48.0	48.9	49.9	50.5	50.8	51.4
11.0-11.9	11.44	275	49.0	1.4	46.9	47.4	47.8	48.3	49.2	50.2	50.7	51.1	51.6
12.0-12.9	12.47	204	49.0	1.4	47.0	47.5	47.9	48.4	49.3	50.3	50.8	51.2	51.7
13.0-13.9	13.47	192	49.0	1.4	47.0	47.5	47.8	48.3	49.3	50.3	50.8	51.2	51.7
14.0-14.9	14.49	186	48.9	1.5	46.8	47.3	47.6	48.1	49.1	50.1	50.7	51.0	51.6
15.0-15.9	15.45	182	48.8	1.5	46.5	47.0	47.3	47.9	48.9	49.9	50.4	50.8	51.4
16.0-16.9	16.45	196	48.7	1.5	46.1	46.7	47.0	47.5	48.6	49.6	50.2	50.6	51.1
17.0-17.9	17.45	191	48.6	1.5	45.9	46.4	46.7	47.3	48.3	49.3	49.9	50.3	50.9
18.0-18.9	18.45	172	48.4	1.5	45.8	46.3	46.6	47.2	48.1	49.1	49.7	50.1	50.6
19.0-19.9	19.43	160	48.3	1.5	45.6	46.1	46.5	47.0	48.0	49.1	49.6	50.0	50.6
20.0-29.9	24.96	1620	47.7	1.5	45.4	45.9	46.3	46.8	47.8	48.8	49.4	49.8	50.3
30.0-39.9	34.72	1452	47.6	1.5	45.2	45.7	46.1	46.6	47.6	48.7	49.3	49.7	50.2
40.0-49.9	44.35	1195	47.7	1.5	45.2	45.7	46.1	46.6	47.6	48.7	49.3	49.7	50.2
50.0-59.9	54.89	835	47.7	1.5	45.4	45.9	46.2	46.8	47.8	48.8	49.4	49.7	50.3
60.0-69.9	64.83	1129	48.1	1.5	45.7	46.2	46.5	47.0	48.0	49.0	49.5	49.9	50.4
70.0-79.9	74.16	798	48.3	1.4	46.0	46.5	46.8	47.3	48.2	49.2	49.7	50.1	50.6
80.0-90.9	84.09	566	48.5	1.4	46.3	46.7	47.1	47.5	48.5	49.4	49.9	50.3	50.8
Females													
2.0-2.9	2.45	584	43.1	1.8	40.3	40.9	41.3	41.9	43.1	44.3	45.0	45.4	46.1
3.0-3.9	3.46	586	44.7	1.8	41.9	42.6	43.0	43.6	44.8	46.0	46.7	47.2	47.8
4.0-4.9	4.43	528	45.9	1.7	43.3	43.8	44.2	44.8	45.9	47.0	47.7	48.1	48.7
5.0-5.9	5.46	543	46.9	1.6	44.2	45.1	45.7	45.7	46.7	47.8	48.4	48.8	49.4
6.0-6.9	6.47	273	47.5	1.6	44.8	45.4	45.7	46.3	47.3	48.4	48.9	49.3	49.9
7.0-7.9	7.44	268	47.9	1.6	45.3	45.8	46.2	46.7	47.8	48.8	49.4	49.8	50.4
8.0-8.9	8.47	247	48.2	1.6	45.7	46.2	46.6	47.2	48.2	49.3	49.9	50.3	50.9
9.0-9.9	9.43	273	48.3	1.6	46.0	46.6	46.9	47.5	48.5	49.6	50.1	50.5	51.1
10.0-10.9	10.43	260	48.4	1.5	46.2	46.8	47.1	47.7	48.7	49.7	50.3	50.7	51.2
11.0-11.9	11.46	288	48.4	1.5	46.3	46.8	47.1	47.6	48.6	49.7	50.2	50.6	51.2
12.0-12.9	12.46	221	48.3	1.5	46.0	46.5	46.9	47.4	48.4	49.5	50.0	50.4	51.0
13.0-13.9	13.45	227	48.2	1.6	45.6	46.1	46.5	47.1	48.1	49.2	49.8	50.2	50.7
14.0-14.9	14.47	216	48.0	1.6	45.3	45.8	46.2	46.7	47.8	48.8	49.4	49.8	50.4
15.0-15.9	15.47	189	47.9	1.6	45.1	45.6	46.0	46.6	47.6	48.6	49.2	49.6	50.2
16.0-16.9	16.46	224	47.8	1.5	45.1	45.7	46.0	46.6	47.6	48.6	49.2	49.6	50.2
17.0-17.9	17.45	213	47.6	1.5	45.1	45.6	46.0	46.5	47.6	48.6	49.2	49.5	50.1
18.0-18.9	18.43	186	47.5	1.5	45.0	45.4	45.9	46.4	47.5	48.5	49.1	49.4	50.0
19.0-19.9	19.48	191	47.4	1.4	45.1	45.5	45.9	46.4	47.3	48.3	48.9	49.2	49.8
20.0-29.9	24.91	1842	47.1	1.5	44.9	45.4	45.7	46.3	47.3	48.3	48.9	49.2	49.8
30.0-39.9	34.85	1837	47.2	1.5	44.7	45.2	45.6	46.1	47.1	48.2	48.7	49.1	49.7
40.0-49.9	44.28	1328	47.2	1.5	44.7	45.2	45.6	46.1	47.1	48.1	48.7	49.1	49.6
50.0-59.9	54.83	979	47.3	1.5	44.9	45.4	45.8	46.3	47.3	48.2	48.8	49.2	49.7
60.0-69.9	64.82	1110	47.7	1.4	45.3	45.8	46.1	46.6	47.6	48.5	49.1	49.4	50.0
70.0-79.9	74.46	893	48.1	1.5	45.7	46.3	46.6	47.1	48.1	49.1	49.6	50.0	50.5
80.0-90.9	84.45	599	48.9	1.6	46.3	46.9	47.2	47.8	48.8	49.9	50.5	50.9	51.5

Table IV.16.

Mean (M), standard deviation (SD), and percentiles of upper arm length (cm) by age for males and females of 2 to 90 years

Age Group (years)	Mean Age (years)	N	M	SD	Percentiles 5th	10th	15th	25th	50th	75th	85th	90th	95th
					Males								
2.0-2.9	2.46	567	18.2	1.2	16.3	16.7	17.0	17.4	18.2	19.1	19.6	20.0	20.5
3.0-3.9	3.45	488	19.5	1.3	17.5	17.9	18.2	18.7	19.5	20.4	20.9	21.3	21.8
4.0-4.9	4.47	544	20.9	1.4	18.7	19.2	19.5	20.0	20.9	21.8	22.4	22.8	23.3
5.0-5.9	5.43	493	22.3	1.5	19.9	20.4	20.8	21.3	22.3	23.3	23.9	24.3	24.9
6.0-6.9	6.45	259	23.8	1.7	21.2	21.8	22.1	22.7	23.8	24.9	25.5	26.0	26.6
7.0-7.9	7.47	271	25.4	1.8	22.5	23.1	23.5	24.1	25.3	26.5	27.2	27.7	28.4
8.0-8.9	8.46	260	26.9	1.7	23.8	24.4	24.8	25.5	26.8	28.1	28.9	29.4	30.2
9.0-9.9	9.50	282	28.4	2.1	25.1	25.8	26.3	27.0	28.3	29.8	30.6	31.1	32.0
10.0-10.9	10.45	288	29.8	2.2	26.3	27.0	27.5	28.3	29.7	31.2	32.0	32.6	33.5
11.0-11.9	11.44	274	31.1	2.3	27.5	28.3	28.8	29.5	31.0	32.6	33.5	34.1	35.0
12.0-12.9	12.47	203	32.4	2.3	28.7	29.5	30.0	30.8	32.3	33.9	34.8	35.5	36.4
13.0-13.9	13.47	188	33.5	2.4	29.8	30.6	31.1	31.9	33.5	35.1	36.0	36.6	37.6
14.0-14.9	14.49	181	34.5	2.4	30.8	31.6	32.1	32.9	34.5	36.1	37.0	37.7	38.6
15.0-15.9	15.45	179	35.4	2.4	31.7	32.4	33.0	33.8	35.3	37.0	37.9	38.5	39.5
16.0-16.9	16.45	194	36.1	2.3	32.4	33.2	33.7	34.5	36.1	37.7	38.6	39.2	40.2
17.0-17.9	17.45	191	36.7	2.1	33.1	33.9	34.4	35.2	36.7	38.3	39.2	39.8	40.7
18.0-18.9	18.45	169	37.2	2.2	33.6	34.4	34.9	35.7	37.2	38.7	39.6	40.2	41.1
19.0-19.9	19.43	156	37.5	2.1	34.0	34.8	35.3	36.0	37.5	39.0	39.9	40.5	41.4
20.0-29.9	24.96	1595	37.8	2.1	34.4	35.1	35.6	36.4	37.8	39.2	40.1	40.6	41.5
30.0-39.9	34.72	1424	37.8	2.2	34.4	35.1	35.6	36.3	37.8	39.3	40.1	40.7	41.5
40.0-49.9	44.35	1171	37.8	2.2	34.3	35.0	35.6	36.3	37.8	39.3	40.1	40.7	41.6
50.0-59.9	54.89	824	37.8	2.2	34.3	35.0	35.5	36.3	37.8	39.3	40.2	40.7	41.6
60.0-69.9	64.83	1116	37.7	2.4	34.1	34.9	35.4	36.2	37.8	39.4	40.3	40.9	41.9
70.0-79.9	74.16	782	37.5	2.2	34.0	34.8	35.3	36.0	37.5	39.0	39.9	40.4	41.3
80.0-90.9	84.09	548	37.5	2.1	34.2	34.9	35.4	36.1	37.5	38.9	39.7	40.3	41.1
					Females								
2.0-2.9	2.45	547	18.1	1.3	16.1	16.5	16.8	17.3	18.1	19.0	19.5	19.9	20.4
3.0-3.9	3.46	563	19.1	1.3	17.0	17.4	17.7	18.2	19.1	20.0	20.5	20.9	21.4
4.0-4.9	4.43	526	20.4	1.4	18.2	18.7	19.0	19.5	20.4	21.4	22.0	22.3	22.9
5.0-5.9	5.46	543	22.1	1.5	19.7	20.2	20.5	21.1	22.1	23.1	23.7	24.2	24.8
6.0-6.9	6.47	275	23.8	1.7	21.2	21.8	22.1	22.7	23.8	25.0	25.6	26.1	26.8
7.0-7.9	7.44	263	25.5	1.8	22.7	23.3	23.7	24.3	25.4	26.7	27.4	27.9	28.6
8.0-8.9	8.47	246	27.1	1.8	24.2	24.8	25.2	25.9	27.1	28.4	29.2	29.7	30.5
9.0-9.9	9.43	267	28.6	2.0	25.4	26.1	26.5	27.2	28.5	29.9	30.7	31.3	32.1
10.0-10.9	10.43	254	29.9	2.1	26.6	27.3	27.8	28.5	29.9	31.3	32.1	32.7	33.5
11.0-11.9	11.46	281	31.0	2.2	27.7	28.4	28.9	29.6	31.0	32.5	33.3	33.9	34.8
12.0-12.9	12.46	216	32.0	2.2	28.6	29.3	29.8	30.5	32.0	33.5	34.3	34.9	35.8
13.0-13.9	13.45	225	32.7	2.2	29.3	30.0	30.5	31.3	32.7	34.2	35.1	35.7	36.6
14.0-14.9	14.47	220	33.3	2.1	29.9	30.6	31.1	31.9	33.3	34.8	35.7	36.3	37.2
15.0-15.9	15.47	188	33.8	2.1	30.4	31.1	31.6	32.3	33.7	35.3	36.1	36.7	37.6
16.0-16.9	16.46	218	34.1	2.2	30.7	31.4	31.9	32.6	34.1	35.6	36.4	37.0	37.8
17.0-17.9	17.45	208	34.3	1.9	30.9	31.6	32.1	32.8	34.2	35.7	36.6	37.1	38.0
18.0-18.9	18.43	181	34.4	2.1	31.0	31.7	32.2	33.0	34.4	35.8	36.7	37.2	38.1
19.0-19.9	19.48	185	34.4	2.1	31.1	31.8	32.3	33.0	34.4	35.9	36.7	37.3	38.1
20.0-29.9	24.91	1812	34.2	2.2	31.0	31.7	32.2	32.9	34.4	35.9	36.7	37.3	38.2
30.0-39.9	34.85	1791	34.4	2.2	30.8	31.6	32.1	32.9	34.4	35.9	36.8	37.4	38.4
40.0-49.9	44.28	1291	34.8	2.1	31.0	31.7	32.2	32.9	34.4	35.9	36.7	37.3	38.2
50.0-59.9	54.83	963	34.8	2.2	31.0	31.7	32.2	32.9	34.4	35.9	36.7	37.3	38.2
60.0-69.9	64.82	1091	34.6	2.3	30.9	31.6	32.1	32.9	34.4	35.9	36.8	37.4	38.3
70.0-79.9	74.46	864	34.5	2.1	31.1	31.8	32.2	33.0	34.4	35.8	36.7	37.2	38.1
80.0-90.9	84.45	571	34.3	2.0	31.2	31.8	32.3	33.0	34.3	35.7	36.5	37.0	37.8

Table IV.17.

Mean (M), standard deviation (SD), and percentiles of biacromial breadth (cm) by age for males and females of 3 to 90 years

Age Group (years)	Mean Age (years)	N	M	SD	5th	10th	15th	25th	50th	75th	85th	90th	95th
								Males					
3.0-3.9	3.45	491	22.5	1.4	20.3	20.8	21.1	21.6	22.5	23.5	24.0	24.4	25.0
4.0-4.9	4.47	545	23.8	1.5	21.6	22.1	22.4	23.0	23.9	25.0	25.6	26.0	26.6
5.0-5.9	5.43	491	24.7	1.7	22.6	23.1	23.5	24.1	25.2	26.4	27.1	27.5	28.2
6.0-6.9	6.45	259	26.1	1.8	23.6	24.2	24.6	25.3	26.5	27.8	28.5	29.0	29.7
7.0-7.9	7.47	271	27.5	1.9	24.8	25.5	25.9	26.5	27.8	29.1	29.8	30.3	31.1
8.0-8.9	8.46	258	29.0	1.9	26.1	26.7	27.1	27.8	29.1	30.4	31.1	31.7	32.4
9.0-9.9	9.50	281	30.7	2.0	27.2	27.9	28.3	29.0	30.4	31.8	32.5	33.1	33.9
10.0-10.9	10.45	286	32.1	2.2	28.1	28.9	29.4	30.1	31.5	33.0	33.9	34.5	35.3
11.0-11.9	11.44	273	33.6	2.4	29.1	29.9	30.4	31.2	32.8	34.4	35.4	36.0	37.0
12.0-12.9	12.47	203	35.0	2.6	30.4	31.2	31.8	32.7	34.3	36.1	37.1	37.7	38.8
13.0-13.9	13.47	188	36.3	2.6	32.0	32.8	33.4	34.3	36.0	37.7	38.7	39.4	40.5
14.0-14.9	14.49	183	37.4	2.5	33.8	34.6	35.2	36.0	37.7	39.4	40.3	41.0	42.0
15.0-15.9	15.45	179	38.4	2.4	35.3	36.1	36.6	37.4	39.0	40.6	41.5	42.2	43.1
16.0-16.9	16.45	195	39.3	2.3	36.2	37.0	37.5	38.3	39.9	41.5	42.4	43.0	43.9
17.0-17.9	17.45	191	40.0	2.3	36.8	37.6	38.1	38.9	40.5	42.0	42.9	43.5	44.5
18.0-18.9	18.45	169	40.7	2.2	37.5	38.3	38.8	39.6	41.1	42.6	43.5	44.1	45.0
19.0-19.9	19.43	156	41.1	2.3	37.5	38.3	38.8	39.6	41.1	42.7	43.6	44.2	45.1
20.0-29.9	24.96	1597	41.3	2.3	37.7	38.5	39.0	39.7	41.2	42.8	43.6	44.2	45.1
30.0-39.9	34.72	1423	41.2	2.3	37.8	38.5	39.1	39.8	41.4	42.9	43.8	44.4	45.3
40.0-49.9	44.35	1172	41.1	2.3	37.7	38.4	39.0	39.8	41.3	42.9	43.8	44.4	45.3
50.0-59.9	54.89	821	41.0	2.3	37.3	38.1	38.6	39.4	41.0	42.6	43.5	44.1	45.0
60.0-69.9	64.83	1118	40.4	2.3	36.8	37.6	38.1	38.9	40.5	42.1	43.0	43.6	44.5
70.0-79.9	74.16	787	39.9	2.3	36.2	37.0	37.5	38.3	39.8	41.4	42.3	42.9	43.8
80.0-90.9	84.09	551	38.8	2.3	35.4	36.1	36.6	37.4	38.9	40.4	41.3	41.9	42.8
								Females					
3.0-3.9	3.46	566	22.5	1.5	20.0	20.5	20.8	21.3	22.3	23.3	23.9	24.2	24.8
4.0-4.9	4.43	526	23.5	1.7	21.1	21.6	22.0	22.6	23.6	24.8	25.4	25.9	26.6
5.0-5.9	5.46	543	24.8	1.6	22.3	22.8	23.2	23.8	24.8	26.0	26.6	27.0	27.7
6.0-6.9	6.47	275	26.2	1.8	23.5	24.1	24.5	25.1	26.3	27.5	28.2	28.7	29.4
7.0-7.9	7.44	264	27.6	2.0	24.5	25.2	25.6	26.3	27.6	28.9	29.7	30.2	31.0
8.0-8.9	8.47	246	29.2	2.1	25.6	26.2	26.7	27.4	28.7	30.2	30.9	31.5	32.3
9.0-9.9	9.43	270	30.5	2.1	26.7	27.4	27.9	28.6	29.9	31.3	32.1	32.7	33.5
10.0-10.9	10.43	254	31.9	2.1	28.2	28.9	29.3	30.0	31.4	32.8	33.6	34.2	35.0
11.0-11.9	11.46	282	33.1	2.2	29.7	30.4	30.9	31.7	33.1	34.6	35.5	36.0	36.9
12.0-12.9	12.46	216	34.1	2.3	31.0	31.8	32.3	33.1	34.6	36.2	37.1	37.7	38.6
13.0-13.9	13.45	225	34.9	2.3	31.9	32.7	33.2	34.0	35.5	37.1	38.0	38.6	39.6
14.0-14.9	14.47	219	35.6	2.2	32.6	33.3	33.8	34.6	36.0	37.5	38.3	38.9	39.8
15.0-15.9	15.47	188	36.2	2.0	33.0	33.7	34.2	34.9	36.2	37.6	38.4	38.9	39.7
16.0-16.9	16.46	218	36.6	2.1	33.3	34.0	34.4	35.1	36.5	37.9	38.7	39.2	40.1
17.0-17.9	17.45	210	36.8	2.1	33.5	34.2	34.6	35.3	36.7	38.1	38.9	39.4	40.2
18.0-18.9	18.43	180	37.0	2.0	33.5	34.2	34.7	35.4	36.7	38.1	38.9	39.4	40.2
19.0-19.9	19.48	186	37.1	2.0	33.6	34.3	34.7	35.4	36.7	38.1	38.8	39.3	40.1
20.0-29.9	24.91	1810	36.8	2.1	33.5	34.2	34.7	35.4	36.8	38.3	39.1	39.6	40.5
30.0-39.9	34.85	1795	36.9	2.2	33.7	34.4	35.0	35.7	37.2	38.7	39.5	40.1	41.0
40.0-49.9	44.28	1295	36.9	2.2	33.7	34.5	35.0	35.8	37.2	38.8	39.6	40.2	41.1
50.0-59.9	54.83	964	36.8	2.2	33.5	34.2	34.8	35.6	37.0	38.6	39.4	40.0	40.9
60.0-69.9	64.82	1093	36.7	2.2	33.1	33.8	34.3	35.1	36.5	38.0	38.9	39.5	40.3
70.0-79.9	74.46	866	35.8	2.1	32.5	33.2	33.7	34.4	35.8	37.2	38.0	38.6	39.4
80.0-90.9	84.45	578	34.7	2.0	31.7	32.3	32.8	33.5	34.8	36.1	36.8	37.4	38.1

Table IV.18.

Mean (M), standard deviation (SD), and percentiles of bi-iliac breadth (cm) by age for males and females of 2 to 90 years

Age Group (years)	Mean Age (years)	N	M	SD	Percentiles								
					5th	10th	15th	25th	50th	75th	85th	90th	95th
Males													
2.0-2.9	2.46	568	15.6	1.1	13.6	13.9	14.1	14.5	15.2	15.9	16.3	16.6	17.1
3.0-3.9	3.45	490	16.0	1.1	14.5	14.8	15.1	15.5	16.2	17.0	17.4	17.7	18.2
4.0-4.9	4.47	546	16.6	1.2	15.0	15.4	15.7	16.1	16.8	17.7	18.1	18.4	18.9
5.0-5.9	5.43	490	17.4	1.3	15.5	15.9	16.2	16.7	17.6	18.5	19.0	19.4	20.0
6.0-6.9	6.45	257	18.3	1.6	16.0	16.5	16.9	17.4	18.4	19.5	20.1	20.6	21.2
7.0-7.9	7.47	271	19.3	1.8	16.5	17.1	17.5	18.1	19.2	20.4	21.1	21.6	22.4
8.0-8.9	8.46	258	20.3	2.0	17.0	17.6	18.0	18.7	19.9	21.3	22.0	22.6	23.4
9.0-9.9	9.50	278	21.3	2.2	17.5	18.1	18.6	19.3	20.7	22.2	23.0	23.6	24.5
10.0-10.9	10.45	286	22.2	2.4	18.0	18.7	19.2	20.0	21.5	23.1	24.1	24.7	25.7
11.0-11.9	11.44	273	23.1	2.6	18.7	19.5	20.0	20.9	22.5	24.3	25.4	26.1	27.2
12.0-12.9	12.47	203	23.9	2.8	19.5	20.4	21.0	21.9	23.7	25.7	26.8	27.6	28.8
13.0-13.9	13.47	188	24.7	2.9	20.5	21.3	22.0	22.9	24.8	26.8	28.0	28.8	30.1
14.0-14.9	14.49	181	25.4	2.9	21.3	22.2	22.8	23.8	25.7	27.7	28.8	29.7	30.9
15.0-15.9	15.45	179	25.9	2.8	22.0	22.8	23.5	24.4	26.2	28.2	29.3	30.1	31.3
16.0-16.9	16.45	194	26.4	2.7	22.4	23.2	23.8	24.7	26.5	28.4	29.5	30.2	31.4
17.0-17.9	17.45	190	26.9	2.8	22.6	23.4	24.0	24.9	26.7	28.6	29.7	30.5	31.6
18.0-18.9	18.45	169	27.2	2.7	23.0	23.8	24.4	25.3	27.0	28.9	29.9	30.6	31.8
19.0-19.9	19.43	155	27.2	2.7	23.1	23.9	24.5	25.3	27.0	28.9	29.9	30.6	31.7
20.0-29.9	24.96	1593	28.3	2.8	23.6	24.4	25.0	25.9	27.7	29.6	30.6	31.4	32.5
30.0-39.9	34.72	1423	28.6	2.8	24.4	25.3	25.9	26.9	28.7	30.6	31.7	32.5	33.6
40.0-49.9	44.35	1169	29.5	2.8	25.2	26.1	26.7	27.6	29.4	31.4	32.5	33.2	34.4
50.0-59.9	54.89	819	30.2	2.8	25.9	26.7	27.3	28.3	30.0	32.0	33.0	33.8	34.9
60.0-69.9	64.83	1105	30.4	2.6	26.4	27.2	27.8	28.7	30.4	32.2	33.3	34.0	35.1
70.0-79.9	74.16	774	30.4	2.4	26.8	27.6	28.1	29.0	30.6	32.3	33.2	33.9	34.9
80.0-90.9	84.09	539	30.6	2.2	27.1	27.8	28.3	29.1	30.5	32.1	32.9	33.5	34.4
Females													
2.0-2.9	2.45	548	15.4	1.3	13.0	13.4	13.7	14.1	15.0	15.9	16.4	16.8	17.3
3.0-3.9	3.46	565	15.8	1.4	13.9	14.3	14.6	15.1	16.0	16.9	17.5	17.9	18.4
4.0-4.9	4.43	527	16.4	1.4	14.7	15.1	15.4	15.9	16.8	17.8	18.3	18.7	19.3
5.0-5.9	5.46	542	17.4	1.5	15.3	15.8	16.1	16.6	17.6	18.7	19.3	19.7	20.4
6.0-6.9	6.47	274	18.4	1.8	15.7	16.3	16.7	17.2	18.4	19.7	20.4	20.9	21.6
7.0-7.9	7.44	261	19.5	2.0	16.2	16.8	17.2	17.9	19.2	20.6	21.4	21.9	22.8
8.0-8.9	8.47	245	20.7	2.2	16.8	17.5	17.9	18.7	20.1	21.6	22.5	23.1	24.0
9.0-9.9	9.43	270	21.7	2.4	17.6	18.3	18.8	19.6	21.1	22.7	23.6	24.2	25.2
10.0-10.9	10.43	254	22.7	2.5	18.6	19.4	19.9	20.7	22.3	24.0	25.0	25.6	26.7
11.0-11.9	11.46	280	23.7	2.6	19.6	20.4	21.0	21.8	23.5	25.4	26.4	27.2	28.3
12.0-12.9	12.46	216	24.5	2.8	20.5	21.4	22.0	22.9	24.7	26.7	27.8	28.5	29.7
13.0-13.9	13.45	224	25.2	2.9	21.2	22.1	22.7	23.7	25.6	27.6	28.8	29.6	30.9
14.0-14.9	14.47	219	25.8	3.0	21.7	22.6	23.2	24.2	26.2	28.3	29.5	30.3	31.6
15.0-15.9	15.47	188	26.3	3.0	21.8	22.8	23.4	24.4	26.4	28.5	29.8	30.6	31.9
16.0-16.9	16.46	218	26.7	3.1	21.8	22.8	23.4	24.4	26.4	28.6	29.8	30.7	32.0
17.0-17.9	17.45	209	27.0	3.2	21.8	22.7	23.4	24.4	26.5	28.7	29.9	30.8	32.2
18.0-18.9	18.43	181	27.2	3.3	21.9	22.9	23.5	24.6	26.6	28.9	30.1	31.0	32.4
19.0-19.9	19.48	187	27.4	3.3	22.1	23.1	23.8	24.8	26.9	29.2	30.4	31.3	32.7
20.0-29.9	24.91	1811	27.7	3.3	22.6	23.6	24.3	25.4	27.5	29.8	31.2	32.1	33.5
30.0-39.9	34.85	1786	28.4	3.4	23.4	24.4	25.2	26.3	28.5	30.9	32.3	33.2	34.7
40.0-49.9	44.28	1292	29.6	3.5	24.0	25.1	25.8	26.9	29.2	31.6	33.0	34.0	35.5
50.0-59.9	54.83	962	29.7	3.4	24.6	25.7	26.4	27.5	29.7	32.1	33.5	34.5	35.9
60.0-69.9	64.82	1079	30.1	3.3	25.1	26.1	26.8	27.9	30.0	32.3	33.6	34.5	35.9
70.0-79.9	74.46	854	30.0	3.1	25.4	26.4	27.0	28.1	30.1	32.2	33.4	34.3	35.6
80.0-90.9	84.45	562	29.8	2.8	25.6	26.5	27.1	28.1	29.9	31.8	32.9	33.7	34.9

Table IV.19.

Mean (M), standard deviation (SD), and percentiles of elbow breadth (mm) by age for males and females of 2 to 90 years

Age Group (years)	Mean Age (years)	N	M	SD	Percentiles								
					5th	10th	15th	25th	50th	75th	85th	90th	95th
Males												
2.0-2.9	2.46	564	44.4	2.8	39.5	40.5	41.1	42.1	44.0	45.9	47.0	47.8	48.9
3.0-3.9	3.45	490	45.1	2.9	40.6	41.5	42.2	43.2	45.2	47.2	48.3	49.1	50.3
4.0-4.9	4.47	547	46.5	3.0	42.0	43.0	43.7	44.8	46.7	48.8	50.0	50.8	52.0
5.0-5.9	5.43	495	48.5	3.3	43.8	44.9	45.6	46.8	49.0	51.3	52.6	53.5	54.8
6.0-6.9	6.45	260	50.8	3.7	45.6	46.8	47.7	49.0	51.5	54.1	55.5	56.5	58.1
7.0-7.9	7.47	272	53.4	4.1	47.2	48.6	49.5	50.9	53.6	56.4	58.0	59.1	60.8
8.0-8.9	8.46	259	55.9	4.4	48.7	50.1	51.1	52.5	55.4	58.3	60.0	61.2	62.9
9.0-9.9	9.50	282	58.6	4.6	50.4	51.8	52.8	54.3	57.3	60.4	62.1	63.3	65.2
10.0-10.9	10.45	288	60.8	4.8	52.2	53.7	54.7	56.3	59.4	62.6	64.4	65.7	67.6
11.0-11.9	11.44	274	63.0	5.0	54.4	56.0	57.1	58.8	62.0	65.4	67.2	68.6	70.5
12.0-12.9	12.47	203	65.0	5.0	57.1	58.7	59.8	61.5	64.8	68.3	70.3	71.6	73.6
13.0-13.9	13.47	189	66.7	4.9	59.7	61.3	62.4	64.1	67.4	70.8	72.7	74.1	76.1
14.0-14.9	14.49	185	68.2	4.7	61.8	63.4	64.5	66.1	69.3	72.6	74.5	75.7	77.7
15.0-15.9	15.45	179	69.4	4.6	63.1	64.6	65.7	67.3	70.3	73.5	75.3	76.5	78.4
16.0-16.9	16.45	194	70.4	4.6	63.6	65.1	66.2	67.7	70.8	73.9	75.7	76.9	78.8
17.0-17.9	17.45	191	71.1	4.7	63.6	65.2	66.2	67.8	70.9	74.1	75.9	77.2	79.1
18.0-18.9	18.45	170	71.7	4.8	63.8	65.3	66.4	68.0	71.1	74.4	76.2	77.4	79.3
19.0-19.9	19.43	158	72.1	4.6	64.3	65.8	66.8	68.4	71.5	74.6	76.4	77.6	79.4
20.0-29.9	24.96	1596	72.2	4.7	64.7	66.2	67.3	68.9	72.0	75.2	77.0	78.2	80.1
30.0-39.9	34.72	1426	71.6	4.7	65.4	67.0	68.1	69.7	72.8	76.1	77.9	79.2	81.1
40.0-49.9	44.35	1176	73.7	4.8	66.0	67.6	68.7	70.4	73.5	76.8	78.7	79.9	81.9
50.0-59.9	54.89	824	74.8	4.9	66.6	68.2	69.3	71.0	74.2	77.5	79.3	80.6	82.6
60.0-69.9	64.83	1120	75.0	4.9	67.1	68.7	69.8	71.5	74.7	78.0	79.8	81.1	83.0
70.0-79.9	74.16	791	74.8	4.8	67.5	69.1	70.2	71.9	75.0	78.3	80.2	81.4	83.3
80.0-90.9	84.09	557	74.8	4.7	67.9	69.5	70.5	72.2	75.3	78.5	80.3	81.6	83.5
Females												
2.0-2.9	2.45	545	41.9	2.9	37.6	38.5	39.2	40.1	42.0	44.0	45.1	45.8	47.0
3.0-3.9	3.46	567	43.4	3.2	39.0	40.0	40.8	41.8	44.0	46.2	47.4	48.3	49.6
4.0-4.9	4.43	525	45.2	3.3	40.0	41.1	41.8	42.9	45.1	47.3	48.6	49.5	50.8
5.0-5.9	5.46	542	47.3	3.6	41.5	42.7	43.5	44.7	47.0	49.4	50.8	51.7	53.2
6.0-6.9	6.47	275	49.5	3.9	43.0	44.3	45.2	46.5	49.0	51.7	53.2	54.3	55.9
7.0-7.9	7.44	264	51.6	4.2	44.5	45.8	46.8	48.2	50.9	53.8	55.4	56.5	58.2
8.0-8.9	8.47	246	53.8	4.3	46.4	47.8	48.7	50.2	53.0	55.9	57.6	58.7	60.5
9.0-9.9	9.43	268	55.6	4.3	48.5	49.9	50.9	52.3	55.1	58.0	59.6	60.8	62.5
10.0-10.9	10.43	256	57.2	4.1	51.0	52.3	53.3	54.7	57.4	60.3	61.9	63.0	64.6
11.0-11.9	11.46	283	58.7	4.1	53.1	54.4	55.4	56.8	59.5	62.3	63.9	65.0	66.7
12.0-12.9	12.46	216	59.9	4.2	54.2	55.6	56.6	58.0	60.8	63.8	65.4	66.5	68.2
13.0-13.9	13.45	225	60.8	4.4	54.5	55.9	56.9	58.4	61.3	64.4	66.1	67.3	69.1
14.0-14.9	14.47	220	61.5	4.5	54.4	55.9	56.9	58.4	61.4	64.5	66.2	67.4	69.2
15.0-15.9	15.47	189	62.1	4.5	54.5	56.0	57.0	58.5	61.5	64.6	66.3	67.5	69.3
16.0-16.9	16.46	217	62.4	4.5	54.7	56.1	57.1	58.7	61.6	64.6	66.3	67.5	69.3
17.0-17.9	17.45	210	62.6	4.5	54.8	56.3	57.3	58.8	61.7	64.8	66.5	67.7	69.5
18.0-18.9	18.43	183	62.6	4.7	54.6	56.2	57.2	58.8	61.8	65.0	66.8	68.1	69.9
19.0-19.9	19.48	187	62.6	4.7	54.8	56.3	57.4	59.0	62.0	65.3	67.1	68.3	70.2
20.0-29.9	24.91	1810	61.9	4.7	54.8	56.4	57.4	59.0	62.1	65.3	67.1	68.3	70.2
30.0-39.9	34.85	1798	63.6	4.8	56.4	58.0	59.1	60.7	63.9	67.2	69.0	70.3	72.3
40.0-49.9	44.28	1302	64.4	4.8	57.5	59.1	60.2	61.9	65.1	68.5	70.4	71.7	73.7
50.0-59.9	54.83	966	65.9	5.0	58.3	59.9	61.0	62.7	65.9	69.3	71.3	72.6	74.6
60.0-69.9	64.82	1094	66.7	5.0	58.5	60.1	61.2	62.9	66.2	69.6	71.5	72.8	74.8
70.0-79.9	74.46	873	66.2	5.0	58.2	59.8	60.9	62.6	65.9	69.3	71.2	72.5	74.5
80.0-90.9	84.45	590	65.2	4.8	57.6	59.2	60.3	61.9	65.0	68.4	70.2	71.5	73.4

Table IV.20.

Mean (M), standard deviation (SD), and percentiles of wrist breadth (mm) by age for males and females of 2 to 90 years

Age Group (years)	Mean Age (years)	N	M	SD	Percentiles								
					5th	10th	15th	25th	50th	75th	85th	90th	95th
Males													
2.0-2.9	2.46	564	36.7	2.4	32.3	33.1	33.6	34.4	36.0	37.7	38.6	39.2	40.2
3.0-3.9	3.45	490	37.4	2.4	34.1	34.9	35.5	36.3	37.9	39.6	40.6	41.2	42.2
4.0-4.9	4.47	547	38.6	2.5	35.2	36.1	36.7	37.5	39.2	41.0	42.0	42.7	43.7
5.0-5.9	5.43	493	40.1	2.8	36.2	37.2	37.8	38.8	40.6	42.6	43.7	44.5	45.6
6.0-6.9	6.45	260	41.9	3.1	37.5	38.5	39.2	40.3	42.3	44.4	45.6	46.5	47.7
7.0-7.9	7.47	272	43.8	3.2	38.9	40.0	40.7	41.8	43.9	46.1	47.3	48.2	49.5
8.0-8.9	8.46	258	45.7	3.3	40.2	41.3	42.0	43.1	45.2	47.5	48.7	49.6	50.9
9.0-9.9	9.50	282	47.6	3.4	41.5	42.6	43.3	44.4	46.6	48.9	50.2	51.1	52.5
10.0-10.9	10.45	288	49.3	3.6	42.6	43.8	44.6	45.8	48.1	50.6	52.0	52.9	54.4
11.0-11.9	11.44	274	50.9	3.9	44.1	45.3	46.2	47.5	50.0	52.7	54.2	55.2	56.8
12.0-12.9	12.47	203	52.5	4.0	46.1	47.4	48.3	49.7	52.3	55.1	56.7	57.8	59.4
13.0-13.9	13.47	189	53.7	3.9	48.3	49.6	50.5	51.9	54.5	57.3	58.8	59.9	61.5
14.0-14.9	14.49	185	54.9	3.6	50.4	51.6	52.5	53.8	56.2	58.8	60.2	61.2	62.7
15.0-15.9	15.45	179	55.8	3.4	51.7	52.8	53.6	54.8	57.0	59.4	60.7	61.6	62.9
16.0-16.9	16.45	194	56.6	3.3	51.8	52.9	53.7	54.9	57.1	59.4	60.7	61.5	62.9
17.0-17.9	17.45	191	57.2	3.3	51.9	53.0	53.8	54.9	57.1	59.3	60.6	61.5	62.8
18.0-18.9	18.45	169	57.3	3.2	52.1	53.2	53.9	55.0	57.1	59.3	60.5	61.3	62.6
19.0-19.9	19.43	158	57.2	3.2	52.3	53.4	54.1	55.2	57.4	59.6	60.8	61.7	63.0
20.0-29.9	24.96	1598	57.8	3.3	52.6	53.7	54.4	55.6	57.8	60.0	61.3	62.1	63.5
30.0-39.9	34.72	1424	58.5	3.4	53.1	54.2	55.0	56.2	58.4	60.7	62.0	62.9	64.3
40.0-49.9	44.35	1175	59.2	3.5	53.5	54.7	55.5	56.7	59.0	61.4	62.7	63.7	65.0
50.0-59.9	54.89	823	60.0	3.6	53.9	55.1	55.9	57.2	59.6	62.0	63.4	64.4	65.8
60.0-69.9	64.83	1121	60.2	3.7	54.3	55.5	56.3	57.6	60.0	62.6	64.0	65.0	66.4
70.0-79.9	74.16	793	60.4	3.8	54.6	55.8	56.7	58.0	60.4	63.0	64.5	65.4	66.9
80.0-90.9	84.09	560	61.0	3.8	54.8	56.1	57.0	58.3	60.8	63.4	64.9	65.9	67.4
Females													
2.0-2.9	2.45	545	34.4	2.3	30.5	31.2	31.8	32.5	34.0	35.6	36.4	37.0	37.9
3.0-3.9	3.46	568	35.8	2.7	31.9	32.8	33.4	34.3	36.1	38.0	39.1	39.8	40.9
4.0-4.9	4.43	527	37.5	2.6	33.7	34.5	35.1	36.0	37.7	39.5	40.5	41.2	42.3
5.0-5.9	5.46	542	39.3	2.8	35.1	36.0	36.6	37.6	39.4	41.3	42.3	43.1	44.2
6.0-6.9	6.47	275	41.1	3.1	36.1	37.1	37.8	38.8	40.8	42.9	44.1	44.9	46.2
7.0-7.9	7.44	262	42.7	3.3	37.2	38.2	38.9	40.0	42.1	44.3	45.6	46.5	47.8
8.0-8.9	8.47	246	44.4	3.3	38.7	39.7	40.4	41.5	43.7	45.9	47.1	48.0	49.3
9.0-9.9	9.43	267	45.7	3.2	40.4	41.4	42.1	43.2	45.3	47.5	48.7	49.6	50.8
10.0-10.9	10.43	256	47.0	3.1	42.3	43.3	44.0	45.1	47.2	49.3	50.5	51.4	52.6
11.0-11.9	11.46	283	48.0	3.2	43.8	44.8	45.6	46.7	48.8	51.0	52.3	53.1	54.4
12.0-12.9	12.46	216	48.9	3.2	44.7	45.8	46.6	47.7	49.8	52.1	53.4	54.2	55.5
13.0-13.9	13.45	225	49.5	3.2	44.9	46.0	46.7	47.8	49.9	52.2	53.4	54.3	55.6
14.0-14.9	14.47	219	50.0	3.3	44.9	46.0	46.7	47.9	50.0	52.3	53.5	54.4	55.7
15.0-15.9	15.47	188	50.3	3.1	45.2	46.2	46.9	48.0	50.0	52.1	53.3	54.1	55.3
16.0-16.9	16.46	217	50.5	3.1	45.3	46.3	47.0	48.0	50.0	52.1	53.2	54.1	55.3
17.0-17.9	17.45	210	50.6	3.1	45.4	46.4	47.1	48.1	50.1	52.2	53.4	54.2	55.4
18.0-18.9	18.43	183	50.6	3.1	45.3	46.3	47.1	48.1	50.2	52.3	53.5	54.3	55.5
19.0-19.9	19.48	187	50.5	3.0	45.5	46.5	47.2	48.2	50.2	52.3	53.4	54.2	55.4
20.0-29.9	24.91	1813	50.3	3.0	45.6	46.6	47.3	48.3	50.3	52.4	53.5	54.3	55.5
30.0-39.9	34.85	1797	50.8	3.1	46.3	47.3	48.0	49.1	51.2	53.3	54.5	55.4	56.6
40.0-49.9	44.28	1299	52.0	3.3	46.8	47.9	48.6	49.8	51.9	54.1	55.4	56.2	57.5
50.0-59.9	54.83	964	52.4	3.3	47.4	48.5	49.2	50.4	52.6	54.9	56.1	57.0	58.4
60.0-69.9	64.82	1093	53.1	3.4	47.8	48.9	49.7	50.8	53.1	55.4	56.7	57.6	59.0
70.0-79.9	74.46	873	53.2	3.4	48.1	49.3	50.0	51.2	53.5	55.8	57.2	58.1	59.4
80.0-90.9	84.45	591	53.7	3.4	48.4	49.5	50.3	51.5	53.8	56.1	57.5	58.4	59.7

Table IV.21.

Mean (M), standard deviation (SD), and percentiles of waist circumference (cm) by age for males and females of 2 to 90 years

Age Group (years)	Mean Age (years)	N	M	SD	Percentiles								
					5th	10th	15th	25th	50th	75th	85th	90th	95th
Males													
2.0-2.9	2.46	560	46.9	2.9	42.3	43.3	43.9	44.9	46.8	48.8	49.9	50.7	51.9
3.0-3.9	3.45	488	48.4	3.6	43.3	44.4	45.2	46.4	48.7	51.2	52.7	53.7	55.2
4.0-4.9	4.47	545	49.9	4.3	44.0	45.3	46.3	47.7	50.5	53.6	55.3	56.6	58.5
5.0-5.9	5.43	491	51.6	4.8	44.5	45.9	46.9	48.4	51.5	54.8	56.8	58.2	60.3
6.0-6.9	6.45	259	53.8	6.0	44.7	46.3	47.4	49.2	52.9	57.2	59.8	61.7	64.8
7.0-7.9	7.47	271	56.2	7.3	45.2	47.1	48.4	50.5	55.0	60.3	63.5	66.0	69.9
8.0-8.9	8.46	259	58.6	7.8	46.6	48.6	50.0	52.2	56.8	62.4	65.8	68.4	72.5
9.0-9.9	9.50	279	61.1	9.6	46.5	48.8	50.4	53.0	58.6	65.5	69.9	73.3	78.8
10.0-10.9	10.45	287	63.4	9.8	49.0	51.3	53.0	55.7	61.5	68.7	73.2	76.7	82.4
11.0-11.9	11.44	273	65.7	10.2	50.9	53.2	55.0	57.7	63.7	71.2	76.0	79.7	85.9
12.0-12.9	12.47	203	68.0	10.5	52.9	55.4	57.2	60.0	66.3	74.0	79.0	82.9	89.3
13.0-13.9	13.47	188	70.1	10.9	55.2	57.7	59.6	62.6	69.0	77.1	82.4	86.4	93.1
14.0-14.9	14.49	181	72.1	11.2	56.1	58.6	60.5	63.6	70.2	78.4	83.7	87.8	94.6
15.0-15.9	15.45	178	73.8	11.4	56.9	59.5	61.4	64.5	71.2	79.5	84.9	89.0	96.0
16.0-16.9	16.45	193	75.5	11.1	59.0	61.7	63.6	66.7	73.3	81.4	86.5	90.3	96.7
17.0-17.9	17.45	188	77.0	10.8	61.7	64.4	66.3	69.4	76.0	83.9	88.9	92.6	98.7
18.0-18.9	18.45	169	78.4	11.1	62.2	64.9	66.9	70.0	76.7	84.8	90.0	93.8	100.1
19.0-19.9	19.43	156	79.6	11.5	62.4	65.2	67.2	70.4	77.2	85.5	90.7	94.6	101.1
20.0-29.9	24.96	1589	84.9	12.2	67.8	70.7	72.9	76.4	83.8	92.8	98.5	102.7	109.8
30.0-39.9	34.72	1417	90.5	12.3	73.8	76.9	79.2	82.8	90.4	99.5	105.2	109.5	116.4
40.0-49.9	44.35	1168	94.5	12.6	76.7	79.9	82.2	85.8	93.5	102.7	108.5	112.8	119.7
50.0-59.9	54.89	819	97.0	11.9	80.2	83.3	85.5	89.0	96.3	105.0	110.3	114.3	120.6
60.0-69.9	64.83	1106	98.7	11.1	83.1	86.1	88.2	91.5	98.5	106.6	111.5	115.1	120.9
70.0-79.9	74.16	767	97.5	11.3	82.1	85.1	87.3	90.6	97.7	106.0	111.0	114.7	120.7
80.0-90.9	84.09	537	95.1	10.4	80.4	83.3	85.3	88.4	95.0	102.6	107.1	110.5	115.9
Females													
2.0-2.9	2.45	544	47.1	3.5	41.7	42.7	43.4	44.5	46.8	49.3	50.7	51.8	53.4
3.0-3.9	3.46	563	49.1	4.4	42.7	43.9	44.8	46.1	48.9	52.0	53.9	55.3	57.4
4.0-4.9	4.43	526	51.0	4.7	43.4	44.7	45.6	47.1	50.0	53.4	55.4	56.8	59.1
5.0-5.9	5.46	541	52.5	5.7	43.4	44.9	45.9	47.6	51.0	55.0	57.5	59.3	62.1
6.0-6.9	6.47	272	54.1	6.8	43.4	45.1	46.3	48.3	52.4	57.3	60.3	62.6	66.3
7.0-7.9	7.44	263	56.7	8.0	44.0	45.9	47.3	49.5	54.1	59.8	63.4	66.1	70.6
8.0-8.9	8.47	245	59.6	8.8	45.6	47.6	49.1	51.5	56.6	62.9	66.9	70.0	75.0
9.0-9.9	9.43	269	61.5	9.2	47.6	49.8	51.3	53.8	59.2	65.9	70.2	73.4	78.8
10.0-10.9	10.43	252	63.7	9.5	50.1	52.3	54.0	56.6	62.2	69.2	73.6	77.0	82.7
11.0-11.9	11.46	280	68.1	10.1	52.5	54.9	56.6	59.3	65.3	72.5	77.2	80.7	86.6
12.0-12.9	12.46	215	71.0	10.6	54.7	57.1	58.9	61.8	68.0	75.7	80.6	84.3	90.5
13.0-13.9	13.45	224	73.4	11.2	56.3	58.9	60.8	63.8	70.3	78.4	83.6	87.5	94.1
14.0-14.9	14.47	219	74.5	11.6	57.6	60.2	62.2	65.3	72.1	80.6	86.0	90.2	97.2
15.0-15.9	15.47	187	75.8	12.0	58.3	61.1	63.1	66.3	73.3	82.1	87.8	92.2	99.5
16.0-16.9	16.46	218	76.0	12.3	58.6	61.5	63.5	66.8	74.1	83.2	89.1	93.6	101.3
17.0-17.9	17.45	204	77.3	12.7	58.7	61.5	63.6	67.0	74.4	83.7	89.8	94.5	102.5
18.0-18.9	18.43	181	78.2	12.9	59.6	62.5	64.6	68.1	75.6	85.1	91.3	96.1	104.2
19.0-19.9	19.48	186	78.4	12.4	61.2	64.0	66.2	69.6	77.0	86.2	92.2	96.8	104.6
20.0-29.9	24.91	1810	82.4	13.8	62.4	65.4	67.7	71.4	79.4	89.5	96.2	101.4	110.1
30.0-39.9	34.85	1785	88.3	15.2	66.8	70.2	72.7	76.7	85.6	96.9	104.3	110.1	120.0
40.0-49.9	44.28	1288	91.5	14.4	71.9	75.3	77.7	81.7	90.4	101.2	108.2	113.5	122.5
50.0-59.9	54.83	962	94.2	14.2	74.9	78.3	80.7	84.7	93.3	103.9	110.7	115.9	124.6
60.0-69.9	64.82	1076	94.9	13.4	76.6	79.9	82.3	86.1	94.3	104.2	110.5	115.3	123.2
70.0-79.9	74.46	852	93.3	13.0	75.8	79.0	81.3	85.1	93.0	102.7	108.8	113.4	121.0
80.0-90.9	84.45	555	89.8	10.8	74.9	77.7	79.8	83.0	89.7	97.6	102.5	106.2	112.1

Postnatal Anthropometric Reference

Table IV.22.

Mean (M), standard deviation (SD), and percentiles of buttocks (hip) circumference (cm) by age for males and females of 2 to 90 years

Age Group (years)	Mean Age (years)	N	M	SD	Percentiles								
					5th	10th	15th	25th	50th	75th	85th	90th	95th
Males													
2.0-2.9	2.46	559	49.8	3.2	44.4	45.5	46.3	47.4	49.5	51.7	52.9	53.7	54.9
3.0-3.9	3.45	488	51.2	3.7	45.4	46.6	47.5	48.8	51.2	53.7	55.1	56.0	57.5
4.0-4.9	4.47	543	53.1	4.1	47.2	48.6	49.5	51.0	53.7	56.6	58.1	59.2	60.8
5.0-5.9	5.43	490	55.7	5.0	48.1	49.7	50.9	52.6	55.9	59.3	61.2	62.5	64.5
6.0-6.9	6.45	258	59.1	5.3	50.4	52.1	53.3	55.1	58.6	62.1	64.1	65.5	67.5
7.0-7.9	7.47	271	62.8	5.6	53.1	54.9	56.2	58.1	61.8	65.6	67.7	69.1	71.2
8.0-8.9	8.46	257	66.5	5.9	56.0	58.0	59.3	61.3	65.2	69.2	71.4	72.9	75.2
9.0-9.9	9.50	279	70.3	6.3	59.1	61.1	62.5	64.7	68.7	72.9	75.3	76.9	79.3
10.0-10.9	10.45	287	73.8	6.9	61.3	63.5	65.1	67.4	71.8	76.5	79.0	80.8	83.4
11.0-11.9	11.44	272	77.1	7.2	64.0	66.4	68.0	70.4	75.1	79.9	82.6	84.4	87.1
12.0-12.9	12.47	203	80.3	7.5	67.1	69.6	71.3	73.8	78.7	83.7	86.5	88.4	91.3
13.0-13.9	13.47	188	83.1	7.8	70.4	72.9	74.6	77.2	82.3	87.6	90.6	92.6	95.8
14.0-14.9	14.49	181	85.6	8.0	73.3	75.9	77.7	80.4	85.6	91.2	94.3	96.5	99.7
15.0-15.9	15.45	177	87.7	8.2	75.3	78.0	79.8	82.6	88.0	93.7	96.9	99.1	102.5
16.0-16.9	16.45	193	89.5	7.9	77.2	79.7	81.5	84.2	89.3	94.8	97.8	99.9	103.1
17.0-17.9	17.45	189	91.1	8.0	78.0	80.5	82.3	84.9	90.1	95.6	98.6	100.7	103.9
18.0-18.9	18.45	169	92.3	8.1	79.2	81.8	83.6	86.3	91.5	97.0	100.1	102.3	105.5
19.0-19.9	19.43	155	93.3	8.1	80.3	83.0	84.8	87.5	92.9	98.5	101.6	103.8	107.1
20.0-29.9	24.96	1588	95.5	8.3	81.3	83.9	85.7	88.5	93.9	99.5	102.7	105.0	108.3
30.0-39.9	34.72	1417	95.9	8.4	83.1	85.8	87.7	90.5	96.0	101.8	105.0	107.3	110.8
40.0-49.9	44.35	1169	97.8	8.6	84.1	86.8	88.7	91.6	97.1	103.1	106.4	108.7	112.2
50.0-59.9	54.89	821	98.0	8.6	84.4	87.2	89.1	91.9	97.5	103.5	106.8	109.1	112.6
60.0-69.9	64.83	1107	97.3	8.4	84.3	87.0	88.8	91.7	97.1	103.0	106.2	108.5	111.9
70.0-79.9	74.16	766	96.7	8.3	83.4	86.0	87.9	90.6	96.1	101.8	105.0	107.3	110.7
80.0-90.9	84.09	536	95.1	8.1	82.4	85.0	86.8	89.5	94.8	100.4	103.5	105.7	109.0
Females													
2.0-2.9	2.45	545	50.8	3.8	45.0	46.2	47.1	48.4	50.8	53.4	54.9	55.9	57.4
3.0-3.9	3.46	561	51.0	4.3	44.1	45.4	46.4	47.8	50.6	53.6	55.2	56.4	58.1
4.0-4.9	4.43	524	52.9	4.9	44.8	46.4	47.5	49.1	52.3	55.7	57.6	58.9	60.9
5.0-5.9	5.46	543	56.1	5.7	46.9	48.6	49.9	51.7	55.4	59.3	61.5	63.1	65.4
6.0-6.9	6.47	272	60.0	6.5	49.6	51.6	53.0	55.1	59.3	63.7	66.3	68.0	70.7
7.0-7.9	7.44	263	64.1	7.2	52.7	54.9	56.4	58.8	63.4	68.4	71.2	73.2	76.2
8.0-8.9	8.47	245	68.6	8.0	56.1	58.6	60.3	62.8	67.9	73.5	76.6	78.8	82.2
9.0-9.9	9.43	268	72.7	8.6	59.4	62.0	63.8	66.6	72.1	78.0	81.4	83.8	87.5
10.0-10.9	10.43	254	76.9	9.1	62.7	65.4	67.4	70.3	76.2	82.5	86.1	88.7	92.6
11.0-11.9	11.46	280	80.7	9.6	65.8	68.7	70.7	73.8	80.0	86.6	90.4	93.1	97.2
12.0-12.9	12.46	216	84.0	9.9	68.6	71.6	73.7	76.9	83.3	90.2	94.1	96.9	101.1
13.0-13.9	13.45	225	87.0	10.2	71.0	74.1	76.3	79.6	86.2	93.2	97.3	100.1	104.4
14.0-14.9	14.47	219	89.5	10.4	73.2	76.4	78.6	81.9	88.6	95.8	99.9	102.8	107.2
15.0-15.9	15.47	187	91.6	10.5	75.0	78.2	80.4	83.9	90.6	97.9	102.0	104.9	109.4
16.0-16.9	16.46	218	93.2	10.6	76.4	79.7	81.9	85.4	92.2	99.5	103.7	106.6	111.1
17.0-17.9	17.45	205	94.5	10.7	77.5	80.8	83.1	86.6	93.4	100.8	105.0	108.0	112.5
18.0-18.9	18.43	181	95.5	10.8	78.4	81.6	83.9	87.4	94.3	101.8	106.0	109.0	113.5
19.0-19.9	19.48	186	96.2	10.8	78.9	82.3	84.6	88.1	95.0	102.5	106.8	109.8	114.4
20.0-29.9	24.91	1810	97.3	11.0	79.9	83.3	85.6	89.2	96.2	103.8	108.1	111.2	115.8
30.0-39.9	34.85	1782	99.7	12.0	81.1	84.7	87.2	91.1	98.8	107.1	111.9	115.3	120.4
40.0-49.9	44.28	1293	102.6	12.5	83.2	87.0	89.6	93.7	101.7	110.3	115.3	118.8	124.2
50.0-59.9	54.83	961	102.3	12.7	83.0	86.8	89.5	93.6	101.8	110.6	115.6	119.2	124.7
60.0-69.9	64.82	1078	100.8	12.4	81.7	85.5	88.1	92.1	100.0	108.6	113.6	117.0	122.4
70.0-79.9	74.46	854	99.2	11.5	80.8	84.3	86.7	90.5	97.8	105.7	110.3	113.4	118.3
80.0-90.9	84.45	557	96.5	11.2	78.6	82.0	84.4	88.0	95.1	102.8	107.2	110.3	115.1

146

Table IV.23.
Mean (M), standard deviation (SD), and percentiles of waist to buttocks ratio by age for males and females of 2 to 90 years

Age Group (years)	Mean Age (years)	N	M	SD	Percentiles								
					5th	10th	15th	25th	50th	75th	85th	90th	95th
Males													
2.0-2.9	2.46	554	0.93	0.1	0.87	0.88	0.90	0.91	0.94	0.98	1.00	1.01	1.03
3.0-3.9	3.45	487	0.92	0.0	0.87	0.89	0.90	0.91	0.94	0.97	0.99	1.00	1.02
4.0-4.9	4.47	543	0.92	0.0	0.86	0.88	0.89	0.90	0.93	0.96	0.98	0.99	1.01
5.0-5.9	5.43	489	0.91	0.0	0.85	0.87	0.88	0.89	0.92	0.95	0.97	0.98	1.00
6.0-6.9	6.45	258	0.90	0.1	0.83	0.85	0.86	0.88	0.91	0.94	0.96	0.97	0.99
7.0-7.9	7.47	271	0.88	0.1	0.82	0.83	0.85	0.86	0.90	0.93	0.95	0.96	0.98
8.0-8.9	8.46	257	0.87	0.1	0.80	0.82	0.83	0.85	0.88	0.92	0.94	0.95	0.98
9.0-9.9	9.50	279	0.86	0.1	0.79	0.80	0.82	0.84	0.87	0.91	0.93	0.95	0.97
10.0-10.9	10.45	287	0.85	0.1	0.77	0.79	0.81	0.83	0.86	0.90	0.92	0.94	0.96
11.0-11.9	11.44	272	0.85	0.1	0.76	0.78	0.80	0.82	0.85	0.89	0.92	0.93	0.95
12.0-12.9	12.47	203	0.84	0.1	0.76	0.78	0.79	0.81	0.85	0.89	0.91	0.92	0.95
13.0-13.9	13.47	188	0.83	0.1	0.75	0.77	0.78	0.80	0.84	0.88	0.90	0.92	0.94
14.0-14.9	14.49	181	0.83	0.1	0.75	0.77	0.78	0.80	0.84	0.88	0.90	0.92	0.94
15.0-15.9	15.45	176	0.83	0.1	0.75	0.77	0.78	0.80	0.84	0.88	0.90	0.91	0.94
16.0-16.9	16.45	192	0.82	0.1	0.75	0.77	0.78	0.80	0.84	0.88	0.90	0.91	0.94
17.0-17.9	17.45	188	0.83	0.1	0.75	0.77	0.78	0.80	0.84	0.88	0.90	0.91	0.94
18.0-18.9	18.45	169	0.84	0.1	0.76	0.78	0.79	0.81	0.84	0.88	0.90	0.92	0.94
19.0-19.9	19.43	155	0.84	0.1	0.76	0.78	0.79	0.81	0.85	0.89	0.91	0.92	0.94
20.0-29.9	24.96	1585	0.88	0.1	0.79	0.81	0.82	0.85	0.88	0.92	0.94	0.95	0.97
30.0-39.9	34.72	1413	0.93	0.1	0.82	0.85	0.87	0.90	0.94	0.98	1.01	1.02	1.04
40.0-49.9	44.35	1167	0.95	0.1	0.85	0.88	0.90	0.92	0.97	1.01	1.03	1.04	1.06
50.0-59.9	54.89	819	0.97	0.1	0.88	0.91	0.92	0.95	0.99	1.03	1.05	1.07	1.09
60.0-69.9	64.83	1103	0.98	0.1	0.89	0.92	0.93	0.96	1.00	1.04	1.07	1.08	1.10
70.0-79.9	74.16	764	0.99	0.1	0.89	0.92	0.93	0.96	1.00	1.05	1.07	1.08	1.11
80.0-90.9	84.09	535	0.98	0.1	0.89	0.91	0.93	0.95	1.00	1.04	1.06	1.08	1.10
Females													
2.0-2.9	2.45	543	0.93	0.1	0.87	0.89	0.90	0.91	0.95	0.98	1.00	1.02	1.04
3.0-3.9	3.46	560	0.92	0.1	0.86	0.88	0.89	0.91	0.94	0.97	0.99	1.00	1.02
4.0-4.9	4.43	523	0.91	0.1	0.85	0.87	0.88	0.90	0.93	0.96	0.98	0.99	1.01
5.0-5.9	5.46	541	0.89	0.1	0.84	0.85	0.86	0.88	0.91	0.94	0.96	0.97	0.99
6.0-6.9	6.47	271	0.88	0.1	0.82	0.84	0.85	0.86	0.89	0.93	0.94	0.96	0.98
7.0-7.9	7.44	263	0.86	0.1	0.80	0.82	0.83	0.85	0.88	0.91	0.93	0.94	0.96
8.0-8.9	8.47	245	0.85	0.1	0.79	0.80	0.81	0.83	0.86	0.90	0.91	0.93	0.95
9.0-9.9	9.43	268	0.83	0.1	0.77	0.79	0.80	0.82	0.85	0.88	0.90	0.92	0.94
10.0-10.9	10.43	252	0.82	0.1	0.75	0.77	0.78	0.80	0.84	0.87	0.89	0.91	0.93
11.0-11.9	11.46	280	0.81	0.1	0.74	0.76	0.77	0.79	0.83	0.86	0.88	0.90	0.92
12.0-12.9	12.46	215	0.80	0.1	0.73	0.75	0.76	0.78	0.82	0.86	0.88	0.89	0.92
13.0-13.9	13.45	224	0.80	0.1	0.72	0.74	0.75	0.77	0.81	0.85	0.87	0.89	0.91
14.0-14.9	14.47	219	0.79	0.1	0.71	0.73	0.75	0.77	0.81	0.85	0.87	0.89	0.91
15.0-15.9	15.47	187	0.79	0.1	0.71	0.73	0.74	0.76	0.81	0.85	0.87	0.89	0.92
16.0-16.9	16.46	218	0.79	0.1	0.71	0.73	0.74	0.76	0.80	0.85	0.87	0.89	0.92
17.0-17.9	17.45	203	0.79	0.1	0.70	0.72	0.74	0.76	0.80	0.85	0.88	0.89	0.92
18.0-18.9	18.43	181	0.79	0.1	0.70	0.72	0.74	0.76	0.81	0.85	0.88	0.90	0.93
19.0-19.9	19.48	186	0.79	0.1	0.70	0.73	0.74	0.76	0.81	0.86	0.88	0.90	0.93
20.0-29.9	24.91	1809	0.82	0.1	0.72	0.74	0.76	0.78	0.83	0.88	0.91	0.93	0.96
30.0-39.9	34.85	1781	0.84	0.1	0.74	0.77	0.78	0.81	0.86	0.91	0.94	0.96	0.99
40.0-49.9	44.28	1288	0.86	0.1	0.76	0.79	0.80	0.83	0.88	0.93	0.96	0.98	1.01
50.0-59.9	54.83	960	0.89	0.1	0.79	0.81	0.83	0.86	0.90	0.96	0.99	1.01	1.04
60.0-69.9	64.82	1074	0.91	0.1	0.81	0.83	0.85	0.88	0.93	0.98	1.01	1.03	1.07
70.0-79.9	74.46	851	0.92	0.1	0.81	0.84	0.85	0.88	0.93	0.98	1.01	1.03	1.06
80.0-90.9	84.45	555	0.91	0.1	0.82	0.84	0.86	0.88	0.93	0.98	1.00	1.02	1.05

Table IV.24.

Mean (M), standard deviation (SD), and percentiles of thigh circumference (cm) by age for males and females of 2 to 90 years

Age Group (years)	Mean Age (years)	N	M	SD	5th	10th	15th	25th	50th	75th	85th	90th	95th
Males													
2.0-2.9	2.46	556	28.0	2.3	24.5	25.2	25.7	26.4	27.9	29.5	30.4	31.1	32.1
3.0-3.9	3.45	487	28.5	2.4	24.8	25.6	26.1	26.9	28.4	30.1	31.1	31.8	32.8
4.0-4.9	4.47	542	29.5	2.8	25.3	26.1	26.7	27.6	29.4	31.3	32.4	33.2	34.4
5.0-5.9	5.43	488	30.9	3.2	25.9	26.8	27.5	28.5	30.6	32.8	34.1	35.1	36.5
6.0-6.9	6.45	259	32.5	3.8	26.7	27.8	28.6	29.8	32.1	34.8	36.3	37.4	39.0
7.0-7.9	7.47	271	34.4	4.3	27.7	29.0	29.8	31.2	33.9	36.9	38.7	39.9	41.8
8.0-8.9	8.46	257	36.3	4.8	28.9	30.2	31.2	32.7	35.7	39.1	41.0	42.4	44.6
9.0-9.9	9.50	279	38.3	5.3	30.2	31.7	32.7	34.4	37.7	41.4	43.5	45.1	47.5
10.0-10.9	10.45	287	40.2	5.6	31.5	33.1	34.2	35.9	39.5	43.4	45.8	47.4	50.0
11.0-11.9	11.44	271	42.0	5.9	32.9	34.5	35.7	37.6	41.3	45.4	47.9	49.6	52.3
12.0-12.9	12.47	202	43.8	6.1	34.4	36.1	37.3	39.3	43.1	47.4	49.9	51.7	54.4
13.0-13.9	13.47	188	45.3	6.2	35.8	37.6	38.8	40.8	44.7	49.0	51.6	53.4	56.2
14.0-14.9	14.49	181	46.7	6.2	37.2	39.0	40.3	42.2	46.2	50.5	53.0	54.8	57.6
15.0-15.9	15.45	176	47.9	6.1	38.5	40.3	41.6	43.5	47.4	51.7	54.2	55.9	58.7
16.0-16.9	16.45	193	48.9	6.0	39.8	41.5	42.7	44.6	48.5	52.7	55.1	56.9	59.5
17.0-17.9	17.45	189	49.8	5.9	40.9	42.6	43.8	45.6	49.4	53.5	55.9	57.6	60.2
18.0-18.9	18.45	169	50.5	5.7	41.7	43.4	44.6	46.4	50.1	54.1	56.4	58.0	60.5
19.0-19.9	19.43	155	51.0	5.6	42.4	44.1	45.3	47.0	50.6	54.5	56.7	58.3	60.7
20.0-29.9	24.96	1584	51.4	5.1	43.8	45.2	46.3	47.9	51.1	54.7	56.9	58.4	60.7
30.0-39.9	34.72	1419	50.9	5.1	43.9	45.3	46.4	48.0	51.2	54.9	57.0	58.5	60.9
40.0-49.9	44.35	1165	51.5	4.9	44.1	45.5	46.6	48.1	51.2	54.7	56.8	58.2	60.5
50.0-59.9	54.89	819	49.8	4.8	42.8	44.2	45.2	46.7	49.8	53.2	55.2	56.7	58.9
60.0-69.9	64.83	1095	48.7	4.7	41.8	43.1	44.1	45.6	48.6	51.9	53.9	55.3	57.5
70.0-79.9	74.16	758	46.9	4.8	39.8	41.2	42.2	43.7	46.7	50.2	52.2	53.7	55.9
80.0-90.9	84.09	522	45.0	4.1	38.9	40.1	40.9	42.2	44.9	47.8	49.6	50.8	52.7
Females													
2.0-2.9	2.45	544	28.3	2.5	24.6	25.3	25.9	26.6	28.2	30.0	31.0	31.8	33.0
3.0-3.9	3.46	562	28.4	3.0	24.0	24.9	25.4	26.3	28.2	30.3	31.6	32.5	33.9
4.0-4.9	4.43	526	29.3	3.4	24.3	25.2	25.9	26.9	29.0	31.5	33.0	34.1	35.9
5.0-5.9	5.46	543	31.0	4.0	25.2	26.2	27.0	28.1	30.6	33.4	35.2	36.5	38.6
6.0-6.9	6.47	274	32.9	4.4	26.5	27.6	28.5	29.7	32.5	35.7	37.7	39.2	41.6
7.0-7.9	7.44	262	34.9	4.9	28.0	29.2	30.1	31.5	34.4	38.0	40.3	41.9	44.6
8.0-8.9	8.47	246	37.2	5.3	29.6	30.9	31.9	33.4	36.6	40.5	43.0	44.8	47.8
9.0-9.9	9.43	267	39.2	5.7	31.1	32.5	33.6	35.2	38.6	42.8	45.4	47.3	50.5
10.0-10.9	10.43	254	41.1	5.9	33.4	34.6	35.6	37.1	40.6	45.2	48.4	51.0	55.8
11.0-11.9	11.46	281	42.9	6.1	34.9	36.3	37.2	38.8	42.4	47.2	50.4	53.1	57.9
12.0-12.9	12.46	214	44.5	6.3	36.3	37.6	38.6	40.3	44.0	48.9	52.2	55.0	59.9
13.0-13.9	13.45	225	45.8	6.4	37.4	38.8	39.9	41.6	45.3	50.3	53.7	56.5	61.5
14.0-14.9	14.47	219	46.9	6.5	38.5	39.9	41.0	42.7	46.5	51.5	54.9	57.7	62.6
15.0-15.9	15.47	185	47.8	6.6	39.3	40.7	41.8	43.5	47.4	52.5	55.9	58.7	63.7
16.0-16.9	16.46	216	48.5	6.6	39.9	41.4	42.4	44.2	48.1	53.2	56.8	59.6	64.6
17.0-17.9	17.45	205	49.1	7.0	39.6	41.3	42.5	44.4	48.6	53.9	57.4	60.0	64.5
18.0-18.9	18.43	180	49.5	7.0	40.0	41.7	42.9	44.8	49.0	54.3	57.7	60.3	64.7
19.0-19.9	19.48	184	49.7	7.0	40.3	41.9	43.1	45.1	49.3	54.6	58.0	60.6	65.0
20.0-29.9	24.91	1809	50.1	7.1	40.5	42.2	43.4	45.3	49.6	54.9	58.3	60.9	65.4
30.0-39.9	34.85	1773	51.1	7.2	41.2	42.9	44.1	46.1	50.5	55.8	59.3	62.0	66.5
40.0-49.9	44.28	1282	51.2	7.2	41.5	43.2	44.5	46.5	50.8	56.3	59.8	62.5	67.0
50.0-59.9	54.83	957	50.7	7.2	41.1	42.8	44.1	46.1	50.4	55.8	59.2	61.9	66.4
60.0-69.9	64.82	1073	49.1	6.9	39.8	41.4	42.6	44.5	48.7	53.9	57.3	59.8	64.2
70.0-79.9	74.46	848	47.6	6.7	38.6	40.2	41.3	43.2	47.2	52.3	55.5	58.0	62.3
80.0-90.9	84.45	547	45.4	6.4	37.0	38.5	39.6	41.4	45.3	50.1	53.3	55.7	59.7

Table IV.25.

Mean (M), standard deviation (SD), and percentiles of triceps skinfold thickness (mm) by age for males and females of 2 to 90 years

Age Group (years)	Mean Age (years)	N	M	SD	Percentiles								
					5th	10th	15th	25th	50th	75th	85th	90th	95th
Males													
2.0-2.9	2.46	550	8.4	2.1	6.0	6.4	6.8	7.4	8.6	10.3	11.3	12.2	13.6
3.0-3.9	3.45	483	8.4	2.2	5.7	6.2	6.6	7.2	8.5	10.2	11.4	12.3	13.9
4.0-4.9	4.47	542	8.5	2.5	5.3	5.8	6.1	6.7	8.1	10.0	11.2	12.2	14.0
5.0-5.9	5.43	492	8.8	3.1	4.9	5.4	5.8	6.4	8.0	10.4	12.0	13.4	16.0
6.0-6.9	6.45	258	9.2	4.0	4.4	5.0	5.4	6.1	8.1	11.0	13.4	15.4	19.4
7.0-7.9	7.47	271	9.6	4.7	4.2	4.7	5.2	6.0	8.1	11.7	14.7	17.4	23.0
8.0-8.9	8.46	259	9.9	5.1	4.2	4.8	5.3	6.2	8.5	12.5	15.9	19.1	26.0
9.0-9.9	9.50	282	10.2	5.3	4.6	5.2	5.8	6.7	9.3	13.7	17.5	21.1	28.7
10.0-10.9	10.45	287	10.4	5.4	5.0	5.7	6.3	7.3	10.1	14.9	19.1	22.9	31.3
11.0-11.9	11.44	274	10.6	5.6	5.2	5.9	6.6	7.7	10.7	15.9	20.4	24.7	34.1
12.0-12.9	12.47	201	10.6	6.0	5.0	5.7	6.3	7.5	10.5	16.0	21.0	25.8	36.6
13.0-13.9	13.47	189	10.7	6.3	4.4	5.2	5.7	6.8	9.8	15.2	20.3	25.4	37.3
14.0-14.9	14.49	179	10.6	6.5	3.9	4.5	5.1	6.0	8.8	13.9	18.8	23.8	35.8
15.0-15.9	15.45	178	10.6	6.3	3.7	4.3	4.8	5.7	8.2	12.9	17.4	21.8	32.5
16.0-16.9	16.45	192	10.5	6.2	3.8	4.4	4.9	5.8	8.4	13.1	17.5	21.9	32.2
17.0-17.9	17.45	190	10.4	6.0	4.0	4.7	5.2	6.1	8.7	13.5	17.8	22.1	32.0
18.0-18.9	18.45	167	10.2	5.9	3.7	4.4	5.0	6.1	8.8	13.2	16.8	19.9	26.0
19.0-19.9	19.43	155	10.1	5.8	3.9	4.6	5.2	6.2	9.0	13.6	17.3	20.5	26.7
20.0-29.9	24.96	1566	9.8	5.1	4.3	5.2	6.0	7.2	10.2	14.4	17.3	19.7	23.6
30.0-39.9	34.72	1408	11.5	5.8	4.7	5.6	6.4	7.7	10.8	15.1	18.1	20.5	24.5
40.0-49.9	44.35	1159	12.1	5.7	5.2	6.2	7.0	8.3	11.5	15.7	18.6	20.9	24.7
50.0-59.9	54.89	817	12.3	5.7	5.4	6.4	7.2	8.5	11.7	15.9	18.8	21.0	24.7
60.0-69.9	64.83	1125	12.5	5.6	5.5	6.5	7.3	8.6	11.6	15.6	18.3	20.4	24.0
70.0-79.9	74.16	821	12.0	5.2	5.5	6.5	7.2	8.5	11.4	15.2	17.8	19.8	23.2
80.0-90.9	84.09	637	11.2	4.8	5.4	6.3	7.0	8.2	10.9	14.5	16.9	18.7	21.8
Females													
2.0-2.9	2.45	536	9.5	2.3	5.9	6.5	6.9	7.6	8.9	10.5	11.5	12.2	13.3
3.0-3.9	3.46	555	9.0	2.6	5.6	6.3	6.7	7.5	9.1	10.9	12.1	12.9	14.2
4.0-4.9	4.43	528	9.1	2.9	5.1	5.8	6.3	7.1	8.9	11.1	12.4	13.4	15.0
5.0-5.9	5.46	541	9.5	3.5	4.9	5.6	6.2	7.1	9.2	11.7	13.3	14.5	16.4
6.0-6.9	6.47	273	10.1	4.1	4.8	5.6	6.2	7.3	9.6	12.5	14.4	15.9	18.2
7.0-7.9	7.44	263	10.9	4.7	4.7	5.6	6.3	7.4	10.0	13.4	15.6	17.2	19.9
8.0-8,9	8 47	245	11.8	5.4	4.8	5.7	6.5	7.7	10.6	14.3	16.8	18.7	21.8
9.0-9.9	9.43	266	12.7	6.0	5.0	6.0	6.8	8.1	11.3	15.4	18.2	20.3	23.7
10.0-10.9	10.43	254	13.6	6.5	5.4	6.5	7.4	8.8	12.2	16.7	19.7	22.0	25.8
11.0-11.9	11.46	281	14.5	6.7	6.0	7.2	8.1	9.7	13.3	18.1	21.3	23.7	27.7
12.0-12.9	12.46	216	15.4	6.8	6.7	8.0	9.0	10.6	14.4	19.4	22.6	25.0	29.1
13.0-13.9	13.45	225	16.1	6.8	7.5	8.8	9.9	11.6	15.5	20.4	23.7	26.1	30.1
14.0-14.9	14.47	218	16.8	6.8	8.3	9.7	10.8	12.5	16.5	21.5	24.8	27.2	31.2
15.0-15.9	15.47	187	17.5	6.9	8.9	10.4	11.5	13.3	17.4	22.6	25.9	28.4	32.5
16.0-16.9	16.46	216	18.0	7.1	9.1	10.6	11.7	13.6	17.8	23.2	26.6	29.2	33.4
17.0-17.9	17.45	202	18.5	7.6	8.8	10.4	11.5	13.5	17.8	23.4	27.0	29.7	34.1
18.0-18.9	18.43	178	18.9	7.7	9.0	10.5	11.7	13.6	17.9	23.5	27.0	29.7	34.0
19.0-19.9	19.48	183	19.3	7.9	9.0	10.5	11.7	13.6	18.0	23.6	27.2	29.9	34.3
20.0-29.9	24.91	1767	20.8	8.0	10.2	12.0	13.4	15.7	20.5	26.3	29.9	32.4	36.6
30.0-39.9	34.85	1702	23.6	8.2	10.8	13.6	15.5	18.4	23.9	29.5	32.6	34.7	37.8
40.0-49.9	44.28	1231	26.0	8.2	12.7	15.5	17.4	20.3	25.7	31.2	34.2	36.3	39.4
50.0-59.9	54.83	930	26.3	7.9	13.6	16.3	18.1	20.9	26.1	31.4	34.2	36.2	39.1
60.0-69.9	64.82	1092	24.2	7.3	12.7	15.3	17.1	19 7	24.7	29.8	32.6	34.5	37.3
70.0-79.9	74.46	903	22.1	7.3	10.4	12.8	14.6	17.1	21.9	26.9	29.6	31.4	34.1
80.0-90.9	84.45	698	17.7	6.9	6.7	8.9	10.5	12.9	17.4	22.0	24.5	26.3	28.8

Table IV.26.

Mean (M), standard deviation (SD), and percentiles of subscapular skinfold thickness (mm) by age for males and females of 2 to 90 years

Age Group (years)	Mean Age (years)	N	M	SD	Percentiles								
					5th	10th	15th	25th	50th	75th	85th	90th	95th
Males													
2.0-2.9	2.46	544	6.2	1.8	3.8	4.2	4.5	5.0	6.0	7.3	8.1	8.7	9.7
3.0-3.9	3.45	483	5.9	1.7	3.5	3.9	4.2	4.7	5.7	7.0	7.7	8.3	9.2
4.0-4.9	4.47	541	5.8	1.8	3.3	3.7	4.0	4.5	5.5	6.8	7.5	8.1	9.1
5.0-5.9	5.43	490	5.7	2.3	2.8	3.2	3.6	4.1	5.4	7.2	8.3	9.1	10.6
6.0-6.9	6.45	258	6.0	2.7	2.6	3.1	3.5	4.1	5.5	7.4	8.7	9.6	11.3
7.0-7.9	7.47	270	6.4	2.9	2.7	3.1	3.5	4.1	5.6	7.6	8.9	9.9	11.6
8.0-8.9	8.46	258	6.8	3.0	2.8	3.3	3.6	4.3	5.8	7.8	9.2	10.3	12.1
9.0-9.9	9.50	276	7.3	3.3	2.9	3.4	3.8	4.5	6.1	8.2	9.7	10.8	12.7
10.0-10.9	10.45	287	7.9	3.6	3.0	3.6	4.0	4.7	6.4	8.6	10.2	11.3	13.3
11.0-11.9	11.44	272	8.9	4.0	3.2	3.8	4.3	5.0	6.8	9.2	10.8	12.0	14.1
12.0-12.9	12.47	200	9.3	4.1	3.5	4.1	4.5	5.3	7.2	9.7	11.4	12.8	15.0
13.0-13.9	13.47	187	9.4	4.2	3.7	4.3	4.8	5.7	7.7	10.4	12.2	13.6	16.0
14.0-14.9	14.49	178	9.0	4.0	3.9	4.6	5.2	6.1	8.2	11.1	13.0	14.5	17.0
15.0-15.9	15.45	177	9.8	4.3	4.2	5.0	5.5	6.5	8.8	11.8	13.9	15.4	18.1
16.0-16.9	16.45	189	10.1	4.4	4.5	5.3	5.9	6.9	9.3	12.6	14.7	16.4	19.2
17.0-17.9	17.45	188	11.5	4.6	5.1	6.0	6.6	7.6	10.0	13.0	15.0	16.6	19.1
18.0-18.9	18.45	168	12.1	4.8	5.5	6.3	7.0	8.1	10.6	13.8	15.9	17.6	20.3
19.0-19.9	19.43	153	12.1	4.8	5.8	6.7	7.4	8.6	11.2	14.6	16.8	18.5	21.4
20.0-29.9	24.96	1551	15.6	5.7	7.0	8.4	9.5	11.2	14.5	18.2	20.4	21.9	24.2
30.0-39.9	34.72	1365	18.4	6.1	8.5	10.6	12.0	14.2	18.2	22.3	24.4	25.9	28.2
40.0-49.9	44.35	1099	19.6	6.3	9.1	11.3	12.8	14.9	19.0	23.1	25.4	26.9	29.1
50.0-59.9	54.89	773	20.0	6.5	9.4	11.7	13.2	15.5	19.8	24.2	26.5	28.2	30.5
60.0-69.9	64.83	1063	20.4	6.5	9.7	12.0	13.6	15.9	20.3	24.6	27.0	28.6	30.9
70.0-79.9	74.16	755	18.8	6.1	8.8	11.0	12.4	14.6	18.6	22.7	24.8	26.3	28.5
80.0-90.9	84.09	535	16.2	5.1	7.8	9.6	10.9	12.7	16.2	19.6	21.5	22.8	24.6
Females													
2.0-2.9	2.45	533	7.1	2.4	3.9	4.4	4.8	5.5	6.9	8.6	9.7	10.5	11.8
3.0-3.9	3.46	554	6.4	2.8	3.0	3.5	3.9	4.6	6.1	8.2	9.5	10.5	12.2
4.0-4.9	4.43	525	6.3	3.1	2.5	3.0	3.4	4.1	5.8	8.1	9.7	10.9	12.9
5.0-5.9	5.46	542	6.5	3.6	2.3	2.8	3.3	4.0	5.9	8.5	10.2	11.7	14.1
6.0-6.9	6.47	272	7.1	4.2	2.3	2.8	3.3	4.1	6.2	9.1	11.2	12.8	15.6
7.0-7.9	7.44	260	7.8	4.7	2.4	3.0	3.5	4.4	6.7	10.0	12.4	14.2	17.4
8.0-8.9	8.47	244	8.7	5.3	2.6	3.3	3.9	4.9	7.4	11.2	13.8	15.9	19.6
9.0-9.9	9.43	265	9.6	5.9	2.9	3.7	4.3	5.4	8.2	12.3	15.2	17.5	21.5
10.0-10.9	10.43	252	10.6	6.4	3.3	4.1	4.8	6.1	9.1	13.6	16.7	19.2	23.5
11.0-11.9	11.46	276	11.6	6.8	3.7	4.7	5.4	6.8	10.1	14.9	18.2	20.8	25.4
12.0-12.9	12.46	214	12.5	7.0	4.2	5.3	6.1	7.5	11.1	16.1	19.5	22.3	26.9
13.0-13.9	13.45	222	13.4	7.3	4.8	5.9	6.8	8.3	12.0	17.2	20.7	23.5	28.3
14.0-14.9	14.47	216	14.2	7.4	5.3	6.5	7.5	9.1	12.9	18.2	21.8	24.7	29.4
15.0-15.9	15.47	181	15.0	7.5	5.9	7.1	8.1	9.8	13.8	19.2	22.8	25.6	30.4
16.0-16.9	16.46	212	15.7	7.5	6.4	7.7	8.8	10.5	14.6	20.0	23.7	26.5	31.2
17.0-17.9	17.45	197	16.3	7.5	6.9	8.3	9.4	11.1	15.3	20.8	24.4	27.3	31.9
18.0-18.9	18.43	173	16.8	7.6	7.4	8.8	9.9	11.7	15.9	21.5	25.2	28.0	32.6
19.0-19.9	19.48	178	17.4	7.6	7.8	9.3	10.4	12.3	16.6	22.2	25.9	28.7	33.4
20.0-29.9	24.91	1689	19.6	7.7	9.6	11.1	12.3	14.2	18.6	24.2	27.8	30.5	34.9
30.0-39.9	34.85	1619	22.9	8.6	9.7	12.4	14.3	17.2	22.8	28.8	32.1	34.3	37.8
40.0-49.9	44.28	1159	25.2	8.7	11.9	14.6	16.5	19.4	25.1	31.0	34.3	36.6	40.0
50.0-59.9	54.83	876	25.0	8.8	11.5	14.3	16.3	19.2	24.9	31.0	34.3	36.6	40.0
60.0-69.9	64.82	1031	23.3	8.4	10.4	13.0	14.9	17.7	23.1	28.9	32.0	34.2	37.5
70.0-79.9	74.46	836	20.1	8.0	7.8	10.2	12.0	14.6	19.8	25.2	28.2	30.3	33.5
80.0-90.9	84.45	557	15.7	6.9	5.1	7.1	8.6	10.8	15.2	19.8	22.4	24.2	26.9

Table IV.27.

Mean (M), standard deviation (SD), and percentiles of sum of triceps and subscapular skinfold thickness (mm) by age for males and females of 2 to 90 years

Age Group (years)	Mean Age (years)	N	M	SD	Percentiles								
					5th	10th	15th	25th	50th	75th	85th	90th	95th
Males													
2.0-2.9	2.46	544	14.8	4.0	9.4	10.4	11.1	12.3	14.8	17.7	19.5	20.8	22.8
3.0-3.9	3.45	482	14.2	3.8	9.0	10.0	10.7	11.7	14.1	16.8	18.4	19.6	21.5
4.0-4.9	4.47	540	14.4	3.9	8.6	9.6	10.3	11.4	13.7	16.4	18.0	19.3	21.2
5.0-5.9	5.43	490	14.8	4.4	8.1	9.1	9.8	10.9	13.4	16.4	18.2	19.5	21.7
6.0-6.9	6.45	258	15.4	6.1	6.8	7.9	8.7	10.1	13.3	17.3	19.9	21.8	25.0
7.0-7.9	7.47	270	16.0	7.1	6.4	7.5	8.5	10.0	13.5	18.1	21.1	23.4	27.2
8.0-8.9	8.46	258	16.7	7.4	6.7	7.9	8.9	10.5	14.2	19.1	22.3	24.7	28.8
9.0-9.9	9.50	276	17.3	7.7	7.3	8.7	9.7	11.5	15.5	20.8	24.3	26.9	31.3
10.0-10.9	10.45	287	17.9	7.9	7.9	9.4	10.5	12.4	16.8	22.5	26.3	29.2	33.9
11.0-11.9	11.44	271	18.5	8.2	8.3	9.8	11.0	13.1	17.7	23.8	27.7	30.8	35.8
12.0-12.9	12.47	199	19.1	8.5	8.3	9.9	11.1	13.1	17.8	24.0	28.0	31.0	36.1
13.0-13.9	13.47	187	19.7	9.7	7.4	8.9	10.2	12.3	17.2	23.9	28.4	31.8	37.6
14.0-14.9	14.49	177	20.2	10.6	6.6	8.2	9.4	11.5	16.5	23.3	28.0	31.6	37.7
15.0-15.9	15.45	177	20.6	10.3	6.9	8.4	9.6	11.6	16.3	22.7	27.0	30.2	35.7
16.0-16.9	16.45	188	21.1	10.0	7.6	9.2	10.4	12.5	17.3	23.7	27.9	31.1	36.6
17.0-17.9	17.45	186	21.5	9.9	8.6	10.4	11.7	13.9	19.0	25.8	30.2	33.6	39.2
18.0-18.9	18.45	167	22.0	9.5	9.7	11.5	12.8	15.1	20.3	27.0	31.4	34.7	40.2
19.0-19.9	19.43	153	22.4	9.4	10.1	12.0	13.3	15.6	20.9	27.6	32.0	35.3	40.7
20.0-29.9	24.96	1537	25.0	9.8	11.7	14.2	16.1	19.0	25.2	32.3	36.5	39.5	44.1
30.0-39.9	34.72	1355	30.0	10.9	13.2	16.5	18.8	22.3	29.2	36.5	40.7	43.5	47.8
40.0-49.9	44.35	1095	31.7	10.5	15.4	18.6	20.8	24.2	30.9	38.0	41.9	44.7	48.9
50.0-59.9	54.89	768	31.9	10.1	16.3	19.5	21.8	25.1	31.8	38.7	42.6	45.3	49.3
60.0-69.9	64.83	1059	31.8	10.1	16.4	19.6	21.9	25.3	32.0	39.0	42.8	45.5	49.6
70.0-79.9	74.16	753	30.9	9.9	15.5	18.7	20.8	24.2	30.6	37.3	41.0	43.6	47.5
80.0-90.9	84.09	535	27.5	8.6	14.0	16.8	18.7	21.6	27.2	32.9	36.1	38.3	41.6
Females													
2.0-2.9	2.45	533	16.8	4.9	9.7	10.8	11.6	12.9	15.8	19.2	21.4	22.9	25.5
3.0-3.9	3.46	554	15.5	4.7	9.3	10.4	11.2	12.6	15.5	19.0	21.1	22.8	25.4
4.0-4.9	4.43	525	15.3	5.7	8.2	9.4	10.4	11.9	15.4	19.7	22.6	24.7	28.2
5.0-5.9	5.46	541	15.9	6.9	7.4	8.7	9.7	11.4	15.3	20.5	23.9	26.6	30.9
6.0-6.9	6.47	272	17.1	8.1	7.1	8.5	9.6	11.4	15.7	21.5	25.4	28.5	33.6
7.0-7.9	7.44	260	18.6	9.2	7.1	8.6	9.8	11.7	16.4	22.9	27.3	30.7	36.6
8.0-8.9	8.47	243	20.4	10.5	7.5	9.1	10.3	12.4	17.6	24.8	29.8	33.6	40.3
9.0-9.9	9.43	264	22.2	11.5	8.0	9.7	11.1	13.4	19.1	27.0	32.4	36.7	43.9
10.0-10.9	10.43	252	24.2	12.3	8.9	10.8	12.3	14.9	21.0	29.6	35.4	40.0	47.9
11.0-11.9	11.46	276	26.1	12.9	10.2	12.3	13.9	16.7	23.4	32.5	38.7	43.6	51.8
12.0-12.9	12.46	214	27.9	13.1	11.8	14.1	15.9	18.9	25.9	35.5	42.0	47.0	55.4
13.0-13.9	13.45	222	29.5	13.1	13.5	15.9	17.8	21.0	28.4	38.3	44.8	49.9	58.4
14.0-14.9	14.47	214	31.0	13.2	15.0	17.5	19.5	22.8	30.4	40.4	47.0	52.0	60.4
15.0-15.9	15.47	181	32.4	13.2	15.7	18.4	20.5	23.9	31.6	41.4	47.7	52.5	60.3
16.0-16.9	16.46	212	33.6	13.4	16.3	19.1	21.2	24.6	32.4	42.2	48.4	53.1	60.8
17.0-17.9	17.45	193	34.6	13.6	16.5	19.5	21.7	25.4	33.4	43.2	49.3	53.8	60.9
18.0-18.9	18.43	173	35.5	14.0	16.4	19.7	22.1	26.0	34.4	44.4	50.4	54.8	61.6
19.0-19.9	19.48	178	36.4	14.4	16.4	19.7	22.1	26.1	34.5	44.6	50.7	55.1	62.0
20.0-29.9	24.91	1671	39.6	15.1	19.1	22.8	25.5	29.8	39.1	50.0	56.6	61.4	68.9
30.0-39.9	34.85	1578	45.4	15.4	24.0	27.8	30.7	35.2	44.7	55.7	62.2	66.9	74.2
40.0-49.9	44.28	1137	50.6	15.5	25.9	31.2	34.8	40.3	50.6	61.2	66.9	70.9	76.7
50.0-59.9	54.83	856	50.6	15.4	25.7	31.1	34.8	40.3	50.7	61.2	66.8	70.7	76.4
60.0-69.9	64.82	1010	47.2	14.4	23.9	29.0	32.4	37.6	47.2	57.0	62.3	65.9	71.3
70.0-79.9	74.46	831	42.1	14.0	19.3	24.2	27.5	32.5	41.8	51.3	56.4	59.9	65.1
80.0-90.9	84.45	554	33.8	12.4	13.4	17.5	20.4	24.6	32.6	40.7	45.1	48.1	52.5

Table IV.28.

Mean (M), standard deviation (SD), and percentiles of suprailiac skinfold thickness (mm) by age for males and females of 2 to 90 years

Age Group (years)	Mean Age (years)	N	M	SD	Percentiles								
					5th	10th	15th	25th	50th	75th	85th	90th	95th
Males													
2.0-2.9	2.46	535	5.2	1.7	2.7	3.1	3.4	3.9	4.9	6.1	6.8	7.3	8.1
3.0-3.9	3.45	481	4.7	1.7	2.4	2.8	3.1	3.6	4.6	5.9	6.6	7.2	8.0
4.0-4.9	4.47	541	4.8	2.4	1.8	2.3	2.7	3.4	4.8	6.6	7.8	8.7	10.0
5.0-5.9	5.43	487	5.3	3.2	1.4	2.0	2.4	3.1	4.8	7.0	8.4	9.5	11.2
6.0-6.9	6.45	257	6.0	4.0	1.2	1.7	2.2	2.9	4.7	7.2	8.8	10.0	12.1
7.0-7.9	7.47	268	6.8	4.8	1.2	1.7	2.2	3.0	5.0	7.7	9.5	10.9	13.2
8.0-8.9	8.46	255	7.6	5.4	1.3	1.9	2.4	3.3	5.5	8.6	10.7	12.3	14.9
9.0-9.9	9.50	277	8.4	5.8	1.5	2.2	2.8	3.8	6.3	9.7	12.0	13.7	16.6
10.0-10.9	10.45	281	9.1	6.0	1.9	2.6	3.3	4.4	7.1	10.7	13.1	14.9	17.9
11.0-11.9	11.44	269	9.7	6.0	2.3	3.1	3.8	5.0	7.8	11.6	14.0	15.9	18.9
12.0-12.9	12.47	200	10.3	6.1	3.1	3.9	4.5	5.6	8.4	12.5	15.5	17.8	22.0
13.0-13.9	13.47	187	10.8	6.4	3.3	4.1	4.7	5.9	8.7	13.0	16.1	18.7	23.1
14.0-14.9	14.49	175	11.3	6.9	3.3	4.1	4.7	5.9	8.9	13.3	16.5	19.1	23.8
15.0-15.9	15.45	175	11.8	7.1	3.3	4.1	4.7	5.9	8.9	13.3	16.6	19.2	23.9
16.0-16.9	16.45	187	12.3	7.4	3.3	4.2	4.9	6.1	9.2	13.7	16.9	19.5	24.0
17.0-17.9	17.45	183	12.8	7.5	3.6	4.6	5.4	6.8	10.3	15.1	18.3	20.7	24.8
18.0-18.9	18.45	164	13.4	6.2	5.3	6.5	7.4	8.9	12.2	16.6	19.4	21.5	24.9
19.0-19.9	19.43	153	14.0	6.3	5.8	6.9	7.8	9.4	12.8	17.1	19.9	22.0	25.5
20.0-29.9	24.96	1548	17.9	7.1	9.1	10.7	12.0	14.0	18.4	24.0	27.4	30.0	34.2
30.0-39.9	34.72	1374	22.1	8.5	9.8	12.1	13.7	16.3	21.6	27.4	30.8	33.2	36.8
40.0-49.9	44.35	1139	22.6	8.4	10.5	12.8	14.5	17.2	22.5	28.5	31.9	34.3	38.0
50.0-59.9	54.89	797	22.2	8.2	10.2	12.5	14.1	16.6	21.8	27.4	30.7	33.0	36.5
60.0-69.9	64.83	1092	20.8	7.6	9.7	11.8	13.4	15.7	20.5	25.9	28.9	31.1	34.4
70.0-79.9	74.16	764	17.7	6.4	8.2	10.0	11.3	13.2	17.3	21.7	24.2	26.0	28.7
80.0-90.9	84.09	537	14.6	5.3	6.8	8.3	9.4	11.0	14.3	18.0	20.1	21.6	23.8
Females													
2.0-2.9	2.45	529	6.4	2.2	3.5	4.0	4.3	4.9	6.3	7.9	8.8	9.6	10.8
3.0-3.9	3.46	554	5.3	2.4	2.3	2.7	3.0	3.6	4.9	6.5	7.6	8.4	9.7
4.0-4.9	4.43	525	5.3	2.4	2.1	2.5	2.8	3.3	4.5	6.1	7.1	7.9	9.2
5.0-5.9	5.46	539	5.9	2.7	2.2	2.7	3.0	3.6	4.9	6.7	7.8	8.7	10.1
6.0-6.9	6.47	272	7.0	3.2	2.6	3.1	3.5	4.2	5.8	7.9	9.2	10.2	11.9
7.0-7.9	7.44	261	8.2	3.8	3.1	3.7	4.2	5.0	6.9	9.4	11.0	12.2	14.2
8.0-8.9	8.47	243	9.6	4.5	3.7	4.4	5.0	6.0	8.2	11.2	13.1	14.5	17.0
9.0-9.9	9.43	266	11.0	5.1	4.2	5.1	5.8	6.9	9.5	12.9	15.1	16.8	19.7
10.0-10.9	10.43	253	12.3	5.6	4.9	5.9	6.6	7.9	10.8	14.6	17.1	18.9	22.1
11.0-11.9	11.46	280	13.5	6.1	5.5	6.5	7.4	8.8	12.0	16.2	18.9	21.0	24.4
12.0-12.9	12.46	210	14.5	6.5	6.0	7.2	8.1	9.6	13.1	17.6	20.5	22.8	26.4
13.0-13.9	13.45	222	15.4	6.9	6.4	7.7	8.7	10.3	14.0	18.8	21.9	24.3	28.2
14.0-14.9	14.47	212	16.1	7.2	6.4	7.8	8.9	10.8	14.8	19.6	22.7	24.9	28.4
15.0-15.9	15.47	183	16.7	7.4	6.4	8.0	9.2	11.2	15.4	20.4	23.4	25.6	29.0
16.0-16.9	16.46	211	17.2	7.6	6.0	7.9	9.3	11.4	15.9	20.9	23.8	25.8	28.9
17.0-17.9	17.45	195	17.5	7.9	6.0	7.9	9.4	11.7	16.3	21.6	24.6	26.7	30.0
18.0-18.9	18.43	175	17.8	8.0	6.1	8.1	9.6	11.9	16.7	22.0	25.1	27.2	30.5
19.0-19.9	19.48	178	18.0	8.1	6.2	8.3	9.8	12.1	17.0	22.4	25.5	27.7	31.1
20.0-29.9	24.91	1733	18.7	9.3	5.7	8.0	9.7	12.4	18.1	24.5	28.2	30.8	34.8
30.0-39.9	34.85	1659	22.0	8.8	9.3	11.8	13.6	16.3	22.0	28.2	31.8	34.3	38.1
40.0-49.9	44.28	1199	25.1	10.1	10.1	12.7	14.6	17.6	23.7	30.4	34.3	37.0	41.1
50.0-59.9	54.83	890	25.3	10.1	10.1	12.7	14.7	17.7	23.8	30.5	34.3	37.1	41.2
60.0-69.9	64.82	1007	23.2	9.3	10.0	12.6	14.5	17.5	23.5	30.1	33.9	36.6	40.7
70.0-79.9	74.46	816	19.4	7.8	8.1	10.3	11.8	14.2	19.2	24.6	27.7	29.9	33.2
80.0-90.9	84.45	549	14.8	5.9	6.0	7.5	8.7	10.4	14.0	18.0	20.3	21.9	24.3

Table IV.29.

Mean (M), standard deviation (SD), and percentiles of thigh skinfold thickness (mm) by age for males and females of 2 to 90 years

Age Group (years)	Mean Age (years)	N	M	SD	Percentiles								
					5th	10th	15th	25th	50th	75th	85th	90th	95th
Males													
2.0-2.9	2.46	538	11.5	2.8	7.3	8.1	8.6	9.5	11.2	13.2	14.4	15.2	16.4
3.0-3.9	3.45	484	10.3	2.8	6.4	7.1	7.7	8.5	10.3	12.4	13.6	14.4	15.7
4.0-4.9	4.47	539	10.1	3.4	5.4	6.2	6.8	7.8	9.9	12.3	13.7	14.8	16.5
5.0-5.9	5.43	484	10.4	4.1	4.7	5.6	6.3	7.4	9.7	12.5	14.2	15.5	17.5
6.0-6.9	6.45	258	11.0	4.9	4.2	5.2	5.9	7.1	9.7	12.9	14.9	16.3	18.7
7.0-7.9	7.47	266	11.6	5.5	4.0	5.0	5.8	7.1	9.9	13.5	15.7	17.4	20.0
8.0-8.9	8.46	251	12.2	5.9	4.2	5.3	6.1	7.5	10.6	14.5	16.9	18.7	21.6
9.0-9.9	9.50	268	12.5	6.0	4.7	5.8	6.7	8.2	11.6	15.8	18.4	20.4	23.5
10.0-10.9	10.45	275	12.7	6.0	5.1	6.4	7.3	8.9	12.5	16.9	19.7	21.8	25.0
11.0-11.9	11.44	253	12.6	6.0	5.2	6.5	7.5	9.2	12.9	17.4	20.3	22.5	25.9
12.0-12.9	12.47	192	12.4	6.2	4.8	6.1	7.0	8.6	12.3	16.9	19.9	22.0	25.5
13.0-13.9	13.47	177	12.1	6.4	4.0	5.2	6.1	7.6	11.1	15.5	18.3	20.4	23.8
14.0-14.9	14.49	169	11.7	6.3	3.4	4.4	5.2	6.5	9.6	13.6	16.1	18.0	21.1
15.0-15.9	15.45	166	11.2	5.9	3.5	4.5	5.2	6.5	9.5	13.3	15.7	17.5	20.4
16.0-16.9	16.45	182	10.8	5.2	3.6	4.5	5.2	6.4	8.9	12.1	14.1	15.6	18.0
17.0-17.9	17.45	180	10.4	4.6	3.7	4.6	5.2	6.2	8.5	11.4	13.1	14.4	16.5
18.0-18.9	18.45	162	10.0	4.7	3.5	4.3	4.9	6.0	8.4	11.3	13.2	14.5	16.7
19.0-19.9	19.43	143	9.8	4.9	3.3	4.2	4.9	6.0	8.5	11.7	13.7	15.2	17.6
20.0-29.9	24.96	1503	10.3	4.7	4.6	5.7	6.6	7.9	11.0	14.7	17.1	18.8	21.6
30.0-39.9	34.72	1364	12.2	5.6	5.1	6.3	7.2	8.7	12.0	16.2	18.7	20.6	23.6
40.0-49.9	44.35	1123	12.3	5.7	5.1	6.3	7.2	8.7	12.0	16.1	18.7	20.6	23.6
50.0-59.9	54.89	800	12.5	5.8	5.0	6.2	7.1	8.6	11.9	16.0	18.6	20.5	23.5
60.0-69.9	64.83	1083	12.2	5.6	4.8	6.0	6.8	8.3	11.5	15.4	17.9	19.7	22.6
70.0-79.9	74.16	746	11.9	5.6	4.7	5.9	6.7	8.2	11.4	15.3	17.8	19.6	22.5
80.0-90.9	84.09	519	11.8	5.3	4.7	5.7	6.5	7.9	10.9	14.6	16.8	18.5	21.2
Females													
2.0-2.9	2.45	531	13.3	3.9	7.4	8.5	9.3	10.5	13.0	15.7	17.3	18.4	20.1
3.0-3.9	3.46	556	12.9	4.0	7.0	8.0	8.8	10.0	12.4	15.2	16.8	17.9	19.6
4.0-4.9	4.43	524	12.9	4.3	6.5	7.6	8.4	9.7	12.3	15.2	16.9	18.2	20.0
5.0-5.9	5.46	541	13.1	4.7	6.3	7.4	8.3	9.6	12.4	15.6	17.5	18.8	20.9
6.0-6.9	6.47	267	13.7	5.1	6.3	7.5	8.4	9.9	12.9	16.3	18.4	19.8	22.1
7.0-7.9	7.44	258	14.4	5.5	6.5	7.8	8.8	10.3	13.5	17.2	19.4	21.0	23.4
8.0-8.9	8.47	232	15.3	5.9	6.8	8.2	9.3	10.9	14.4	18.4	20.7	22.4	25.0
9.0-9.9	9.43	261	16.2	6.2	7.3	8.8	9.9	11.6	15.3	19.5	22.0	23.8	26.6
10.0-10.9	10.43	238	17.3	6.5	7.9	9.5	10.6	12.5	16.4	20.8	23.4	25.3	28.2
11.0-11.9	11.46	255	18.3	6.7	8.6	10.3	11.5	13.4	17.5	22.1	24.8	26.7	29.7
12.0-12.9	12.46	183	19.3	6.9	9.3	11.1	12.3	14.3	18.5	23.3	26.0	28.0	31.1
13.0-13.9	13.45	197	20.3	7.0	10.1	11.9	13.2	15.3	19.5	24.4	27.2	29.2	32.3
14.0-14.9	14.47	193	21.2	7.0	10.9	12.7	14.1	16.2	20.5	25.4	28.2	30.2	33.3
15.0-15.9	15.47	160	22.0	7.0	11.7	13.5	14.9	17.0	21.4	26.2	29.1	31.1	34.2
16.0-16.9	16.46	191	22.7	7.0	12.4	14.3	15.6	17.8	22.1	27.0	29.8	31.9	35.0
17.0-17.9	17.45	164	23.3	7.0	13.0	14.9	16.3	18.4	22.8	27.7	30.5	32.5	35.5
18.0-18.9	18.43	156	23.8	7.0	13.6	15.5	16.9	19.0	23.4	28.2	31.0	33.0	36.0
19.0-19.9	19.48	155	24.2	6.9	14.0	16.0	17.4	19.5	23.9	28.7	31.5	33.5	36.5
20.0-29.9	24.91	1491	25.6	7.2	14.0	16.4	18.1	20.6	25.3	30.2	32.8	34.6	37.3
30.0-39.9	34.85	1327	28.0	8.1	15.2	17.9	19.8	22.7	28.1	33.7	36.7	38.8	41.9
40.0-49.9	44.28	951	30.7	8.9	16.3	19.3	21.3	24.3	30.1	36.1	39.3	41.5	44.8
50.0-59.9	54.83	702	30.3	8.6	17.0	20.0	22.0	25.1	30.9	36.8	40.1	42.3	45.6
60.0-69.9	64.82	908	29.1	8.0	16.8	19.6	21.5	24.3	29.7	35.3	38.3	40.4	43.5
70.0-79.9	74.46	739	28.6	8.0	16.2	18.9	20.8	23.6	29.0	34.5	37.5	39.6	42.6
80.0-90.9	84.45	509	26.4	7.8	14.2	16.9	18.8	21.5	26.8	32.2	35.1	37.1	40.1

Table IV.30

Mean (M), standard deviation (SD), and percentiles of sum of triceps, subscapular, suprailiac, and thigh skinfold thickness (mm) by age for males and females of 2 to 90 years

Age Group (years)	Mean Age (years)	N	M	SD	Percentiles								
					5th	10th	15th	25th	50th	75th	85th	90th	95th
Males													
2.0-2.9	2.46	525	31.6	10.0	16.9	19.6	21.6	24.7	30.9	37.9	41.9	44.7	49.1
3.0-3.9	3.45	477	29.3	8.6	16.4	18.9	20.6	23.3	28.7	34.7	38.2	40.6	44.3
4.0-4.9	4.47	537	29.1	10.2	14.2	16.8	18.8	21.8	28.0	35.0	39.1	41.9	46.4
5.0-5.9	5.43	482	30.1	10.8	14.0	16.8	18.7	21.9	28.3	35.5	39.7	42.6	47.2
6.0-6.9	6.45	256	31.9	11.5	14.3	17.1	19.2	22.4	29.1	36.5	40.9	44.0	48.8
7.0-7.9	7.47	265	33.8	14.8	12.3	15.5	18.0	21.9	30.1	39.6	45.2	49.2	55.5
8.0-8.9	8.46	250	35.6	15.6	12.7	16.1	18.6	22.6	31.2	41.0	46.8	51.0	57.4
9.0-9.9	9.50	266	37.3	16.3	13.1	16.6	19.2	23.4	32.2	42.4	48.4	52.8	59.4
10.0-10.9	10.45	272	38.5	20.1	10.6	14.6	17.6	22.5	33.2	45.8	53.4	58.9	67.5
11.0-11.9	11.44	252	39.5	20.8	10.8	14.8	17.9	23.0	34.0	47.1	54.9	60.6	69.5
12.0-12.9	12.47	189	40.3	21.1	11.1	15.2	18.4	23.6	34.8	48.1	56.1	61.9	70.9
13.0-13.9	13.47	174	40.9	21.1	11.6	15.8	18.9	24.2	35.5	48.9	57.0	62.8	71.9
14.0-14.9	14.49	166	41.3	21.0	12.2	16.4	19.6	24.9	36.2	49.6	57.7	63.5	72.5
15.0-15.9	15.45	163	41.7	20.7	12.8	17.1	20.4	25.6	37.0	50.3	58.3	64.0	73.0
16.0-16.9	16.45	178	42.2	20.3	13.6	17.9	21.2	26.5	37.8	51.0	58.9	64.6	73.5
17.0-17.9	17.45	174	42.7	20.0	14.5	18.9	22.2	27.5	38.7	51.9	59.7	65.3	74.0
18.0-18.9	18.45	158	43.4	19.7	15.5	19.9	23.2	28.5	39.8	52.9	60.6	66.2	74.8
19.0-19.9	19.43	141	44.3	19.7	16.3	20.8	24.2	29.6	41.0	54.2	62.0	67.6	76.3
20.0-29.9	24.96	1456	52.4	20.6	20.0	26.2	30.5	37.1	49.9	63.4	70.9	76.1	83.9
30.0-39.9	34.72	1296	62.0	23.0	24.9	31.7	36.5	43.7	57.8	72.6	80.8	86.5	95.0
40.0-49.9	44.35	1057	64.2	22.4	29.3	36.4	41.4	48.9	63.4	78.7	87.1	92.9	101.6
50.0-59.9	54.89	748	66.1	20.9	33.2	39.9	44.5	51.6	65.2	79.4	87.2	92.6	100.7
60.0-69.9	64.83	1024	65.1	20.0	33.2	39.5	44.0	50.7	63.5	76.9	84.3	89.4	97.1
70.0-79.9	74.16	720	61.2	19.9	29.9	36.2	40.7	47.3	60.2	73.7	81.2	86.3	94.0
80.0-90.9	84.09	511	54.2	16.8	28.0	33.5	37.3	43.1	54.2	65.7	72.1	76.5	83.1
Females													
2.0-2.9	2.45	522	36.1	8.9	23.2	25.5	27.2	29.9	35.4	41.7	45.5	48.2	52.5
3.0-3.9	3.46	550	33.9	10.0	19.6	22.1	23.8	26.7	32.7	39.7	44.0	47.2	52.1
4.0-4.9	4.43	519	33.7	11.8	17.3	19.9	21.8	25.0	31.7	40.0	45.1	48.8	54.8
5.0-5.9	5.46	537	35.0	13.7	16.3	19.1	21.2	24.6	32.3	41.7	47.7	52.1	59.3
6.0-6.9	6.47	265	37.4	15.6	16.4	19.4	21.7	25.5	34.0	44.7	51.5	56.6	64.9
7.0-7.9	7.44	258	40.3	17.3	17.1	20.4	22.9	27.1	36.5	48.4	56.0	61.7	71.0
8.0-8.9	8.47	231	44.0	19.1	18.6	22.2	24.9	29.5	39.8	53.0	61.4	67.7	77.9
9.0-9.9	9.43	258	47.6	20.4	20.3	24.3	27.2	32.2	43.3	57.5	66.5	73.3	84.3
10.0-10.9	10.43	238	51.4	21.5	22.6	26.9	30.1	35.4	47.2	62.2	71.7	78.9	90.4
11.0-11.9	11.46	253	55.2	22.3	25.3	29.8	33.2	38.8	51.2	66.8	76.7	84.0	95.9
12.0-12.9	12.46	181	58.8	22.7	28.1	32.8	36.4	42.2	55.1	71.0	81.0	88.5	100.4
13.0-13.9	13.45	196	62.0	22.7	31.0	35.9	39.6	45.6	58.7	74.8	84.8	92.2	104.1
14.0-14.9	14.47	191	65.0	22.6	34.0	39.0	42.8	48.9	62.1	78.2	88.1	95.4	107.1
15.0-15.9	15.47	157	67.6	22.3	36.8	41.9	45.8	51.9	65.2	81.1	90.9	98.0	109.5
16.0-16.9	16.46	189	69.8	22.0	39.3	44.6	48.4	54.6	67.8	83.5	93.2	100.2	111.4
17.0-17.9	17.45	163	71.6	21.7	41.5	46.8	50.7	56.9	70.1	85.6	95.1	102.0	112.9
18.0-18.9	18.43	155	73.2	21.5	43.4	48.7	52.6	58.8	72.0	87.4	96.8	103.6	114.4
19.0-19.9	19.48	154	74.5	21.4	45.0	50.3	54.3	60.5	73.6	89.1	98.4	105.1	115.8
20.0-29.9	24.91	1451	78.7	23.2	46.1	52.3	56.8	63.8	78.3	94.9	104.7	111.7	122.5
30.0-39.9	34.85	1276	88.3	23.3	50.9	58.8	64.2	72.3	87.7	103.4	112.1	118.0	126.8
40.0-49.9	44.28	897	98.9	25.8	57.8	66.4	72.3	81.2	98.1	115.4	124.8	131.3	140.9
50.0-59.9	54.83	655	98.4	25.8	56.7	65.7	71.8	80.9	98.2	115.6	125.1	131.6	141.3
60.0-69.9	64.82	860	95.0	23.9	56.8	65.1	70.9	79.4	95.5	111.8	120.7	126.7	135.7
70.0-79.9	74.46	716	86.2	23.2	49.2	57.2	62.8	71.0	86.5	102.3	110.9	116.7	125.4
80.0-90.9	84.45	496	74.2	21.8	39.1	46.6	51.7	59.4	73.9	88.6	96.6	102.1	110.2

Table IV.31.

Mean (M), standard deviation (SD), and percentiles of mid-upper arm circumference (cm) by age for males and females of 2 to 90 years

Age Group (years)	Mean Age (years)	N	M	SD	Percentiles								
					5th	10th	15th	25th	50th	75th	85th	90th	95th
Males													
2.0-2.9	2.46	570	16.2	1.2	14.2	14.5	14.8	15.2	16.0	16.8	17.2	17.5	17.9
3.0-3.9	3.45	487	16.5	1.4	14.4	14.8	15.2	15.6	16.6	17.5	18.0	18.3	18.9
4.0-4.9	4.47	545	16.9	1.6	14.4	14.9	15.3	15.8	16.9	18.0	18.6	19.0	19.6
5.0-5.9	5.43	494	17.4	1.9	14.4	15.0	15.4	16.1	17.3	18.5	19.2	19.7	20.4
6.0-6.9	6.45	259	18.1	2.2	14.5	15.2	15.7	16.5	17.9	19.4	20.2	20.7	21.5
7.0-7.9	7.47	271	18.9	2.5	14.8	15.6	16.2	17.0	18.7	20.4	21.3	21.9	22.9
8.0-8.9	8.46	258	19.9	2.8	15.2	16.1	16.7	17.7	19.5	21.4	22.4	23.1	24.2
9.0-9.9	9.50	282	20.9	3.1	15.6	16.6	17.3	18.4	20.4	22.4	23.6	24.4	25.6
10.0-10.9	10.45	288	22.0	3.4	16.1	17.2	17.9	19.1	21.2	23.5	24.8	25.6	26.9
11.0-11.9	11.44	273	23.1	3.7	16.7	17.9	18.7	20.0	22.3	24.8	26.2	27.1	28.5
12.0-12.9	12.47	203	24.2	4.0	17.5	18.8	19.7	21.1	23.6	26.3	27.8	28.8	30.4
13.0-13.9	13.47	188	25.3	4.2	18.5	19.9	20.8	22.3	25.0	27.8	29.4	30.5	32.1
14.0-14.9	14.49	181	26.4	4.2	19.7	21.1	22.0	23.5	26.2	29.1	30.7	31.8	33.4
15.0-15.9	15.45	179	27.3	4.0	20.9	22.2	23.1	24.5	27.2	29.9	31.4	32.5	34.0
16.0-16.9	16.45	193	28.2	3.8	22.1	23.3	24.2	25.5	28.0	30.5	31.9	32.9	34.3
17.0-17.9	17.45	190	29.1	3.7	23.1	24.4	25.2	26.5	28.9	31.4	32.8	33.7	35.2
18.0-18.9	18.45	169	29.8	3.8	23.9	25.2	26.1	27.5	30.0	32.7	34.2	35.2	36.7
19.0-19.9	19.43	155	30.4	3.8	24.5	25.8	26.7	28.0	30.5	33.1	34.5	35.5	36.9
20.0-29.9	24.96	1595	31.6	3.6	26.1	27.3	28.2	29.4	31.8	34.2	35.6	36.5	37.8
30.0-39.9	34.72	1424	32.2	3.8	26.3	27.6	28.5	29.8	32.3	34.9	36.3	37.3	38.7
40.0-49.9	44.35	1173	33.2	3.9	26.9	28.2	29.1	30.5	33.0	35.7	37.1	38.1	39.6
50.0-59.9	54.89	828	32.7	3.8	26.6	27.9	28.8	30.1	32.6	35.2	36.6	37.6	39.0
60.0-69.9	64.83	1130	32.0	3.5	26.5	27.6	28.5	29.7	32.0	34.4	35.7	36.5	37.9
70.0-79.9	74.16	827	30.6	3.5	25.1	26.2	27.1	28.3	30.6	32.9	34.2	35.1	36.4
80.0-90.9	84.09	638	28.9	3.4	23.5	24.7	25.5	26.7	28.9	31.2	32.5	33.4	34.7
Females													
2.0-2.9	2.45	546	16.4	1.3	13.8	14.3	14.6	15.0	15.9	16.8	17.3	17.6	18.1
3.0-3.9	3.46	563	16.2	1.5	14.1	14.6	15.0	15.5	16.5	17.5	18.1	18.5	19.1
4.0-4.9	4.43	526	16.5	1.7	14.1	14.7	15.1	15.6	16.7	17.9	18.6	19.0	19.7
5.0-5.9	5.46	542	17.3	2.0	14.3	14.9	15.4	16.0	17.4	18.8	19.6	20.2	21.0
6.0-6.9	6.47	274	18.2	2.5	14.4	15.1	15.7	16.5	18.1	19.8	20.8	21.5	22.5
7.0-7.9	7.44	263	19.3	2.9	14.6	15.4	16.0	16.9	18.7	20.7	21.8	22.6	23.8
8.0-8.9	8.47	246	20.4	3.2	15.0	15.9	16.5	17.5	19.5	21.6	22.9	23.7	25.1
9.0-9.9	9.43	268	21.4	3.4	15.7	16.7	17.3	18.4	20.4	22.7	24.0	25.0	26.4
10.0-10.9	10.43	254	22.5	3.5	16.7	17.7	18.5	19.6	21.8	24.2	25.6	26.5	28.0
11.0-11.9	11.46	281	23.5	3.7	17.8	18.9	19.6	20.8	23.2	25.7	27.2	28.3	29.9
12.0-12.9	12.46	216	24.3	3.9	18.7	19.8	20.6	21.9	24.4	27.1	28.7	29.8	31.6
13.0-13.9	13.45	224	25.1	4.0	19.3	20.5	21.3	22.6	25.2	28.1	29.7	30.9	32.7
14.0-14.9	14.47	220	25.7	4.1	19.7	21.0	21.8	23.1	25.8	28.7	30.4	31.6	33.4
15.0-15.9	15.47	188	26.3	4.2	20.1	21.3	22.2	23.5	26.2	29.2	30.9	32.1	33.9
16.0-16.9	16.46	218	26.7	4.3	20.3	21.6	22.5	23.8	26.6	29.6	31.3	32.5	34.4
17.0-17.9	17.45	208	27.1	4.3	20.4	21.6	22.5	23.9	26.6	29.6	31.4	32.6	34.5
18.0-18.9	18.43	182	27.4	4.5	20.3	21.6	22.5	23.9	26.7	29.8	31.6	32.8	34.8
19.0-19.9	19.48	184	27.7	4.4	20.5	21.8	22.7	24.0	26.8	29.8	31.5	32.8	34.7
20.0-29.9	24.91	1817	28.6	4.7	21.4	22.7	23.7	25.2	28.1	31.4	33.3	34.6	36.7
30.0-39.9	34.85	1790	30.4	4.9	23.1	24.6	25.6	27.1	30.3	33.7	35.7	37.1	39.3
40.0-49.9	44.28	1293	31.9	5.0	24.2	25.6	26.6	28.2	31.4	34.8	36.8	38.2	40.4
50.0-59.9	54.83	971	32.0	5.1	24.4	25.9	27.0	28.6	31.9	35.4	37.5	38.9	41.2
60.0-69.9	64.82	1124	31.6	4.8	24.3	25.7	26.7	28.3	31.4	34.7	36.7	38.1	40.2
70.0-79.9	74.46	915	30.2	4.6	23.1	24.5	25.4	26.9	29.9	33.1	35.0	36.3	38.4
80.0-90.9	84.45	705	27.9	4.3	21.5	22.7	23.6	25.0	27.8	30.9	32.7	33.9	35.8

Table IV.32.

Mean (M), standard deviation (SD), and percentiles of total mid-upper arm area (cm^2) by age for males and females of 2 to 90 years

Age Group (years)	Mean Age (years)	N	M	SD	Percentiles								
					5th	10th	15th	25th	50th	75th	85th	90th	95th
Males													
2.0-2.9	2.46	570	21.4	3.1	16.1	17.1	17.7	18.8	20.7	22.8	23.9	24.7	25.9
3.0-3.9	3.45	487	22.3	3.9	16.3	17.5	18.4	19.7	22.2	24.9	26.5	27.5	29.1
4.0-4.9	4.47	545	23.3	4.7	16.2	17.6	18.6	20.2	23.2	26.5	28.3	29.6	31.5
5.0-5.9	5.43	494	24.6	5.6	16.0	17.7	18.9	20.7	24.2	28.0	30.2	31.7	34.0
6.0-6.9	6.45	259	26.6	6.8	16.1	18.1	19.5	21.7	26.0	30.6	33.3	35.2	38.1
7.0-7.9	7.47	271	29.2	8.3	16.6	18.9	20.6	23.2	28.3	34.0	37.3	39.6	43.1
8.0-8.9	8.46	258	32.2	9.8	17.3	20.0	21.9	24.9	30.9	37.5	41.3	44.0	48.1
9.0-9.9	9.50	282	36.0	11.4	18.4	21.4	23.5	26.9	33.7	41.2	45.6	48.7	53.4
10.0-10.9	10.45	288	39.8	13.0	19.5	22.9	25.3	29.0	36.6	45.1	50.0	53.4	58.7
11.0-11.9	11.44	273	44.0	14.9	21.0	24.8	27.5	31.7	40.4	50.1	55.8	59.7	65.9
12.0-12.9	12.47	203	48.6	17.1	22.8	27.2	30.3	35.2	45.4	56.8	63.4	68.0	75.3
13.0-13.9	13.47	188	53.0	19.1	25.0	29.9	33.5	39.1	50.7	63.7	71.3	76.6	84.9
14.0-14.9	14.49	181	57.5	20.2	28.1	33.4	37.3	43.4	55.8	69.8	77.9	83.7	92.6
15.0-15.9	15.45	179	61.6	20.0	32.0	37.4	41.3	47.4	59.8	73.6	81.6	87.2	95.9
16.0-16.9	16.45	193	65.5	18.8	36.9	42.2	45.9	51.7	63.4	76.3	83.6	88.8	96.8
17.0-17.9	17.45	190	69.2	18.2	41.6	46.9	50.7	56.4	67.9	80.5	87.6	92.7	100.3
18.0-18.9	18.45	169	72.4	19.5	43.0	48.7	52.7	58.9	71.3	84.8	92.5	98.0	106.3
19.0-19.9	19.43	155	75.2	20.3	43.8	49.5	53.6	59.9	72.6	86.4	94.3	99.9	108.3
20.0-29.9	24.96	1595	83.9	21.2	50.0	56.0	60.3	66.8	79.9	94.0	102.1	107.8	116.4
30.0-39.9	34.72	1424	85.4	20.3	55.6	61.8	66.1	72.8	86.0	100.2	108.3	114.0	122.6
40.0-49.9	44.35	1173	89.5	19.8	58.1	64.0	68.2	74.5	87.0	100.5	108.1	113.4	121.5
50.0-59.9	54.89	828	87.4	18.9	58.9	64.7	68.8	75.0	87.3	100.4	107.9	113.1	121.0
60.0-69.9	64.83	1130	83.8	18.3	55.7	61.2	65.1	71.1	82.9	95.5	102.7	107.7	115.3
70.0-79.9	74.16	827	76.7	17.5	50.1	55.4	59.1	64.7	75.9	88.0	94.8	99.6	106.9
80.0-90.9	84.09	638	68.1	16.0	44.1	48.9	52.3	57.5	67.9	79.0	85.4	89.8	96.6
Females													
2.0-2.9	2.45	546	22.4	3.8	15.4	16.4	17.1	18.2	20.4	22.9	24.4	25.4	27.0
3.0-3.9	3.46	563	21.1	4.2	15.8	17.0	17.9	19.2	22.0	25.1	27.0	28.3	30.4
4.0-4.9	4.43	526	21.8	4.8	15.8	17.1	18.1	19.6	22.8	26.4	28.6	30.1	32.6
5.0-5.9	5.46	542	24.0	6.2	15.9	17.5	18.7	20.5	24.4	29.0	31.8	33.9	37.1
6.0-6.9	6.47	274	27.0	8.0	16.1	18.0	19.4	21.6	26.4	32.2	35.8	38.4	42.6
7.0-7.9	7.44	263	30.5	9.8	16.5	18.6	20.2	22.8	28.3	35.2	39.5	42.7	47.8
8.0-8.9	8.47	246	34.5	11.6	17.6	19.9	21.7	24.6	30.8	38.6	43.5	47.2	53.1
9.0-9.9	9.43	268	38.2	12.8	19.4	22.0	24.0	27.1	34.0	42.6	47.9	52.0	58.5
10.0-10.9	10.43	254	42.0	13.8	22.1	25.0	27.2	30.7	38.4	47.8	53.8	58.2	65.4
11.0-11.9	11.46	281	45.6	15.0	25.1	28.4	30.8	34.8	43.4	54.1	60.8	65.8	73.9
12.0-12.9	12.46	216	48.9	16.2	27.7	31.4	34.1	38.5	48.2	60.1	67.6	73.2	82.3
13.0-13.9	13.45	224	51.8	17.1	29.8	33.8	36.7	41.4	51.9	64.7	72.8	78.8	88.6
14.0-14.9	14.47	220	54.4	18.0	31.2	35.3	38.4	43.3	54.2	67.7	76.1	82.4	92.7
15.0-15.9	15.47	188	56.6	18.7	32.1	36.3	39.4	44.4	55.5	69.3	78.0	84.5	95.1
16.0-16.9	16.46	218	58.6	19.4	32.6	36.8	39.9	45.1	56.3	70.3	79.2	85.8	96.6
17.0-17.9	17.45	208	60.2	20.4	32.7	37.0	40.3	45.6	57.3	71.9	81.2	88.1	99.5
18.0-18.9	18.43	182	61.6	21.2	32.9	37.4	40.7	46.2	58.3	73.5	83.2	90.5	102.4
19.0-19.9	19.48	184	62.9	21.7	33.6	38.2	41.6	47.2	59.7	75.3	85.2	92.7	104.9
20.0-29.9	24.91	1817	67.6	23.3	36.1	41.1	44.8	50.9	64.2	80.9	91.4	99.3	112.1
30.0-39.9	34.85	1790	76.4	27.4	40.1	45.8	50.2	57.3	73.1	93.0	105.6	115.1	130.7
40.0-49.9	44.28	1293	83.5	27.2	47.0	53.0	57.6	64.9	80.9	100.6	113.0	122.2	137.1
50.0-59.9	54.83	971	84.3	27.7	47.3	53.4	58.0	65.5	81.9	102.0	114.7	124.1	139.4
60.0-69.9	64.82	1124	82.0	26.0	47.2	53.1	57.5	64.6	80.1	99.0	110.8	119.6	133.8
70.0-79.9	74.46	915	74.8	23.8	42.6	48.0	52.0	58.4	72.5	89.8	100.6	108.6	121.5
80.0-90.9	84.45	705	63.9	19.7	37.6	42.2	45.6	51.0	62.9	77.4	86.4	93.0	103.8

156

Table IV.33.

Mean (M), standard deviation (SD), and percentiles of mid-upper arm muscle area (cm^2) by age for males and females of 2 to 90 years

Age Group (years)	Mean Age (years)	N	M	SD	Percentiles								
					5th	10th	15th	25th	50th	75th	85th	90th	95th
Males													
2.0-2.9	2.46	548	14.7	2.2	11.4	12.0	12.5	13.2	14.5	16.0	16.9	17.5	18.5
3.0-3.9	3.45	481	16.4	2.5	12.4	13.1	13.7	14.5	16.1	17.9	18.9	19.6	20.7
4.0-4.9	4.47	542	17.4	2.8	13.0	13.8	14.3	15.2	16.9	18.8	19.9	20.7	21.9
5.0-5.9	5.43	492	18.2	3.1	13.6	14.5	15.1	16.1	18.1	20.3	21.6	22.5	23.9
6.0-6.9	6.45	258	19.3	3.6	14.6	15.6	16.3	17.4	19.8	22.4	23.9	25.0	26.7
7.0-7.9	7.47	271	20.8	3.9	15.8	16.9	17.7	19.0	21.5	24.4	26.2	27.4	29.3
8.0-8.9	8.46	257	22.8	4.3	17.0	18.2	19.1	20.5	23.2	26.4	28.2	29.5	31.6
9.0-9.9	9.50	282	25.6	5.0	18.2	19.6	20.5	22.0	25.1	28.6	30.7	32.2	34.5
10.0-10.9	10.45	287	28.6	5.9	19.3	20.9	22.0	23.7	27.2	31.3	33.7	35.5	38.2
11.0-11.9	11.44	272	32.1	7.2	20.8	22.6	23.9	25.9	30.2	35.0	38.0	40.1	43.4
12.0-12.9	12.47	201	36.1	8.0	23.1	25.2	26.7	29.1	34.1	40.0	43.5	46.0	50.1
13.0-13.9	13.47	188	40.0	9.4	26.3	28.6	30.3	33.0	38.7	45.3	49.2	52.1	56.6
14.0-14.9	14.49	179	44.1	9.8	30.3	32.9	34.7	37.7	43.7	50.7	54.9	58.0	62.7
15.0-15.9	15.45	177	47.9	9.5	34.3	37.0	38.9	42.0	48.3	55.6	59.9	63.0	67.8
16.0-16.9	16.45	191	51.6	10.4	37.6	40.5	42.6	45.8	52.5	60.1	64.6	67.9	72.9
17.0-17.9	17.45	188	55.0	11.2	40.0	43.1	45.3	48.8	56.0	64.2	69.0	72.5	78.0
18.0-18.9	18.45	167	58.0	11.7	42.0	45.2	47.5	51.2	58.6	67.1	72.2	75.8	81.5
19.0-19.9	19.43	154	60.6	12.2	42.6	45.8	48.2	51.8	59.4	68.0	73.1	76.7	82.5
20.0-29.9	24.96	1564	64.5	13.4	45.2	48.8	51.4	55.4	63.8	73.4	79.1	83.2	89.6
30.0-39.9	34.72	1405	66.6	13.5	48.7	52.4	55.2	59.4	68.1	78.1	84.0	88.3	95.0
40.0-49.9	44.35	1158	69.9	12.8	49.8	53.5	56.2	60.5	69.1	79.0	84.8	89.0	95.6
50.0-59.9	54.89	815	67.4	12.6	49.7	53.3	55.8	59.7	67.8	76.9	82.3	86.1	92.1
60.0-69.9	64.83	1122	64.8	12.4	46.8	50.2	52.7	56.5	64.4	73.3	78.6	82.4	88.3
70.0-79.9	74.16	820	59.5	11.1	43.5	46.5	48.8	52.2	59.2	67.2	71.8	75.2	80.4
80.0-90.9	84.09	635	52.7	10.1	38.1	40.9	42.9	46.0	52.4	59.6	63.9	66.9	71.7
Females													
2.0-2.9	2.45	534	15.0	2.2	10.9	11.5	12.0	12.6	14.0	15.5	16.4	17.0	18.0
3.0-3.9	3.46	554	14.7	2.4	11.9	12.6	13.1	13.9	15.5	17.2	18.3	19.0	20.1
4.0-4.9	4.43	526	15.3	2.6	12.7	13.5	14.1	15.0	16.8	18.9	20.1	20.9	22.2
5.0-5.9	5.46	540	16.8	3.1	13.2	14.1	14.7	15.7	17.8	20.1	21.5	22.5	24.0
6.0-6.9	6.47	272	18.8	3.6	13.6	14.6	15.4	16.5	18.8	21.4	22.9	24.0	25.8
7.0-7.9	7.44	263	20.9	4.2	14.0	15.1	15.8	17.1	19.6	22.4	24.1	25.3	27.3
8.0-8.9	8.47	245	23.2	4.5	14.6	15.7	16.6	17.9	20.7	23.8	25.7	27.1	29.2
9.0-9.9	9.43	266	25.4	5.6	15.7	17.0	17.9	19.4	22.5	26.1	28.2	29.7	32.2
10.0-10.9	10.43	254	27.6	5.5	17.7	19.2	20.3	21.9	25.5	29.5	32.0	33.7	36.5
11.0-11.9	11.46	281	29.7	6.5	20.2	21.9	23.2	25.1	29.1	33.8	36.6	38.6	41.8
12.0-12.9	12.46	216	31.5	6.9	22.6	24.5	25.9	28.0	32.5	37.7	40.8	43.1	46.6
13.0-13.9	13.45	224	33.1	7.3	24.3	26.3	27.8	30.1	35.0	40.5	43.9	46.3	50.1
14.0-14.9	14.47	218	34.5	7.6	25.1	27.2	28.7	31.1	36.1	41.9	45.3	47.8	51.8
15.0-15.9	15.47	187	35.6	8.0	25.1	27.2	28.7	31.2	36.2	42.1	45.6	48.2	52.2
16.0-16.9	16.46	216	36.6	8.2	24.9	27.1	28.6	31.0	36.1	41.9	45.4	48.0	52.0
17.0-17.9	17.45	202	37.4	8.6	24.7	26.8	28.4	30.9	36.1	42.1	45.8	48.4	52.6
18.0-18.9	18.43	178	38.0	8.7	24.9	27.0	28.6	31.1	36.3	42.4	46.0	48.7	52.9
19.0-19.9	19.48	182	38.5	8.8	25.3	27.5	29.1	31.6	36.9	43.0	46.7	49.4	53.6
20.0-29.9	24.91	1766	39.9	9.1	26.4	28.7	30.3	32.9	38.4	44.7	48.6	51.3	55.7
30.0-39.9	34.85	1698	42.3	10.5	27.4	30.0	31.9	34.9	41.3	48.8	53.4	56.7	62.0
40.0-49.9	44.28	1227	44.8	11.3	29.0	31.8	33.9	37.1	44.1	52.2	57.2	60.9	66.7
50.0-59.9	54.83	928	45.7	11.7	28.8	31.7	33.7	37.0	44.1	52.4	57.4	61.2	67.1
60.0-69.9	64.82	1092	45.1	11.7	28.1	30.9	32.9	36.2	43.1	51.2	56.2	59.9	65.7
70.0-79.9	74.46	899	43.7	11.3	27.5	30.2	32.2	35.3	42.1	50.1	54.9	58.5	64.2
80.0-90.9	84.45	696	41.0	10.5	26.2	28.8	30.7	33.7	40.1	47.6	52.2	55.6	61.0

Table IV.34.

Mean (M), standard deviation (SD), and percentiles of mid-upper arm fat area (cm^2) by age for males and females of 2 to 90 years

Age Group (years)	Mean Age (years)	N	M	SD	Percentiles								
					5th	10th	15th	25th	50th	75th	85th	90th	95th
						Males							
2.0-2.9	2.46	548	6.5	1.6	4.2	4.6	4.9	5.4	6.4	7.5	8.2	8.7	9.5
3.0-3.9	3.45	481	6.8	2.1	3.9	4.3	4.7	5.3	6.5	8.0	8.9	9.6	10.6
4.0-4.9	4.47	542	6.2	2.1	3.6	4.1	4.5	5.1	6.4	8.1	9.1	9.9	11.2
5.0-5.9	5.43	492	6.4	2.7	3.3	3.8	4.2	4.9	6.6	8.7	10.0	11.1	12.8
6.0-6.9	6.45	258	6.9	3.5	2.9	3.5	3.9	4.8	6.7	9.5	11.3	12.8	15.2
7.0-7.9	7.47	271	7.8	4.5	2.7	3.3	3.9	4.8	7.1	10.3	12.6	14.4	17.6
8.0-8.9	8.46	257	8.8	5.2	2.8	3.5	4.1	5.1	7.7	11.5	14.1	16.2	19.9
9.0-9.9	9.50	282	9.7	5.7	3.3	4.1	4.8	5.9	8.9	13.2	16.2	18.6	22.8
10.0-10.9	10.45	287	10.6	6.3	3.7	4.7	5.4	6.8	10.1	15.0	18.4	21.2	25.9
11.0-11.9	11.44	272	11.4	6.9	4.0	5.0	5.9	7.4	11.1	16.6	20.6	23.7	29.2
12.0-12.9	12.47	201	12.1	7.7	3.9	5.0	5.9	7.5	11.5	17.6	21.9	25.5	31.7
13.0-13.9	13.47	188	12.7	8.4	3.6	4.7	5.6	7.2	11.3	17.5	22.0	25.8	32.3
14.0-14.9	14.49	179	13.1	8.8	3.4	4.4	5.3	6.8	10.8	16.8	21.2	24.8	31.2
15.0-15.9	15.45	177	13.5	8.8	3.5	4.5	5.3	6.8	10.6	16.4	20.6	24.0	29.9
16.0-16.9	16.45	191	13.8	8.5	3.9	5.0	5.8	7.4	11.2	16.9	20.9	24.2	29.9
17.0-17.9	17.45	188	14.0	8.4	4.4	5.5	6.4	8.0	12.1	18.0	22.2	25.6	31.4
18.0-18.9	18.45	167	14.2	8.8	4.4	5.6	6.6	8.3	12.6	19.0	23.6	27.2	33.7
19.0-19.9	19.43	154	14.4	8.5	4.9	6.1	7.1	8.9	13.3	19.7	24.3	27.9	34.1
20.0-29.9	24.96	1564	15.5	8.3	6.1	7.5	8.7	10.6	15.3	21.8	26.2	29.7	35.6
30.0-39.9	34.72	1405	18.0	9.0	7.4	9.0	10.2	12.4	17.4	24.3	28.9	32.5	38.5
40.0-49.9	44.35	1158	18.2	8.9	7.7	9.3	10.5	12.7	17.7	24.5	29.1	32.6	38.6
50.0-59.9	54.89	815	18.4	8.7	8.0	9.6	10.8	12.9	17.9	24.6	29.0	32.4	38.1
60.0-69.9	64.83	1122	18.4	8.4	8.3	9.8	11.1	13.1	17.9	24.2	28.4	31.6	36.9
70.0-79.9	74.16	820	17.7	8.4	7.5	9.0	10.2	12.2	16.9	23.1	27.2	30.4	35.8
80.0-90.9	84.09	635	15.9	7.2	7.0	8.3	9.3	11.1	15.0	20.2	23.7	26.3	30.7
						Females							
2.0-2.9	2.45	534	7.6	2.3	3.4	4.1	4.6	5.3	6.7	8.1	8.8	9.3	10.1
3.0-3.9	3.46	554	6.7	2.2	3.3	4.1	4.6	5.4	6.8	8.3	9.1	9.7	10.5
4.0-4.9	4.43	526	6.7	2.7	2.3	3.1	3.7	4.6	6.3	8.0	9.0	9.6	10.6
5.0-5.9	5.46	540	7.4	3.4	2.0	3.1	3.8	4.9	7.0	9.2	10.4	11.2	12.4
6.0-6.9	6.47	272	8.6	4.2	1.8	3.1	4.0	5.4	8.0	10.7	12.2	13.2	14.7
7.0-7.9	7.44	263	9.9	5.1	1.8	3.3	4.4	6.0	9.2	12.4	14.2	15.4	17.2
8.0-8.9	8.47	245	11.5	6.1	1.8	3.6	4.9	6.9	10.6	14.4	16.5	18.0	20.1
9.0-9.9	9.43	266	13.0	7.0	2.0	4.0	5.5	7.7	12.0	16.4	18.8	20.4	22.9
10.0-10.9	10.43	254	14.6	7.9	2.2	4.5	6.2	8.6	13.4	18.4	21.1	22.9	25.7
11.0-11.9	11.46	281	16.2	8.6	2.6	5.1	6.9	9.6	14.9	20.3	23.3	25.3	28.4
12.0-12.9	12.46	216	17.6	9.3	3.0	5.7	7.7	10.6	16.3	22.1	25.3	27.5	30.8
13.0-13.9	13.45	224	19.0	9.8	3.5	6.4	8.5	11.6	17.6	23.8	27.2	29.5	33.0
14.0-14.9	14.47	218	20.2	10.1	4.1	7.1	9.3	12.6	18.8	25.3	28.9	31.3	34.9
15.0-15.9	15.47	187	21.2	10.4	4.4	7.7	10.0	13.4	20.0	26.6	30.3	32.7	36.4
16.0-16.9	16.46	216	22.2	10.6	5.0	8.4	10.8	14.3	21.0	27.8	31.5	34.1	37.8
17.0-17.9	17.45	202	23.0	10.8	5.5	9.0	11.5	15.1	21.9	28.9	32.7	35.2	39.1
18.0-18.9	18.43	178	23.7	10.9	6.1	9.6	12.1	15.7	22.7	29.8	33.7	36.3	40.2
19.0-19.9	19.48	182	24.4	11.0	6.5	10.2	12.7	16.4	23.5	30.7	34.6	37.3	41.3
20.0-29.9	24.91	1766	27.1	11.9	7.7	11.8	14.6	18.8	26.6	34.5	38.8	41.7	46.0
30.0-39.9	34.85	1698	32.3	13.7	10.1	15.0	18.3	23.3	32.6	42.0	47.1	50.5	55.6
40.0-49.9	44.28	1227	37.1	12.9	16.2	20.9	24.1	28.9	37.7	46.6	51.4	54.6	59.4
50.0-59.9	54.83	928	37.7	13.2	16.3	21.1	24.4	29.2	38.2	47.2	52.0	55.3	60.1
60.0-69.9	64.82	1092	34.2	12.7	13.9	18.9	22.3	27.2	36.3	45.4	50.3	53.6	58.5
70.0-79.9	74.46	899	30.3	11.9	10.7	14.9	17.7	21.8	29.6	37.5	41.8	44.6	48.9
80.0-90.9	84.45	696	23.1	9.0	8.4	11.6	13.7	16.9	22.8	28.8	32.0	34.2	37.5

Table IV.35.

Mean (M), standard deviation (SD), and percentiles of mid-upper arm fat index (arm fat area/total arm area x 100) by age for males and females of 2 to 90 years

Age Group (years)	Mean Age (years)	N	M	SD	Percentiles								
					5th	10th	15th	25th	50th	75th	85th	90th	95th
Males													
2.0-2.9	2.46	548	30.6	5.0	23.0	24.4	25.5	27.0	30.2	33.7	35.7	37.2	39.4
3.0-3.9	3.45	481	28.4	4.7	22.0	23.4	24.4	25.9	28.9	32.3	34.2	35.6	37.8
4.0-4.9	4.47	542	27.5	4.6	21.0	22.4	23.3	24.8	27.8	31.1	33.0	34.4	36.6
5.0-5.9	5.43	492	27.4	5.4	19.4	20.8	21.9	23.5	26.8	30.6	32.8	34.4	36.9
6.0-6.9	6.45	258	27.6	6.5	17.5	19.1	20.3	22.1	25.9	30.4	33.1	35.0	38.1
7.0-7.9	7.47	271	27.8	7.5	16.3	18.0	19.2	21.2	25.5	30.6	33.7	36.0	39.6
8.0-8.9	8.46	257	27.8	8.0	16.1	17.8	19.2	21.3	25.8	31.3	34.7	37.2	41.2
9.0-9.9	9.50	282	27.6	8.1	16.5	18.4	19.8	22.0	26.8	32.5	36.1	38.8	43.0
10.0-10.9	10.45	287	27.2	8.0	16.7	18.7	20.2	22.5	27.6	33.6	37.3	39.9	44.2
11.0-11.9	11.44	272	26.4	8.1	16.4	18.4	19.9	22.4	27.6	33.9	37.8	40.6	45.1
12.0-12.9	12.47	201	25.5	8.4	14.9	16.9	18.4	20.9	26.2	32.7	36.7	39.6	44.4
13.0-13.9	13.47	188	24.4	8.7	12.8	14.7	16.1	18.4	23.5	29.8	33.7	36.7	41.4
14.0-14.9	14.49	179	23.2	8.7	10.7	12.4	13.6	15.7	20.3	26.1	29.7	32.4	36.8
15.0-15.9	15.45	177	22.0	8.3	9.5	11.0	12.1	14.0	18.1	23.3	26.6	29.0	33.0
16.0-16.9	16.45	191	20.9	7.8	9.3	10.7	11.8	13.6	17.5	22.4	25.5	27.9	31.6
17.0-17.9	17.45	188	19.8	7.3	9.7	11.2	12.4	14.2	18.3	23.4	26.6	29.0	32.9
18.0-18.9	18.45	167	18.9	7.3	9.7	11.2	12.4	14.4	18.7	24.1	27.6	30.1	34.3
19.0-19.9	19.43	154	18.2	7.1	9.8	11.4	12.7	14.7	19.1	24.7	28.3	30.9	35.2
20.0-29.9	24.96	1564	18.7	6.7	9.9	11.6	12.9	14.9	19.2	24.2	27.2	29.4	32.8
30.0-39.9	34.72	1405	21.5	6.8	12.0	13.8	15.1	17.1	21.4	26.3	29.3	31.4	34.6
40.0-49.9	44.35	1158	21.4	7.1	11.8	13.6	14.9	17.0	21.5	26.6	29.6	31.8	35.2
50.0-59.9	54.89	815	21.4	6.9	11.9	13.7	15.0	17.0	21.3	26.2	29.2	31.3	34.5
60.0-69.9	64.83	1122	22.1	6.8	12.3	14.0	15.2	17.2	21.4	26.1	28.9	30.9	34.1
70.0-79.9	74.16	820	22.3	6.7	12.7	14.4	15.7	17.6	21.7	26.4	29.1	31.1	34.1
80.0-90.9	84.09	635	22.2	6.2	13.2	14.9	16.1	17.9	21.8	26.1	28.7	30.5	33.4
Females													
2.0-2.9	2.45	534	32.4	5.6	23.1	24.9	26.2	28.2	31.8	35.6	37.7	39.2	41.3
3.0-3.9	3.46	554	31.3	5.0	23.7	25.2	26.2	27.8	31.1	34.6	36.6	38.0	40.2
4.0-4.9	4.43	526	30.8	5.4	22.5	24.0	25.2	26.9	30.3	34.1	36.2	37.8	40.1
5.0-5.9	5.46	540	30.6	6.0	21.6	23.3	24.5	26.4	30.1	34.3	36.7	38.4	41.1
6.0-6.9	6.47	272	30.8	6.6	20.5	22.6	24.0	26.1	30.4	34.9	37.4	39.1	41.8
7.0-7.9	7.44	263	31.2	7.1	19.7	22.1	23.7	26.1	30.7	35.5	38.2	40.0	42.8
8.0-8.9	8.47	245	31.7	7.5	18.4	21.3	23.2	26.0	31.0	35.9	38.5	40.2	42.7
9.0-9.9	9.43	266	32.3	7.6	18.5	21.5	23.4	26.3	31.3	36.3	38.8	40.6	43.1
10.0-10.9	10.43	254	33.0	8.1	18.2	21.3	23.4	26.4	31.7	36.9	39.6	41.5	44.1
11.0-11.9	11.46	281	33.7	8.0	19.1	22.2	24.2	27.1	32.3	37.4	40.1	41.9	44.5
12.0-12.9	12.46	216	34.3	7.8	20.3	23.2	25.2	28.1	33.2	38.2	40.8	42.6	45.2
13.0-13.9	13.45	224	35.0	7.9	21.0	24.0	26.1	29.0	34.4	39.6	42.3	44.1	46.8
14.0-14.9	14.47	218	35.6	7.7	22.5	25.5	27.5	30.5	35.7	40.9	43.6	45.4	48.0
15.0-15.9	15.47	187	36.1	7.7	23.1	26.1	28.2	31.2	36.5	41.7	44.5	46.3	49.0
16.0-16.9	16.46	216	36.6	8.1	22.7	25.9	28.0	31.1	36.7	42.1	44.9	46.8	49.6
17.0-17.9	17.45	202	37.0	8.1	23.0	26.2	28.3	31.3	36.9	42.2	45.1	46.9	49.7
18.0-18.9	18.43	178	37.4	8.2	23.1	26.3	28.4	31.5	37.0	42.4	45.2	47.1	49.9
19.0-19.9	19.48	182	37.7	8.3	23.2	26.4	28.5	31.6	37.1	42.5	45.4	47.3	50.1
20.0-29.9	24.91	1766	39.2	8.5	24.7	28.1	30.3	33.5	39.3	45.0	47.9	49.9	52.9
30.0-39.9	34.85	1698	41.9	8.6	27.7	31.2	33.5	36.8	42.8	48.6	51.7	53.8	56.8
40.0-49.9	44.28	1227	44.3	8.0	31.1	34.3	36.4	39.4	44.9	50.3	53.1	55.0	57.8
50.0-59.9	54.83	928	43.8	7.8	30.7	33.8	35.8	38.8	44.2	49.5	52.3	54.1	56.9
60.0-69.9	64.82	1092	41.1	7.4	28.7	31.6	33.5	36.3	41.4	46.3	48.9	50.7	53.2
70.0-79.9	74.46	899	39.3	7.3	27.0	29.9	31.8	34.6	39.6	44.5	47.1	48.8	51.3
80.0-90.9	84.45	696	34.4	6.8	22.7	25.3	27.1	29.7	34.4	38.9	41.3	42.9	45.3

Postnatal Anthropometric Reference

Table IV.36.

Mean (M), standard deviation (SD), and percentiles of fat-free mass (kg) by age for males and females of 12 to 90 years

Age Group (years)	Mean Age (years)	N	M	SD	Percentiles								
					5th	10th	15th	25th	50th	75th	85th	90th	95th
Males													
12.0-12.9	12.47	185	38.0	8.0	24.5	27.2	29.1	31.9	37.1	42.3	45.2	47.1	50.0
13.0-13.9	13.47	177	44.4	9.0	30.0	33.0	35.1	38.3	44.2	50.4	53.7	56.0	59.4
14.0-14.9	14.49	168	49.1	9.1	35.0	38.1	40.3	43.5	49.7	55.9	59.3	61.7	65.2
15.0-15.9	15.45	169	52.1	8.9	37.4	40.3	42.3	45.3	51.0	57.0	60.3	62.6	66.1
16.0-16.9	16.45	178	54.3	8.7	39.5	42.2	44.2	47.1	52.7	58.5	61.7	64.0	67.3
17.0-17.9	17.45	184	55.7	8.6	41.3	44.2	46.2	49.2	54.8	60.6	63.7	65.9	69.1
18.0-18.9	18.45	162	56.5	8.9	41.9	44.9	47.0	50.1	56.0	61.9	65.2	67.4	70.8
19.0-19.9	19.43	156	57.0	8.6	43.3	45.9	47.7	50.5	56.0	61.9	65.2	67.5	71.1
20.0-29.9	24.96	1552	58.0	9.1	43.5	46.2	48.2	51.1	56.9	63.1	66.7	69.2	73.0
30.0-39.9	34.72	1387	60.7	10.3	43.8	47.0	49.3	52.7	59.2	66.2	70.0	72.7	76.8
40.0-49.9	44.35	1155	61.3	10.1	44.9	48.0	50.2	53.6	60.0	66.8	70.6	73.3	77.2
50.0-59.9	54.89	793	61.6	9.8	45.3	48.4	50.5	53.8	60.0	66.6	70.3	72.9	76.7
60.0-69.9	64.83	1055	59.4	9.3	44.5	47.5	49.6	52.7	58.8	65.1	68.7	71.2	74.9
70.0-79.9	74.16	724	57.0	9.0	42.6	45.4	47.5	50.5	56.3	62.5	65.9	68.3	71.8
80.0-90.9	84.09	505	53.7	8.0	41.2	43.8	45.5	48.2	53.4	58.9	61.9	64.0	67.2
Females													
12.0-12.9	12.46	204	37.4	5.7	29.0	30.5	31.6	33.3	36.8	40.9	43.4	45.2	48.2
13.0-13.9	13.45	210	38.7	5.6	30.2	31.7	32.8	34.5	37.9	42.0	44.4	46.2	49.0
14.0-14.9	14.47	198	39.6	5.9	30.6	32.1	33.2	34.9	38.4	42.6	45.1	46.9	49.8
15.0-15.9	15.47	160	40.2	5.5	31.7	33.2	34.2	35.9	39.3	43.2	45.5	47.2	49.9
16.0-16.9	16.46	188	40.6	5.6	31.9	33.4	34.5	36.1	39.6	43.5	45.9	47.6	50.4
17.0-17.9	17.45	181	40.9	5.6	32.5	34.0	35.1	36.8	40.2	44.3	46.7	48.4	51.2
18.0-18.9	18.43	147	41.1	5.9	32.7	34.2	35.4	37.1	40.8	45.0	47.6	49.4	52.4
19.0-19.9	19.48	159	41.3	5.9	32.8	34.3	35.5	37.3	40.9	45.2	47.8	49.7	52.7
20.0-29.9	24.91	1511	42.3	6.3	32.7	34.4	35.5	37.4	41.2	45.6	48.3	50.3	53.4
30.0-39.9	34.85	1634	44.4	7.1	33.6	35.4	36.7	38.8	43.0	48.1	51.2	53.4	57.0
40.0-49.9	44.28	1250	44.9	7.1	34.4	36.2	37.5	39.6	43.9	49.0	52.1	54.3	58.0
50.0-59.9	54.83	910	44.7	7.0	34.3	36.1	37.4	39.4	43.7	48.7	51.8	54.0	57.6
60.0-69.9	64.82	1031	43.0	6.4	33.3	34.9	36.1	38.0	41.9	46.4	49.2	51.2	54.4
70.0-79.9	74.46	818	41.9	6.1	32.0	33.5	34.7	36.4	40.1	44.3	46.8	48.7	51.7
80.0-90.9	84.45	521	38.9	5.2	31.3	32.7	33.7	35.3	38.5	42.3	44.5	46.1	48.6

Table IV.37.

Mean (M), standard deviation (SD), and percentiles of fat-free mass index (kg/m^2) by age for males and females of 12 to 90 years

Age Group	Mean Age				Percentiles								
(years)	(years)	N	M	SD	5th	10th	15th	25th	50th	75th	85th	90th	95th
Males													
12.0-12.9	12.08	185	15.9	2.0	12.7	13.3	13.7	14.3	15.6	16.9	17.7	18.3	19.2
13.0-13.9	13.08	177	16.7	2.2	13.2	13.8	14.3	14.9	16.3	17.8	18.7	19.3	20.3
14.0-14.9	14.08	168	17.3	2.3	13.9	14.6	15.1	15.8	17.2	18.8	19.8	20.4	21.4
15.0-15.9	15.08	169	17.7	2.3	14.1	14.7	15.2	15.9	17.3	18.9	19.9	20.6	21.6
16.0-16.9	16.08	178	18.1	2.3	14.2	14.9	15.3	16.1	17.5	19.1	20.0	20.7	21.7
17.0-17.9	17.08	184	18.3	2.3	14.8	15.5	15.9	16.7	18.1	19.7	20.6	21.3	22.3
18.0-18.9	18.08	162	18.5	2.5	14.8	15.5	16.0	16.8	18.3	20.0	21.0	21.8	22.9
19.0-19.9	19.00	156	18.8	2.5	14.9	15.6	16.1	16.9	18.4	20.2	21.2	21.9	23.0
20.0-29.9	21.00	1552	19.0	2.5	15.2	15.9	16.4	17.2	18.8	20.6	21.7	22.4	23.5
30.0-39.9	30.92	1387	19.8	2.7	15.6	16.3	16.9	17.7	19.4	21.3	22.4	23.2	24.5
40.0-49.9	40.75	1155	20.1	2.7	15.9	16.7	17.2	18.1	19.8	21.7	22.8	23.6	24.8
50.0-59.9	51.08	793	20.2	2.7	16.1	16.9	17.5	18.3	20.1	22.0	23.1	23.9	25.1
60.0-69.9	60.83	1055	19.9	2.6	16.2	16.9	17.4	18.2	19.9	21.7	22.7	23.5	24.6
70.0-79.9	70.83	724	19.4	2.5	15.5	16.3	16.8	17.6	19.1	20.9	21.9	22.6	23.7
80.0-90.9	80.50	505	18.7	2.3	15.3	15.9	16.4	17.2	18.6	20.2	21.1	21.8	22.8
Females													
12.0-12.9	12.08	204	15.3	1.6	12.8	13.2	13.5	13.9	14.8	16.0	16.7	17.2	18.1
13.0-13.9	13.06	210	15.2	1.6	12.8	13.2	13.5	13.9	14.9	16.1	16.8	17.4	18.3
14.0-14.9	14.08	198	15.3	1.7	12.8	13.2	13.5	14.0	15.0	16.2	17.0	17.6	18.6
15.0-15.9	15.08	160	15.3	1.7	12.8	13.2	13.5	14.0	15.0	16.3	17.1	17.8	18.8
16.0-16.9	16.08	188	15.4	1.8	12.8	13.3	13.6	14.1	15.1	16.5	17.3	18.0	19.1
17.0-17.9	17.08	181	15.5	1.8	12.9	13.3	13.6	14.1	15.2	16.6	17.5	18.2	19.3
18.0-18.9	18.08	147	15.6	1.9	12.9	13.3	13.7	14.2	15.3	16.7	17.7	18.4	19.6
19.0-19.9	19.07	159	15.8	2.0	12.9	13.4	13.7	14.2	15.4	16.9	17.8	18.6	19.8
20.0-29.9	21.00	1511	16.1	2.1	13.0	13.5	13.8	14.4	15.6	17.1	18.2	19.0	20.3
30.0-39.9	30.92	1634	16.7	2.4	13.4	14.0	14.4	15.0	16.4	18.2	19.4	20.3	21.9
40.0-49.9	40.58	1250	17.2	2.5	13.8	14.3	14.7	15.4	16.9	18.7	19.9	20.9	22.5
50.0-59.9	50.75	910	17.2	2.4	14.0	14.5	14.9	15.5	16.9	18.7	19.9	20.8	22.4
60.0-69.9	61.00	1031	17.0	2.2	13.9	14.4	14.8	15.4	16.7	18.4	19.5	20.4	21.9
70.0-79.9	70.67	818	16.8	2.1	13.8	14.3	14.6	15.2	16.5	18.1	19.2	20.0	21.4
80.0-90.9	80.58	521	16.2	1.7	13.8	14.2	14.5	15.0	16.0	17.3	18.1	18.7	19.7

Table IV.38

Mean (M), standard deviation (SD), and percentiles of total body fat mass (kg) by age for males and females of 12 to 90 years

Age Group (years)	Mean Age (years)	N	M	SD	Percentiles								
					5th	10th	15th	25th	50th	75th	85th	90th	95th
Males													
12.0-12.9	12.47	185	11.25	7.7	2.9	3.7	4.3	5.5	8.7	13.8	17.7	21.1	27.1
13.0-13.9	13.47	177	11.59	7.9	2.9	3.7	4.3	5.5	8.8	13.9	17.9	21.2	27.4
14.0-14.9	14.49	168	12.20	8.1	3.3	4.2	4.9	6.2	9.6	15.1	19.2	22.7	29.1
15.0-15.9	15.45	169	12.92	8.1	3.8	4.8	5.6	7.0	10.6	16.3	20.5	24.0	30.4
16.0-16.9	16.45	178	13.75	7.7	4.5	5.4	6.2	7.6	11.0	16.1	19.8	22.8	28.0
17.0-17.9	17.45	184	14.60	6.9	5.9	7.0	7.9	9.3	12.8	17.5	20.8	23.4	27.8
18.0-18.9	18.45	162	15.42	7.3	6.4	7.6	8.5	10.1	13.9	19.2	22.9	25.8	30.7
19.0-19.9	19.43	156	16.17	7.4	7.1	8.3	9.3	11.0	14.9	20.3	24.0	26.8	31.8
20.0-29.9	24.96	1552	19.00	8.7	7.6	9.2	10.5	12.6	17.4	23.3	27.2	30.0	34.6
30.0-39.9	34.72	1387	20.57	8.4	8.9	10.9	12.3	14.6	19.6	25.4	28.9	31.4	35.3
40.0-49.9	44.35	1155	21.90	8.7	9.5	11.5	13.0	15.4	20.4	26.2	29.7	32.3	36.2
50.0-59.9	54.89	793	22.12	8.0	10.6	12.6	14.0	16.3	21.1	26.6	29.9	32.2	35.9
60.0-69.9	64.83	1055	21.87	7.4	11.2	13.0	14.4	16.5	21.0	26.1	29.1	31.2	34.5
70.0-79.9	74.16	724	20.09	6.8	10.5	12.3	13.5	15.6	19.8	24.5	27.4	29.4	32.5
80.0-90.9	84.09	505	17.99	5.9	9.5	11.0	12.1	13.9	17.5	21.7	24.1	25.8	28.5
Females													
12.0-12.9	12.46	204	15.05	7.5	4.6	6.2	7.4	9.4	13.6	18.6	21.5	23.6	26.9
13.0-13.9	13.45	210	17.15	7.7	5.8	7.5	8.8	10.8	15.0	19.9	22.8	24.8	28.0
14.0-14.9	14.47	198	18.68	8.3	6.6	8.5	9.9	12.1	16.8	22.2	25.3	27.6	31.1
15.0-15.9	15.47	160	19.77	9.1	6.4	8.3	9.8	12.1	17.0	22.7	26.1	28.5	32.2
16.0-16.9	16.46	188	20.54	10.0	6.0	8.1	9.6	12.1	17.3	23.4	27.0	29.6	33.6
17.0-17.9	17.45	181	21.10	10.3	6.4	8.5	10.1	12.7	18.3	24.8	28.6	31.4	35.7
18.0-18.9	18.43	147	21.53	10.4	6.4	8.9	10.7	13.5	19.5	26.2	30.1	32.8	37.0
19.0-19.9	19.48	159	21.91	10.5	6.5	9.0	10.8	13.7	19.7	26.5	30.4	33.1	37.4
20.0-29.9	24.91	1511	23.79	10.4	8.0	10.5	12.3	15.1	21.0	27.5	31.3	33.9	38.0
30.0-39.9	34.85	1634	27.70	12.1	7.9	11.5	14.1	17.8	25.1	32.6	36.7	39.5	43.7
40.0-49.9	44.28	1250	29.34	11.4	10.1	14.0	16.6	20.5	27.7	34.9	38.8	41.4	45.3
50.0-59.9	54.83	910	29.83	10.5	12.0	15.7	18.1	21.8	28.5	35.3	38.9	41.4	45.1
60.0-69.9	64.82	1031	28.19	9.9	11.4	14.7	17.0	20.4	26.7	33.1	36.5	38.8	42.2
70.0-79.9	74.46	818	25.78	9.0	10.6	13.7	15.8	18.9	24.7	30.6	33.7	35.8	39.0
80.0-90.9	84.45	521	21.73	7.5	9.1	11.7	13.5	16.1	20.9	25.8	28.4	30.2	32.8

Table IV.39.
Mean (M), standard deviation (SD), and percentiles of total fat mass index (kg of fat/m^2) by age for males and females of 12 to 90 years

Age Group (years)	Mean Age (years)	N	M	SD	Percentiles								
					5th	10th	15th	25th	50th	75th	85th	90th	95th
Males													
12.0-12.9	12.08	185	4.73	3.0	1.34	1.65	1.91	2.38	3.61	5.57	7.08	8.36	10.73
13.0-13.9	13.08	177	4.32	2.8	1.22	1.52	1.76	2.21	3.39	5.30	6.79	8.06	10.43
14.0-14.9	14.08	168	4.23	2.6	1.23	1.52	1.76	2.18	3.29	5.05	6.40	7.54	9.65
15.0-15.9	15.08	169	4.33	2.6	1.26	1.54	1.78	2.19	3.28	4.99	6.29	7.38	9.39
16.0-16.9	16.08	178	4.56	2.4	1.60	1.91	2.16	2.60	3.69	5.30	6.47	7.42	9.12
17.0-17.9	17.08	184	4.86	2.3	2.03	2.38	2.66	3.14	4.29	5.91	7.06	7.97	9.56
18.0-18.9	18.08	162	5.18	2.4	2.13	2.52	2.82	3.33	4.53	6.18	7.29	8.16	9.64
19.0-19.9	19.00	156	5.47	2.5	2.20	2.60	2.91	3.43	4.66	6.33	7.47	8.35	9.85
20.0-29.9	21.00	1552	6.02	2.7	2.34	2.89	3.30	3.98	5.48	7.29	8.40	9.21	10.50
30.0-39.9	30.92	1387	6.80	2.7	2.83	3.54	4.05	4.85	6.50	8.33	9.39	10.14	11.29
40.0-49.9	40.75	1155	7.17	2.6	3.23	3.92	4.42	5.20	6.78	8.53	9.54	10.25	11.33
50.0-59.9	51.08	793	7.28	2.6	3.40	4.09	4.59	5.38	6.96	8.70	9.70	10.40	11.48
60.0-69.9	60.83	1055	7.33	2.5	3.52	4.18	4.66	5.40	6.89	8.52	9.45	10.11	11.11
70.0-79.9	70.83	724	6.84	2.2	3.52	4.16	4.62	5.33	6.75	8.30	9.19	9.81	10.76
80.0-90.9	80.50	505	6.27	2.0	3.21	3.78	4.20	4.83	6.12	7.52	8.32	8.88	9.74
Females													
12.0-12.9	12.08	204	6.15	2.8	2.66	3.15	3.53	4.17	5.67	7.68	9.03	10.08	11.84
13.0-13.9	13.06	210	6.70	3.1	2.77	3.29	3.69	4.37	5.97	8.13	9.58	10.71	12.61
14.0-14.9	14.08	198	7.15	3.3	2.89	3.43	3.86	4.58	6.27	8.57	10.13	11.33	13.37
15.0-15.9	15.08	160	7.50	3.5	3.00	3.57	4.01	4.77	6.55	8.98	10.62	11.90	14.06
16.0-16.9	16.08	188	7.79	3.7	3.11	3.70	4.17	4.95	6.82	9.36	11.08	12.42	14.69
17.0-17.9	17.08	181	8.04	3.8	3.22	3.83	4.32	5.14	7.08	9.72	11.51	12.91	15.27
18.0-18.9	18.08	147	8.28	3.9	3.32	3.96	4.46	5.31	7.32	10.06	11.92	13.36	15.81
19.0-19.9	19.07	159	8.50	4.0	3.43	4.09	4.61	5.48	7.55	10.37	12.28	13.77	16.29
20.0-29.9	21.00	1511	8.92	4.2	3.64	4.34	4.88	5.80	7.97	10.93	12.93	14.49	17.12
30.0-39.9	30.92	1634	10.70	4.6	4.70	5.52	6.15	7.20	9.66	12.92	15.09	16.76	19.55
40.0-49.9	40.58	1250	11.20	4.4	5.52	6.38	7.05	8.14	10.64	13.87	15.97	17.58	20.23
50.0-59.9	50.75	910	11.57	4.3	5.95	6.82	7.47	8.55	10.96	14.03	16.01	17.50	19.95
60.0-69.9	61.00	1031	11.16	4.0	5.92	6.74	7.37	8.38	10.65	13.50	15.32	16.69	18.94
70.0-79.9	70.67	818	10.39	3.6	5.58	6.34	6.92	7.86	9.95	12.57	14.24	15.50	17.55
80.0-90.9	80.58	521	9.07	3.1	5.09	5.77	6.28	7.11	8.96	11.25	12.72	13.81	15.60

Table IV.40.

Mean (M), standard deviation (SD), and percentiles of percent body fat (%) by age for males and females of 12 to 90 years

Age Group (years)	Mean Age (years)	N	M	SD	Percentiles								
					5th	10th	15th	25th	50th	75th	85th	90th	95th
Males													
12.0-12.9	12.47	185	20.78	8.0	10.1	11.6	12.8	14.8	19.2	24.9	28.6	31.4	36.0
13.0-13.9	13.47	177	19.28	7.7	9.0	10.5	11.6	13.4	17.5	23.0	26.5	29.2	33.7
14.0-14.9	14.49	168	18.66	7.7	8.3	9.6	10.7	12.4	16.4	21.7	25.2	27.8	32.3
15.0-15.9	15.45	169	18.67	6.8	9.7	11.1	12.2	13.9	17.9	22.8	26.0	28.4	32.4
16.0-16.9	16.45	178	19.06	6.5	10.3	11.7	12.7	14.4	18.1	22.7	25.7	27.9	31.5
17.0-17.9	17.45	184	19.70	6.0	11.1	12.6	13.7	15.5	19.1	23.4	25.9	27.7	30.5
18.0-18.9	18.45	162	20.44	6.0	11.5	13.1	14.3	16.1	19.8	23.9	26.3	28.0	30.6
19.0-19.9	19.43	156	21.18	5.9	12.0	13.6	14.8	16.6	20.3	24.2	26.5	28.1	30.6
20.0-29.9	24.96	1552	23.94	6.2	13.1	15.2	16.6	18.7	22.6	26.6	28.7	30.2	32.4
30.0-39.9	34.72	1387	24.33	5.8	14.4	16.8	18.4	20.6	24.7	28.5	30.5	31.9	33.8
40.0-49.9	44.35	1155	25.48	5.5	16.0	18.3	19.7	21.9	25.7	29.4	31.3	32.6	34.5
50.0-59.9	54.89	793	25.61	5.6	16.7	18.7	20.1	22.2	26.0	29.7	31.8	33.1	35.2
60.0-69.9	64.83	1055	25.54	5.3	16.5	18.7	20.1	22.1	25.8	29.4	31.2	32.5	34.3
70.0-79.9	74.16	724	25.38	5.3	16.3	18.4	19.8	21.9	25.5	29.0	30.9	32.1	33.9
80.0-90.9	84.09	505	24.42	5.0	15.8	17.9	19.2	21.2	24.7	28.0	29.8	31.0	32.7
Females													
12.0-12.9	12.46	204	26.95	7.7	15.2	17.6	19.3	21.9	27.0	32.4	35.4	37.5	40.6
13.0-13.9	13.45	210	28.94	7.7	16.7	19.0	20.7	23.3	28.2	33.4	36.3	38.3	41.4
14.0-14.9	14.47	198	30.36	6.6	20.4	22.6	24.1	26.4	30.8	35.4	37.9	39.7	42.3
15.0-15.9	15.47	160	31.33	6.7	20.5	22.7	24.2	26.5	30.8	35.4	37.9	39.6	42.3
16.0-16.9	16.46	188	31.98	6.9	20.6	22.8	24.3	26.6	31.0	35.6	38.2	39.9	42.6
17.0-17.9	17.45	181	32.41	7.4	20.7	23.1	24.7	27.2	32.0	37.1	39.9	41.8	44.7
18.0-18.9	18.43	147	32.71	7.7	20.6	23.0	24.8	27.3	32.3	37.5	40.4	42.5	45.5
19.0-19.9	19.48	159	32.94	7.6	20.9	23.4	25.1	27.6	32.6	37.8	40.7	42.7	45.6
20.0-29.9	24.91	1511	33.96	8.4	20.5	23.4	25.5	28.4	34.1	39.8	42.9	45.0	48.1
30.0-39.9	34.85	1634	36.69	8.1	21.4	25.3	27.8	31.2	36.9	42.2	44.9	46.6	49.2
40.0-49.9	44.28	1250	37.83	7.5	23.2	26.9	29.3	32.4	37.8	42.6	45.0	46.6	48.9
50.0-59.9	54.83	910	38.49	7.1	24.6	28.3	30.5	33.6	38.8	43.4	45.7	47.2	49.3
60.0-69.9	64.82	1031	38.23	7.0	24.5	28.0	30.2	33.2	38.3	42.7	45.0	46.4	48.5
70.0-79.9	74.46	818	36.79	6.5	24.4	27.7	29.7	32.5	37.2	41.4	43.5	44.9	46.9
80.0-90.9	84.45	521	34.62	6.1	22.6	25.7	27.5	30.1	34.5	38.4	40.3	41.6	43.4

LIST OF FIGURES: SMOOTHED ANTHROPOMETRIC REFERENCE

Figure IV.21. Percentiles of Percent Total Leg Length (%) for Males Ranging from 2 to 20 Years.

Figure IV.22. Percentiles of Percent Total Leg Length (%) for Females Ranging from 2 to 20 Years.

Figure IV.23. Percentiles of Percent Lower Leg Length (%) for Males Ranging from 2 to 20 Years.

Figure IV.24. Percentiles of Percent Lower Leg Length (%) for Females Ranging from 2 to 20 Years.

Figure IV.25. Percentiles of Triceps Skinfold Thickness (mm) for Males Ranging from 2 to 20 Years.

Figure IV.26. Percentiles of Triceps Skinfold Thickness (mm) for Females Ranging from 2 to 20 Years.

Figure IV.27. Percentiles of Subscapular Skinfold Thickness (mm) for Males Ranging from 2 to 20 Years.

Figure IV.28. Percentiles of Subscapular Skinfold Thickness (mm) for Females Ranging from 2 to 20 Years.

Figure IV.29. Percentiles of Mid-Upper Arm Muscle Area (cm^2) for Males Ranging in Age from 2 to 20 Years.

Figure IV.30. Percentiles of Mid-Upper Arm Muscle Area (cm^2) for Females Ranging in Age from 2 to 20 Years.

Figure IV.31. Percentiles of Waist Circumference in Centimeters (cm) and Inches (in.) for Males Ranging in Age from 2 to 20 Years.

Figure IV.32. Percentiles of Waist Circumference in Centimeters (cm) and Inches (in.) for Females Ranging in Age from 2 to 20 Years.

Figure IV.33. Percentiles of Fat-Free Mass (kg) for Males Ranging in Age from 20 to 90 Years.

Figure IV.34. Percentiles of Fat-Free Mass (kg) for Females Ranging in Age from 20 to 90 Years.

Figure IV.35. Percentiles of Fat-Free Mass Index (kg/m^2) for Males Ranging in Age from 20 to 90 Years.

Figure IV.36. Percentiles of Fat-Free Mass Index (kg/m^2) for Females Ranging in Age from 20 to 90 Years.

Figure IV.37. Percentiles of Percent Body Fat (%) for Males Ranging in Age from 20 to 90 Years.

Figure IV.38. Percentiles of Percent Body Fat (%) for Females Ranging in Age from 20 to 90 Years.

Figure IV.39. Percentiles of Fat Mass Index (kg/m^2) for Males Ranging in Age from 20 to 90 Years.

Figure IV.40. Percentiles of Fat Mass Index (kg/m^2) for Females Ranging in Age from 20 to 90 Years.

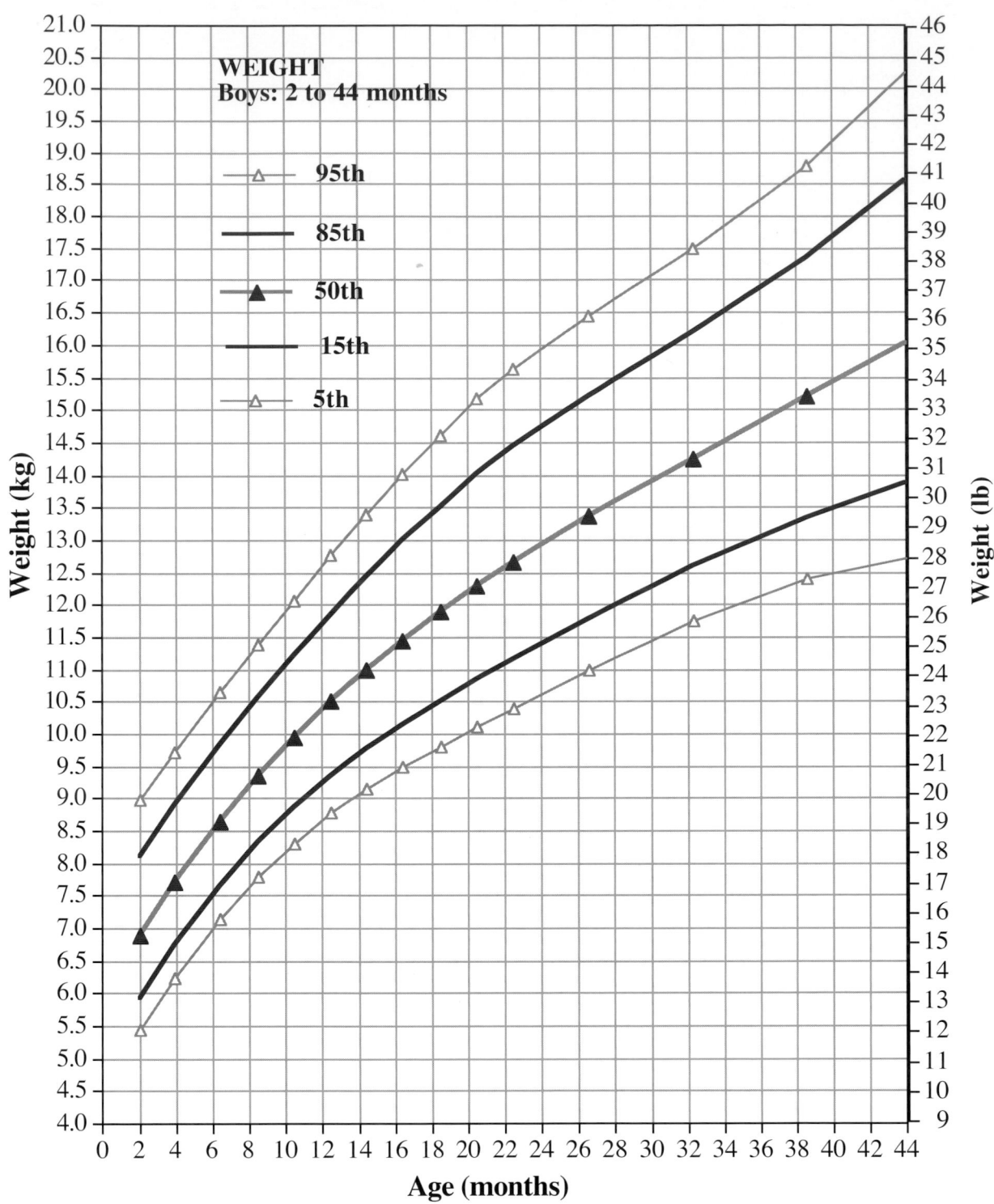

Figure IV.7. Percentiles of Weight in Kilograms (kg) and Pounds (lb.) by Age for Boys Ranging in Age from 2 to 44 Months.

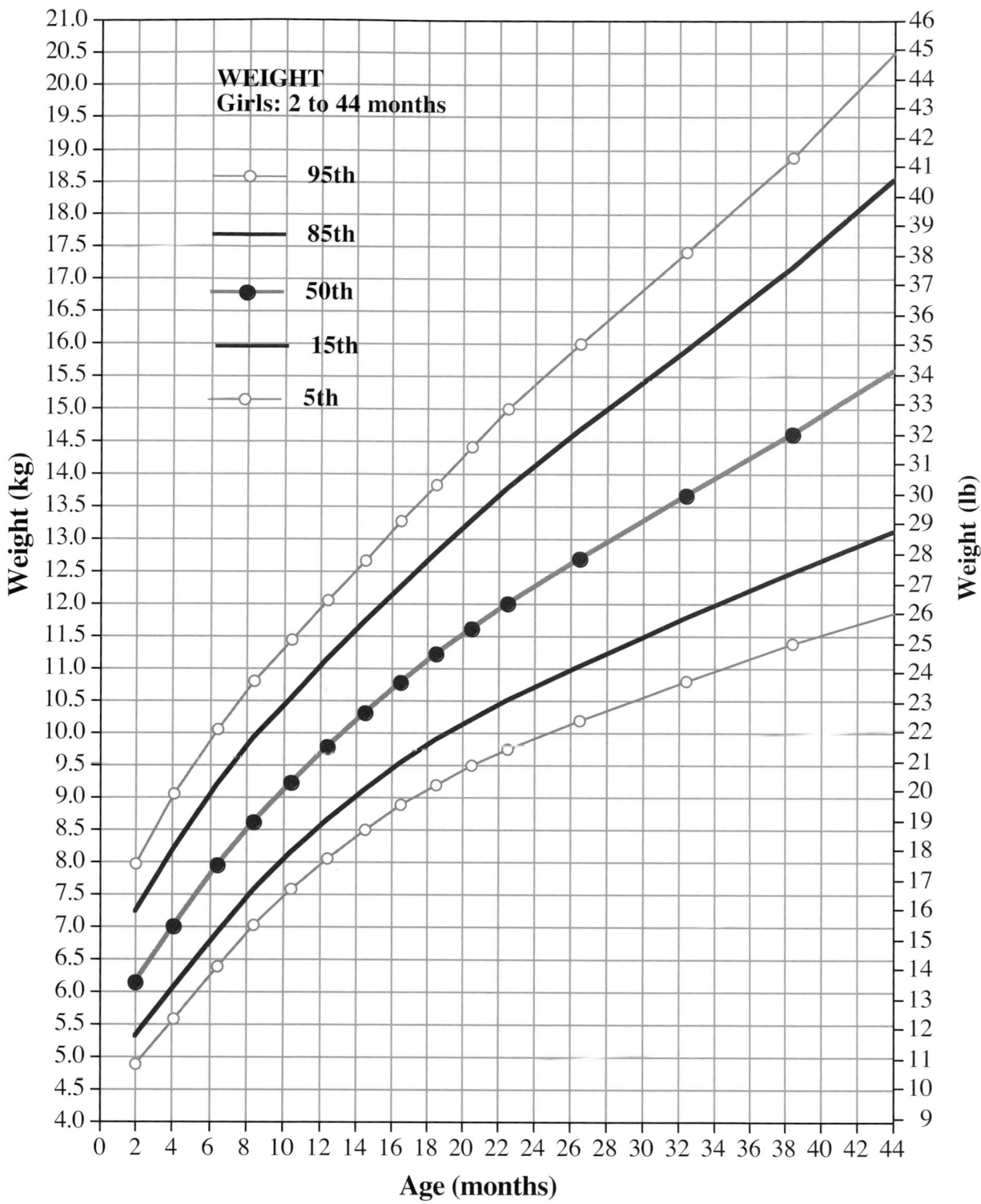

Figure IV.8. Percentiles of Weight in Kilograms (kg) and Pounds (lb.) by Age for Girls Ranging in Age from 2 to 44 Months.

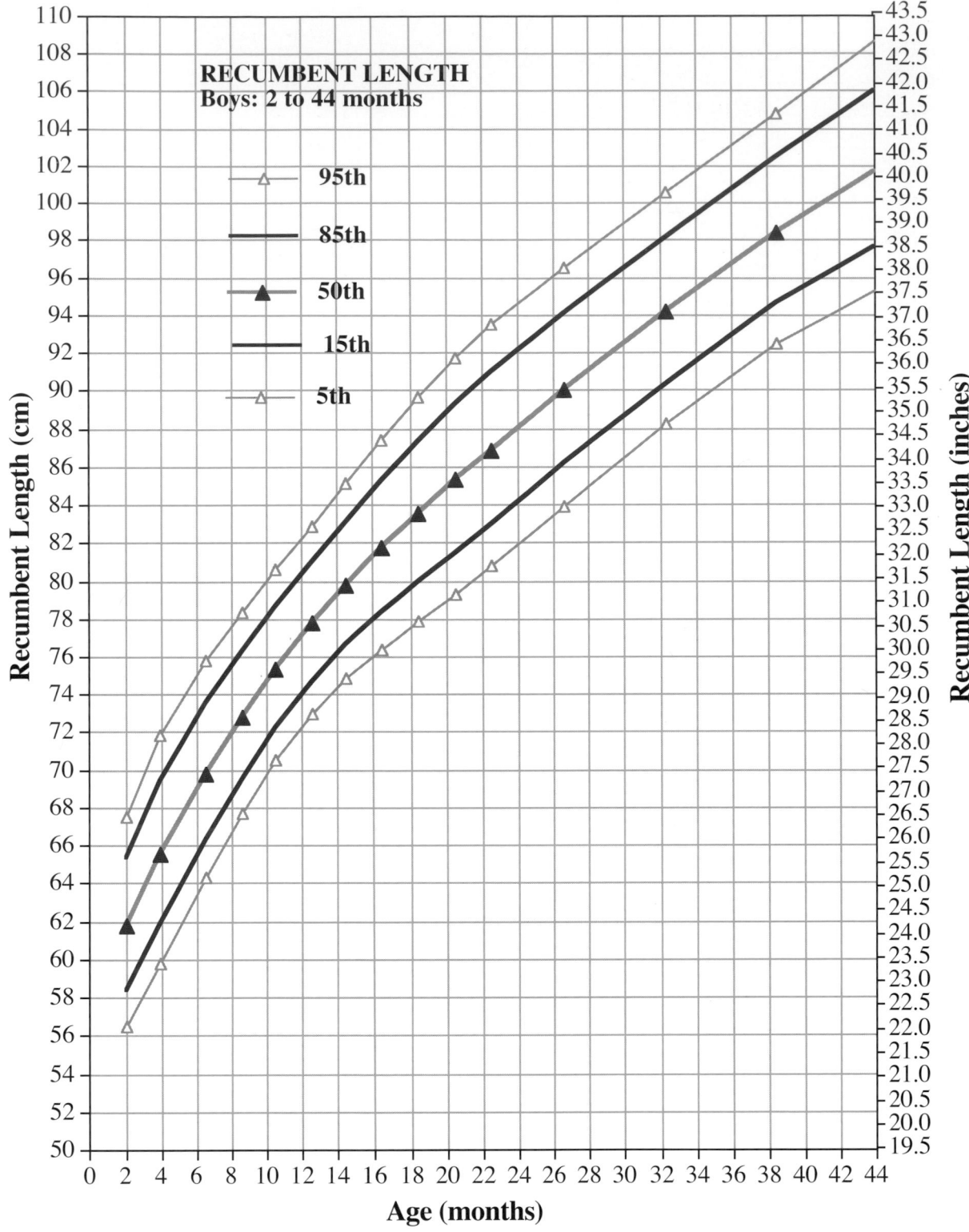

Figure IV.9. Percentiles of Recumbent Length in Centimeters (cm) and Inches (in.) by Age for Boys Ranging in Age from 2 to 44 Months.

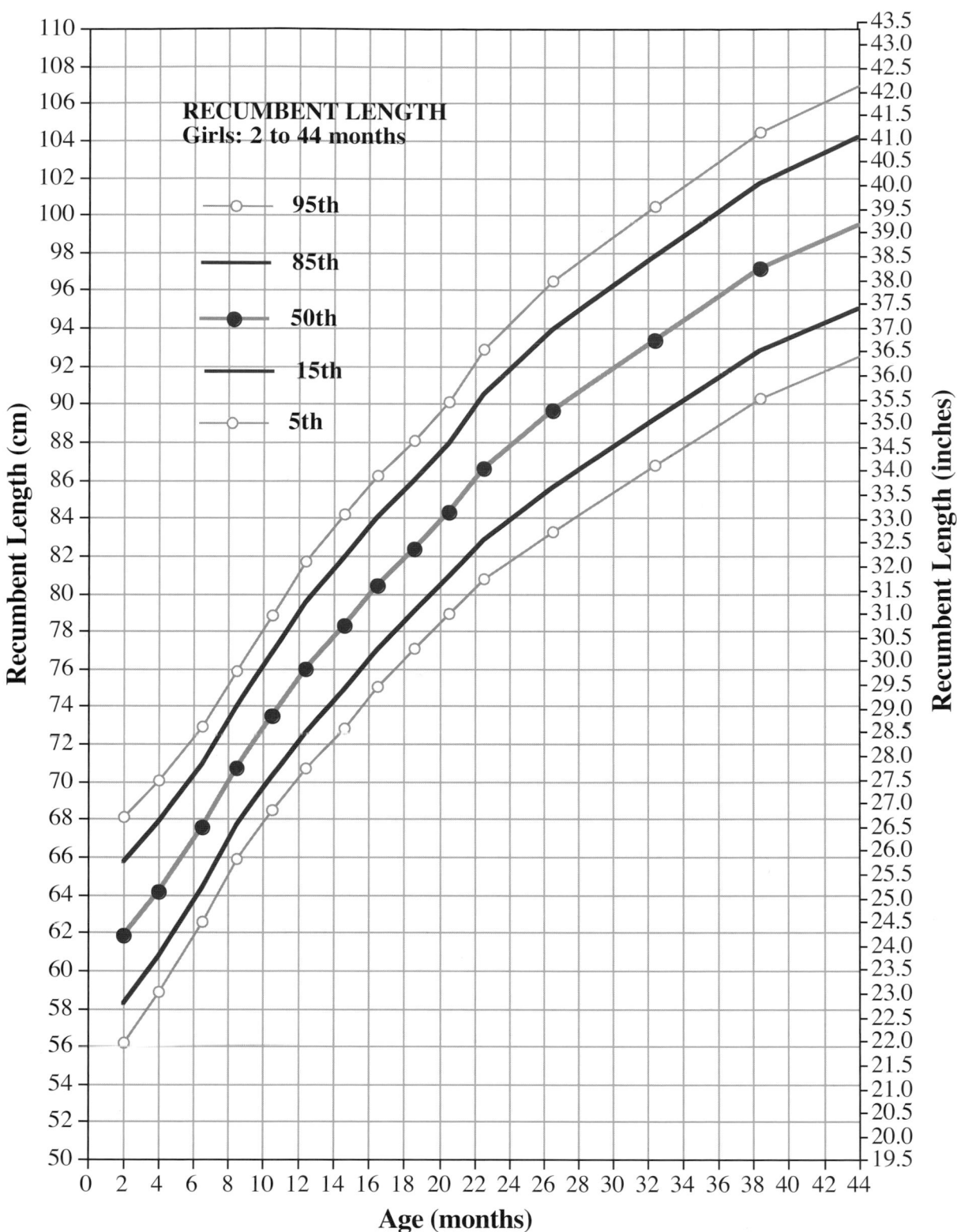

Figure IV.10. Percentiles of Recumbent Length in Centimeters (cm) and Inches (in.) by Age for Girls Ranging in Age from 2 to 44 Months.

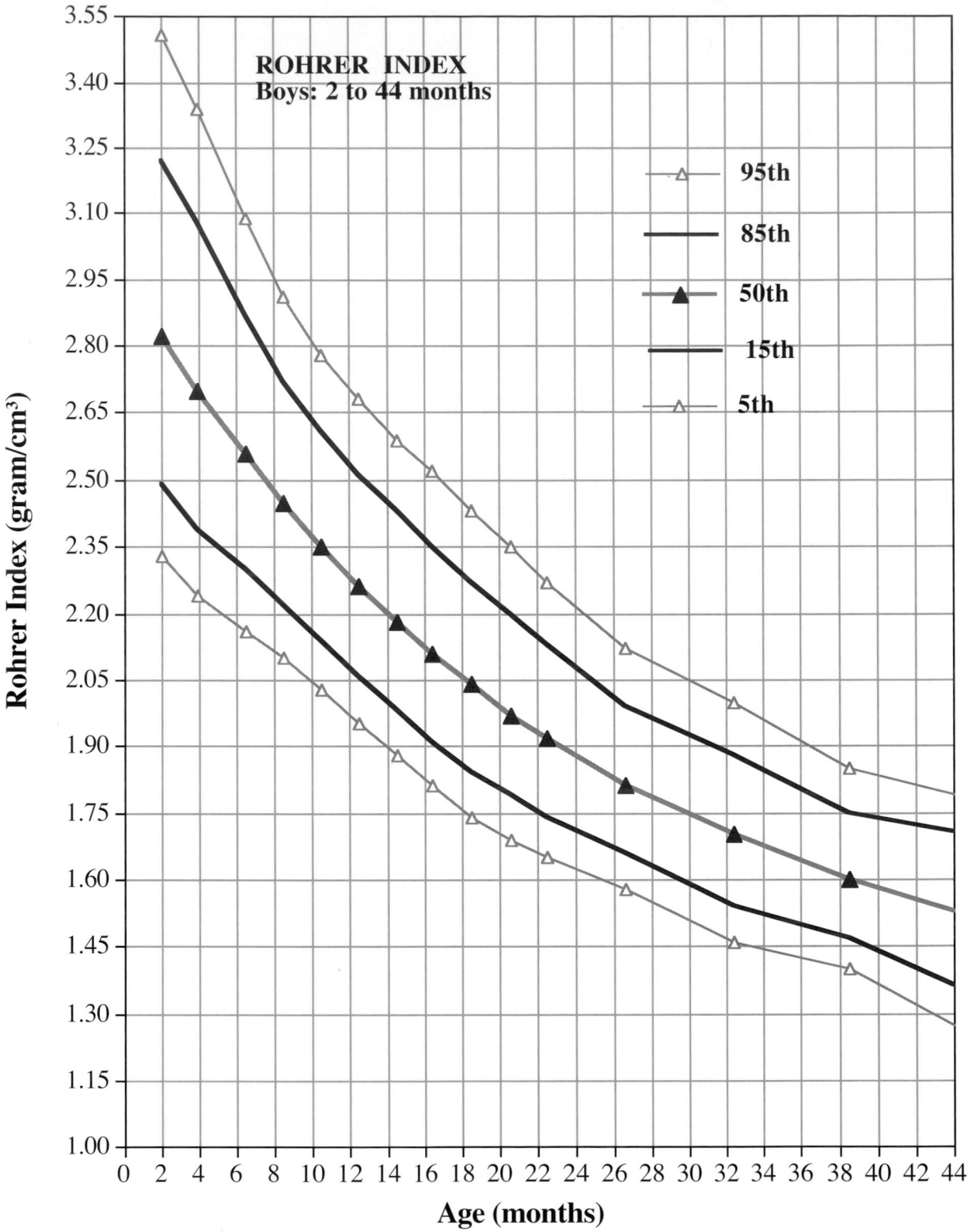

Figure IV.11. Percentiles of Rohrer Index (gram/cm^3) by Age for Boys Ranging in Age from 2 to 44 Months.

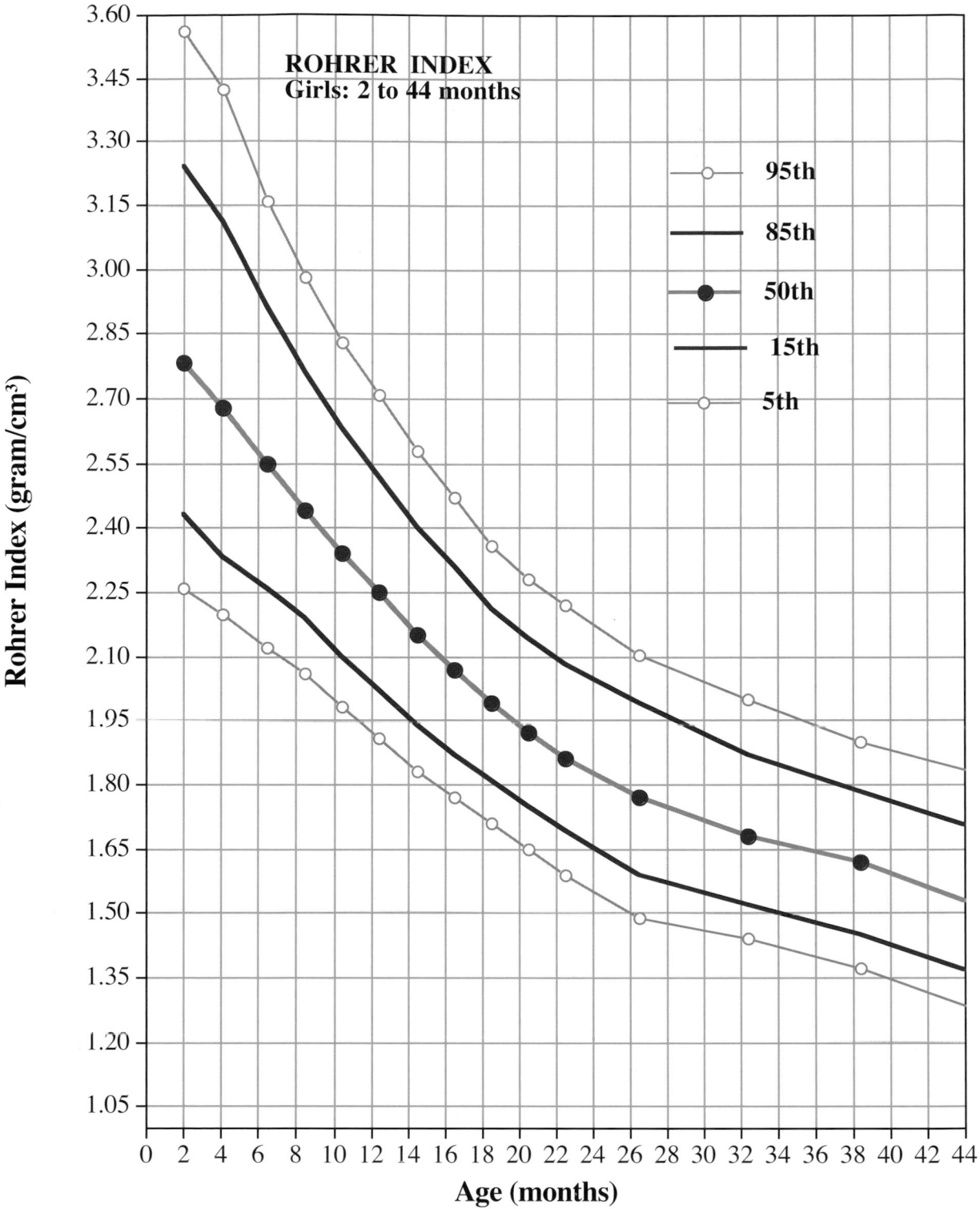

Figure IV.12. Percentiles of Rohrer Index (gram/cm^3) by Age for Girls Ranging in Age from 2 to 44 Months.

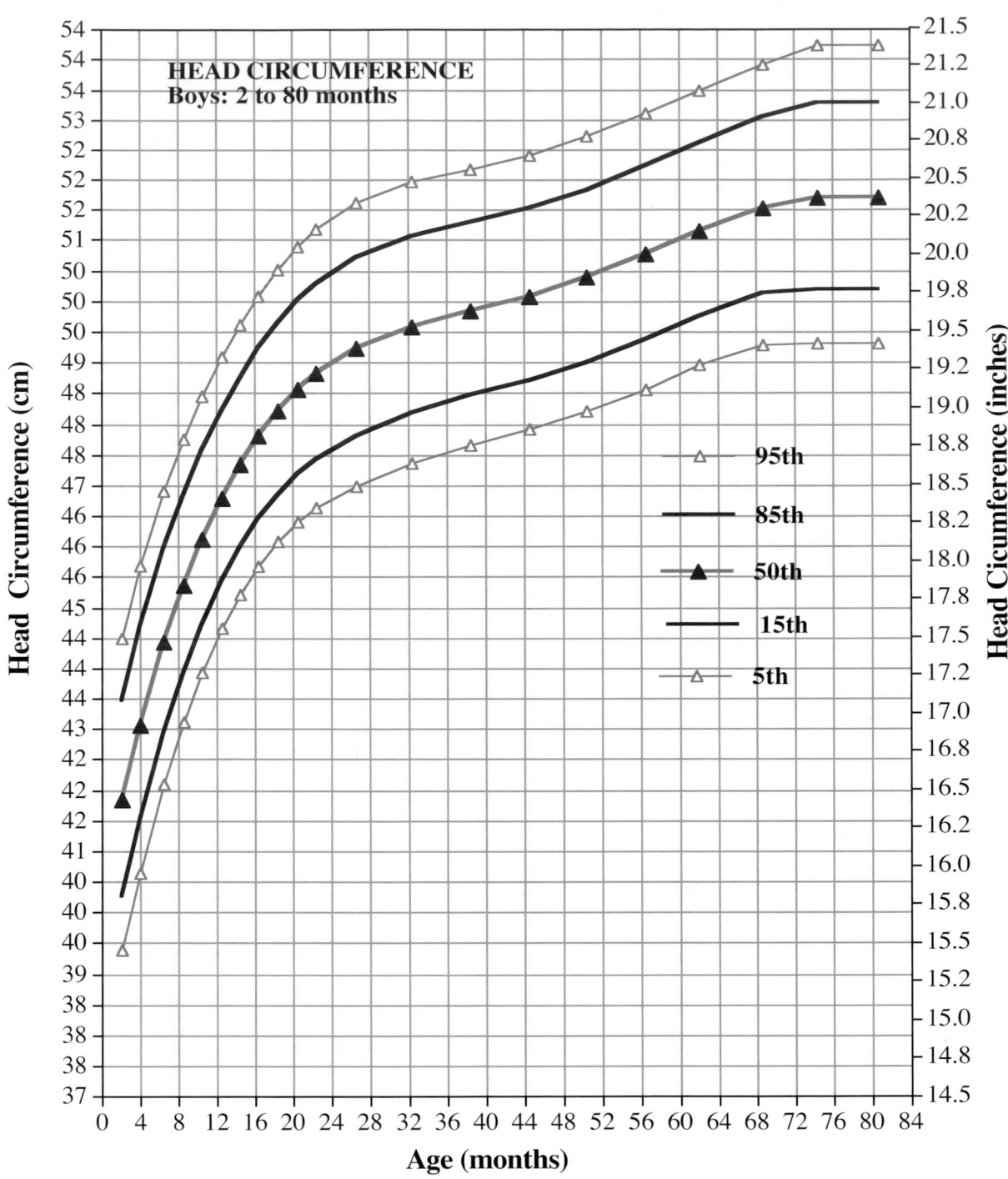

Figure IV.13. Percentiles of Head Circumference in Centimeters (cm) and Inches (in.) by Age for Boys Ranging in Age from 2 to 80 Months.

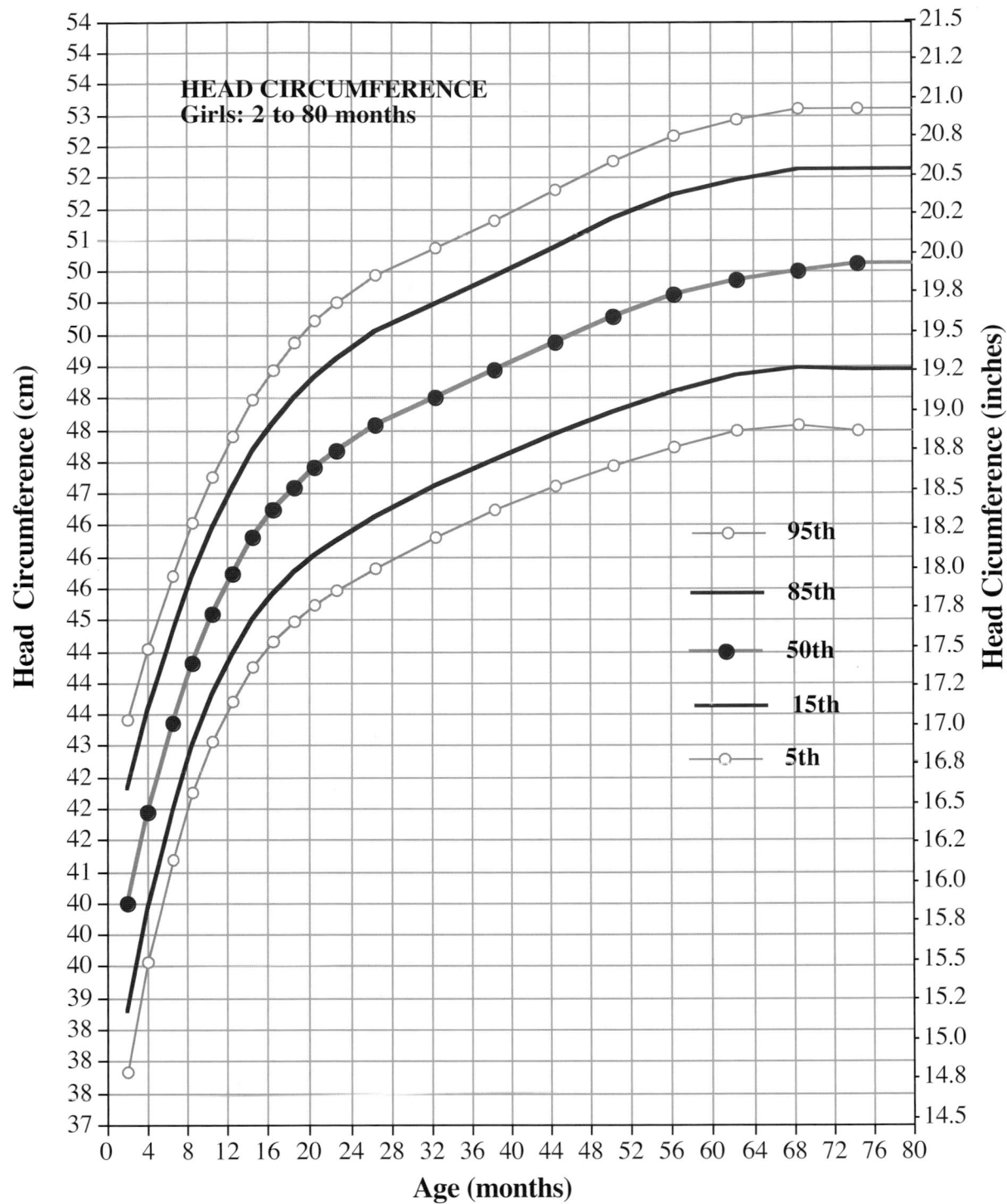

Figure IV.14. Percentiles of Head Circumference in Centimeters (cm) and Inches (in.) by Age for Girls Ranging in Age from 2 to 80 Months.

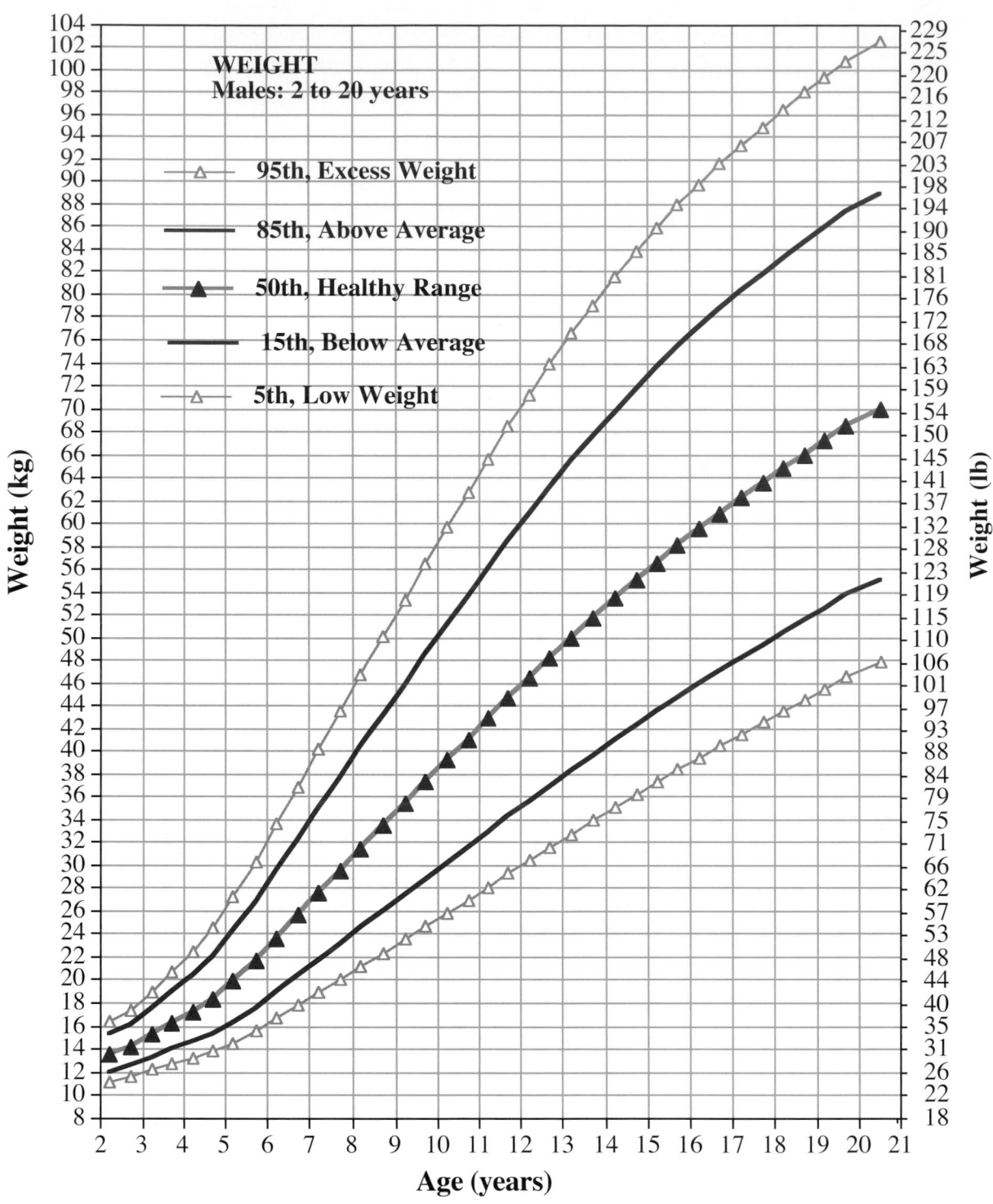

Figure IV.15. Percentiles of Weight in Kilograms (kg) and Pounds (lb.) for Males Ranging in Age from 2 to 20 Years.

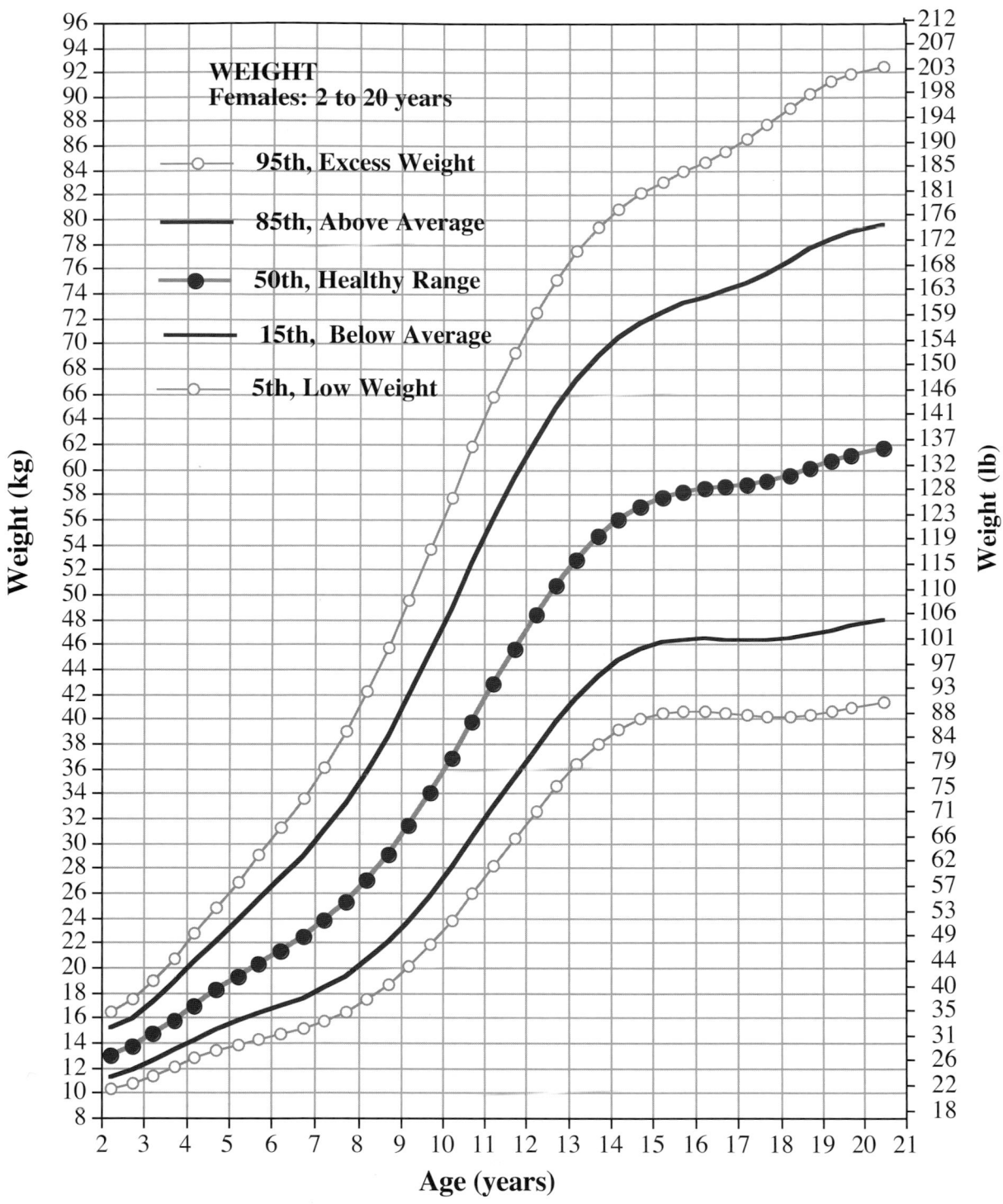

Figure IV.16. Percentiles of Weight in Kilograms (kg) and Pounds (lb.) for Females Ranging in Age from 2 to 20 Years.

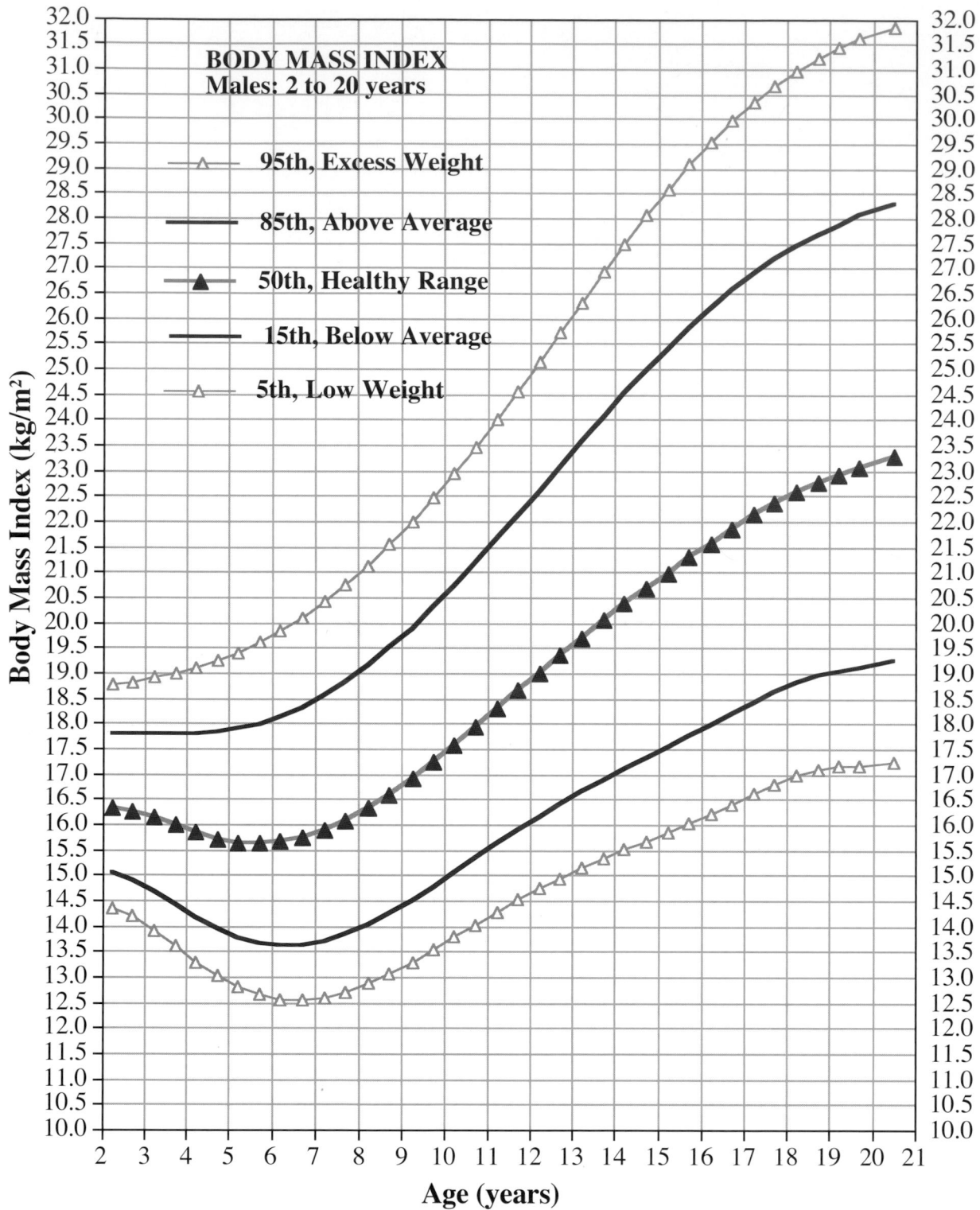

Figure IV.17. Percentiles of Body Mass Index (kg/m²) for Males Ranging in Age from 2 to 20 Years.

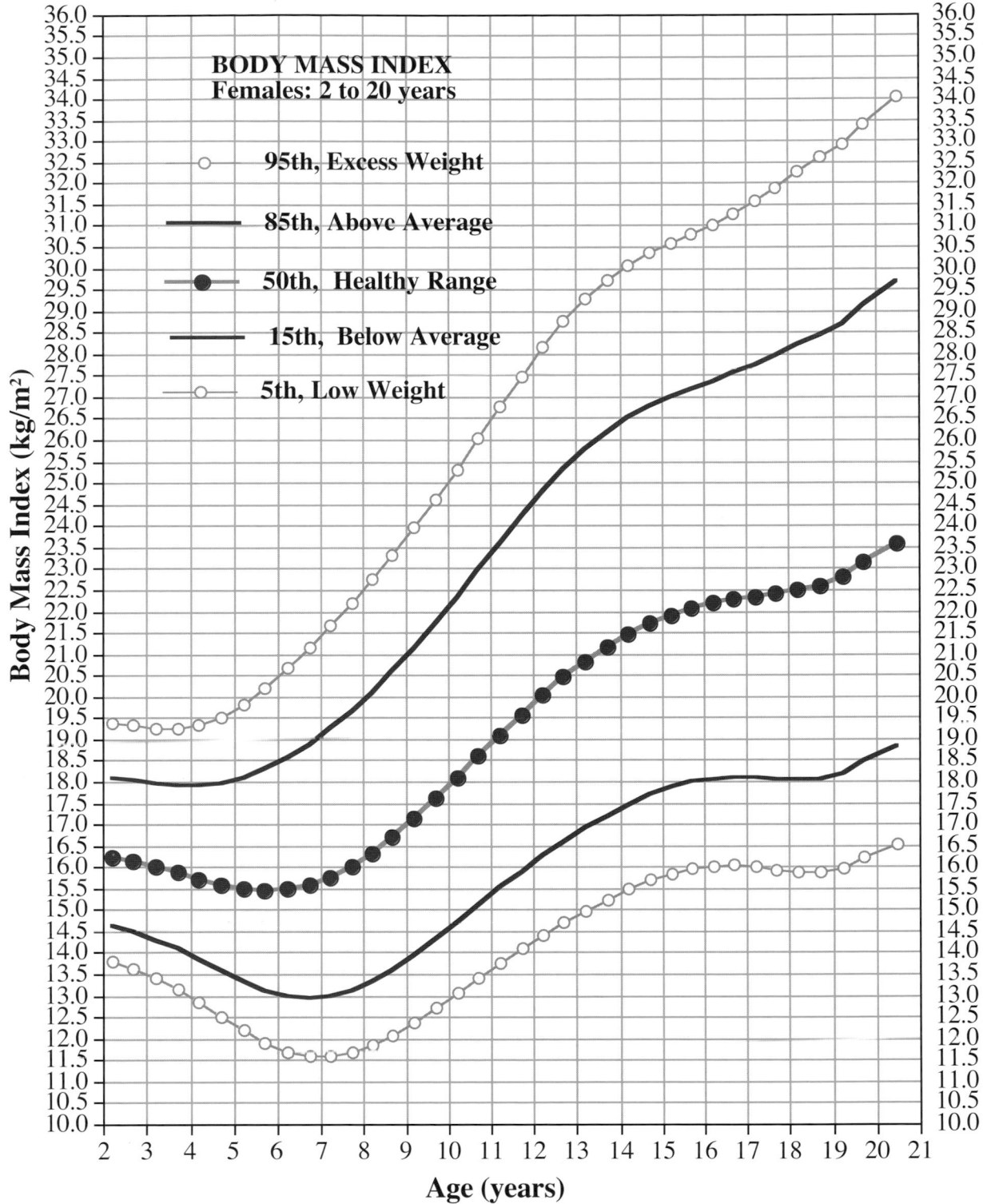

Figure IV.18. Percentiles of Body Mass Index (kg/m^2) for Females Ranging in Age from 2 to 20 Years.

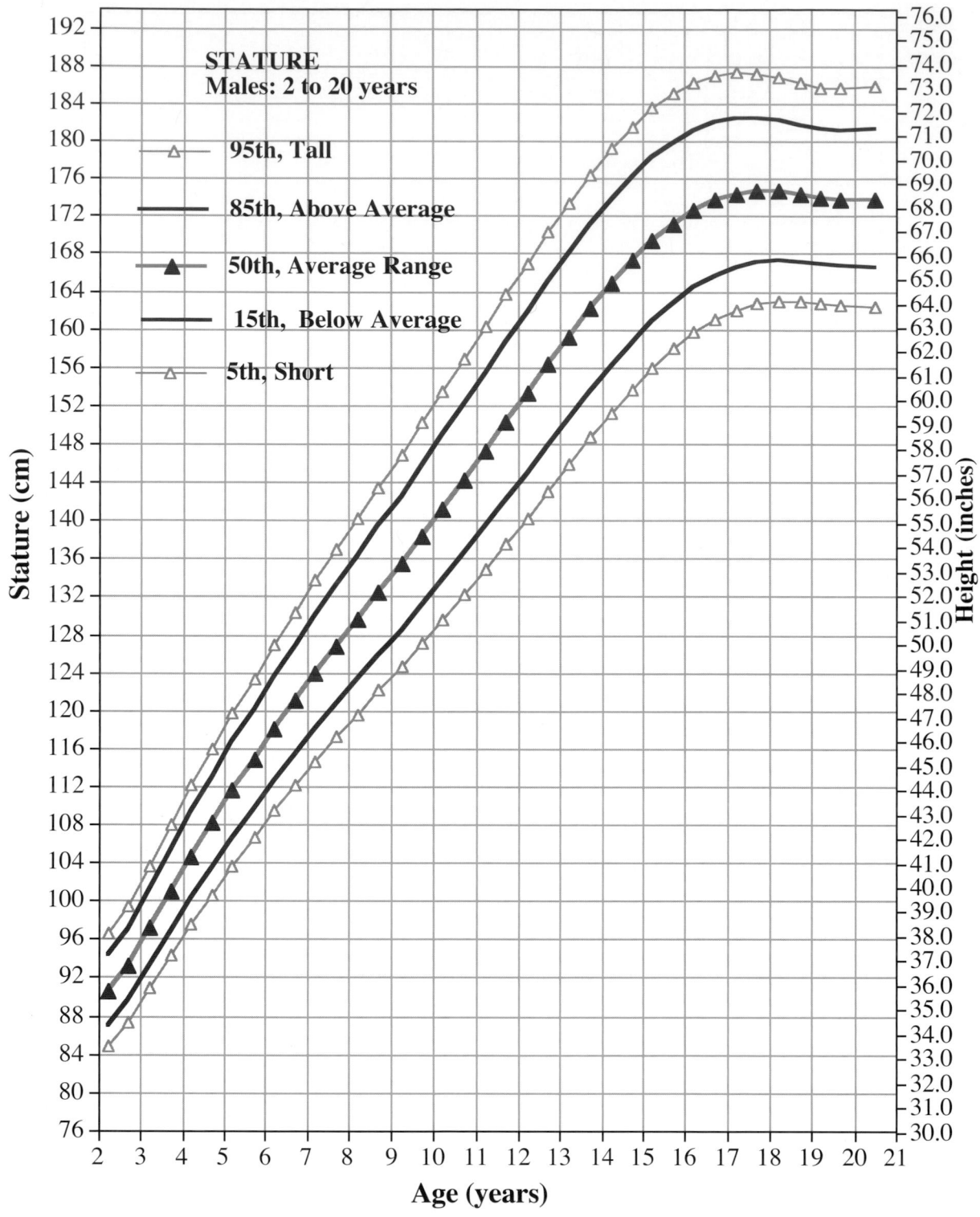

Figure IV.19. Percentiles of Stature in Centimeters (cm) and Inches (in.) for Males Ranging in Age from 2 to 20 Years.

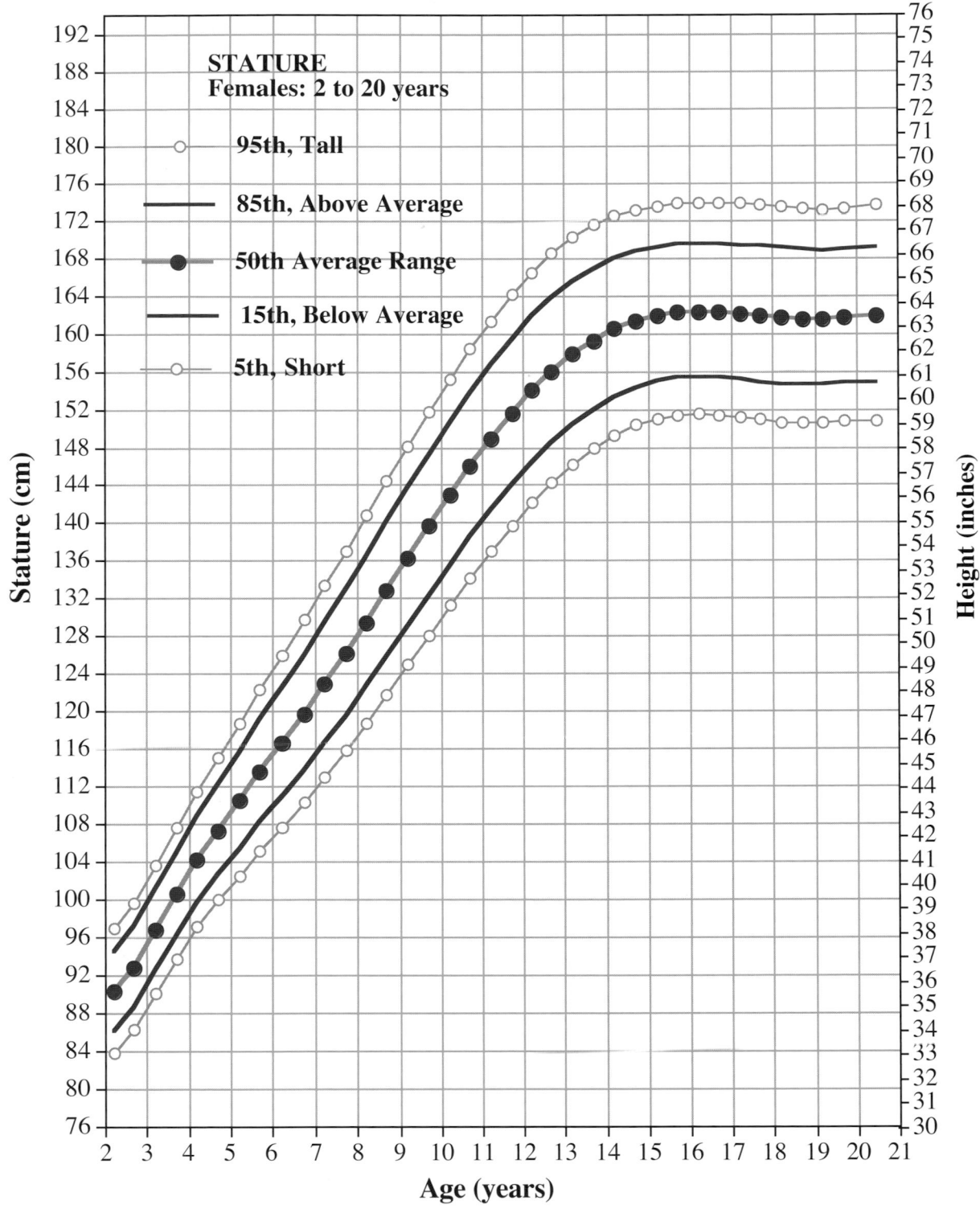

Figure IV.20. Percentiles of Stature in Centimeters (cm) and Inches (in.) for Females Ranging in Age from 2 to 20 Years.

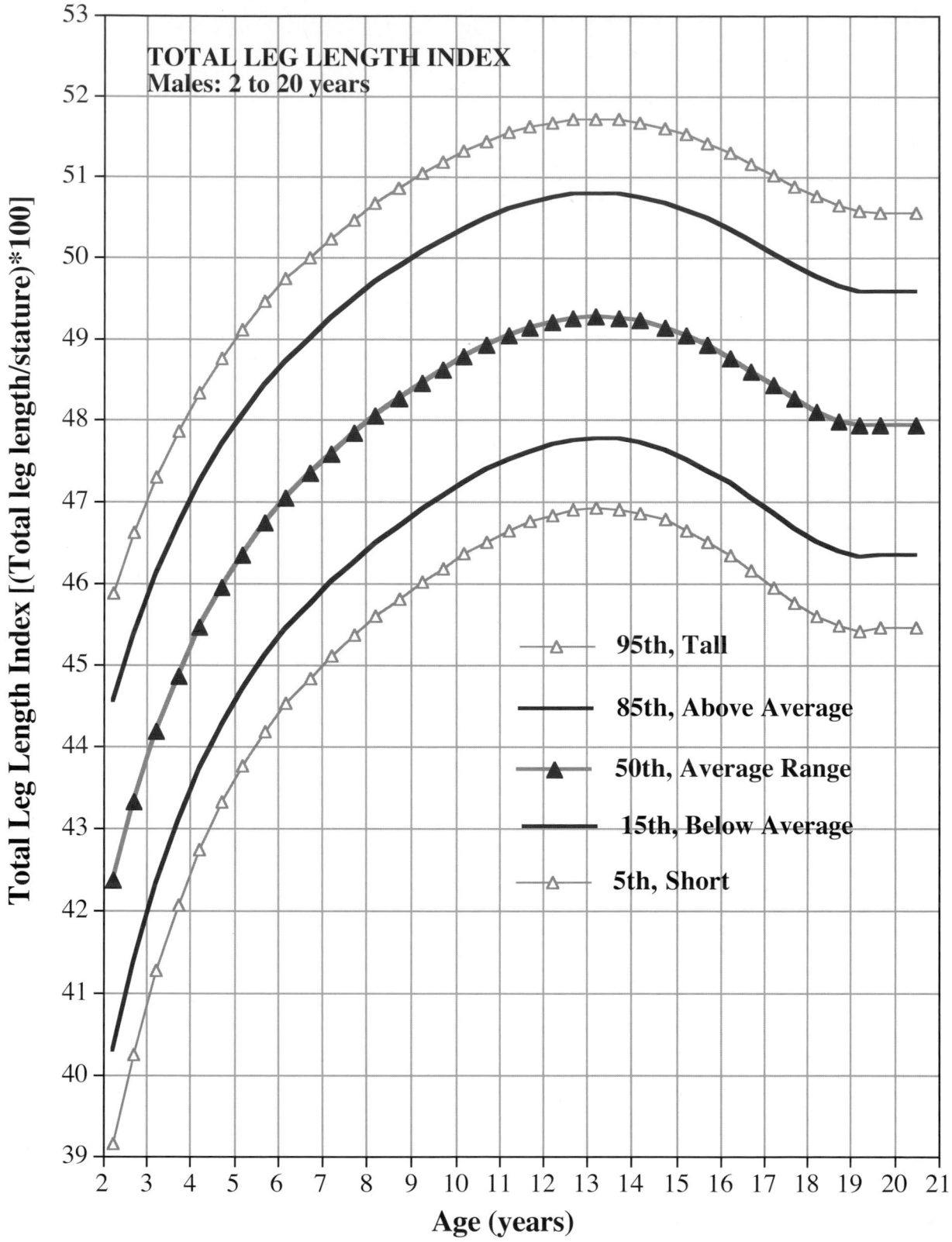

Figure IV.21. Percentiles of Percent Total Leg Length (%) for Males Ranging from 2 to 20 Years.

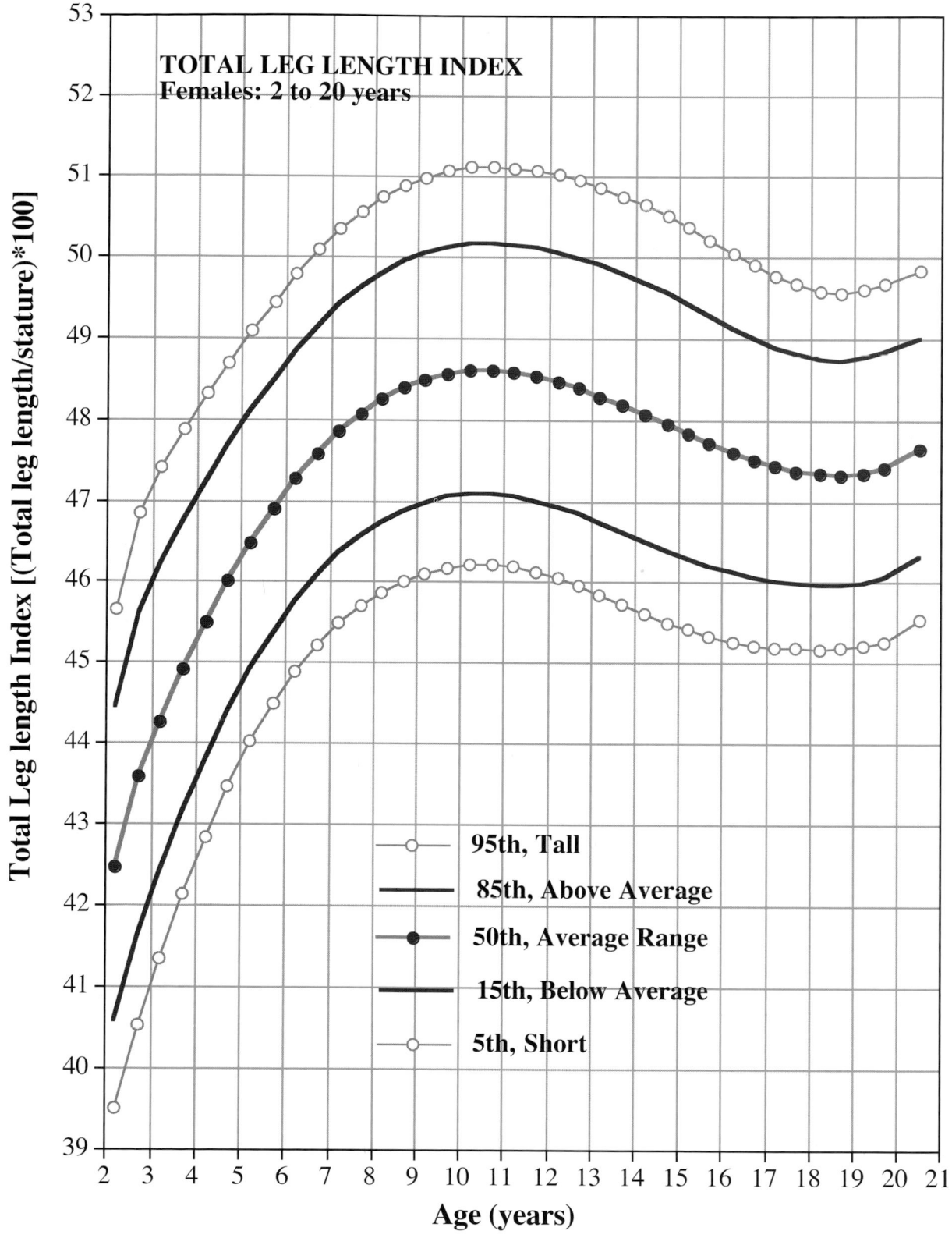

Figure IV.22. Percentiles of Percent Total Leg Length (%) for Females Ranging from 2 to 20 Years.

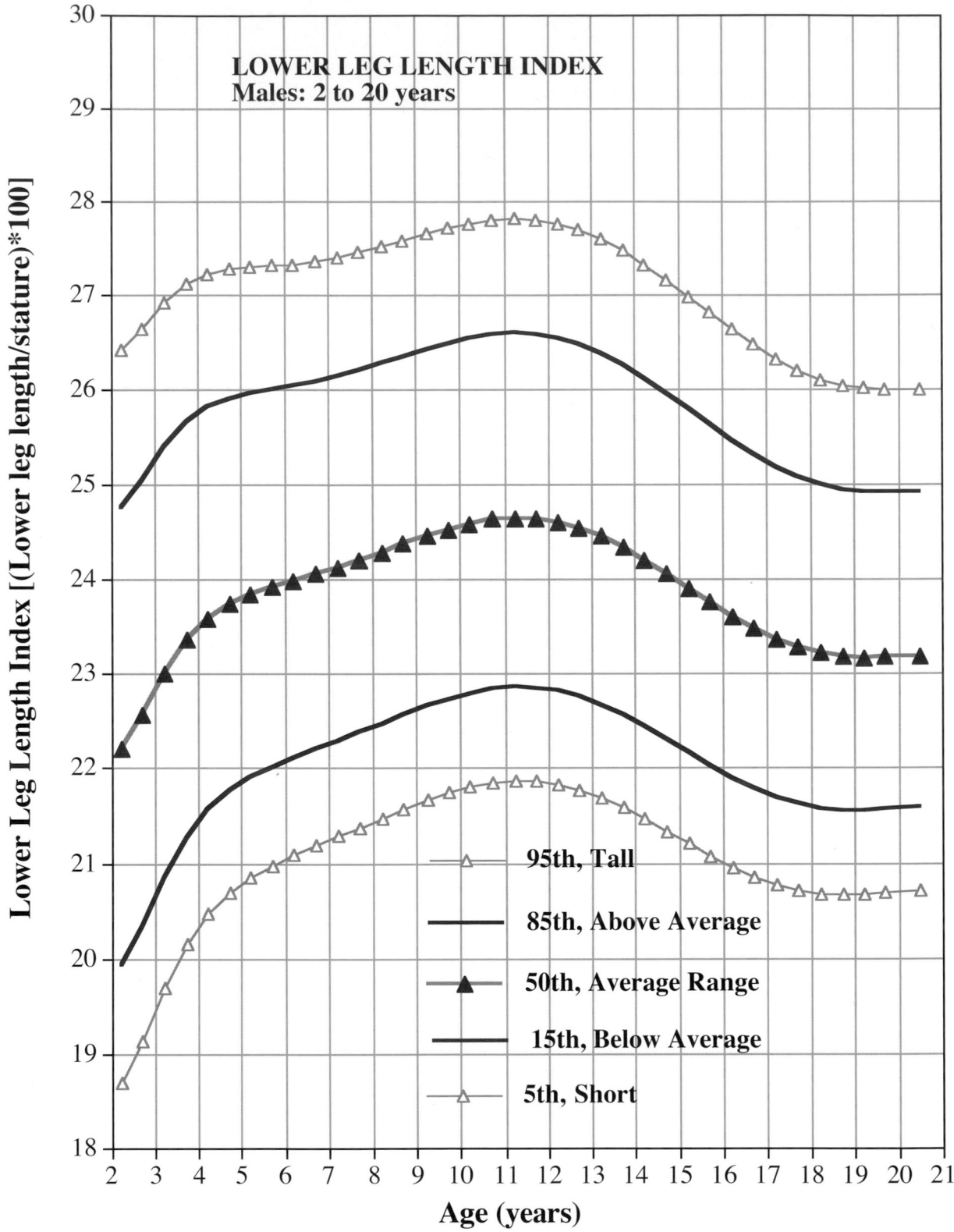

Figure IV.23. Percentiles of Percent Lower Leg Length (%) for Males Ranging from 2 to 20 Years.

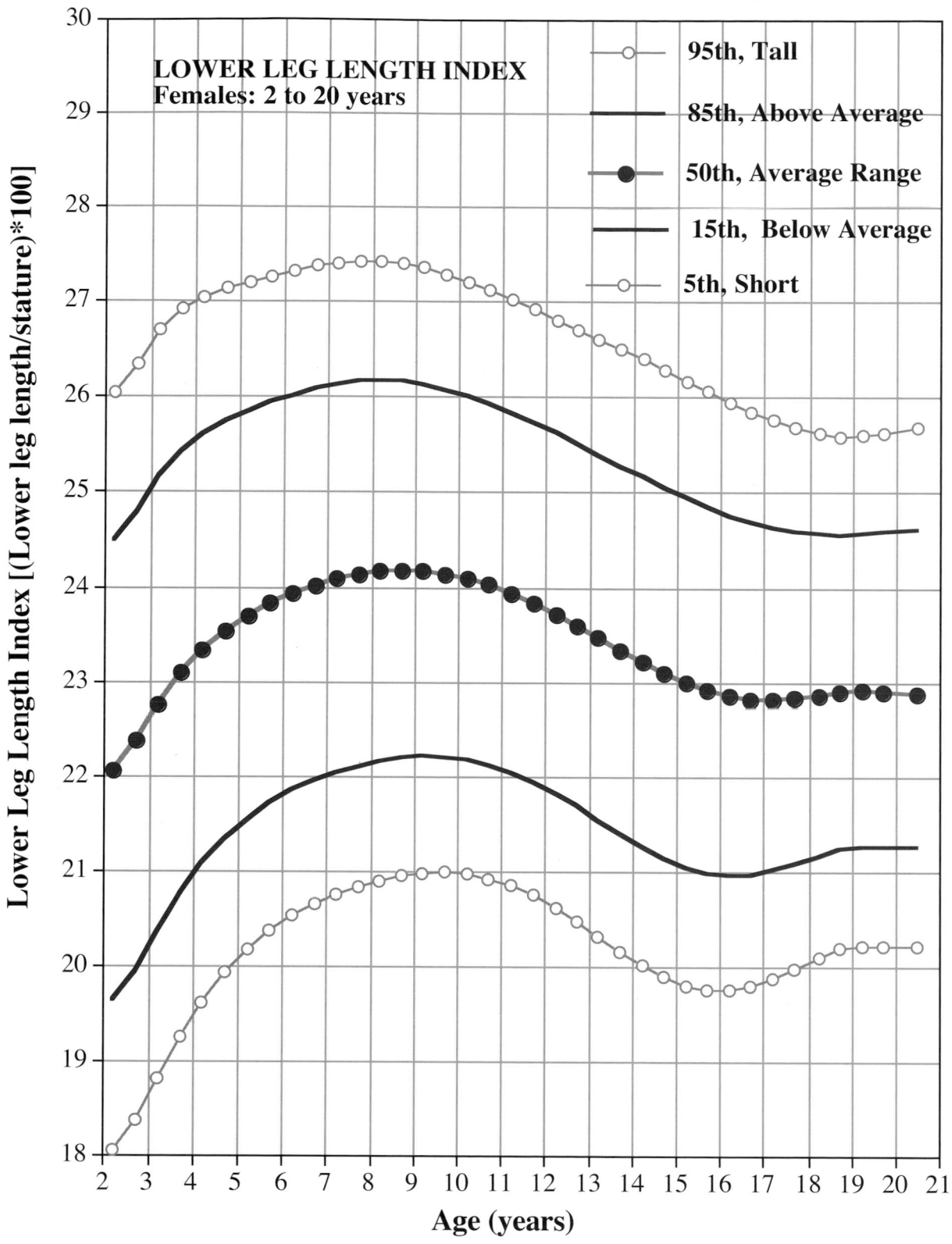

Figure IV.24. Percentiles of Percent Lower Leg Length (%) for Females Ranging from 2 to 20 Years.

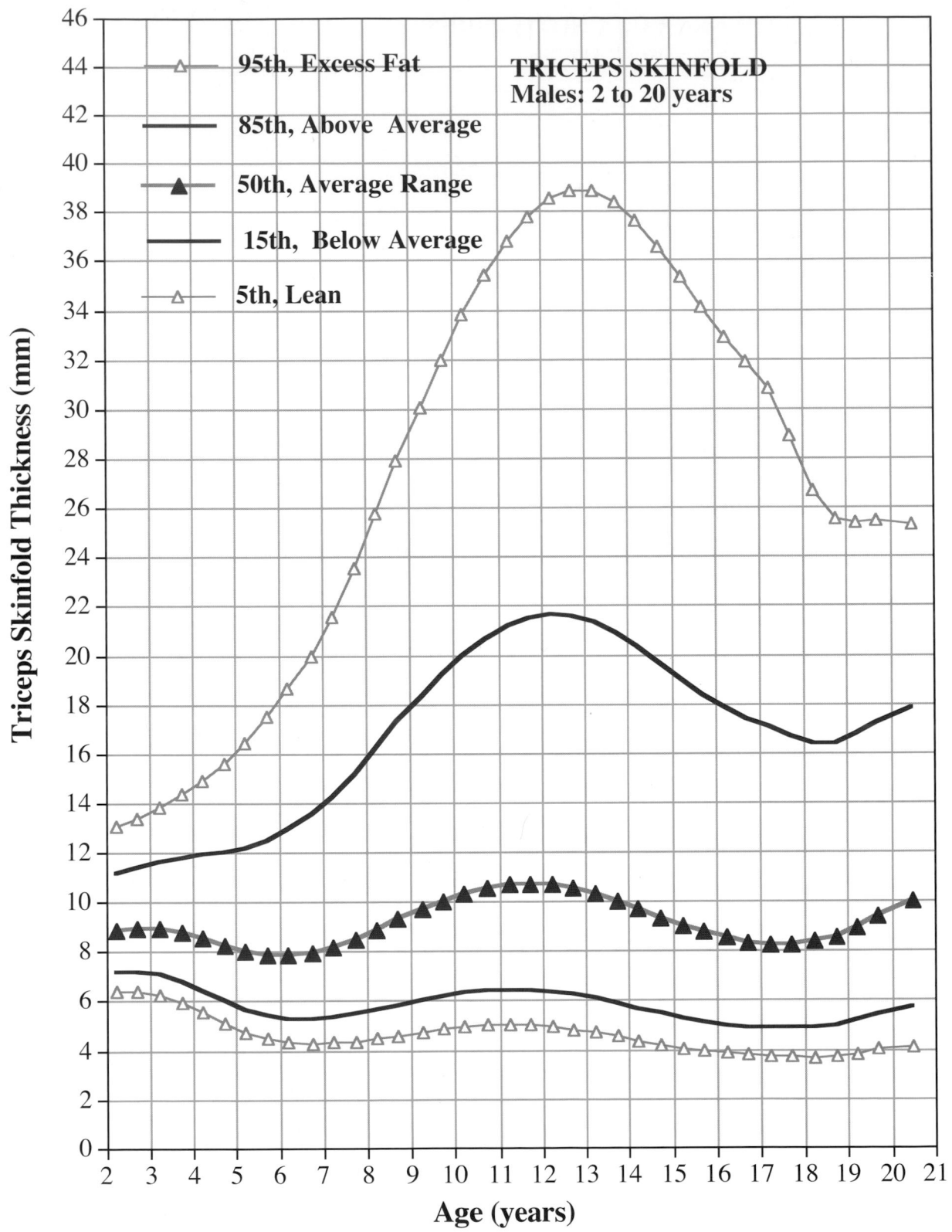

Figure IV.25. Percentiles of Triceps Skinfold Thickness (mm) for Males Ranging from 2 to 20 Years.

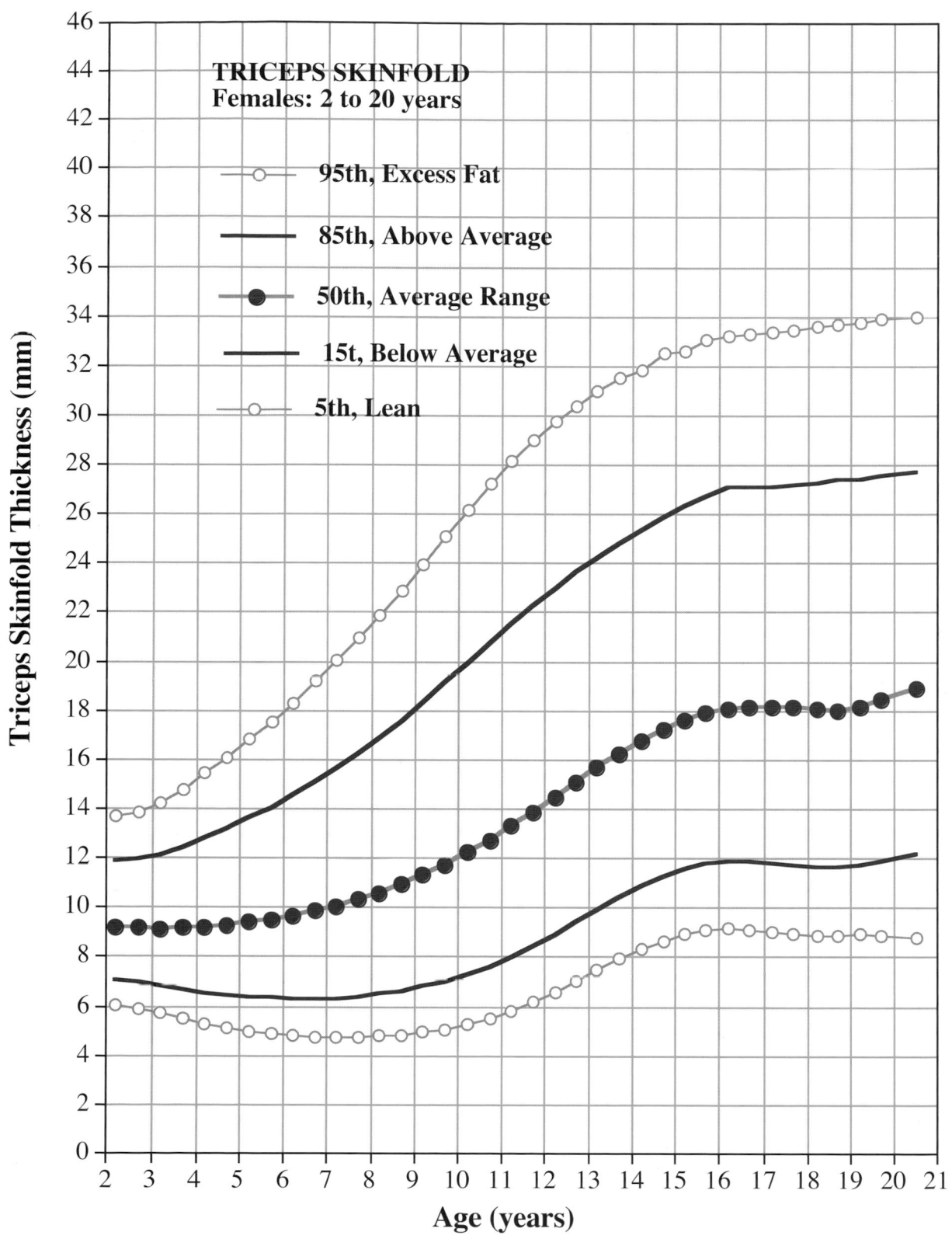

Figure IV.26. Percentiles of Triceps Skinfold Thickness (mm) for Females Ranging from 2 to 20 Years.

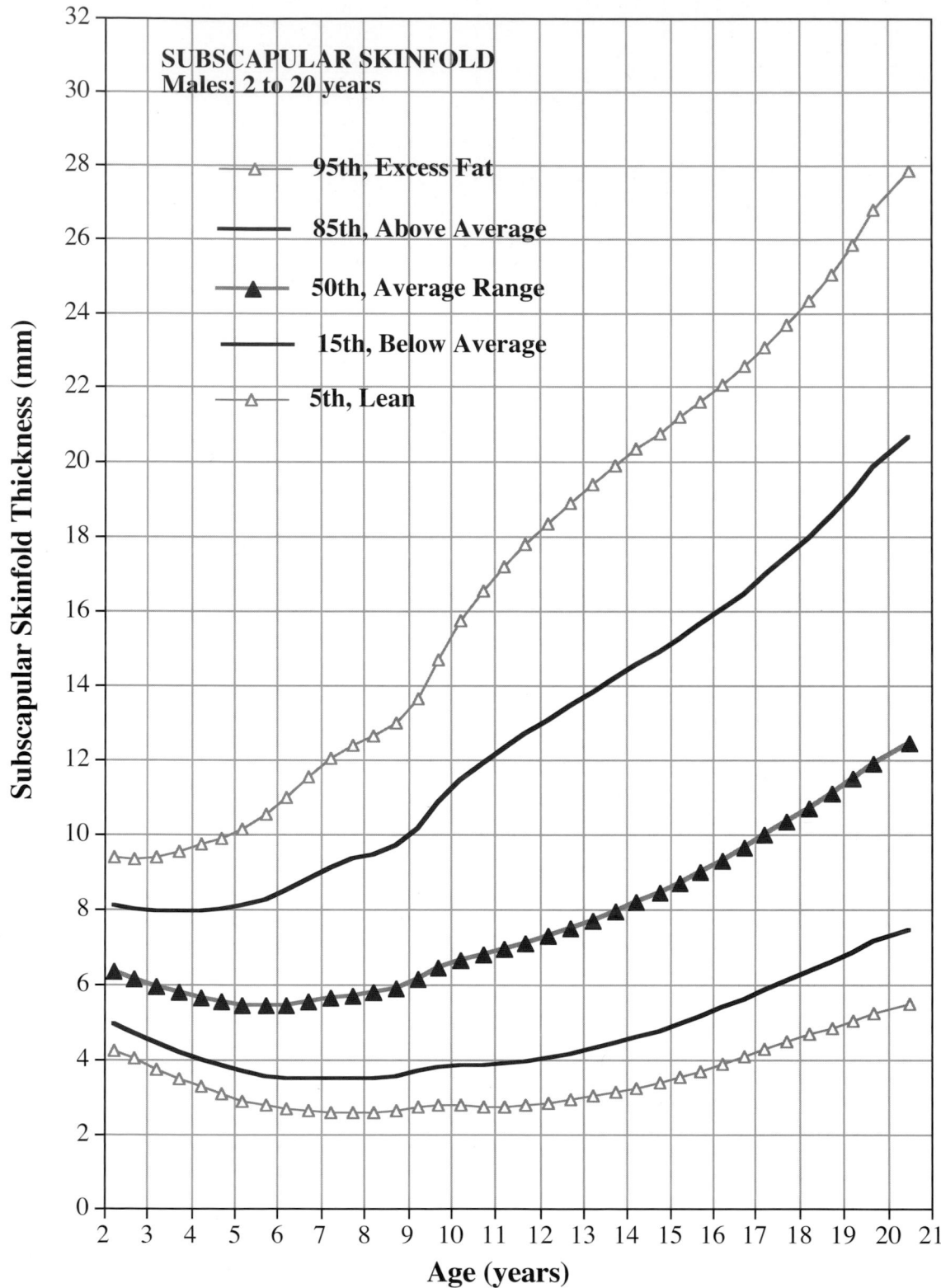

Figure IV.27. Percentiles of Subscapular Skinfold Thickness (mm) for Males Ranging from 2 to 20 Years.

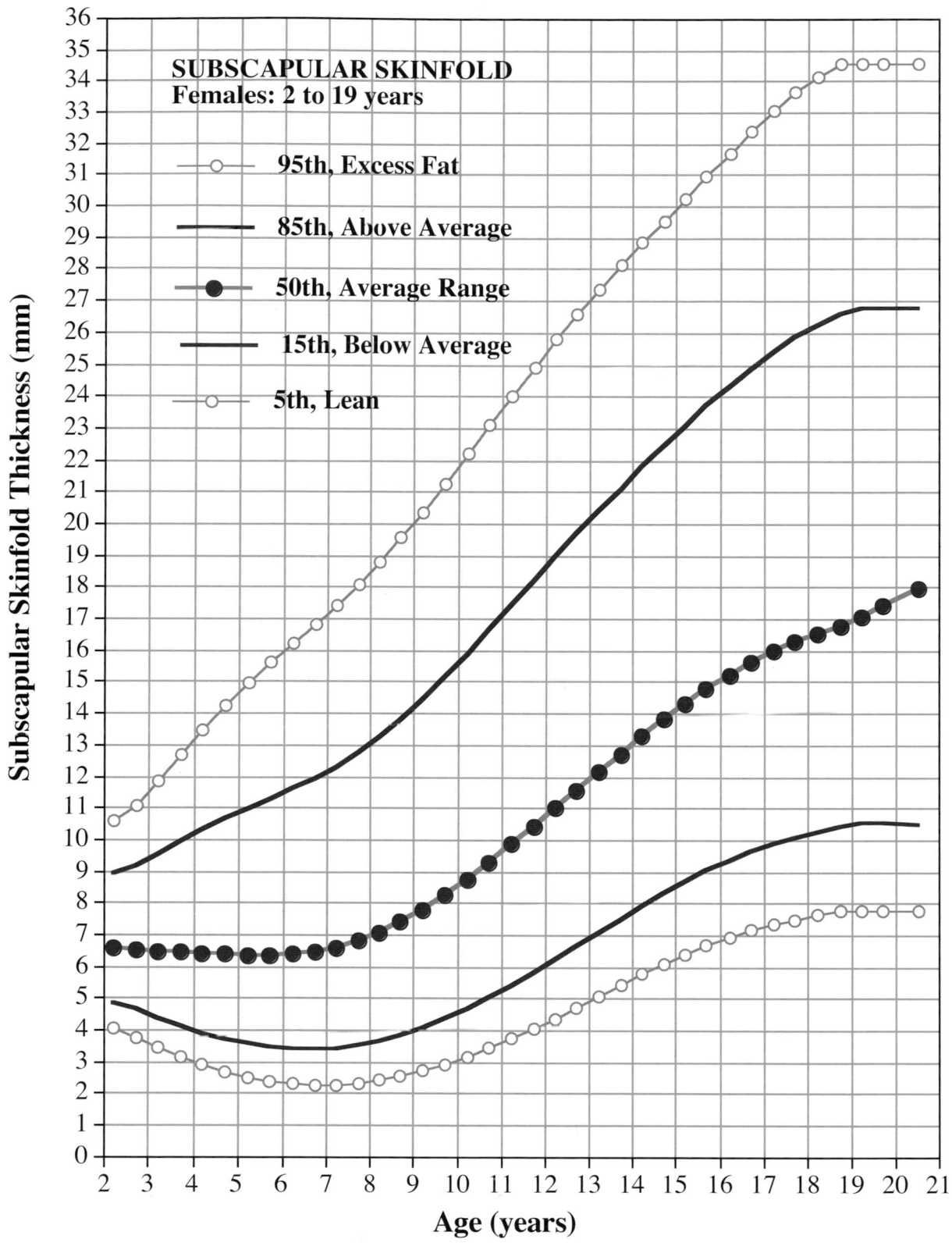

Figure IV.28. Percentiles of Subscapular Skinfold Thickness (mm) for Females Ranging from 2 to 20 Years.

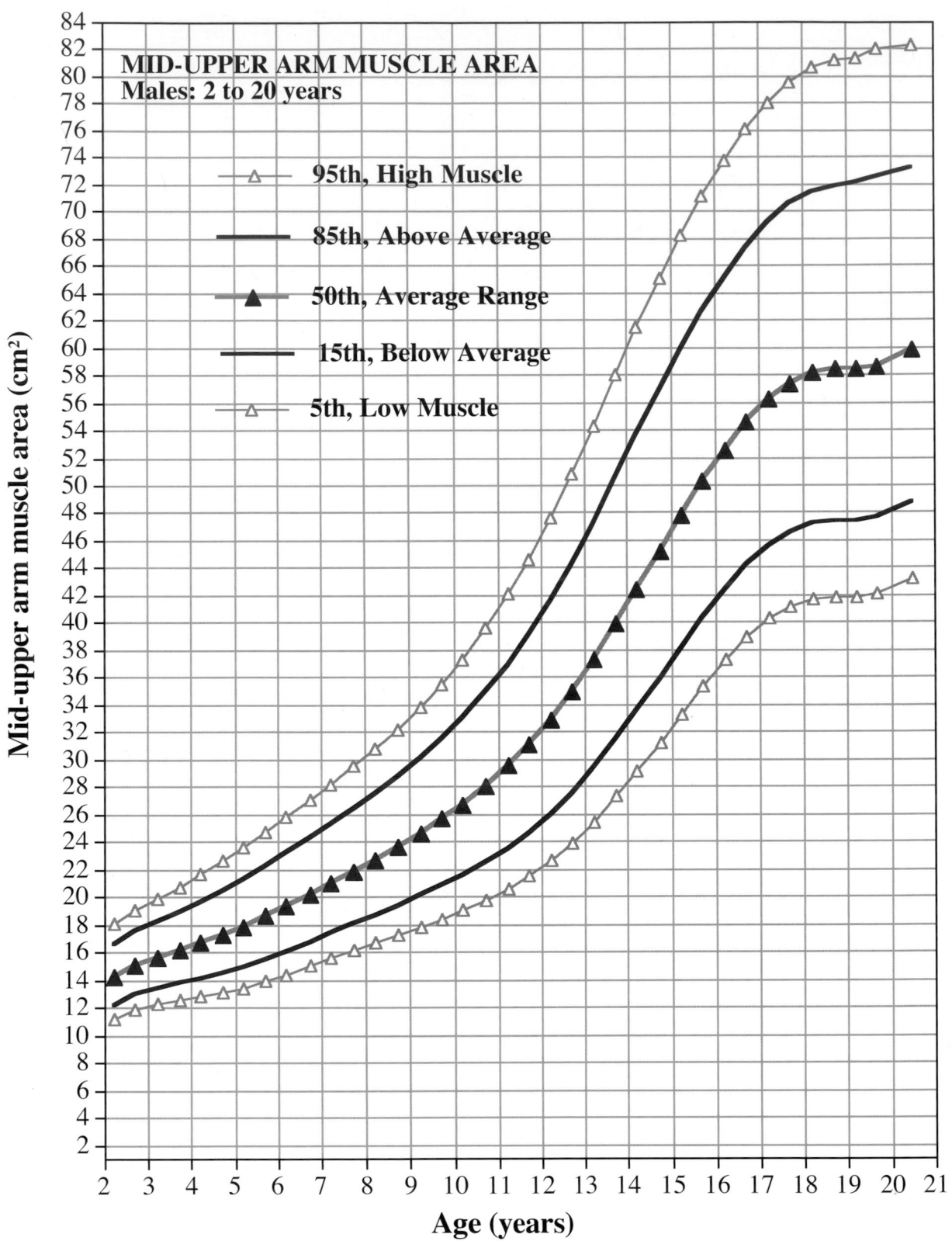

Figure IV.29. Percentiles of Mid-Upper Arm Muscle Area (cm²) for Males Ranging in Age from 2 to 20 Years.

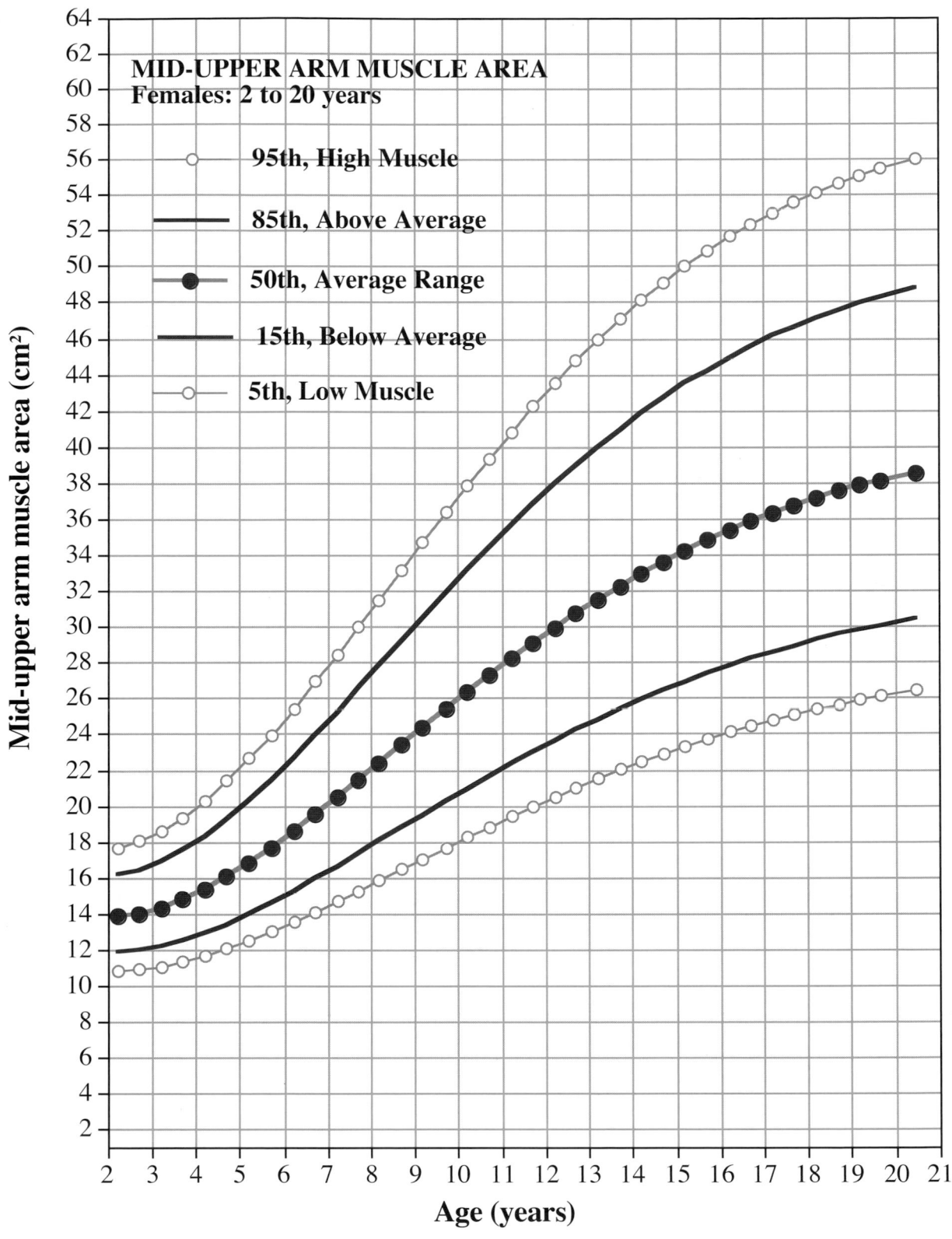

Figure IV.30. Percentiles of Mid-Upper Arm Muscle Area (cm²) for Females Ranging in Age from 2 to 20 Years.

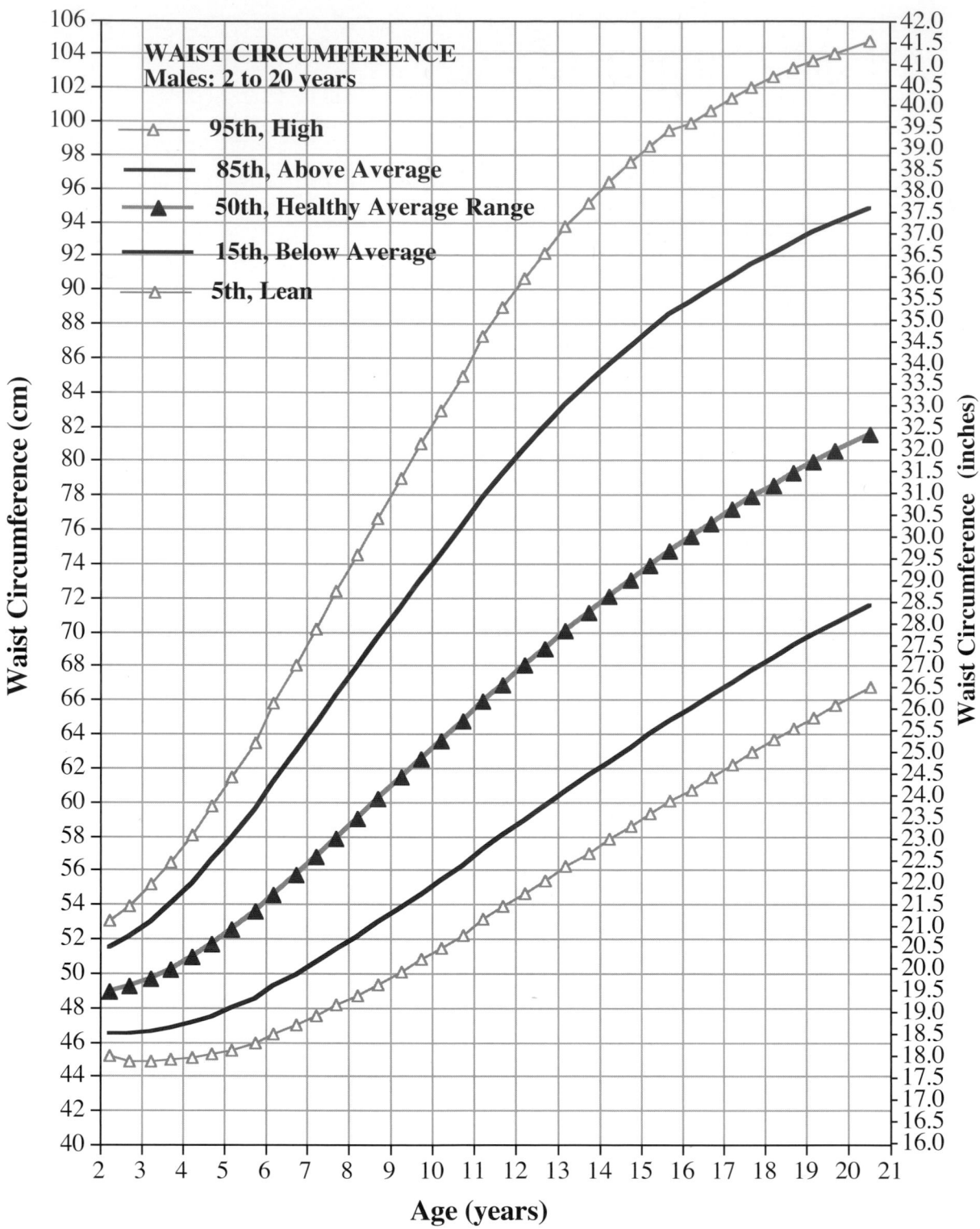

Figure IV.31. Percentiles of Waist Circumference in Centimeters (cm) and Inches (in.) for Males Ranging in Age from 2 to 20 Years.

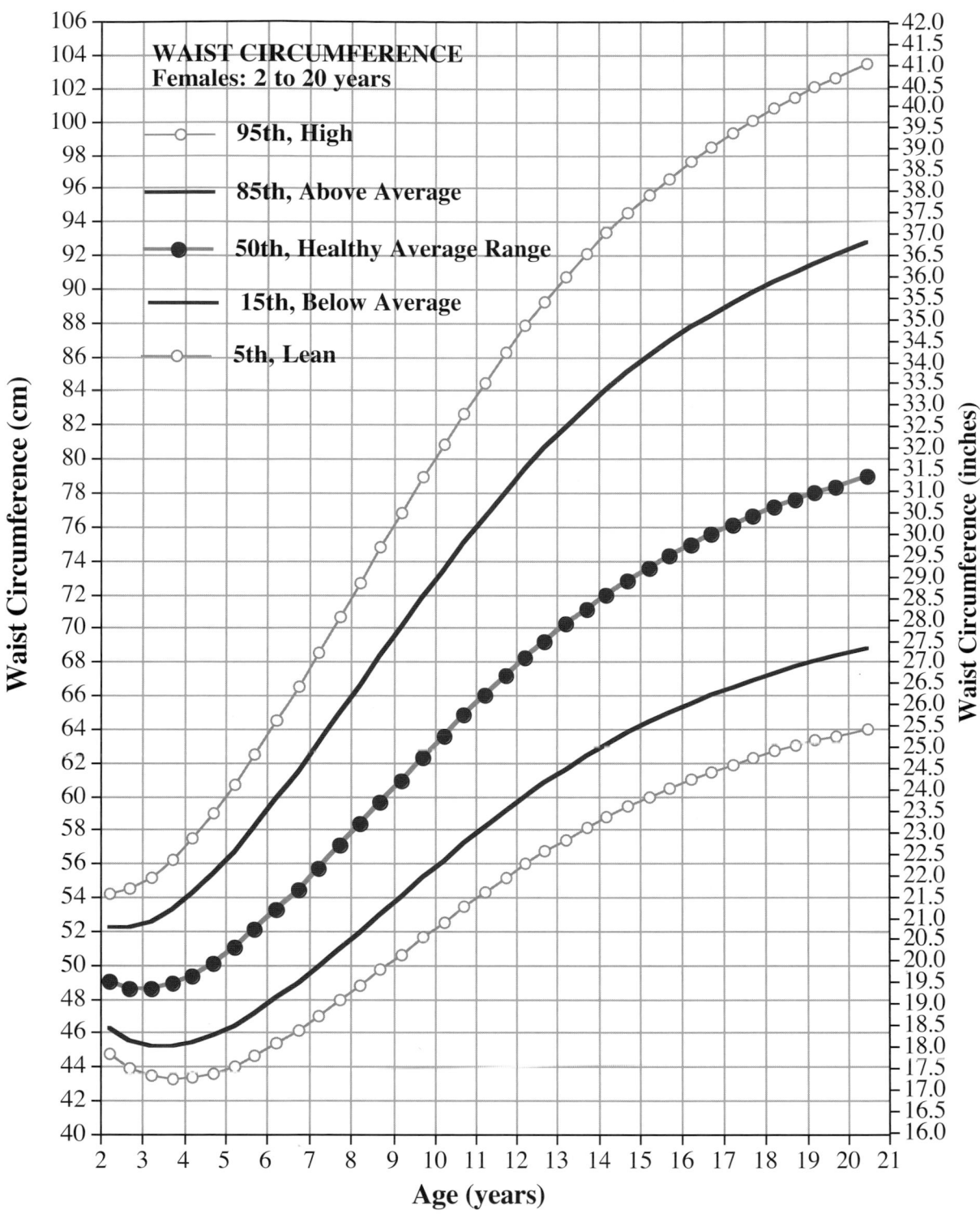

Figure IV.32. Percentiles of Waist Circumference in Centimeters (cm) and Inches (in.) for Females Ranging in Age from 2 to 20 Years.

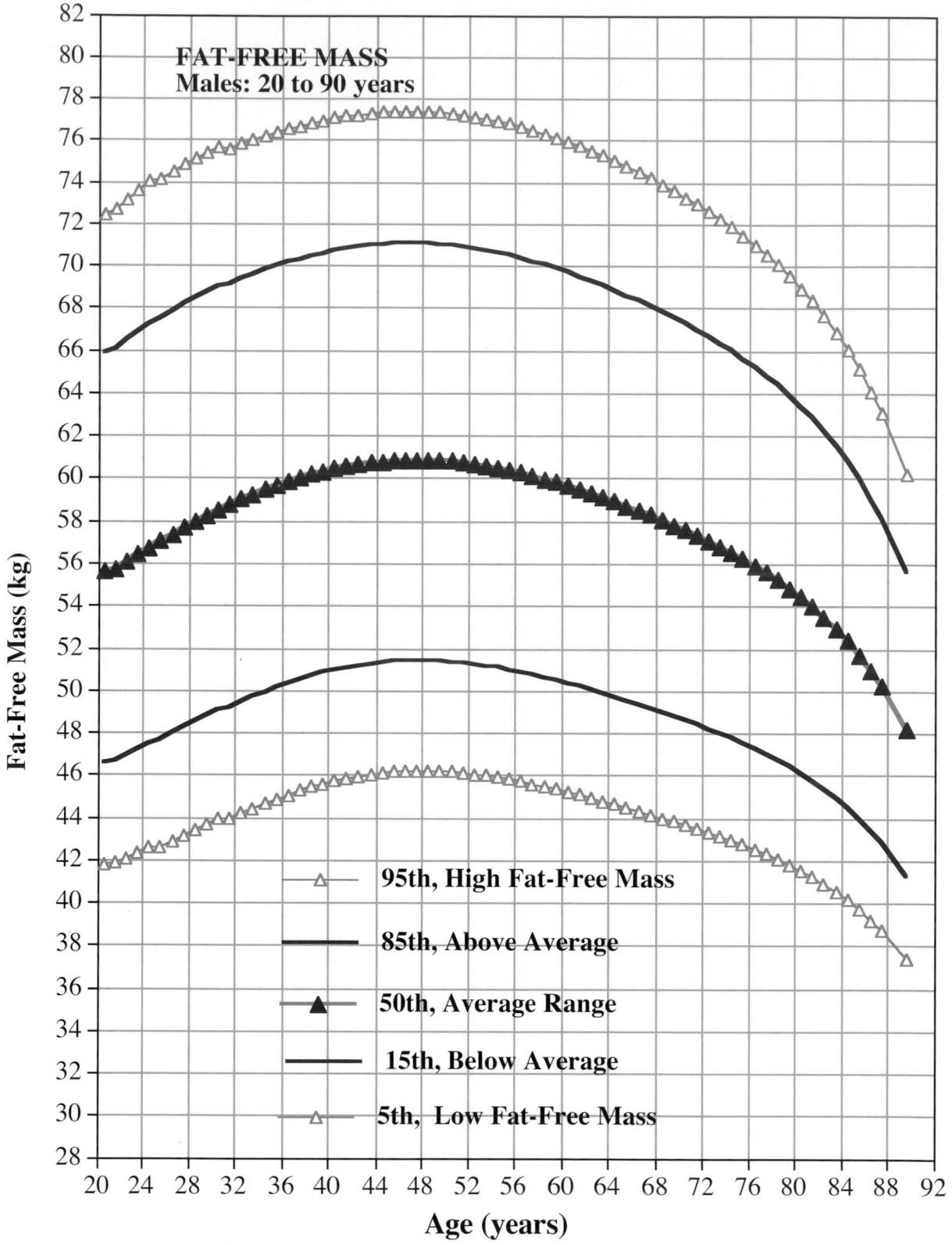

Figure IV.33. Percentiles of Fat-Free Mass (kg) for Males Ranging in Age from 20 to 90 Years.

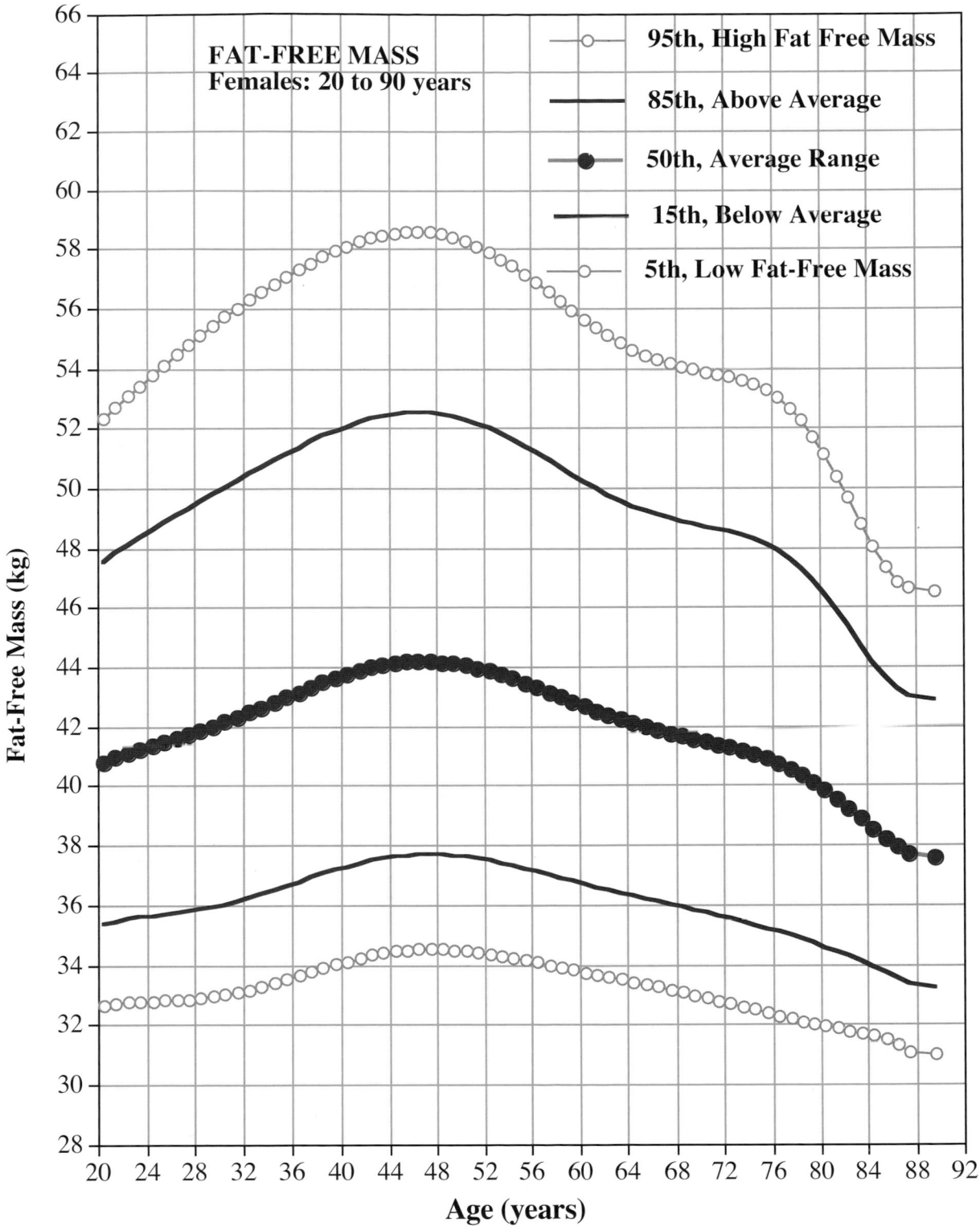

Figure IV.34. Percentiles of Fat-Free Mass (kg) for Females Ranging in Age from 20 to 90 Years.

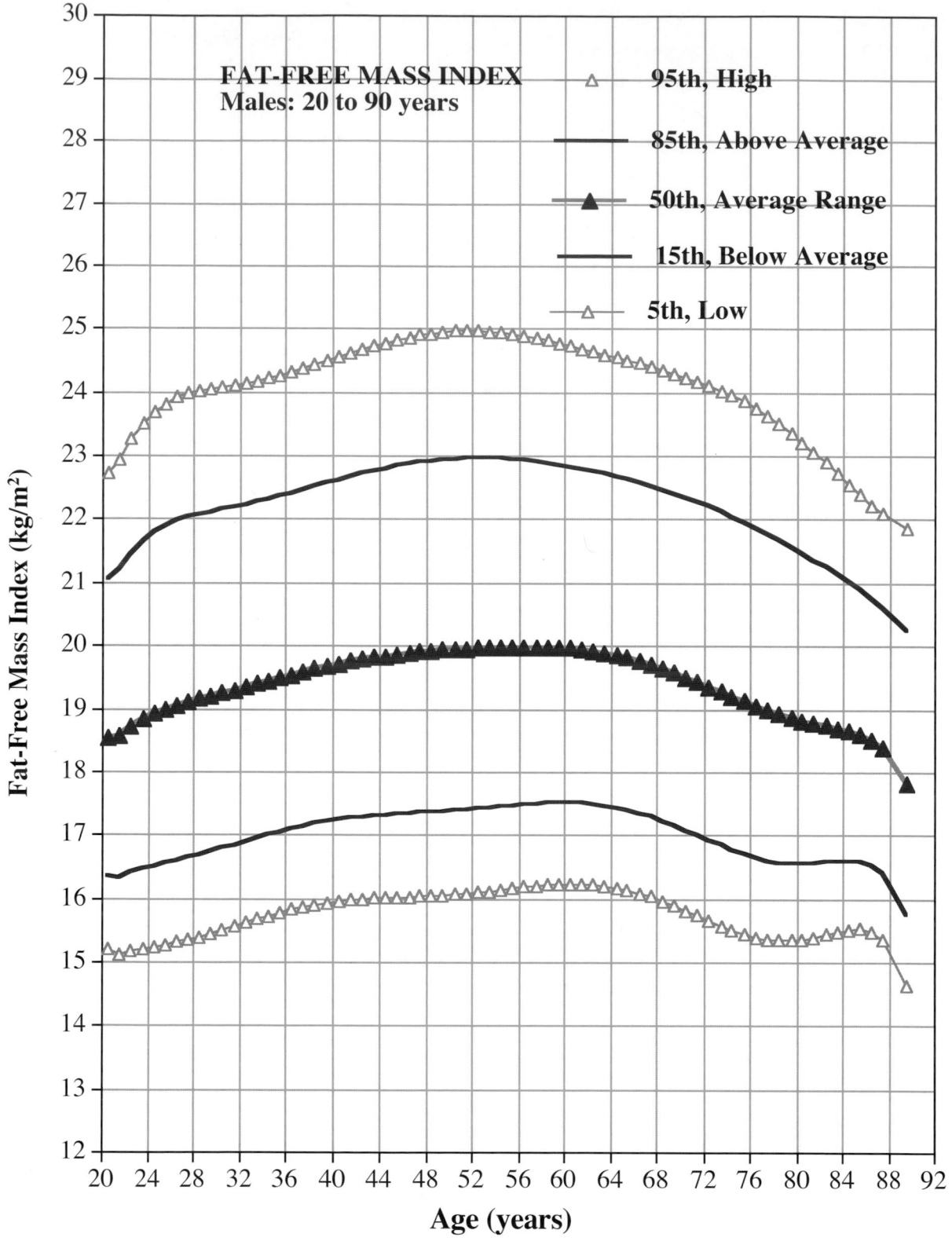

Figure IV.35. Percentiles of Fat-Free Mass Index (kg/m^2) for Males Ranging in Age from 20 to 90 Years.

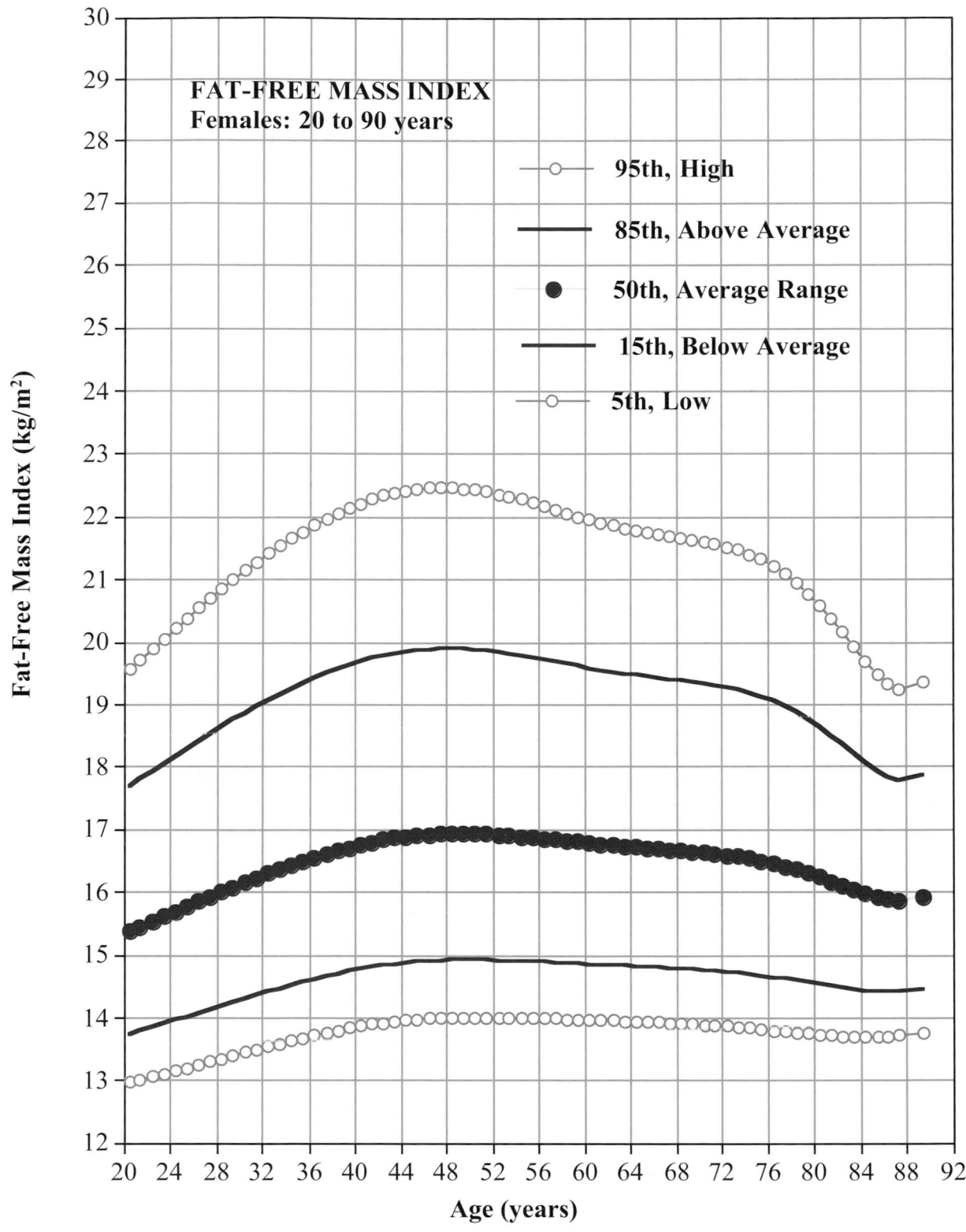

Figure IV.36. Percentiles of Fat-Free Mass Index (kg/m²) for Females Ranging in Age from 20 to 90 Years.

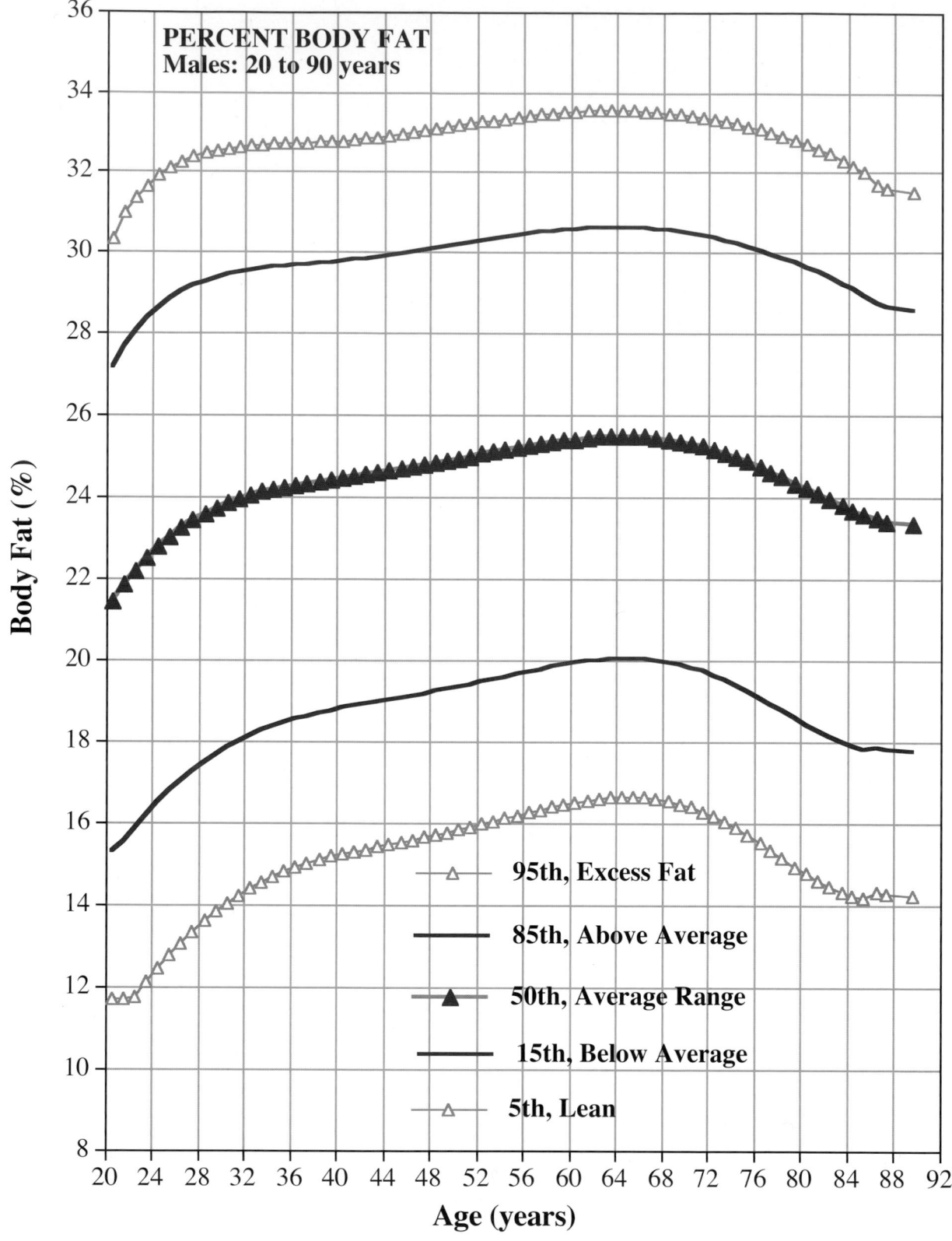

Figure IV.37. Percentiles of Percent Body Fat (%) for Males Ranging in Age from 20 to 90 Years.

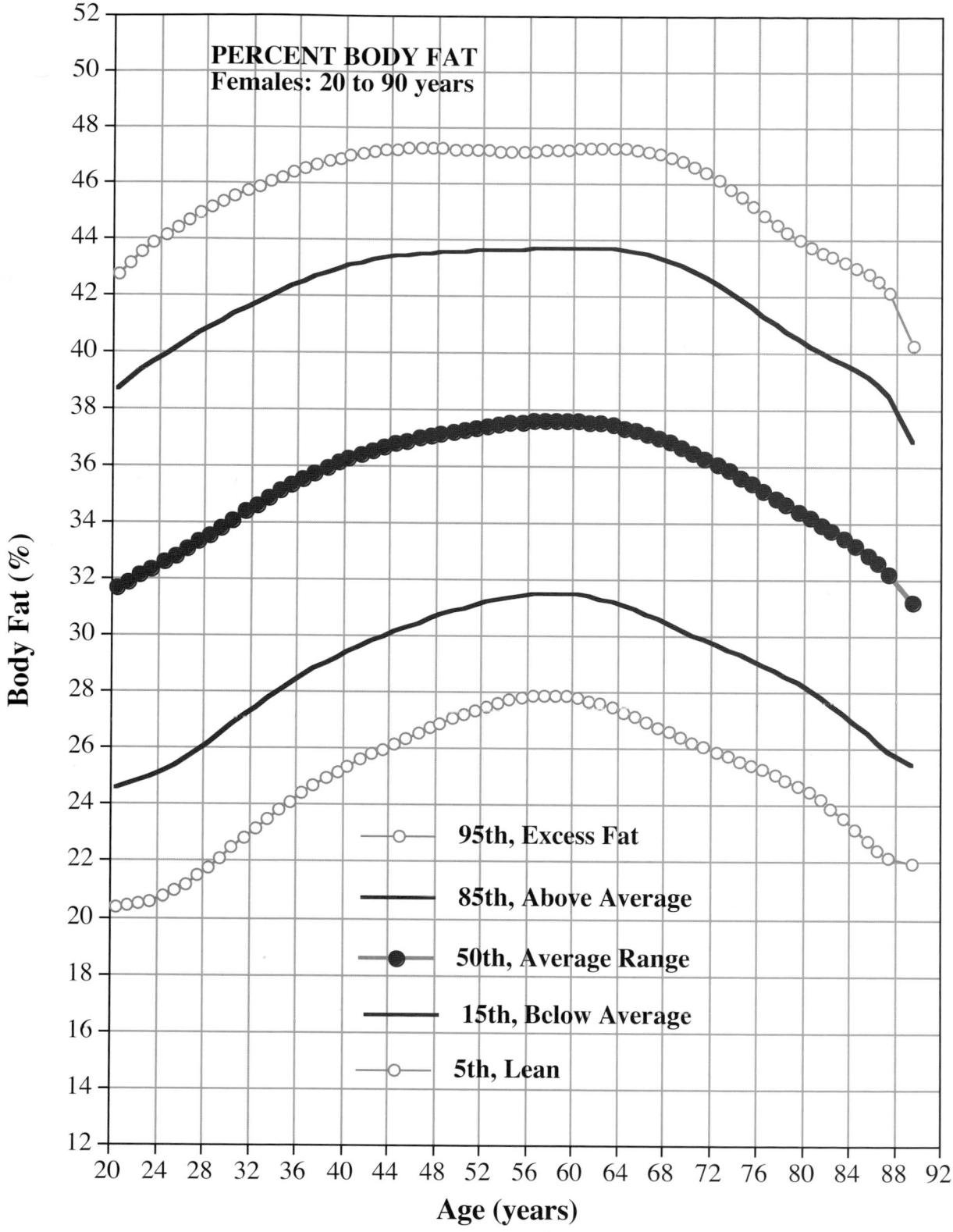

Figure IV.38. Percentiles of Percent Body Fat (%) for Females Ranging in Age from 20 to 90 Years.

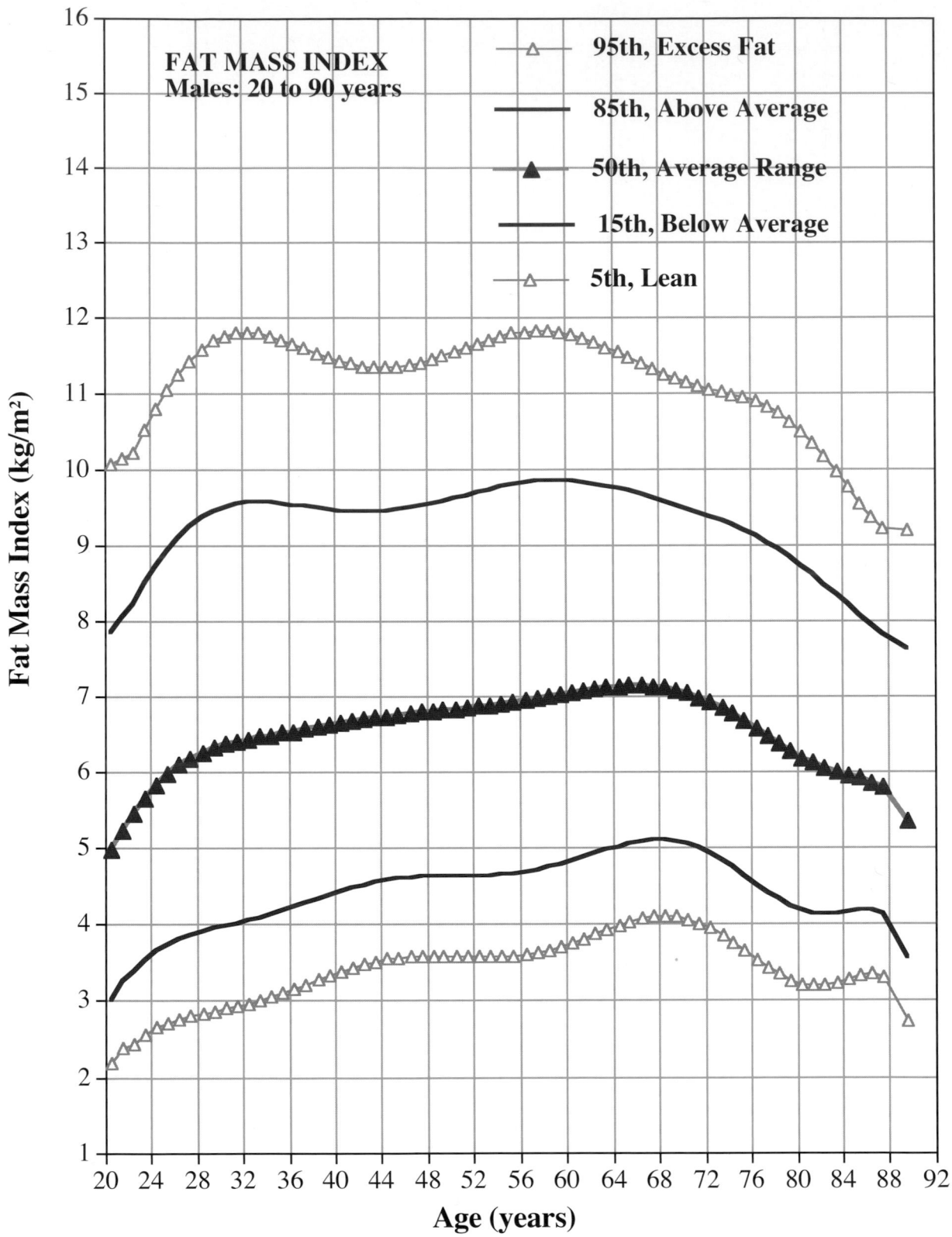

Figure IV.39. Percentiles of Fat Mass Index (kg/m²) for Males Ranging in Age from 20 to 90 Years.

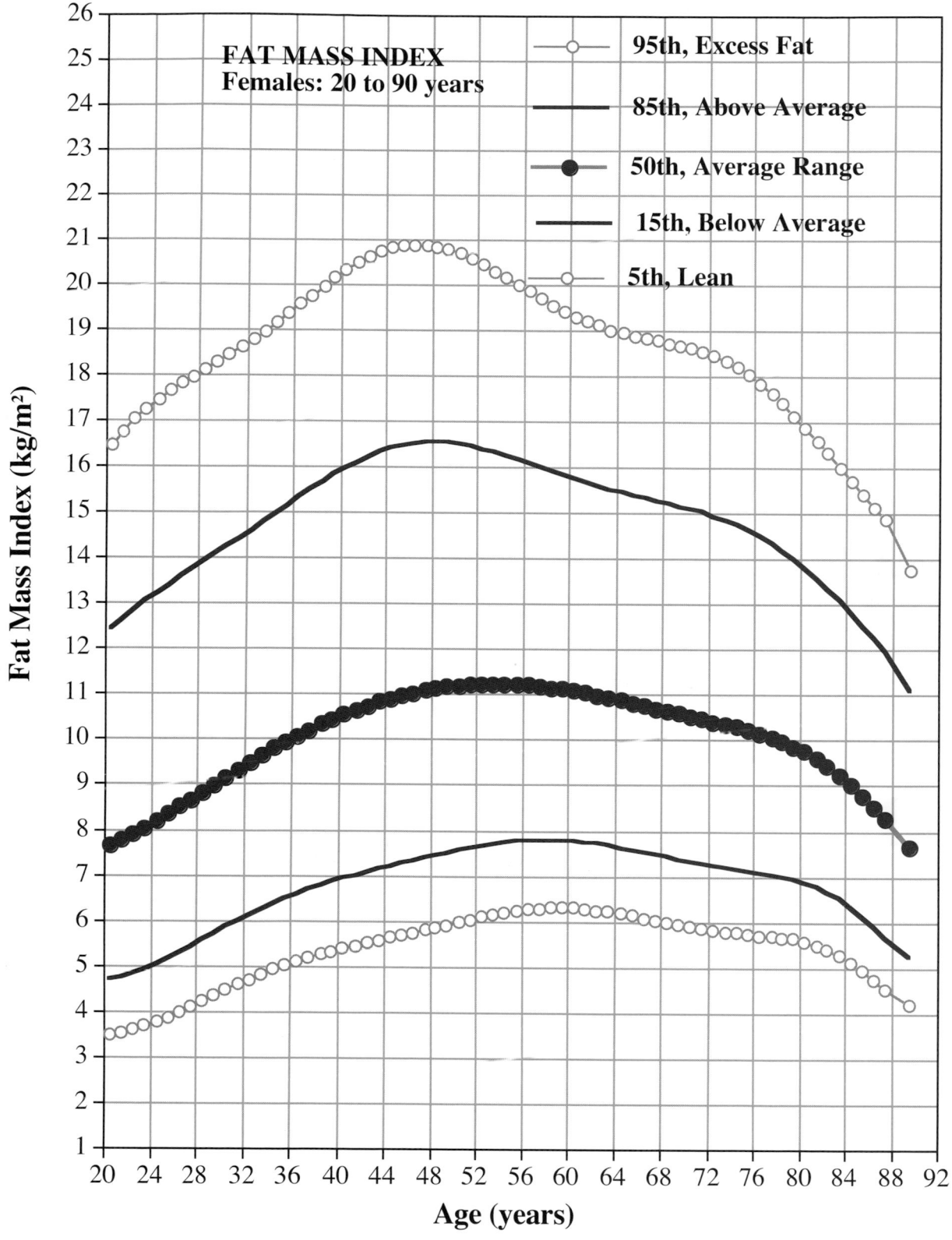

Figure IV.40. Percentiles of Fat Mass Index (kg/m²) for Females Ranging in Age from 20 to 90 Years.

LITERATURE CITED

1. Cole, T. J. 1990. The LMS method for constructing normalized growth standards. Eur. J. of Clin. Nutr., 44:45-60.

2. http://www.cdc.gov/nchs/about/major/nhanes/growthcharts/datafiles.htm.

3. Flegal, K. M. 1999. Curve smoothing and transformations in the development of growth curves. Am. J. Clin. Nutr. [Suppl] 70:163-65.

4. StatView, version 5.0. Abacus Concepts, Berkeley, CA, USA.

5. Cricket Graph III.Version 1.5.3. Computer Associates International, Inc., Islandia, NY 11788-2000.

6. National Health and Nutrition Examination Survey. Anthropometric Reference Data, United States, 1988-1994. Available online at:

   http://www.cdc.gov/nchs/about/major/nhanes/Anthropometric%20Measures.htm.

CHAPTER V
THE CENTERS FOR DISEASE CONTROL AND THE WORLD HEALTH ORGANIZATION GROWTH STANDARDS

CHAPTER V

THE CENTERS FOR DISEASE CONTROL AND THE WORLD HEALTH ORGANIZATION GROWTH STANDARDS

THE 2000 CDC GROWTH CHARTS FROM BIRTH TO 20 YEARS

In 1977 the National Center for Health Statistics (NCHS) of the United States developed the growth charts as a clinical tool for health professionals to determine if the growth of a child is adequate. Then, in 2000 the Centers for Disease Control (CDC) published the revised growth charts for children ranging from 2 to 20 years (1). Most of the data used to construct the 2000 charts comes from the National Health and Nutrition Examination Survey (NHANES), which has periodically collected height and weight and other health information on the American population since the early 1960's. The revised growth charts contain a mix of both breast- and formula-fed infants in the U.S. population. In addition, the revised growth charts include the body mass index, which can be used to judge whether an individual's weight is appropriate for their height for children beginning at 2 years of age.

The CDC growth charts include information of weight, recumbent length, and weight-for-length for children from 2 to 36 months and weight, stature, and body mass index by age for children from 2 to 20 years of age. These references are presented in **Tables V.1** to **V.11** and provide the skew factor (L), mean (M), and coefficients of variation (S), referred to as LMS parameters, and the smoothed percentiles. **Figures V.1** to **V.14** present the growth charts published by the CDC (1).

LIST OF TABLES: CDC GROWTH STANDARDS

Source: http://www.cdc.gov/growthcharts/

Table V.7c. LMS parameters and smoothed percentiles of weight (kg)-for-age in months for girls from 2 to 20 years.

Table V.8a. LMS parameters and smoothed percentiles of stature (cm)-for-age in months for boys from 2 to 20 years.

Table V.8b. LMS parameters and smoothed percentiles of stature (cm)-for-age in months for boys from 2 to 20 years.

Table V.8c. LMS parameters and smoothed percentiles of stature (cm)-for-age in months for boys from 2 to 20 years.

Table V.9a. LMS parameters and smoothed percentiles of stature (cm)-for-age in months for girls from 2 to 20 years.

Table V.9b. LMS parameters and smoothed percentiles of stature (cm)-for-age in months for girls from 2 to 20 years.

Table V.9c. LMS parameters and smoothed percentiles of stature (cm)-for-age in months for girls from 2 to 20 years.

Table V.10a. LMS parameters and smoothed percentiles of body mass index (kg/m^2)-for-age in months for boys from 2 to 20 years.

Table V.10b. LMS parameters and smoothed percentiles of body mass index (kg/m^2)-for-age in months for boys from 2 to 20 years.

Table V.10c. LMS parameters and smoothed percentiles of body mass index (kg/m^2)-for-age in months for boys from 2 to 20 years.

Table V.11a. LMS parameters and smoothed percentiles of body mass index (kg/m^2)-for-age in months for girls from 2 to 20 years.

Table V.11b. LMS parameters and smoothed percentiles of body mass index (kg/m^2)-for-age in months for girls from 2 to 20 years.

Table V.11c. LMS parameters and smoothed percentiles of body mass index (kg/m^2)-for-age in months for girls from 2 to 20 years.

CDC Growth Standards

Table V.1.

LMS parameters and smoothed percentiles of weight (kg)-for-age for boys and girls from birth to 36 months

Age Group (months)	L	M	S	Percentiles								
				3rd	5th	10th	25th	50th	75th	90th	95th	97th
Boys												
0.0	1.8152	3.5302	0.1524	2.4	2.5	2.8	3.2	3.5	3.9	4.2	4.3	4.4
0.5	1.5475	4.0031	0.1460	2.8	3.0	3.2	3.6	4.0	4.4	4.7	4.9	5.0
1.5	1.0688	4.8795	0.1365	3.6	3.8	4.0	4.4	4.9	5.3	5.7	6.0	6.1
2.5	0.6960	5.6729	0.1297	4.3	4.5	4.8	5.2	5.7	6.2	6.6	6.9	7.1
3.5	0.4198	6.3914	0.1247	5.0	5.2	5.4	5.9	6.4	6.9	7.5	7.8	8.0
4.5	0.2199	7.0418	0.1210	5.6	5.7	6.0	6.5	7.0	7.6	8.2	8.6	8.8
5.5	0.0775	7.6304	0.1183	6.1	6.3	6.6	7.0	7.6	8.3	8.9	9.3	9.5
6.5	-0.0219	8.1630	0.1162	6.6	6.7	7.0	7.5	8.2	8.8	9.5	9.9	10.2
7.5	-0.0894	8.6448	0.1145	7.0	7.2	7.5	8.0	8.6	9.3	10.0	10.5	10.7
8.5	-0.1334	9.0811	0.1132	7.4	7.6	7.9	8.4	9.1	9.8	10.5	11.0	11.3
9.5	-0.1601	9.4765	0.1122	7.7	7.9	8.2	8.8	9.5	10.2	11.0	11.4	11.7
10.5	-0.1743	9.8353	0.1114	8.0	8.2	8.5	9.1	9.8	10.6	11.4	11.8	12.2
11.5	-0.1797	10.1615	0.1107	8.3	8.5	8.8	9.4	10.2	11.0	11.7	12.2	12.6
12.5	-0.1793	10.4589	0.1101	8.5	8.8	9.1	9.7	10.5	11.3	12.1	12.6	12.9
13.5	-0.1752	10.7306	0.1097	8.8	9.0	9.3	10.0	10.7	11.6	12.4	12.9	13.2
14.5	-0.1693	10.9799	0.1093	9.0	9.2	9.6	10.2	11.0	11.8	12.7	13.2	13.5
15.5	-0.1631	11.2096	0.1090	9.2	9.4	9.8	10.4	11.2	12.1	12.9	13.4	13.8
16.5	-0.1577	11.4221	0.1087	9.3	9.6	10.0	10.6	11.4	12.3	13.1	13.7	14.1
17.5	-0.1540	11.6198	0.1085	9.5	9.7	10.1	10.8	11.6	12.5	13.4	13.9	14.3
18.5	-0.1528	11.8048	0.1083	9.7	9.9	10.3	11.0	11.8	12.7	13.6	14.1	14.5
19.5	-0.1545	11.9790	0.1082	9.8	10.1	10.4	11.1	12.0	12.9	13.8	14.3	14.7
20.5	-0.1595	12.1440	0.1081	9.9	10.2	10.6	11.3	12.1	13.1	14.0	14.5	14.9
21.5	-0.1682	12.3015	0.1081	10.1	10.3	10.7	11.4	12.3	13.2	14.2	14.7	15.1
22.5	-0.1806	12.4528	0.1081	10.2	10.5	10.9	11.6	12.5	13.4	14.3	14.9	15.3
23.5	-0.1967	12.5991	0.1081	10.3	10.6	11.0	11.7	12.6	13.6	14.5	15.1	15.5
24.5	-0.2165	12.7415	0.1082	10.4	10.7	11.1	11.9	12.7	13.7	14.7	15.3	15.7
25.5	-0.2398	12.8810	0.1083	10.6	10.8	11.2	12.0	12.9	13.9	14.8	15.5	15.9
26.5	-0.2663	13.0184	0.1084	10.7	10.9	11.4	12.1	13.0	14.0	15.0	15.6	16.1
27.5	-0.2958	13.1545	0.1086	10.8	11.1	11.5	12.2	13.2	14.2	15.2	15.8	16.2
28.5	-0.3277	13.2899	0.1088	10.9	11.2	11.6	12.4	13.3	14.3	15.3	16.0	16.4
29.5	-0.3618	13.4252	0.1091	11.0	11.3	11.7	12.5	13.4	14.5	15.5	16.2	16.6
30.5	-0.3976	13.5609	0.1094	11.1	11.4	11.8	12.6	13.6	14.6	15.7	16.3	16.8
31.5	-0.4345	13.6974	0.1097	11.2	11.5	12.0	12.7	13.7	14.8	15.8	16.5	17.0
32.5	-0.4722	13.8350	0.1101	11.4	11.6	12.1	12.9	13.8	14.9	16.0	16.7	17.2
33.5	-0.5101	13.9742	0.1105	11.5	11.7	12.2	13.0	14.0	15.1	16.2	16.9	17.4
34.5	-0.5479	14.1150	0.1109	11.6	11.9	12.3	13.1	14.1	15.2	16.4	17.1	17.6
35.5	-0.5851	14.2578	0.1114	11.7	12.0	12.4	13.2	14.3	15.4	16.5	17.3	17.8
36.0	-0.6033	14.3299	0.1116	11.8	12.0	12.5	13.3	14.3	15.5	16.6	17.4	17.9
Girls												
0.0	1.5092	3.3992	0.1421	2.4	2.5	2.7	3.1	3.4	3.7	4.0	4.2	4.3
0.5	1.3579	3.7975	0.1381	2.8	2.9	3.1	3.4	3.8	4.1	4.5	4.6	4.7
1.5	1.1055	4.5448	0.1317	3.4	3.5	3.8	4.1	4.5	4.9	5.3	5.5	5.7
2.5	0.9026	5.2306	0.1269	4.0	4.2	4.4	4.8	5.2	5.7	6.1	6.3	6.5
3.5	0.7341	5.8600	0.1230	4.5	4.7	5.0	5.4	5.9	6.4	6.8	7.1	7.3
4.5	0.5902	6.4376	0.1198	5.1	5.2	5.5	5.9	6.4	7.0	7.5	7.8	8.0
5.5	0.4644	6.9679	0.1172	5.5	5.7	6.0	6.4	7.0	7.5	8.1	8.4	8.6
6.5	0.3522	7.4549	0.1149	6.0	6.1	6.4	6.9	7.5	8.0	8.6	9.0	9.2
7.5	0.2505	7.9024	0.1129	6.4	6.5	6.8	7.3	7.9	8.5	9.1	9.5	9.7
8.5	0.1572	8.3142	0.1113	6.7	6.9	7.2	7.7	8.3	9.0	9.6	10.0	10.2
9.5	0.0709	8.6934	0.1099	7.1	7.2	7.5	8.1	8.7	9.4	10.0	10.4	10.7
10.5	-0.0097	9.0433	0.1087	7.4	7.6	7.9	8.4	9.0	9.7	10.4	10.8	11.1
11.5	-0.0853	9.3666	0.1077	7.7	7.9	8.2	8.7	9.4	10.1	10.8	11.2	11.5
12.5	-0.1564	9.6661	0.1068	7.9	8.1	8.4	9.0	9.7	10.4	11.1	11.6	11.9
13.5	-0.2236	9.9442	0.1062	8.2	8.4	8.7	9.3	9.9	10.7	11.4	11.9	12.2
14.5	-0.2870	10.2033	0.1057	8.4	8.6	8.9	9.5	10.2	11.0	11.7	12.2	12.5
15.5	-0.3470	10.4454	0.1053	8.6	8.8	9.2	9.7	10.4	11.2	12.0	12.5	12.8
16.5	-0.4037	10.6725	0.1051	8.8	9.0	9.4	10.0	10.7	11.5	12.3	12.8	13.1
17.5	-0.4572	10.8864	0.1051	9.0	9.2	9.6	10.2	10.9	11.7	12.5	13.0	13.4
18.5	-0.5077	11.0887	0.1051	9.2	9.4	9.7	10.3	11.1	11.9	12.7	13.3	13.7
19.5	-0.5552	11.2809	0.1053	9.3	9.6	9.9	10.5	11.3	12.1	13.0	13.5	13.9
20.5	-0.5999	11.4644	0.1056	9.5	9.7	10.1	10.7	11.5	12.3	13.2	13.8	14.2
21.5	-0.6419	11.6404	0.1060	9.6	9.9	10.2	10.9	11.6	12.5	13.4	14.0	14.4
22.5	-0.6811	11.8101	0.1065	9.8	10.0	10.4	11.0	11.8	12.7	13.6	14.2	14.6
23.5	-0.7179	11.9745	0.1071	9.9	10.1	10.5	11.2	12.0	12.9	13.8	14.5	14.9
24.5	-0.7522	12.1346	0.1077	10.0	10.3	10.6	11.3	12.1	13.1	14.0	14.7	15.1
25.5	-0.7842	12.2910	0.1085	10.2	10.4	10.8	11.4	12.3	13.3	14.2	14.9	15.4
26.5	-0.8141	12.4447	0.1093	10.3	10.5	10.9	11.6	12.6	13.4	14.4	15.1	15.6
27.5	-0.8419	12.5962	0.1101	10.4	10.6	11.0	11.7	12.6	13.6	14.6	15.3	15.8
28.5	-0.8679	12.7462	0.1111	10.5	10.8	11.1	11.9	12.7	13.8	14.8	15.6	16.0
29.5	-0.8921	12.8952	0.1120	10.6	10.9	11.3	12.0	12.9	13.9	15.0	15.8	16.3
30.5	-0.9147	13.0436	0.1130	10.7	11.0	11.4	12.1	13.0	14.1	15.2	16.0	16.5
31.5	-0.9359	13.1918	0.1141	10.8	11.1	11.5	12.2	13.2	14.3	15.4	16.2	16.8
32.5	-0.9557	13.3402	0.1151	11.0	11.2	11.6	12.4	13.3	14.5	15.6	16.4	17.0
33.5	-0.9744	13.4891	0.1162	11.1	11.3	11.7	12.5	13.5	14.6	15.8	16.7	17.2
34.5	-0.9920	13.6388	0.1173	11.2	11.4	11.9	12.6	13.6	14.8	16.0	16.9	17.5
35.5	-1.0086	13.7894	0.1184	11.3	11.5	12.0	12.8	13.8	15.0	16.3	17.1	17.7
36.0	-1.0167	13.8651	0.1189	11.3	11.6	12.0	12.8	13.9	15.1	16.4	17.2	17.9

Table V.2.

LMS parameters and smoothed percentiles of recumbent length (cm)-for-age for boys and girls from birth to 36 months

Age Group (months)	L	M	S	Percentiles								
				3rd	5th	10th	25th	50th	75th	90th	95th	97th
Boys												
0.0	1.2670	49.9889	0.0531	45.0	45.6	46.6	48.2	50.0	51.7	53.3	54.2	54.8
0.5	0.5112	52.6960	0.0487	48.0	48.6	49.5	51.0	52.7	54.4	56.0	56.9	57.6
1.5	-0.4522	56.6284	0.0441	52.3	52.8	53.6	55.0	56.6	58.3	59.9	60.9	61.6
2.5	-0.9906	59.6090	0.0418	55.3	55.8	56.6	58.0	59.6	61.3	62.9	63.9	64.6
3.5	-1.2858	62.0770	0.0405	57.8	58.3	59.1	60.5	62.1	63.8	65.5	66.5	67.2
4.5	-1.4303	64.2169	0.0396	59.9	60.4	61.2	62.6	64.2	66.0	67.7	68.7	69.4
5.5	-1.4766	66.1253	0.0391	61.7	62.2	63.0	64.5	66.1	67.9	69.6	70.7	71.4
6.5	-1.4568	67.8602	0.0388	63.4	63.9	64.7	66.2	67.9	69.7	71.4	72.5	73.2
7.5	-1.3919	69.4591	0.0386	64.9	65.4	66.2	67.7	69.5	71.3	73.1	74.2	74.9
8.5	-1.2957	70.9480	0.0385	66.3	66.8	67.7	69.2	70.9	72.8	74.6	75.7	76.5
9.5	-1.1779	72.3459	0.0385	67.5	68.1	69.0	70.5	72.3	74.3	76.1	77.2	78.0
10.5	-1.0453	73.6667	0.0386	68.7	69.3	70.2	71.8	73.7	75.6	77.5	78.6	79.4
11.5	-0.9028	74.9213	0.0386	69.9	70.5	71.4	73.0	74.9	76.9	78.8	79.9	80.7
12.5	-0.7539	76.1184	0.0387	71.0	71.6	72.5	74.2	76.1	78.1	80.0	81.2	82.0
13.5	-0.6013	77.2648	0.0388	72.0	72.6	73.6	75.3	77.3	79.3	81.2	82.4	83.2
14.5	-0.4468	78.3662	0.0389	73.0	73.6	74.6	76.4	78.4	80.4	82.4	83.6	84.4
15.5	-0.2920	79.4273	0.0391	73.9	74.6	75.6	77.4	79.4	81.5	83.5	84.7	85.5
16.5	-0.1378	80.4521	0.0392	74.8	75.5	76.6	78.4	80.5	82.6	84.6	85.8	86.6
17.5	0.0148	81.4438	0.0393	75.7	76.4	77.5	79.3	81.4	83.6	85.6	86.8	87.6
18.5	0.1653	82.4054	0.0395	76.5	77.2	78.4	80.3	82.4	84.6	86.6	87.9	88.7
19.5	0.3133	83.3394	0.0396	77.3	78.1	79.2	81.2	83.3	85.6	87.6	88.8	89.7
20.5	0.4585	84.2478	0.0398	78.1	78.9	80.1	82.0	84.2	86.5	88.6	89.8	90.6
21.5	0.6005	85.1327	0.0399	78.9	79.7	80.9	82.9	85.1	87.4	89.5	90.7	91.6
22.5	0.7394	85.9956	0.0401	79.6	80.4	81.6	83.7	86.0	88.3	90.4	91.7	92.5
23.5	0.8750	86.8382	0.0402	80.4	81.2	82.4	84.5	86.8	89.2	91.3	92.6	93.4
24.5	1.0072	87.6616	0.0404	81.1	81.9	83.2	85.3	87.7	90.0	92.2	93.4	94.3
25.5	0.8373	88.4525	0.0406	81.8	82.6	83.9	86.1	88.5	90.9	93.0	94.3	95.2
26.5	0.6815	89.2233	0.0407	82.5	83.4	84.6	86.8	13.0	91.7	93.9	95.2	96.1
27.5	0.5388	89.9755	0.0408	83.2	84.1	85.4	87.5	90.0	92.4	94.7	96.1	96.9
28.5	0.4077	90.7104	0.0409	83.9	84.8	86.1	88.2	90.7	93.2	95.5	96.9	97.8
29.5	0.2868	91.4291	0.0410	84.6	85.5	86.8	89.0	91.4	94.0	96.3	97.7	98.6
30.5	0.1745	92.1324	0.0410	85.3	86.1	87.4	89.6	92.1	94.7	97.0	98.5	99.4
31.5	0.0694	92.8213	0.0409	86.0	86.8	88.1	90.3	92.8	95.4	97.8	99.2	100.2
32.5	-0.0297	93.4964	0.0409	86.6	87.5	88.8	91.0	93.5	96.1	98.5	100.0	100.9
33.5	-0.1243	94.1585	0.0408	87.3	88.1	89.4	91.6	94.2	96.8	99.2	100.7	101.7
34.5	-0.2153	94.8082	0.0408	87.9	88.8	90.0	92.3	94.8	97.4	99.9	101.4	102.4
35.5	-0.3039	95.4464	0.0407	88.6	89.4	90.7	92.9	95.4	98.1	100.5	102.1	103.1
36.5	-0.3909	96.0736	0.0405	89.2	90.0	91.3	93.5	96.1	98.7	101.2	102.7	103.7
Girls												
0.0	-1.2960	49.2864	0.0501	45.2	45.6	46.4	47.7	49.3	51.0	52.6	53.7	54.4
0.5	-0.8092	51.6836	0.0468	47.5	48.0	48.8	50.1	51.7	53.3	54.9	55.9	56.6
1.5	-0.0508	55.2861	0.0434	51.0	51.5	52.3	53.7	55.3	56.9	58.4	59.3	59.9
2.5	0.4769	58.0938	0.0417	53.7	54.2	55.1	56.5	58.1	59.7	61.2	62.1	62.7
3.5	0.8433	60.4598	0.0407	55.9	56.5	57.4	58.8	60.5	62.1	63.6	64.5	65.1
4.5	1.0976	62.5367	0.0401	57.9	58.5	59.4	60.9	62.5	64.2	65.7	66.6	67.2
5.5	1.2725	64.4063	0.0397	59.6	60.2	61.1	62.7	64.4	66.1	67.6	68.5	69.1
6.5	1.3904	66.1184	0.0394	61.2	61.8	62.8	64.4	66.1	67.8	69.4	70.3	70.9
7.5	1.4667	67.7057	0.0393	62.7	63.3	64.3	65.9	67.7	69.5	71.0	72.0	72.6
8.5	1.5123	69.1912	0.0392	64.0	64.7	65.7	67.4	69.2	71.0	72.6	73.5	74.1
9.5	1.5350	70.5916	0.0392	65.3	66.0	67.0	68.7	70.6	72.4	74.1	75.0	75.6
10.5	1.5404	71.9196	0.0392	66.6	67.2	68.3	70.0	71.9	73.8	75.4	76.4	77.1
11.5	1.5329	73.1850	0.0393	67.7	68.4	69.5	71.3	73.2	75.1	76.8	77.8	78.4
12.5	1.5155	74.3956	0.0394	68.8	69.5	70.6	72.4	74.4	76.3	78.1	79.1	79.7
13.5	1.4908	75.5579	0.0395	69.9	70.6	71.7	73.6	75.6	77.5	79.3	80.3	81.0
14.5	1.4605	76.6769	0.0396	70.9	71.7	72.8	74.6	76.7	78.7	80.5	81.5	82.2
15.5	1.4260	77.7570	0.0397	71.9	72.7	73.8	75.7	77.8	79.8	81.6	82.7	83.4
16.5	1.3885	78.8020	0.0398	72.9	73.6	74.8	76.7	78.8	80.9	82.7	83.8	84.6
17.5	1.3488	79.8149	0.0399	73.8	74.6	75.7	77.7	79.8	81.9	83.8	84.9	85.7
18.5	1.3076	80.7985	0.0400	74.7	75.5	76.7	78.6	80.8	83.0	84.9	86.0	86.8
19.5	1.2654	81.7551	0.0402	75.6	76.4	77.6	79.6	81.8	83.9	85.9	87.1	87.8
20.5	1.2226	82.6868	0.0403	76.4	77.2	78.4	80.5	82.7	84.9	86.9	88.1	88.8
21.5	1.1796	83.5953	0.0404	77.3	78.1	79.3	81.3	83.6	85.8	87.9	89.1	89.9
22.5	1.1366	84.4823	0.0406	78.1	78.9	80.1	82.2	84.5	86.8	88.8	90.0	90.8
23.5	1.0937	85.3492	0.0407	78.8	79.7	80.9	83.0	85.3	87.7	89.8	91.0	91.8
24.5	1.0513	86.1973	0.0409	79.6	80.4	81.7	83.8	86.2	88.5	90.7	91.9	92.7
25.5	1.0420	87.0903	0.0411	80.4	81.2	82.5	84.7	87.1	89.5	91.6	92.9	93.8
26.5	1.0126	87.9571	0.0413	81.2	82.0	83.3	85.5	13.0	90.4	92.6	93.9	94.7
27.5	0.9705	88.7960	0.0415	81.9	82.8	84.1	86.3	88.8	91.3	93.5	94.8	95.7
28.5	0.9211	89.6055	0.0416	82.7	83.5	84.9	87.1	89.6	92.1	94.4	95.7	96.6
29.5	0.8682	90.3848	0.0417	83.4	84.3	85.6	87.9	90.4	92.9	95.2	96.6	97.4
30.5	0.8145	91.1334	0.0418	84.1	85.0	86.3	88.6	91.1	93.7	96.0	97.4	98.3
31.5	0.7620	91.8515	0.0418	84.8	85.6	87.0	89.3	91.9	94.4	96.8	98.2	99.1
32.5	0.7117	92.5396	0.0418	85.4	86.3	87.7	90.0	92.5	95.1	97.5	98.9	99.8
33.5	0.6643	93.1985	0.0419	86.0	86.9	88.3	90.6	93.2	95.8	98.2	99.6	100.6
34.5	0.6203	93.8295	0.0419	86.6	87.5	88.9	91.2	93.8	96.5	98.9	100.3	101.3
35.5	0.5796	94.4338	0.0420	87.2	88.1	89.5	91.8	94.4	97.1	99.5	101.0	101.9
36.5	0.5420	95.0134	0.0420	87.7	88.6	90.0	92.4	95.0	97.7	100.1	101.6	102.6

Table V.3a.

LMS parameters and smoothed percentiles of weight (kg)-for-recumbent length (cm) for boys from birth to 36 months

Length Group (cm)	L	M	S	Percentiles								
				3rd	5th	10th	25th	50th	75th	90th	95th	97th
45.0	1.44904	2.28976	0.14924	1.60	1.69	1.83	2.05	2.29	2.52	2.71	2.82	2.90
45.5	1.31794	2.38617	0.14479	1.70	1.79	1.93	2.15	2.39	2.62	2.82	2.94	3.01
46.5	1.04173	2.5871	0.13655	1.92	2.00	2.13	2.35	2.59	2.82	3.04	3.17	3.25
47.5	0.75662	2.79795	0.12916	2.14	2.22	2.34	2.56	2.80	3.04	3.27	3.41	3.50
48.5	0.47262	3.01768	0.12259	2.36	2.44	2.56	2.77	3.02	3.27	3.51	3.66	3.76
49.5	0.19746	3.24523	0.1168	2.59	2.67	2.79	3.00	3.25	3.51	3.76	3.92	4.02
50.5	-0.06327	3.47957	0.11173	2.82	2.90	3.02	3.23	3.48	3.75	4.02	4.19	4.30
51.5	-0.30566	3.71974	0.10732	3.06	3.13	3.25	3.46	3.72	4.00	4.28	4.46	4.58
52.5	-0.52721	3.96484	0.10347	3.29	3.37	3.49	3.70	3.96	4.26	4.55	4.74	4.87
53.5	-0.72636	4.21403	0.10014	3.53	3.61	3.73	3.95	4.21	4.52	4.82	5.02	5.16
54.5	-0.90238	4.46656	0.09725	3.77	3.85	3.97	4.19	4.47	4.78	5.10	5.31	5.45
55.5	-1.05513	4.72173	0.09474	4.01	4.09	4.21	4.44	4.72	5.04	5.38	5.60	5.75
56.5	-1.18493	4.9789	0.09256	4.25	4.33	4.46	4.69	4.98	5.31	5.66	5.89	6.05
57.5	-1.29253	5.2375	0.09067	4.49	4.57	4.70	4.94	5.24	5.58	5.94	6.18	6.35
58.5	-1.37897	5.49701	0.08902	4.73	4.81	4.94	5.19	5.50	5.85	6.22	6.47	6.65
59.5	-1.44556	5.75694	0.08759	4.97	5.05	5.19	5.44	5.76	6.12	6.51	6.77	6.95
60.5	-1.4938	6.01687	0.08634	5.20	5.29	5.43	5.69	6.02	6.39	6.79	7.06	7.25
61.5	-1.52533	6.2764	0.08525	5.44	5.53	5.67	5.94	6.28	6.67	7.07	7.35	7.54
62.5	-1.54184	6.5352	0.08428	5.67	5.76	5.91	6.19	6.54	6.94	7.35	7.64	7.84
63.5	-1.5451	6.79294	0.08343	5.90	6.00	6.15	6.44	6.79	7.20	7.64	7.93	8.13
64.5	-1.53686	7.04937	0.08268	6.13	6.23	6.39	6.68	7.05	7.47	7.91	8.21	8.42
65.5	-1.51879	7.30425	0.08201	6.36	6.46	6.63	6.93	7.30	7.74	8.19	8.49	8.71
66.5	-1.49249	7.55738	0.0814	6.58	6.69	6.86	7.17	7.56	8.00	8.46	8.77	8.99
67.5	-1.45949	7.80861	0.08085	6.81	6.91	7.09	7.41	7.81	8.27	8.74	9.05	9.27
68.5	-1.42117	8.05781	0.08035	7.03	7.14	7.32	7.65	8.06	8.53	9.01	9.33	9.55
69.5	-1.37884	8.30489	0.07989	7.24	7.36	7.55	7.88	8.30	8.78	9.27	9.60	9.83
70.5	-1.33363	8.5498	0.07946	7.46	7.58	7.77	8.12	8.55	9.04	9.54	9.87	10.10
71.5	-1.28661	8.79252	0.07907	7.67	7.80	7.99	8.35	8.79	9.29	9.80	10.14	10.37
72.5	-1.23867	9.03305	0.0787	7.89	8.01	8.21	8.58	9.03	9.54	10.06	10.40	10.64
73.5	-1.19067	9.27145	0.07836	8.09	8.22	8.43	8.81	9.27	9.79	10.32	10.66	10.90
74.5	-1.14332	9.50777	0.07804	8.30	8.43	8.65	9.03	9.51	10.04	10.57	10.92	11.16
75.5	-1.09726	9.74213	0.07773	8.51	8.64	8.86	9.26	9.74	10.28	10.83	11.18	11.43
76.5	-1.05308	9.97464	0.07745	8.71	8.85	9.08	9.48	9.97	10.53	11.08	11.44	11.68
77.5	-1.01129	10.2055	0.07719	8.91	9.06	9.29	9.70	10.21	10.77	11.33	11.69	11.94
78.5	-0.97236	10.4348	0.07695	9.11	9.26	9.50	9.92	10.43	11.01	11.57	11.94	12.20
79.5	-0.93671	10.6627	0.07673	9.31	9.46	9.71	10.14	10.66	11.24	11.82	12.20	12.45
80.5	-0.90472	10.8896	0.07653	9.51	9.67	9.91	10.35	10.89	11.48	12.07	12.45	12.71
81.5	-0.87678	11.1156	0.07635	9.71	9.87	10.12	10.57	11.12	11.72	12.31	12.70	12.96
82.5	-0.85322	11.341	0.07619	9.91	10.07	10.33	10.78	11.34	11.95	12.56	12.95	13.21
83.5	-0.83438	11.566	0.07606	10.10	10.27	10.53	11.00	11.57	12.19	12.80	13.20	13.47
84.5	-0.82058	11.791	0.07595	10.30	10.47	10.74	11.21	11.79	12.42	13.05	13.45	13.73
85.5	-0.81215	12.0161	0.07587	10.50	10.67	10.94	11.43	12.02	12.66	13.30	13.71	13.98
86.5	-0.80939	12.2417	0.07581	10.70	10.87	11.15	11.64	12.24	12.90	13.55	13.96	14.24
87.5	-0.81264	12.4682	0.07579	10.90	11.07	11.36	11.86	12.47	13.14	13.80	14.22	14.51
88.5	-0.82219	12.6957	0.07579	11.09	11.27	11.56	12.08	12.70	13.38	14.05	14.48	14.77
89.5	-0.83835	12.9246	0.07583	11.30	11.48	11.77	12.29	12.92	13.62	14.30	14.74	15.04
90.5	-0.86145	13.1552	0.07589	11.50	11.68	11.98	12.51	13.16	13.86	14.56	15.01	15.32
91.5	-0.89177	13.3878	0.07599	11.70	11.89	12.19	12.73	13.39	14.11	14.82	15.28	15.60
92.5	-0.92962	13.6227	0.07612	11.91	12.10	12.41	12.96	13.62	14.36	15.09	15.56	15.88
93.5	-0.97527	13.8603	0.07628	12.12	12.31	12.62	13.18	13.86	14.61	15.36	15.84	16.18
94.5	-1.02899	14.1007	0.07647	12.33	12.53	12.84	13.41	14.10	14.87	15.64	16.13	16.48
95.5	-1.09102	14.3442	0.07669	12.55	12.75	13.07	13.64	14.34	15.13	15.92	16.43	16.78
96.5	-1.16157	14.5912	0.07694	12.76	12.97	13.29	13.87	14.59	15.39	16.20	16.73	17.10
97.5	-1.24082	14.8418	0.07721	12.99	13.19	13.52	14.11	14.84	15.66	16.49	17.04	17.42
98.5	-1.32888	15.0963	0.07752	13.21	13.42	13.75	14.35	15.10	15.94	16.79	17.36	17.75
99.5	-1.42581	15.3549	0.07784	13.44	13.65	13.99	14.60	15.35	16.22	17.10	17.69	18.10
100.5	-1.53158	15.6179	0.07818	13.68	13.89	14.23	14.85	15.62	16.50	17.41	18.02	18.45
101.5	-1.64608	15.8854	0.07854	13.92	14.13	14.47	15.10	15.89	16.79	17.73	18.37	18.81
102.5	-1.76908	16.1576	0.07891	14.16	14.38	14.72	15.36	16.16	17.09	18.06	18.72	19.19
103.5	-1.90022	16.4347	0.07928	14.41	14.63	14.98	15.62	16.43	17.39	18.40	19.09	19.58

Table V.3b.

LMS parameters and smoothed percentiles of weight (kg)-for-recumbent length (cm) for girls from birth to 36 months

Length Group (cm)	L	M	S	Percentiles								
				3rd	5th	10th	25th	50th	75th	90th	95th	97th
45.0	0.66684	2.3054	0.16897	1.61	1.70	1.82	2.05	2.31	2.57	2.82	2.97	3.08
45.5	0.69962	2.40326	0.15765	1.72	1.81	1.93	2.15	2.40	2.66	2.90	3.05	3.15
46.5	0.74792	2.60602	0.13939	1.95	2.03	2.15	2.36	2.61	2.85	3.08	3.22	3.31
47.5	0.75175	2.81711	0.12584	2.17	2.25	2.37	2.58	2.82	3.06	3.28	3.41	3.50
48.5	0.69133	3.03536	0.11589	2.40	2.47	2.60	2.80	3.04	3.28	3.50	3.63	3.72
49.5	0.55911	3.25969	0.10865	2.62	2.70	2.82	3.02	3.26	3.50	3.73	3.87	3.96
50.5	0.36155	3.48922	0.1034	2.85	2.93	3.05	3.25	3.49	3.74	3.97	4.12	4.21
51.5	0.11644	3.7232	0.0996	3.08	3.16	3.27	3.48	3.72	3.98	4.23	4.38	4.48
52.5	-0.15251	3.96103	0.09683	3.31	3.38	3.50	3.71	3.96	4.23	4.49	4.65	4.76
53.5	-0.42148	4.20227	0.0948	3.54	3.61	3.73	3.95	4.20	4.48	4.76	4.94	5.06
54.5	-0.67139	4.44648	0.09332	3.77	3.84	3.96	4.18	4.45	4.74	5.04	5.23	5.36
55.5	-0.88997	4.69322	0.09225	3.99	4.07	4.19	4.42	4.69	5.00	5.32	5.52	5.67
56.5	-1.07184	4.94203	0.09147	4.22	4.30	4.43	4.66	4.94	5.27	5.60	5.82	5.98
57.5	-1.21667	5.1924	0.09092	4.45	4.53	4.66	4.89	5.19	5.53	5.89	6.12	6.29
58.5	-1.32736	5.44383	0.09053	4.67	4.75	4.89	5.13	5.44	5.80	6.17	6.43	6.60
59.5	-1.40826	5.69581	0.09025	4.89	4.98	5.12	5.37	5.70	6.07	6.46	6.73	6.92
60.5	-1.46405	5.94789	0.09002	5.11	5.20	5.35	5.61	5.95	6.34	6.75	7.03	7.23
61.5	-1.49911	6.19964	0.08982	5.33	5.43	5.58	5.85	6.20	6.61	7.03	7.33	7.53
62.5	-1.5172	6.4507	0.08962	5.55	5.65	5.80	6.09	6.45	6.87	7.32	7.62	7.84
63.5	-1.52148	6.70074	0.08939	5.77	5.87	6.03	6.33	6.70	7.14	7.60	7.91	8.14
64.5	-1.51448	6.94949	0.08913	5.99	6.09	6.25	6.56	6.95	7.40	7.88	8.20	8.43
65.5	-1.4982	7.19674	0.08882	6.20	6.31	6.48	6.80	7.20	7.66	8.15	8.49	8.72
66.5	-1.47423	7.44231	0.08846	6.41	6.52	6.70	7.03	7.44	7.92	8.43	8.77	9.01
67.5	-1.44381	7.68607	0.08805	6.63	6.74	6.92	7.26	7.69	8.18	8.69	9.04	9.29
68.5	-1.40796	7.92791	0.08758	6.84	6.95	7.14	7.49	7.93	8.43	8.96	9.31	9.56
69.5	-1.36752	8.16778	0.08706	7.05	7.17	7.36	7.72	8.17	8.68	9.22	9.58	9.83
70.5	-1.32324	8.40567	0.0865	7.25	7.38	7.58	7.95	8.41	8.93	9.48	9.84	10.10
71.5	-1.27583	8.64157	0.0859	7.46	7.59	7.80	8.17	8.64	9.18	9.73	10.10	10.36
72.5	-1.22601	8.87552	0.08526	7.67	7.80	8.01	8.40	8.88	9.42	9.98	10.35	10.61
73.5	-1.17456	9.10759	0.08461	7.87	8.01	8.22	8.62	9.11	9.66	10.23	10.60	10.86
74.5	-1.12232	9.33787	0.08393	8.07	8.21	8.44	8.84	9.34	9.90	10.47	10.85	11.11
75.5	-1.0703	9.56645	0.08325	8.28	8.42	8.65	9.06	9.57	10.14	10.71	11.09	11.35
76.5	-1.01962	9.79348	0.08257	8.48	8.62	8.86	9.28	9.79	10.37	10.95	11.34	11.60
77.5	-0.97154	10.0191	0.08191	8.68	8.83	9.07	9.49	10.02	10.60	11.19	11.58	11.84
78.5	-0.9275	10.2435	0.08127	8.88	9.03	9.27	9.71	10.24	10.84	11.43	11.81	12.08
79.5	-0.88905	10.4668	0.08066	9.08	9.23	9.48	9.93	10.47	11.07	11.67	12.05	12.32
80.5	-0.85784	10.6892	0.0801	9.28	9.43	9.69	10.14	10.69	11.30	11.90	12.29	12.56
81.5	-0.8356	10.9109	0.07959	9.48	9.64	9.89	10.35	10.91	11.53	12.14	12.53	12.80
82.5	-0.82401	11.1321	0.07914	9.67	9.84	10.10	10.57	11.13	11.76	12.38	12.78	13.05
83.5	-0.82467	11.3531	0.07876	9.87	33.69	10.30	10.78	11.35	11.99	12.61	13.02	13.30
84.5	-0.83902	11.5741	0.07846	10.07	10.24	10.51	10.99	11.57	12.22	12.86	13.27	13.55
85.5	-0.86819	11.7952	0.07824	10.27	10.44	10.71	11.20	11.80	12.45	13.10	13.52	13.81
86.5	-0.91299	12.0169	0.07811	10.47	10.64	10.92	11.41	12.02	12.68	13.35	13.78	14.07
87.5	-0.97373	12.2393	0.07806	10.67	10.84	11.13	11.63	12.24	12.92	13.60	14.04	14.34
88.5	-1.05024	12.4628	0.0781	10.87	11.05	11.33	11.84	12.46	13.16	13.85	14.31	14.62
89.5	-1.14175	12.6876	0.07823	11.07	11.25	11.54	12.05	12.69	13.40	14.11	14.58	14.91
90.5	-1.24694	12.9141	0.07845	11.28	11.46	11.75	12.27	12.91	13.64	14.38	14.87	15.20
91.5	-1.36388	13.1426	0.07876	11.48	11.66	11.96	12.49	13.14	13.89	14.65	15.16	15.51
92.5	-1.49024	13.3735	0.07914	11.69	11.87	12.17	12.70	13.37	14.14	14.93	15.46	15.82
93.5	-1.6232	13.6072	0.07959	11.90	12.08	12.38	12.92	13.61	14.39	15.21	15.76	16.15
94.5	-1.75975	13.8441	0.08012	12.11	12.30	12.60	13.15	13.84	14.65	15.50	16.08	16.49
95.5	-1.89672	14.0846	0.08072	12.33	12.51	12.82	13.37	14.08	14.92	15.80	16.41	16.85
96.5	-2.03108	14.3293	0.08137	12.54	12.73	13.04	13.60	14.33	15.19	16.11	16.75	17.21
97.5	-2.15999	14.5784	0.08209	12.76	12.95	13.26	13.84	14.58	15.46	16.43	17.10	17.59
98.5	-2.28099	14.8325	0.08287	12.98	13.17	13.49	14.07	14.83	15.75	16.75	17.46	17.98
99.5	-2.39213	15.0919	0.0837	13.20	13.40	13.72	14.31	15.09	16.04	17.08	17.83	18.39
100.5	-2.49199	15.3572	0.08458	13.43	13.63	13.95	14.56	15.36	16.33	17.43	18.22	18.81
101.5	-2.57969	15.6285	0.08551	13.66	13.86	14.19	14.81	15.63	16.64	17.78	18.61	19.24
102.5	-2.65492	15.9064	0.08649	13.89	14.10	14.43	15.07	15.91	16.95	18.14	19.02	19.68
103.5	-2.71778	16.191	0.0875	14.13	14.34	14.68	15.33	16.19	17.27	18.51	19.43	20.14

Table V.4.

LMS parameters and smoothed percentiles of head circumference (cm)-for-age for boys and girls from birth to 36 months

Age Group (months)	L	M	S	3rd	5th	10th	25th	50th	75th	90th	95th	97th
							Boys					
0.0	4.4278	35.8137	0.0522	31.5	32.1	33.1	34.5	35.8	37.0	38.0	38.5	38.9
0.5	4.3109	37.1936	0.0473	33.3	33.8	34.7	35.9	37.2	38.3	39.2	39.8	40.1
1.5	3.8696	39.2074	0.0409	35.8	36.3	37.0	38.1	39.2	40.2	41.1	41.6	41.9
2.5	3.3056	40.6523	0.0370	37.6	38.0	38.6	39.6	40.7	41.6	42.5	43.0	43.3
3.5	2.7206	41.7652	0.0344	38.9	39.3	39.9	40.8	41.8	42.7	43.5	44.0	44.3
4.5	2.1680	42.6612	0.0325	40.0	40.3	40.8	41.7	42.7	43.6	44.4	44.9	45.2
5.5	1.6755	43.4049	0.0311	40.8	41.1	41.7	42.5	43.4	44.3	45.1	45.6	45.9
6.5	1.2552	44.0361	0.0300	41.5	41.8	42.3	43.1	44.0	44.9	45.7	46.2	46.5
7.5	0.9105	44.5810	0.0292	42.1	42.4	42.9	43.7	44.6	45.5	46.3	46.7	47.0
8.5	0.6395	45.0576	0.0287	42.7	43.0	43.4	44.2	45.1	45.9	46.7	47.2	47.5
9.5	0.4370	45.4791	0.0282	43.1	43.4	43.9	44.6	45.5	46.3	47.1	47.6	47.9
10.5	0.2963	45.8551	0.0279	43.5	43.8	44.2	45.0	45.9	46.7	47.5	48.0	48.3
11.5	0.2101	46.1930	0.0277	43.8	44.1	44.6	45.3	46.2	47.1	47.9	48.3	48.7
12.5	0.1711	46.4985	0.0276	44.1	44.4	44.9	45.6	46.5	47.4	48.2	48.6	49.0
13.5	0.1724	46.7764	0.0275	44.4	44.7	45.1	45.9	46.8	47.7	48.5	48.9	49.3
14.5	0.2074	47.0302	0.0275	44.6	44.9	45.4	46.2	47.0	47.9	48.7	49.2	49.5
15.5	0.2702	47.2630	0.0276	44.9	45.2	45.6	46.4	47.3	48.1	49.0	49.4	49.8
16.5	0.3558	47.4772	0.0277	45.0	45.3	45.8	46.6	47.5	48.4	49.2	49.7	50.0
17.5	0.4594	47.6750	0.0278	45.2	45.5	46.0	46.8	47.7	48.6	49.4	49.9	50.2
18.5	0.5772	47.8582	0.0279	45.4	45.7	46.2	47.0	47.9	48.8	49.6	50.1	50.4
19.5	0.7058	48.0282	0.0281	45.5	45.8	46.3	47.1	48.0	48.9	49.8	50.3	50.6
20.5	0.8423	48.1864	0.0283	45.6	46.0	46.4	47.3	48.2	49.1	49.9	50.4	50.8
21.5	0.9843	48.3338	0.0285	45.7	46.1	46.6	47.4	48.3	49.3	50.1	50.6	50.9
22.5	1.1296	48.4714	0.0287	45.8	46.2	46.7	47.5	48.5	49.4	50.3	50.8	51.1
23.5	1.2767	48.6001	0.0290	45.9	46.3	46.8	47.6	48.6	49.5	50.4	50.9	51.2
24.5	1.4241	48.7206	0.0292	46.0	46.4	46.9	47.8	48.7	49.7	50.5	51.0	51.4
25.5	1.5706	48.8337	0.0295	46.1	46.4	47.0	47.9	48.8	49.8	50.7	51.2	51.5
26.5	1.7154	48.9398	0.0298	46.1	46.5	47.0	47.9	48.9	49.9	50.8	51.3	51.6
27.5	1.8577	49.0395	0.0301	46.2	46.6	47.1	48.0	49.0	50.0	50.9	51.4	51.7
28.5	1.9968	49.1332	0.0303	46.2	46.6	47.2	48.1	49.1	50.1	51.0	51.5	51.9
29.5	2.1324	49.2215	0.0306	46.3	46.7	47.2	48.2	49.2	50.2	51.1	51.6	52.0
30.5	2.2641	49.3046	0.0309	46.3	46.7	47.3	48.3	49.3	50.3	51.2	51.7	52.1
31.5	2.3917	49.3829	0.0312	46.4	46.7	47.3	48.3	49.4	50.4	51.3	51.8	52.2
32.5	2.5149	49.4568	0.0316	46.4	46.8	47.4	48.4	49.5	50.5	51.4	51.9	52.3
33.5	2.6337	49.5264	0.0319	46.4	46.8	47.4	48.4	49.5	50.6	51.5	52.0	52.4
34.5	2.7479	49.5922	0.0322	46.4	46.8	47.5	48.5	49.6	50.6	51.6	52.1	52.4
35.5	2.8577	49.6542	0.0325	46.4	46.9	47.5	48.5	49.7	50.7	51.6	52.2	52.5
36.0	2.9109	49.6839	0.0327	46.4	46.9	47.5	48.6	49.7	50.8	51.7	52.2	52.6
							Girls					
0.0	1.2987	34.7116	0.0469	31.9	32.3	32.8	33.7	34.7	35.9	37.0	37.7	38.1
0.5	-1.4403	36.0345	0.0430	33.4	33.7	34.2	35.0	36.0	37.1	38.2	38.8	39.3
1.5	-1.5810	37.9767	0.0381	35.5	35.8	36.2	37.0	38.0	39.0	40.0	40.6	41.0
2.5	-1.5931	39.3801	0.0351	37.0	37.3	37.7	38.5	39.4	40.3	41.3	41.8	42.2
3.5	-1.5215	40.4677	0.0331	38.1	38.4	38.8	39.6	40.5	41.4	42.3	42.8	43.2
4.5	-1.3946	41.3484	0.0317	39.0	39.3	39.7	40.5	41.3	42.3	43.1	43.6	44.0
5.5	-1.2317	42.0834	0.0307	39.8	40.1	40.5	41.2	42.1	43.0	43.8	44.3	44.7
6.5	-1.0466	42.7103	0.0300	40.4	40.7	41.1	41.9	42.7	43.6	44.4	44.9	45.3
7.5	-0.8489	43.2543	0.0294	41.0	41.3	41.7	42.4	43.3	44.1	44.9	45.4	45.8
8.5	-0.6458	43.7325	0.0290	41.4	41.7	42.2	42.9	43.7	44.6	45.4	45.9	46.2
9.5	-0.4422	44.1574	0.0287	41.9	42.1	42.6	43.3	44.2	45.0	45.8	46.3	46.6
10.5	-0.2416	44.5384	0.0285	42.2	42.5	42.9	43.7	44.5	45.4	46.2	46.7	47.0
11.5	-0.0467	44.8824	0.0284	42.6	42.8	43.3	44.0	44.9	45.8	46.5	47.0	47.3
12.5	0.1410	45.1951	0.0283	42.8	43.1	43.6	44.3	45.2	46.1	46.9	47.3	47.7
13.5	0.3204	45.4808	0.0283	43.1	43.4	43.9	44.6	45.5	46.4	47.1	47.6	47.9
14.5	0.4908	45.7431	0.0283	43.3	43.6	44.1	44.9	45.7	46.6	47.4	47.9	48.2
15.5	0.6519	45.9849	0.0283	43.6	43.9	44.3	45.1	46.0	46.9	47.7	48.1	48.5
16.5	0.8037	46.2086	0.0284	43.8	44.1	44.5	45.3	46.2	47.1	47.9	48.4	48.7
17.5	0.9463	46.4162	0.0285	43.9	44.2	44.7	45.5	46.4	47.3	48.1	48.6	48.9
18.5	1.0798	46.6095	0.0286	44.1	44.4	44.9	45.7	46.6	47.5	48.3	48.8	49.1
19.5	1.2046	46.7899	0.0287	44.3	44.6	45.1	45.9	46.8	47.7	48.5	49.0	49.3
20.5	1.3211	46.9586	0.0288	44.4	44.7	45.2	46.0	47.0	47.9	48.7	49.2	49.5
21.5	1.4296	47.1168	0.0290	44.5	44.8	45.4	46.2	47.1	48.0	48.9	49.3	49.7
22.5	1.5306	47.2654	0.0291	44.6	45.0	45.5	46.3	47.3	48.2	49.0	49.5	49.8
23.5	1.6245	47.4052	0.0293	44.7	45.1	45.6	46.5	47.4	48.3	49.2	49.7	50.0
24.5	1.7117	47.5369	0.0295	44.8	45.2	45.7	46.6	47.5	48.5	49.3	49.8	50.1
25.5	1.7926	47.6612	0.0297	44.9	45.3	45.8	46.7	47.7	48.6	49.4	49.9	50.3
26.5	1.8676	47.7787	0.0299	45.0	45.4	45.9	46.8	47.8	48.7	49.6	50.1	50.4
27.5	1.9370	47.8898	0.0301	45.1	45.5	46.0	46.9	47.9	48.9	49.7	50.2	50.5
28.5	2.0014	47.9951	0.0303	45.2	45.5	46.1	47.0	48.0	49.0	49.8	50.3	50.7
29.5	2.0609	48.0949	0.0305	45.2	45.6	46.2	47.1	48.1	49.1	49.9	50.4	50.8
30.5	2.1159	48.1896	0.0307	45.3	45.7	46.3	47.2	48.2	49.2	50.0	50.6	50.9
31.5	2.1667	48.2796	0.0309	45.4	45.7	46.3	47.3	48.3	49.3	50.2	50.7	51.0
32.5	2.2136	48.3651	0.0311	45.4	45.8	46.4	47.3	48.4	49.4	50.3	50.8	51.1
33.5	2.2569	48.4465	0.0314	45.5	45.9	46.4	47.4	48.4	49.5	50.3	50.9	51.2
34.5	2.2968	48.5240	0.0316	45.5	45.9	46.5	47.5	48.5	49.5	50.4	51.0	51.3
35.5	2.3336	48.5978	0.0318	45.6	46.0	46.6	47.5	48.6	49.6	50.5	51.1	51.4
36.0	2.3508	48.6334	0.0319	45.6	46.0	46.6	47.6	48.6	49.7	50.6	51.1	51.4

Table V.5a.

LMS parameters and smoothed percentiles of weight (kg)-for-stature (cm) for boys from 2 to 10 years

Length Group (cm)	L	M	S	3rd	5th	10th	25th	50th	75th	85th	90th	95th	97th
77.0	-0.9993	10.2744	0.0771	8.97	9.12	9.35	9.77	10.27	10.84	11.17	11.40	11.77	12.02
77.5	-0.9799	10.3890	0.0770	9.07	9.22	9.46	9.88	10.39	10.96	11.29	11.53	11.89	12.15
78.5	-0.9436	10.6172	0.0768	9.27	9.42	9.66	10.09	10.62	11.20	11.53	11.77	12.15	12.40
79.5	-0.9108	10.8443	0.0766	9.47	9.63	9.87	10.31	10.84	11.43	11.78	12.02	12.40	12.65
80.5	-0.8820	11.0705	0.0764	9.67	9.83	10.08	10.53	11.07	11.67	12.02	12.26	12.65	12.91
81.5	-0.8576	11.2960	0.0762	9.87	10.03	10.28	10.74	11.30	11.91	12.26	12.51	12.90	13.16
82.5	-0.8378	11.5210	0.0761	10.06	10.23	10.49	10.96	11.52	12.14	12.50	12.75	13.15	13.42
83.5	-0.8229	11.7460	0.0760	10.26	10.43	10.70	11.17	11.75	12.38	12.74	13.00	13.40	13.67
84.5	-0.8134	11.9711	0.0759	10.46	10.63	10.90	11.39	11.97	12.61	12.98	13.25	13.66	13.93
85.5	-0.8095	12.1966	0.0758	10.66	10.83	11.11	11.60	12.20	12.85	13.23	13.50	13.91	14.19
86.5	-0.8115	12.4228	0.0758	10.86	11.03	11.31	11.82	12.42	13.09	13.47	13.75	14.17	14.45
87.5	-0.8198	12.6501	0.0758	11.05	11.23	11.52	12.03	12.65	13.33	13.72	14.00	14.43	14.72
88.5	-0.8346	12.8787	0.0758	11.26	11.44	11.73	12.25	12.88	13.57	13.97	14.25	14.69	14.99
89.5	-0.8563	13.1089	0.0759	11.46	11.64	11.94	12.47	13.11	13.81	14.22	14.51	14.96	15.26
90.5	-0.8851	13.3411	0.0760	11.66	11.85	12.15	12.69	13.34	14.06	14.48	14.77	15.23	15.54
91.5	-0.9214	13.5756	0.0761	11.87	12.06	12.37	12.91	13.58	14.31	14.73	15.04	15.51	15.83
92.5	-0.9655	13.8125	0.0762	12.08	12.27	12.58	13.14	13.81	14.56	15.00	15.31	15.79	16.12
93.5	-1.0176	14.0523	0.0764	12.29	12.48	12.80	13.36	14.05	14.82	15.26	15.58	16.08	16.41
94.5	-1.0779	14.2952	0.0766	12.50	12.70	13.02	13.59	14.30	15.08	15.53	15.86	16.37	16.72
95.5	-1.1468	14.5415	0.0769	12.72	12.92	13.25	13.83	14.54	15.34	15.81	16.14	16.67	17.03
96.5	-1.2243	14.7913	0.0772	12.94	13.15	13.47	14.06	14.79	15.61	16.09	16.44	16.98	17.35
97.5	-1.3106	15.0451	0.0775	13.17	13.37	13.70	14.30	15.05	15.88	16.38	16.73	17.30	17.68
98.5	-1.4057	15.3029	0.0778	13.40	13.60	13.94	14.55	15.30	16.16	16.67	17.04	17.62	18.03
99.5	-1.5097	15.5649	0.0781	13.63	13.84	14.18	14.80	15.56	16.44	16.97	17.35	17.95	18.38
100.5	-1.6225	15.8315	0.0785	13.87	14.08	14.42	15.05	15.83	16.73	17.27	17.67	18.30	18.74
101.5	-1.7438	16.1028	0.0788	14.11	14.33	14.67	15.30	16.10	17.03	17.59	18.00	18.65	19.12
102.5	-1.8734	16.3789	0.0792	14.36	14.58	14.93	15.57	16.38	17.33	17.91	18.33	19.02	19.50
103.5	-2.0106	16.6600	0.0796	14.62	14.83	15.18	15.83	16.66	17.63	18.23	18.67	19.39	19.91
104.5	-2.1550	16.9463	0.0799	14.88	15.09	15.45	16.10	16.95	17.95	18.57	19.03	19.78	20.32
105.5	-2.3055	17.2380	0.0803	15.14	15.36	15.72	16.38	17.24	18.26	18.91	19.39	20.18	20.75
106.5	-2.4610	17.5352	0.0806	15.41	15.63	15.99	16.66	17.54	18.59	19.26	19.76	20.59	21.20
107.5	-2.6203	17.8381	0.0810	15.69	15.91	16.27	16.95	17.84	18.92	19.61	20.13	21.01	21.66
108.5	-2.7818	18.1469	0.0813	15.98	16.20	16.56	17.24	18.15	19.26	19.98	20.52	21.45	22.15
109.5	-2.9436	18.4619	0.0816	16.27	16.49	16.85	17.54	18.46	19.60	20.35	20.92	21.90	22.64
110.5	-3.1039	18.7832	0.0819	16.56	16.78	17.15	17.85	18.78	19.96	20.73	21.33	22.36	23.16
111.5	-3.2605	19.1110	0.0821	16.86	17.09	17.46	18.16	19.11	20.32	21.11	21.74	22.84	23.69
112.5	-3.4113	19.4457	0.0824	17.17	17.40	17.77	18.48	19.45	20.68	21.51	22.17	23.33	24.24
113.5	-3.5543	19.7874	0.0827	17.48	33.69	18.09	18.81	19.79	21.06	21.92	22.60	23.83	24.81
114.5	-3.6876	20.1364	0.0830	17.80	18.03	18.41	19.14	20.14	21.44	22.33	23.05	24.34	25.40
115.5	-3.8096	20.4926	0.0833	18.12	18.35	18.74	19.48	20.49	21.83	22.75	23.50	24.87	26.01
116.5	-3.9190	20.8563	0.0836	18.45	18.68	19.07	19.82	20.86	22.23	23.19	23.97	25.41	26.63
117.5	-4.0149	21.2275	0.0840	18.78	19.02	19.41	20.17	21.23	22.64	23.63	24.44	25.97	27.28
118.5	-4.0967	21.6061	0.0845	19.12	19.36	19.75	20.53	21.61	23.06	24.08	24.93	26.54	27.94
119.5	-4.1642	21.9920	0.0850	19.45	19.70	20.10	20.89	21.99	23.48	24.54	25.43	27.12	28.62
120.5	-4.2174	22.3851	0.0856	19.80	20.04	20.45	21.26	22.39	23.92	25.02	25.94	27.72	29.31
121.5	-4.2568	22.7852	0.0863	20.14	20.39	20.81	21.63	22.79	24.36	25.50	26.46	28.33	30.03

Table V.5b.

LMS parameters and smoothed percentiles of weight (kg)-for-stature (cm) for girls from 2 to 10 years

Length Group (cm)	L	M	S	3rd	5th	10th	25th	50th	75th	85th	90th	95th	97th
77.0	-0.9578	10.0865	0.0817	8.74	8.89	9.13	9.56	10.09	10.67	11.02	11.26	11.65	11.91
77.5	-0.9359	10.1987	0.0814	8.84	8.99	9.23	9.67	10.20	10.79	11.14	11.38	11.77	12.03
78.5	-0.8962	10.4222	0.0808	9.04	9.19	9.44	9.88	10.42	11.02	11.37	11.62	12.01	12.27
79.5	-0.8634	10.6447	0.0802	9.24	9.39	9.65	10.10	10.64	11.25	11.60	11.85	12.25	12.51
80.5	-0.8393	10.8666	0.0797	9.44	9.60	9.85	10.31	10.87	11.48	11.84	12.09	12.49	12.75
81.5	-0.8254	11.0879	0.0792	9.63	9.80	10.06	10.52	11.09	11.71	12.07	12.33	12.73	13.00
82.5	-0.8235	11.3089	0.0788	9.83	10.00	10.26	10.74	11.31	11.94	12.31	12.57	12.97	13.25
83.5	-0.8350	11.5299	0.0785	10.03	10.20	10.47	10.95	11.53	12.17	12.54	12.81	13.22	13.50
84.5	-0.8611	11.7510	0.0783	10.23	10.40	10.67	11.16	11.75	12.40	12.78	13.05	13.47	13.75
85.5	-0.9028	11.9725	0.0781	10.43	10.60	10.88	11.37	11.97	12.64	13.02	13.30	13.72	14.02
86.5	-0.9603	12.1948	0.0781	10.63	10.80	11.08	11.58	12.19	12.87	13.27	13.55	13.99	14.29
87.5	-1.0337	12.4180	0.0781	10.83	11.01	11.29	11.80	12.42	13.11	13.51	13.80	14.25	14.56
88.5	-1.1223	12.6425	0.0782	11.03	11.21	11.50	12.01	12.64	13.35	13.76	14.06	14.53	14.85
89.5	-1.2249	12.8687	0.0784	11.24	11.42	11.71	12.23	12.87	13.59	14.02	14.33	14.81	15.14
90.5	-1.3397	13.0968	0.0787	11.44	11.62	11.91	12.44	13.10	13.84	14.28	14.60	15.10	15.45
91.5	-1.4643	13.3272	0.0791	11.65	11.83	12.13	12.66	13.33	14.09	14.54	14.87	15.40	15.76
92.5	-1.5962	13.5603	0.0795	11.86	12.04	12.34	12.88	13.56	14.34	14.81	15.15	15.70	16.09
93.5	-1.7323	13.7965	0.0800	12.07	12.25	12.55	13.10	13.80	14.60	15.09	15.45	16.02	16.42
94.5	-1.8694	14.0362	0.0806	12.28	12.47	12.77	13.33	14.04	14.86	15.37	15.74	16.35	16.77
95.5	-2.0046	14.2800	0.0812	12.50	12.69	12.99	13.56	14.28	15.13	15.66	16.05	16.68	17.14
96.5	-2.1348	14.5282	0.0819	12.72	12.91	13.21	13.79	14.53	15.41	15.96	16.36	17.03	17.51
97.5	-2.2575	14.7812	0.0827	12.94	13.13	13.44	14.02	14.78	15.69	16.26	16.68	17.39	17.90
98.5	-2.3708	15.0396	0.0835	13.16	13.35	13.67	14.26	15.04	15.98	16.57	17.02	17.76	18.31
99.5	-2.4730	15.3036	0.0844	13.39	13.58	13.90	14.51	15.30	16.27	16.89	17.36	18.14	18.72
100.5	-2.5631	15.5738	0.0853	13.62	13.81	14.14	14.76	15.57	16.57	17.22	17.71	18.53	19.15
101.5	-2.6409	15.8503	0.0863	13.85	14.05	14.38	15.01	15.85	16.88	17.55	18.06	18.94	19.59
102.5	-2.7062	16.1336	0.0873	14.08	14.29	14.63	15.28	16.13	17.20	17.90	18.43	19.35	20.05
103.5	-2.7595	16.4238	0.0883	14.32	14.53	14.88	15.54	16.42	17.53	18.25	18.81	19.77	20.51
104.5	-2.8016	16.7212	0.0894	14.57	14.78	15.14	15.82	16.72	17.86	18.61	19.20	20.21	20.99
105.5	-2.8334	17.0260	0.0905	14.82	15.04	15.40	16.09	17.03	18.21	18.99	19.60	20.66	21.48
106.5	-2.8560	17.3384	0.0915	15.07	15.30	15.67	16.38	17.34	18.56	19.37	20.00	21.11	21.97
107.5	-2.8706	17.6584	0.0926	15.33	15.56	15.94	16.67	17.66	18.92	19.76	20.42	21.57	22.48
108.5	-2.8783	17.9862	0.0936	15.60	15.83	16.22	16.97	17.99	19.28	20.15	20.84	22.04	22.99
109.5	-2.8804	18.3218	0.0946	15.87	16.11	16.51	17.28	18.32	19.66	20.56	21.27	22.52	23.51
110.5	-2.8779	18.6652	0.0955	16.15	16.40	16.81	17.59	18.67	20.04	20.97	21.71	23.01	24.04
111.5	-2.8717	19.0165	0.0964	16.43	16.69	17.11	17.92	19.02	20.44	21.39	22.15	23.50	24.56
112.5	-2.8628	19.3755	0.0971	16.73	16.99	17.42	18.25	19.38	20.83	21.82	22.60	23.99	25.09
113.5	-2.8519	19.7423	0.0978	17.03	17.29	17.74	18.58	19.74	21.24	22.25	23.05	24.48	25.62
114.5	-2.8398	20.1167	0.0983	17.34	17.61	18.06	18.93	20.12	21.65	22.69	23.51	24.98	26.14
115.5	-2.8268	20.4986	0.0986	17.66	33.69	18.40	19.29	20.50	22.07	23.13	23.97	25.47	26.66
116.5	-2.8135	20.8879	0.0988	17.99	18.27	18.74	19.65	20.89	22.49	23.57	24.43	25.96	27.17
117.5	-2.7999	21.2844	0.0988	18.33	18.62	19.10	20.02	21.28	22.91	24.01	24.89	26.44	27.67
118.5	-2.7861	21.6878	0.0986	18.68	18.97	19.46	20.40	21.69	23.34	24.46	25.34	26.91	28.16
119.5	-2.7718	22.0980	0.0982	19.04	19.34	19.84	20.79	22.10	23.78	24.90	25.80	27.38	28.62
120.5	-2.7564	22.5147	0.0975	19.41	19.71	20.22	21.19	22.51	24.21	25.35	26.24	27.83	29.07
121.5	-2.7385	22.9377	0.0966	19.79	20.10	20.62	21.60	22.94	24.64	25.79	26.68	28.26	29.49

Table V.6a.

LMS parameters and smoothed percentiles of weight (kg)-for-age in months for boys from 2 to 20 years

Age Group (months)	L	M	S	Percentiles								
				3rd	5th	10th	25th	50th	75th	90th	95th	97th
24.0	-0.2062	12.6708	0.1081	10.38	10.64	11.05	11.79	12.67	13.64	14.58	15.19	15.60
24.5	-0.2165	12.7415	0.1082	10.44	10.70	11.11	11.85	12.74	13.71	14.67	15.28	15.69
25.5	-0.2398	12.8810	0.1083	10.56	10.82	11.24	11.98	12.88	13.87	14.83	15.45	15.87
26.5	-0.2663	13.0184	0.1084	10.67	10.94	11.36	12.11	13.02	14.02	15.00	15.63	16.06
27.5	-0.2958	13.1545	0.1086	10.79	11.05	11.48	12.23	13.15	14.17	15.16	15.80	16.24
28.5	-0.3277	13.2899	0.1088	10.90	11.17	11.60	12.36	13.29	14.31	15.33	15.98	16.43
29.5	-0.3618	13.4252	0.1091	11.01	11.28	11.71	12.48	13.43	14.46	15.50	16.16	16.62
30.5	-0.3976	13.5609	0.1094	11.13	11.40	11.83	12.61	13.56	14.62	15.66	16.34	16.81
31.5	-0.4345	13.6974	0.1097	11.24	11.51	11.95	12.74	13.70	14.77	15.84	16.53	17.00
32.5	-0.4722	13.8350	0.1101	11.36	11.63	12.07	12.86	13.84	14.92	16.01	16.72	17.20
33.5	-0.5101	13.9742	0.1105	11.47	11.75	12.19	12.99	13.97	15.08	16.19	16.91	17.41
34.5	-0.5479	14.1150	0.1109	11.59	11.86	12.31	13.12	14.12	15.24	16.37	17.11	17.61
35.5	-0.5851	14.2578	0.1114	11.70	11.98	12.43	13.25	14.26	15.40	16.55	17.31	17.83
36.5	-0.6213	14.4026	0.1119	11.82	12.10	12.55	13.38	14.40	15.56	16.74	17.51	18.05
37.5	-0.6563	14.5496	0.1124	11.94	12.22	12.68	13.51	14.55	15.73	16.93	17.72	18.27
38.5	-0.6897	14.6989	0.1130	12.06	12.34	12.80	13.65	14.70	15.90	17.12	17.93	18.50
39.5	-0.7214	14.8505	0.1136	12.18	12.46	12.93	13.78	14.85	16.07	17.32	18.15	18.73
40.5	-0.7512	15.0045	0.1142	12.30	12.59	13.06	13.92	15.00	16.24	17.52	18.37	18.96
41.5	-0.7789	15.1608	0.1148	12.42	12.71	13.19	14.06	15.16	16.42	17.73	18.60	19.20
42.5	-0.8045	15.3194	0.1155	12.54	12.84	13.32	14.20	15.32	16.60	17.93	18.83	19.45
43.5	-0.8280	15.4803	0.1162	12.66	12.96	13.45	14.35	15.48	16.79	18.15	19.06	19.70
44.5	-0.8494	15.6434	0.1169	12.79	13.09	13.59	14.49	15.64	16.97	18.36	19.30	19.95
45.5	-0.8687	15.8087	0.1176	12.91	13.22	13.72	14.64	15.81	17.16	18.58	19.54	20.21
46.5	-0.8860	15.9761	0.1184	13.04	13.35	13.86	14.79	15.98	17.36	18.80	19.78	20.47
47.5	-0.9015	16.1455	0.1192	13.16	13.48	13.99	14.94	16.15	17.55	19.03	20.03	20.74
48.5	-0.9152	16.3168	0.1200	13.29	13.61	14.13	15.09	16.32	17.75	19.26	20.28	21.01
49.5	-0.9274	16.4899	0.1208	13.42	13.74	14.27	15.24	16.49	17.95	19.49	20.54	21.28
50.5	-0.9381	16.6647	0.1216	13.55	13.87	14.41	15.40	16.66	18.15	19.72	20.80	21.56
51.5	-0.9475	16.8411	0.1224	13.68	14.01	14.55	15.55	16.84	18.35	19.96	21.06	21.83
52.5	-0.9558	17.0190	0.1232	13.80	14.14	14.69	15.71	17.02	18.56	20.20	21.32	22.12
53.5	-0.9631	17.1984	0.1240	13.93	14.28	14.83	15.87	17.20	18.77	20.44	21.58	22.40
54.5	-0.9696	17.3791	0.1249	14.06	14.41	14.98	16.03	17.38	18.98	20.68	21.85	22.69
55.5	-0.9755	17.5610	0.1257	14.20	14.55	15.12	16.19	17.56	19.19	20.93	22.12	22.98
56.5	-0.9809	17.7440	0.1266	14.33	14.68	15.26	16.35	17.74	19.40	21.17	22.40	23.27
57.5	-0.9860	17.9281	0.1274	14.46	14.82	15.41	16.51	17.93	19.61	21.42	22.67	23.56
58.5	-0.9909	18.1132	0.1282	14.59	14.96	15.56	16.67	18.11	19.83	21.67	22.95	23.86
59.5	-0.9956	18.2991	0.1291	14.72	15.09	15.70	16.83	18.30	20.04	21.92	23.23	24.16
60.5	-1.0005	18.4859	0.1299	14.86	15.23	15.85	17.00	18.49	20.26	22.18	23.51	24.46
61.5	-1.0054	18.6735	0.1307	14.99	15.37	16.00	17.16	18.67	20.48	22.43	23.79	24.77
62.5	-1.0106	18.8618	0.1315	15.13	15.51	16.14	17.33	18.86	20.70	22.69	24.08	25.07
63.5	-1.0161	19.0508	0.1323	15.26	15.65	16.29	17.49	19.05	20.92	22.95	24.36	25.38
64.5	-1.0219	19.2404	0.1331	15.40	33.69	16.44	17.66	19.24	21.14	23.21	24.65	25.69
65.5	-1.0282	19.4306	0.1339	15.53	15.93	16.59	17.82	19.43	21.36	23.47	24.94	26.01
66.5	-1.0350	19.6214	0.1347	15.67	16.07	16.74	17.99	19.62	21.59	23.73	25.24	26.32
67.5	-1.0424	19.8127	0.1354	15.81	16.22	16.89	18.16	19.81	21.81	23.99	25.53	26.64
68.5	-1.0503	20.0046	0.1362	15.94	16.36	17.04	18.32	20.00	22.03	24.26	25.83	26.96
69.5	-1.0587	20.1970	0.1370	16.08	16.50	17.19	18.49	20.20	22.26	24.53	26.12	27.28
70.5	-1.0677	20.3900	0.1377	16.22	16.65	17.35	18.66	20.39	22.49	24.79	26.43	27.61
71.5	-1.0773	20.5836	0.1384	16.36	16.79	17.50	18.83	20.58	22.71	25.06	26.73	27.94
72.5	-1.0875	20.7777	0.1391	16.50	16.94	17.65	19.00	20.78	22.94	25.33	27.03	28.27
73.5	-1.0982	20.9724	0.1399	16.65	17.08	17.81	19.17	20.97	23.17	25.61	27.34	28.61
74.5	-1.1093	21.1678	0.1406	16.79	17.23	17.96	19.34	21.17	23.40	25.88	27.65	28.94
75.5	-1.1210	21.3638	0.1413	16.93	17.38	18.12	19.51	21.36	23.63	26.15	27.96	29.29
76.5	-1.1330	21.5606	0.1419	17.08	17.53	18.27	19.69	21.56	23.86	26.43	28.28	29.63
77.5	-1.1454	21.7581	0.1426	17.22	17.68	18.43	19.86	21.76	24.09	26.71	28.59	29.98
78.5	-1.1581	21.9564	0.1433	17.37	17.83	18.59	20.03	21.96	24.33	26.99	28.91	30.33
79.5	-1.1711	22.1557	0.1440	17.51	17.98	18.75	20.21	22.16	24.56	27.28	29.24	30.69
80.5	-1.1841	22.3558	0.1447	17.66	18.13	18.91	20.38	22.36	24.80	27.56	29.56	31.05
81.5	-1.1973	22.5570	0.1453	17.81	18.28	19.07	20.56	22.56	25.04	27.85	29.89	31.41
82.5	-1.2105	22.7593	0.1460	17.96	18.43	19.23	20.74	22.76	25.28	28.14	30.23	31.78
83.5	-1.2236	22.9627	0.1467	18.11	18.59	19.39	20.92	22.96	25.52	28.43	30.56	32.15
84.5	-1.2365	23.1674	0.1473	18.26	18.74	19.55	21.09	23.17	25.76	28.73	30.90	32.53
85.5	-1.2492	23.3734	0.1480	18.41	18.90	19.71	21.27	23.37	26.00	29.02	31.24	32.91
86.5	-1.2616	23.5809	0.1487	18.56	19.05	19.88	21.46	23.58	26.25	29.32	31.59	33.29
87.5	-1.2735	23.7898	0.1494	18.71	19.21	20.04	21.64	23.79	26.50	29.63	31.94	33.68
88.5	-1.2850	24.0003	0.1501	18.86	19.37	20.21	21.82	24.00	26.75	29.93	32.30	34.08
89.5	-1.2960	24.2125	0.1508	19.02	19.53	20.38	22.01	24.21	27.00	30.24	32.66	34.48
90.5	-1.3063	24.4265	0.1515	19.17	19.69	20.55	22.19	24.43	27.26	30.56	33.02	34.88
91.5	-1.3159	24.6423	0.1522	19.33	19.85	20.71	22.38	24.64	27.52	30.87	33.39	35.29
92.5	-1.3248	24.8601	0.1529	19.48	20.01	20.89	22.57	24.86	27.78	31.19	33.76	35.71
93.5	-1.3329	25.0799	0.1537	19.64	20.17	21.06	22.76	25.08	28.04	31.52	34.13	36.13
94.5	-1.3401	25.3019	0.1544	19.80	20.33	21.23	22.95	25.30	28.31	31.84	34.51	36.55
95.5	-1.3464	25.5261	0.1552	19.96	20.50	21.40	23.14	25.53	28.57	32.17	34.90	36.98

Table V.6b.
LMS parameters and smoothed percentiles of weight (kg)-for-age in months for boys from 2 to 20 years

Age Group (months)	L	M	S	Percentiles								
				3rd	5th	10th	25th	50th	75th	90th	95th	97th
96.5	-1.3518	25.7526	0.1560	20.11	20.66	21.58	23.34	25.75	28.85	32.51	35.29	37.42
97.5	-1.3563	25.9815	0.1568	20.27	20.83	21.75	23.54	25.98	29.12	32.85	35.68	37.86
98.5	-1.3597	26.2128	0.1576	20.43	20.99	21.93	23.74	26.21	29.40	33.19	36.08	38.31
99.5	-1.3622	26.4468	0.1584	20.59	21.16	22.11	23.94	26.45	29.68	33.54	36.49	38.76
100.5	-1.3636	26.6834	0.1593	20.76	21.33	22.29	24.14	26.68	29.97	33.89	36.90	39.22
101.5	-1.3640	26.9227	0.1601	20.92	21.50	22.47	24.34	26.92	30.26	34.25	37.31	39.68
102.5	-1.3635	27.1649	0.1610	21.08	21.67	22.65	24.55	27.16	30.55	34.61	37.73	40.15
103.5	-1.3619	27.4099	0.1619	21.25	21.84	22.83	24.76	27.41	30.85	34.98	38.16	40.62
104.5	-1.3593	27.6580	0.1628	21.41	22.01	23.02	24.97	27.66	31.15	35.35	38.59	41.10
105.5	-1.3557	27.9090	0.1638	21.58	22.18	23.20	25.18	27.91	31.46	35.73	39.02	41.58
106.5	-1.3512	28.1632	0.1647	21.74	22.36	23.39	25.39	28.16	31.77	36.11	39.46	42.07
107.5	-1.3458	28.4206	0.1657	21.91	22.53	23.58	25.61	28.42	32.08	36.49	39.91	42.57
108.5	-1.3394	28.6813	0.1667	22.08	22.71	23.77	25.83	28.68	32.40	36.89	40.36	43.07
109.5	-1.3322	28.9453	0.1676	22.25	22.89	23.96	26.05	28.95	32.72	37.28	40.82	43.57
110.5	-1.3241	29.2127	0.1686	22.42	23.07	24.16	26.28	29.21	33.05	37.68	41.28	44.08
111.5	-1.3153	29.4836	0.1697	22.59	23.25	24.35	26.50	29.48	33.38	38.09	41.74	44.59
112.5	-1.3057	29.7580	0.1707	22.76	23.43	24.55	26.73	29.76	33.71	38.50	42.22	45.11
113.5	-1.2954	30.0360	0.1717	22.93	23.61	24.75	26.96	30.04	34.05	38.92	42.69	45.63
114.5	-1.2844	30.3177	0.1727	23.11	23.80	24.95	27.20	30.32	34.40	39.34	43.17	46.16
115.5	-1.2728	30.6031	0.1738	23.29	23.98	25.15	27.44	30.60	34.74	39.76	43.66	46.69
116.5	-1.2605	30.8923	0.1748	23.46	24.17	25.36	27.68	30.89	35.10	40.19	44.15	47.23
117.5	-1.2478	31.1853	0.1758	23.64	24.36	25.57	27.92	31.19	35.46	40.63	44.64	47.77
118.5	-1.2345	31.4823	0.1769	23.82	24.55	25.78	28.17	31.48	35.82	41.07	45.14	48.32
119.5	-1.2208	31.7831	0.1779	24.01	24.75	25.99	28.42	31.78	36.19	41.52	45.65	48.86
120.5	-1.2067	32.0880	0.1789	24.19	24.94	26.21	28.67	32.09	36.56	41.97	46.16	49.42
121.5	-1.1922	32.3969	0.1799	24.38	25.14	26.43	28.93	32.40	36.94	42.42	46.67	49.97
122.5	-1.1774	32.7099	0.1810	24.57	25.34	26.65	29.18	32.71	37.32	42.88	47.19	50.53
123.5	-1.1622	33.0270	0.1820	24.76	25.55	26.87	29.45	33.03	37.70	43.35	47.71	51.09
124.5	-1.1469	33.3484	0.1829	24.95	25.75	27.10	29.71	33.35	38.09	43.82	48.23	51.66
125.5	-1.1313	33.6739	0.1839	25.15	25.96	27.32	29.98	33.67	38.49	44.29	48.76	52.22
126.5	-1.1155	34.0036	0.1848	25.35	26.17	27.56	30.26	34.00	38.89	44.77	49.30	52.79
127.5	-1.0997	34.3377	0.1858	25.55	26.39	27.79	30.53	34.34	39.29	45.25	49.83	53.37
128.5	-1.0837	34.6760	0.1867	25.75	26.60	28.03	30.82	34.68	39.70	45.74	50.37	53.94
129.5	-1.0676	35.0186	0.1876	25.96	26.82	28.27	31.10	35.02	40.12	46.23	50.91	54.52
130.5	-1.0515	35.3656	0.1884	26.17	27.04	28.52	31.39	35.37	40.53	46.73	51.46	55.10
131.5	-1.0354	35.7169	0.1892	26.38	27.27	28.77	31.68	35.72	40.96	47.22	52.01	55.68
132.5	-1.0193	36.0726	0.1900	26.60	27.50	29.02	31.98	36.07	41.38	47.73	52.56	56.26
133.5	-1.0032	36.4327	0.1908	26.82	27.73	29.28	32.28	36.43	41.81	48.23	53.11	56.84
134.5	-0.9873	36.7970	0.1915	27.04	27.97	29.54	32.58	36.80	42.25	48.74	53.66	57.43
135.5	-0.9714	37.1658	0.1922	27.26	28.21	29.80	32.89	37.17	42.69	49.25	54.22	58.02
136.5	-0.9557	37.5388	0.1929	27.49	28.45	30.07	33.21	37.54	43.13	49.77	54.78	58.60
137.5	-0.9401	37.9162	0.1935	27.73	28.70	30.34	33.52	37.92	43.58	50.28	55.34	59.19
138.5	-0.9247	38.2978	0.1941	27.96	28.95	30.62	33.85	38.30	44.03	50.80	55.90	59.78
139.5	-0.9095	38.6836	0.1946	28.21	29.21	30.90	34.17	38.68	44.49	51.33	56.47	60.37
140.5	-0.8944	39.0736	0.1951	28.45	29.47	31.18	34.50	39.07	44.94	51.85	57.03	60.96
141.5	-0.8797	39.4678	0.1955	28.70	29.73	31.47	34.84	39.47	45.41	52.38	57.60	61.54
142.5	-0.8652	39.8660	0.1959	28.95	30.00	31.76	35.18	39.87	45.87	52.91	58.17	62.13
143.5	-0.8509	40.2683	0.1963	29.21	30.27	32.06	35.52	40.27	46.34	53.44	58.74	62.72
144.5	-0.8370	40.6744	0.1966	29.47	30.55	32.36	35.87	40.67	46.81	53.98	59.30	63.31
145.5	-0.8233	41.0844	0.1969	29.74	30.83	32.67	36.22	41.08	47.29	54.51	59.87	63.90
146.5	-0.8100	41.4982	0.1971	30.01	31.12	32.98	36.58	41.50	47.76	55.05	60.44	64.48
147.5	-0.7970	41.9155	0.1972	30.29	31.41	33.29	36.94	41.92	48.24	55.59	61.01	65.07
148.5	-0.7844	42.3364	0.1974	30.57	31.70	33.61	37.30	42.34	48.73	56.12	61.58	65.65
149.5	-0.7721	42.7607	0.1974	30.85	32.00	33.94	37.67	42.76	49.21	56.66	62.15	66.24
150.5	-0.7603	43.1883	0.1975	31.14	32.31	34.26	38.04	43.19	49.70	57.20	62.72	66.82
151.5	-0.7488	43.6190	0.1974	31.43	32.62	34.60	38.42	43.62	50.19	57.74	63.28	67.40
152.5	-0.7378	44.0526	0.1974	31.73	32.93	34.93	38.80	44.05	50.68	58.29	63.85	67.98
153.5	-0.7272	44.4890	0.1973	32.03	33.25	35.27	39.18	44.49	51.17	58.83	64.41	68.56
154.5	-0.7170	44.9281	0.1971	32.34	33.57	35.62	39.57	44.93	51.67	59.37	64.98	69.13
155.5	-0.7074	45.3696	0.1969	32.65	33.89	35.97	39.96	45.37	52.16	59.91	65.54	69.71
156.5	-0.6982	45.8134	0.1967	32.97	34.22	36.32	40.36	45.81	52.66	60.45	66.10	70.28
157.5	-0.6895	46.2592	0.1964	33.29	34.56	36.68	40.75	46.26	53.15	60.99	66.66	70.85
158.5	-0.6813	46.7068	0.1960	33.61	34.90	37.04	41.15	46.71	53.65	61.53	67.22	71.42
159.5	-0.6737	47.1561	0.1957	33.94	35.24	37.40	41.56	47.16	54.15	62.06	67.78	71.98
160.5	-0.6666	47.6067	0.1953	34.28	35.59	37.77	41.96	47.61	54.64	62.60	68.33	72.54
161.5	-0.6601	48.0585	0.1948	34.61	35.94	38.14	42.37	48.06	55.14	63.13	68.89	73.11
162.5	-0.6541	48.5111	0.1943	34.95	36.29	38.52	42.78	48.51	55.64	63.67	69.44	73.66
163.5	-0.6488	48.9644	0.1938	35.30	36.65	38.89	43.19	48.96	56.13	64.20	69.99	74.22
164.5	-0.6441	49.4181	0.1933	35.65	37.01	39.27	43.60	49.42	56.63	64.73	70.53	74.78
165.5	-0.6401	49.8719	0.1927	36.00	37.37	39.65	44.02	49.87	57.12	65.25	71.07	75.33
166.5	-0.6367	50.3255	0.1921	36.35	37.74	40.04	44.43	50.33	57.61	65.78	71.61	75.87
167.5	-0.6339	50.7786	0.1915	36.71	38.10	40.42	44.85	50.78	58.10	66.30	72.15	76.42
168.5	-0.6319	51.2310	0.1908	37.07	38.48	40.81	45.27	51.23	58.59	66.82	72.69	76.96
169.5	-0.6305	51.6823	0.1901	37.44	38.85	41.20	45.69	51.68	59.08	67.33	73.22	77.50

Table V.6c.
LMS parameters and smoothed percentiles of weight (kg)-for-age in months for boys from 2 to 20 years

Age Group (months)	L	M	S	Percentiles								
				3rd	5th	10th	25th	50th	75th	90th	95th	97th
170.5	-0.6299	52.1323	0.1894	37.80	39.22	41.59	46.10	52.13	59.56	67.85	73.75	78.04
171.5	-0.6300	52.5806	0.1887	38.17	39.60	41.98	46.52	52.58	60.04	68.36	74.27	78.58
172.5	-0.6309	53.0270	0.1880	38.54	39.98	42.37	46.94	53.03	60.52	68.86	74.79	79.11
173.5	-0.6325	53.4711	0.1872	38.91	40.36	42.77	47.35	53.47	60.99	69.36	75.31	79.64
174.5	-0.6349	53.9126	0.1864	39.28	40.74	43.16	47.77	53.91	61.46	69.86	75.83	80.16
175.5	-0.6381	54.3513	0.1857	39.66	41.12	43.55	48.18	54.35	61.93	70.35	76.34	80.68
176.5	-0.6420	54.7868	0.1849	40.03	41.50	43.94	48.59	54.79	62.39	70.84	76.84	81.20
177.5	-0.6468	55.2188	0.1841	40.40	41.88	44.33	49.00	55.22	62.85	71.33	77.35	81.72
178.5	-0.6523	55.6470	0.1833	40.78	42.26	44.72	49.41	55.65	63.30	71.81	77.84	82.23
179.5	-0.6586	56.0712	0.1825	41.15	42.64	45.11	49.81	56.07	63.75	72.28	78.34	82.74
180.5	-0.6656	56.4910	0.1817	41.52	43.02	45.50	50.21	56.49	64.19	72.75	78.83	83.24
181.5	-0.6734	56.9061	0.1809	41.89	43.39	45.88	50.61	56.91	64.63	73.22	79.31	83.74
182.5	-0.6820	57.3163	0.1801	42.26	43.76	46.26	51.00	57.32	65.06	73.67	79.79	84.24
183.5	-0.6913	57.7214	0.1793	42.63	44.14	46.64	51.39	57.72	65.49	74.13	80.27	84.73
184.5	-0.7013	58.1210	0.1785	43.00	44.51	47.01	51.78	58.12	65.91	74.57	80.74	85.22
185.5	-0.7119	58.5149	0.1777	43.36	44.87	47.38	52.16	58.51	66.32	75.02	81.20	85.70
186.5	-0.7232	58.9029	0.1769	43.72	45.23	47.75	52.53	58.90	66.73	75.45	81.66	86.18
187.5	-0.7351	59.2848	0.1761	44.08	45.59	48.11	52.90	59.28	67.13	75.88	82.11	86.66
188.5	-0.7476	59.6603	0.1754	44.43	45.95	48.47	53.27	59.66	67.53	76.30	82.56	87.13
189.5	-0.7606	60.0293	0.1746	44.78	46.30	48.82	53.63	60.03	67.91	76.72	83.00	87.59
190.5	-0.7740	60.3916	0.1739	45.12	46.64	49.17	53.98	60.39	68.29	77.13	83.44	88.05
191.5	-0.7878	60.7470	0.1732	45.46	46.98	49.51	54.33	60.75	68.66	77.53	83.87	88.50
192.5	-0.8020	61.0954	0.1725	45.79	47.32	49.85	54.67	61.10	69.03	77.92	84.29	88.95
193.5	-0.8164	61.4366	0.1718	46.12	47.64	50.18	55.00	61.44	69.39	78.31	84.71	89.40
194.5	-0.8311	61.7706	0.1711	46.44	47.97	50.50	55.32	61.77	69.74	78.69	85.12	89.83
195.5	-0.8459	62.0972	0.1705	46.76	48.28	50.82	55.64	62.10	70.08	79.06	85.52	90.26
196.5	-0.8608	62.4164	0.1698	47.07	48.59	51.13	55.96	62.42	70.42	79.43	85.92	90.68
197.5	-0.8757	62.7281	0.1692	47.37	48.90	51.43	56.26	62.73	70.74	79.79	86.30	91.10
198.5	-0.8904	63.0323	0.1687	47.67	49.19	51.73	56.56	63.03	71.06	80.13	86.68	91.51
199.5	-0.9051	63.3289	0.1681	47.96	49.48	52.02	56.85	63.33	71.38	80.48	87.06	91.91
200.5	-0.9195	63.6180	0.1676	48.24	49.76	52.30	57.13	63.62	71.68	80.81	87.42	92.30
201.5	-0.9335	63.8996	0.1670	48.51	50.04	52.57	57.41	63.90	71.98	81.14	87.78	92.68
202.5	-0.9473	64.1737	0.1666	48.78	50.30	52.84	57.68	64.17	72.27	81.46	88.13	93.06
203.5	-0.9605	64.4403	0.1661	49.04	50.56	53.09	57.94	64.44	72.55	81.77	88.46	93.42
204.5	-0.9732	64.6996	0.1656	49.29	50.81	53.35	58.19	64.70	72.82	82.07	88.80	93.78
205.5	-0.9854	64.9516	0.1652	49.53	51.05	53.59	58.43	64.95	73.09	82.36	89.12	94.13
206.5	-0.9969	65.1965	0.1648	49.76	51.29	53.82	58.67	65.20	73.35	82.65	89.43	94.46
207.5	-1.0077	65.4344	0.1644	49.99	51.51	54.05	58.90	65.43	73.60	82.93	89.73	94.79
208.5	-1.0178	65.6654	0.1641	50.21	51.73	54.27	59.13	65.67	73.85	83.20	90.03	95.11
209.5	-1.0270	65.8897	0.1638	50.42	51.94	54.49	59.34	65.89	74.09	83.46	90.31	95.41
210.5	-1.0354	66.1075	0.1634	50.62	52.15	54.69	59.55	66.11	74.32	83.71	90.59	95.71
211.5	-1.0429	66.3190	0.1631	50.82	52.35	54.89	59.76	66.32	74.54	83.96	90.86	95.99
212.5	-1.0495	66.5244	0.1629	51.01	52.54	55.08	59.96	66.52	74.76	84.20	91.11	96.27
213.5	-1.0552	66.7239	0.1626	51.19	52.72	55.27	60.15	66.72	74.97	84.43	91.36	96.53
214.5	-1.0598	66.9178	0.1624	51.36	52.89	55.45	60.33	66.92	75.18	84.65	91.60	96.78
215.5	-1.0635	67.1064	0.1621	51.53	53.06	55.62	60.51	67.11	75.38	84.87	91.83	97.02
216.5	-1.0662	67.2899	0.1619	51.69	53.23	55.79	60.69	67.29	75.58	85.08	92.05	97.25
217.5	-1.0679	67.4686	0.1617	51.85	53.38	55.95	60.85	67.47	75.76	85.28	92.26	97.46
218.5	-1.0686	67.6428	0.1615	51.99	53.54	56.11	61.02	67.64	75.95	85.47	92.46	97.67
219.5	-1.0683	67.8128	0.1614	52.14	53.68	56.26	61.18	67.81	76.13	85.66	92.65	97.86
220.5	-1.0669	67.9788	0.1612	52.28	53.82	56.40	61.33	67.98	76.31	85.84	92.84	98.04
221.5	-1.0646	68.1411	0.1610	52.41	53.96	56.54	61.49	68.14	76.48	86.02	93.01	98.22
222.5	-1.0613	68.3000	0.1609	52.54	54.09	56.68	61.63	68.30	76.65	86.19	93.18	98.38
223.5	-1.0571	68.4558	0.1607	52.66	54.22	56.82	61.78	68.46	76.81	86.36	93.34	98.53
224.5	-1.0520	68.6087	0.1606	52.78	54.34	56.95	61.92	68.61	76.97	86.52	93.49	98.68
225.5	-1.0460	68.7589	0.1605	52.90	54.46	57.07	62.06	68.76	77.13	86.67	93.64	98.82
226.5	-1.0392	68.9065	0.1603	53.01	54.58	57.20	62.19	68.91	77.28	86.83	93.78	98.94
227.5	-1.0316	69.0518	0.1602	53.11	54.69	57.32	62.33	69.05	77.44	86.97	93.92	99.07
228.5	-1.0233	69.1947	0.1601	53.22	54.80	57.43	62.46	69.19	77.59	87.12	94.05	99.19
229.5	-1.0144	69.3353	0.1601	53.32	54.91	57.55	62.58	69.34	77.73	87.26	94.18	99.30
230.5	-1.0050	69.4735	0.1599	53.41	55.01	57.66	62.71	69.47	77.88	87.40	94.31	99.41
231.5	-0.9951	69.6093	0.1599	53.50	55.10	57.76	62.83	69.61	78.02	87.54	94.44	99.53
232.5	-0.9850	69.7423	0.1599	53.59	55.20	57.86	62.95	69.74	78.17	87.68	94.57	99.64
233.5	-0.9747	69.8722	0.1600	53.67	55.28	57.96	63.06	69.87	78.31	87.82	94.70	99.75
234.5	-0.9644	69.9987	0.1600	53.75	55.36	58.05	63.17	70.00	78.45	87.97	94.83	99.88
235.5	-0.9543	70.1210	0.1601	53.81	55.44	58.14	63.27	70.12	78.59	88.11	94.97	100.01
236.5	-0.9446	70.2386	0.1603	53.87	55.51	58.22	63.37	70.24	78.72	88.26	95.11	100.15
237.5	-0.9354	70.3504	0.1605	53.93	55.56	58.29	63.46	70.35	78.86	88.41	95.27	100.30
238.5	-0.9271	70.4555	0.1608	53.97	55.61	58.35	63.54	70.46	78.99	88.56	95.44	100.48
239.5	-0.9197	70.5525	0.1612	53.99	55.65	58.39	63.61	70.55	79.12	88.72	95.62	100.67
240.0	-0.9165	70.5976	0.1615	54.00	55.66	58.41	63.64	70.60	79.18	88.81	95.71	100.78

216

Table V.7a.

LMS parameters and smoothed percentiles of weight (kg)-for-age in months for girls from 2 to 20 years

Age Group (months)	L	M	S	Percentiles								
				3rd	5th	10th	25th	50th	75th	90th	95th	97th
24.0	-0.7353	12.0550	0.1074	9.99	10.21	10.57	11.23	12.06	12.99	13.94	14.57	15.00
24.5	-0.7522	12.1346	0.1077	10.05	10.27	10.64	11.31	12.13	13.08	14.04	14.68	15.12
25.5	-0.7842	12.2910	0.1085	10.17	10.40	10.77	11.45	12.29	13.25	14.24	14.90	15.35
26.5	-0.8141	12.4447	0.1093	10.29	10.52	10.90	11.59	12.44	13.43	14.44	15.11	15.58
27.5	-0.8419	12.5962	0.1101	10.41	10.64	11.02	11.72	12.60	13.60	14.64	15.33	15.82
28.5	-0.8679	12.7462	0.1111	10.52	10.76	11.15	11.85	12.75	13.77	14.84	15.55	16.05
29.5	-0.8921	12.8952	0.1120	10.63	10.87	11.27	11.99	12.90	13.94	15.04	15.77	16.28
30.5	-0.9147	13.0436	0.1130	10.74	10.99	11.38	12.12	13.04	14.12	15.24	15.99	16.52
31.5	-0.9359	13.1918	0.1141	10.85	11.10	11.50	12.25	13.19	14.29	15.44	16.21	16.76
32.5	-0.9557	13.3402	0.1151	10.96	11.21	11.62	12.38	13.34	14.46	15.64	16.44	17.00
33.5	-0.9744	13.4891	0.1162	11.06	11.32	11.74	12.51	13.49	14.63	15.84	16.67	17.25
34.5	-0.9920	13.6388	0.1173	11.17	11.43	11.86	12.64	13.64	14.81	16.05	16.90	17.49
35.5	-1.0086	13.7894	0.1184	11.28	11.54	11.97	12.77	13.79	14.99	16.26	17.13	17.74
36.5	-1.0245	13.9411	0.1195	11.39	11.66	12.09	12.90	13.94	15.16	16.47	17.36	18.00
37.5	-1.0396	14.0941	0.1206	11.50	11.77	12.21	13.04	14.09	15.34	16.68	17.60	18.25
38.5	-1.0540	14.2484	0.1217	11.61	11.88	12.33	13.17	14.25	15.53	16.90	17.84	18.51
39.5	-1.0679	14.4043	0.1228	11.72	12.00	12.45	13.31	14.40	15.71	17.11	18.08	18.78
40.5	-1.0814	14.5617	0.1239	11.83	12.11	12.58	13.44	14.56	15.89	17.33	18.33	19.04
41.5	-1.0944	14.7206	0.1249	11.94	12.23	12.70	13.58	14.72	16.08	17.55	18.58	19.31
42.5	-1.1070	14.8812	0.1260	12.06	12.35	12.83	13.72	14.88	16.27	17.78	18.83	19.59
43.5	-1.1193	15.0434	0.1270	12.17	12.47	12.95	13.86	15.04	16.46	18.00	19.08	19.86
44.5	-1.1314	15.2072	0.1280	12.29	12.59	13.08	14.00	15.21	16.65	18.23	19.34	20.14
45.5	-1.1431	15.3726	0.1290	12.41	12.71	13.21	14.15	15.37	16.85	18.46	19.60	20.42
46.5	-1.1547	15.5396	0.1300	12.53	12.84	13.34	14.29	15.54	17.04	18.70	19.86	20.71
47.5	-1.1660	15.7082	0.1309	12.65	12.96	13.48	14.44	15.71	17.24	18.93	20.13	21.00
48.5	-1.1770	15.8782	0.1318	12.77	13.09	13.61	14.59	15.88	17.44	19.17	20.39	21.29
49.5	-1.1879	16.0498	0.1327	12.90	13.22	13.75	14.74	16.05	17.64	19.41	20.66	21.58
50.5	-1.1985	16.2228	0.1336	13.02	13.35	13.88	14.89	16.22	17.85	19.65	20.93	21.87
51.5	-1.2089	16.3972	0.1344	13.15	13.48	14.02	15.05	16.40	18.05	19.89	21.21	22.17
52.5	-1.2190	16.5729	0.1352	13.28	13.61	14.16	15.20	16.57	18.26	20.13	21.48	22.47
53.5	-1.2288	16.7499	0.1360	13.41	13.75	14.30	15.36	16.75	18.46	20.38	21.76	22.77
54.5	-1.2383	16.9283	0.1368	13.54	13.88	14.44	15.51	16.93	18.67	20.63	22.04	23.08
55.5	-1.2475	17.1078	0.1376	13.67	14.02	14.59	15.67	17.11	18.88	20.88	22.32	23.38
56.5	-1.2564	17.2886	0.1383	13.80	14.15	14.73	15.83	17.29	19.09	21.13	22.60	23.69
57.5	-1.2649	17.4705	0.1391	13.94	14.29	14.88	15.99	17.47	19.30	21.38	22.89	24.00
58.5	-1.2729	17.6536	0.1398	14.07	14.43	15.02	16.15	17.65	19.52	21.63	23.17	24.31
59.5	-1.2805	17.8378	0.1405	14.21	14.57	15.17	16.31	17.84	19.73	21.89	23.46	24.63
60.5	-1.2877	18.0231	0.1412	14.34	14.71	15.32	16.47	18.02	19.95	22.15	23.75	24.94
61.5	-1.2943	18.2096	0.1419	14.48	14.85	15.47	16.64	18.21	20.17	22.40	24.04	25.26
62.5	-1.3004	18.3971	0.1426	14.62	14.99	15.62	16.80	18.40	20.39	22.66	24.34	25.58
63.5	-1.3060	18.5857	0.1433	14.75	15.13	15.77	16.97	18.59	20.61	22.93	24.63	25.91
64.5	-1.3109	18.7754	0.1439	14.89	15.28	15.92	17.14	18.78	20.83	23.19	24.93	26.23
65.5	-1.3153	18.9663	0.1446	15.03	15.42	16.07	17.30	18.97	21.05	23.46	25.23	26.56
66.5	-1.3190	19.1583	0.1453	15.17	15.56	16.22	17.47	19.16	21.28	23.72	25.53	26.89
67.5	-1.3220	19.3515	0.1460	15.31	15.71	16.37	17.64	19.35	21.50	23.99	25.83	27.22
68.5	-1.3244	19.5459	0.1467	15.45	15.85	16.53	17.81	19.55	21.73	24.26	26.14	27.55
69.5	-1.3261	19.7415	0.1474	15.59	16.00	16.68	17.98	19.74	21.96	24.54	26.45	27.89
70.5	-1.3270	19.9384	0.1481	15.73	16.14	16.83	18.15	19.94	22.19	24.81	26.76	28.23
71.5	-1.3273	20.1367	0.1489	15.87	16.29	16.99	18.33	20.14	22.43	25.09	27.08	28.58
72.5	-1.3268	20.3364	0.1496	16.01	16.44	17.14	18.50	20.34	22.66	25.37	27.39	28.92
73.5	-1.3255	20.5375	0.1503	16.15	16.58	17.30	18.67	20.54	22.90	25.65	27.71	29.27
74.5	-1.3236	20.7401	0.1511	16.29	16.73	17.46	18.85	20.74	23.14	25.94	28.04	29.62
75.5	-1.3209	20.9444	0.1519	16.44	16.88	17.61	19.03	20.94	23.38	26.23	28.36	29.98
76.5	-1.3175	21.1503	0.1527	16.58	17.03	17.77	19.20	21.15	23.63	26.52	28.69	30.34
77.5	-1.3133	21.3580	0.1535	16.72	17.17	17.93	19.38	21.36	23.87	26.82	29.03	30.70
78.5	-1.3085	21.5675	0.1543	16.86	17.32	18.09	19.56	21.57	24.12	27.11	29.36	31.07
79.5	-1.3029	21.7789	0.1552	17.01	17.47	18.25	19.74	21.78	24.37	27.42	29.70	31.44
80.5	-1.2967	21.9923	0.1560	17.15	17.62	18.41	19.93	21.99	24.63	27.72	30.05	31.82
81.5	-1.2899	22.2079	0.1569	17.29	17.77	18.57	20.11	22.21	24.88	28.03	30.40	32.20
82.5	-1.2824	22.4256	0.1578	17.44	17.92	18.73	20.30	22.43	25.15	28.34	30.75	32.58
83.5	-1.2742	22.6456	0.1588	17.58	18.08	18.90	20.48	22.65	25.41	28.66	31.11	32.97
84.5	-1.2655	22.8680	0.1597	17.73	18.23	19.06	20.67	22.87	25.68	28.98	31.47	33.37
85.5	-1.2563	23.0929	0.1607	17.87	18.38	19.23	20.86	23.09	25.95	29.30	31.84	33.77
86.5	-1.2465	23.3204	0.1616	18.02	18.54	19.40	21.05	23.32	26.22	29.63	32.21	34.17
87.5	-1.2363	23.5505	0.1626	18.17	18.69	19.56	21.25	23.55	26.50	29.97	32.59	34.58
88.5	-1.2256	23.7834	0.1636	18.32	18.85	19.73	21.44	23.78	26.78	30.31	32.97	35.00
89.5	-1.2144	24.0192	0.1647	18.47	19.01	19.91	21.64	24.02	27.06	30.65	33.36	35.42
90.5	-1.2029	24.2579	0.1657	18.62	19.16	20.08	21.84	24.26	27.35	31.00	33.75	35.85
91.5	-1.1910	24.4996	0.1667	18.77	19.32	20.25	22.05	24.50	27.64	31.35	34.15	36.28
92.5	-1.1788	24.7445	0.1678	18.92	19.49	20.43	22.25	24.74	27.94	31.71	34.55	36.72
93.5	-1.1664	24.9926	0.1689	19.08	19.65	20.61	22.46	24.99	28.24	32.07	34.96	37.16
94.5	-1.1537	25.2440	0.1700	19.23	19.81	20.79	22.67	25.24	28.55	32.44	35.38	37.61
95.5	-1.1408	25.4988	0.1710	19.39	19.98	20.97	22.88	25.50	28.86	32.82	35.80	38.07

Table V.7b.

LMS parameters and smoothed percentiles of weight (kg)-for-age in months for girls from 2 to 20 years

Age Group (months)	L	M	S	Percentiles								
				3rd	5th	10th	25th	50th	75th	90th	95th	97th
96.5	-1.1277	25.7570	0.1721	19.54	20.15	21.15	23.09	25.76	29.17	33.19	36.23	38.54
97.5	-1.1145	26.0187	0.1732	19.70	20.31	21.34	23.31	26.02	29.49	33.58	36.66	39.00
98.5	-1.1012	26.2840	0.1744	19.87	20.49	21.52	23.53	26.28	29.81	33.97	37.10	39.48
99.5	-1.0879	26.5530	0.1755	20.03	20.66	21.71	23.76	26.55	30.14	34.36	37.54	39.96
100.5	-1.0745	26.8256	0.1766	20.19	20.83	21.91	23.98	26.83	30.47	34.77	38.00	40.45
101.5	-1.0612	27.1019	0.1777	20.36	21.01	22.10	24.21	27.10	30.81	35.17	38.45	40.95
102.5	-1.0478	27.3820	0.1788	20.53	21.19	22.30	24.44	27.38	31.15	35.58	38.92	41.45
103.5	-1.0346	27.6659	0.1799	20.70	21.37	22.50	24.68	27.67	31.50	36.00	39.39	41.95
104.5	-1.0215	27.9537	0.1810	20.87	21.56	22.70	24.92	27.95	31.85	36.42	39.86	42.47
105.5	-1.0085	28.2452	0.1820	21.05	21.74	22.91	25.16	28.25	32.20	36.85	40.34	42.99
106.5	-0.9957	28.5406	0.1831	21.23	21.93	23.11	25.40	28.54	32.56	37.29	40.83	43.51
107.5	-0.9831	28.8398	0.1842	21.41	22.12	23.32	25.65	28.84	32.93	37.72	41.32	44.04
108.5	-0.9707	29.1429	0.1852	21.59	22.32	23.54	25.90	29.14	33.29	38.17	41.82	44.58
109.5	-0.9585	29.4498	0.1862	21.77	22.51	23.75	26.16	29.45	33.67	38.62	42.32	45.13
110.5	-0.9466	29.7605	0.1872	21.96	22.71	23.97	26.41	29.76	34.04	39.07	42.83	45.67
111.5	-0.9350	30.0749	0.1882	22.15	22.91	24.20	26.68	30.07	34.43	39.53	43.35	46.23
112.5	-0.9238	30.3931	0.1892	22.34	23.12	24.42	26.94	30.39	34.81	39.99	43.86	46.79
113.5	-0.9128	30.7149	0.1901	22.54	23.33	24.65	27.21	30.71	35.20	40.46	44.39	47.35
114.5	-0.9022	31.0403	0.1910	22.74	23.54	24.88	27.48	31.04	35.60	40.93	44.92	47.92
115.5	-0.8920	31.3693	0.1919	22.94	23.75	25.11	27.75	31.37	36.00	41.41	45.45	48.50
116.5	-0.8821	31.7017	0.1928	23.14	23.97	25.35	28.03	31.70	36.40	41.89	45.99	49.07
117.5	-0.8727	32.0374	0.1936	23.35	24.19	25.59	28.31	32.04	36.80	42.38	46.53	49.66
118.5	-0.8636	32.3765	0.1944	23.56	24.41	25.84	28.59	32.38	37.21	42.86	47.07	50.24
119.5	-0.8550	32.7187	0.1952	23.78	24.64	26.08	28.88	32.72	37.62	43.36	47.62	50.84
120.5	-0.8469	33.0639	0.1959	23.99	24.87	26.33	29.17	33.06	38.04	43.85	48.18	51.43
121.5	-0.8392	33.4121	0.1967	24.21	25.10	26.58	29.46	33.41	38.46	44.35	48.73	52.03
122.5	-0.8319	33.7630	0.1973	24.43	25.33	26.84	29.76	33.76	38.88	44.85	49.29	52.63
123.5	-0.8252	34.1166	0.1980	24.66	25.57	27.10	30.06	34.12	39.30	45.35	49.85	53.23
124.5	-0.8189	34.4727	0.1986	24.89	25.81	27.36	30.36	34.47	39.73	45.86	50.41	53.83
125.5	-0.8131	34.8312	0.1991	25.12	26.05	27.62	30.66	34.83	40.15	46.36	50.98	54.44
126.5	-0.8079	35.1918	0.1996	25.35	26.30	27.89	30.97	35.19	40.58	46.87	51.54	55.05
127.5	-0.8031	35.5544	0.2001	25.59	26.55	28.16	31.28	35.55	41.02	47.38	52.11	55.66
128.5	-0.7989	35.9188	0.2006	25.83	26.80	28.43	31.59	35.92	41.45	47.89	52.68	56.27
129.5	-0.7952	36.2849	0.2010	26.07	27.06	28.71	31.90	36.28	41.88	48.41	53.25	56.88
130.5	-0.7920	36.6524	0.2014	26.32	27.31	28.98	32.22	36.65	42.32	48.92	53.82	57.50
131.5	-0.7894	37.0211	0.2017	26.57	27.57	29.26	32.53	37.02	42.75	49.43	54.39	58.11
132.5	-0.7874	37.3909	0.2020	26.82	27.84	29.54	32.85	37.39	43.19	49.94	54.96	58.72
133.5	-0.7859	37.7615	0.2022	27.07	28.10	29.83	33.17	37.76	43.62	50.45	55.53	59.33
134.5	-0.7849	38.1327	0.2024	27.33	28.37	30.11	33.49	38.13	44.06	50.97	56.09	59.94
135.5	-0.7846	38.5043	0.2026	27.59	28.64	30.40	33.82	38.50	44.49	51.47	56.66	60.55
136.5	-0.7848	38.8761	0.2027	27.85	28.91	30.69	34.14	38.88	44.93	51.98	57.22	61.16
137.5	-0.7855	39.2477	0.2028	28.11	29.18	30.98	34.47	39.25	45.36	52.49	57.78	61.76
138.5	-0.7869	39.6191	0.2028	28.38	29.46	31.27	34.79	39.62	45.79	52.99	58.34	62.36
139.5	-0.7889	39.9900	0.2029	28.65	29.74	31.57	35.12	39.99	46.22	53.49	58.90	62.96
140.5	-0.7914	40.3601	0.2028	28.92	30.02	31.86	35.44	40.36	46.65	53.99	59.45	63.56
141.5	-0.7945	40.7292	0.2027	29.19	30.30	32.16	35.77	40.73	47.07	54.49	60.00	64.15
142.5	-0.7983	41.0970	0.2026	29.46	30.58	32.46	36.10	41.10	47.50	54.98	60.55	64.74
143.5	-0.8026	41.4634	0.2025	29.74	30.87	32.76	36.42	41.46	47.92	55.47	61.09	65.32
144.5	-0.8076	41.8280	0.2023	30.02	31.15	33.05	36.75	41.83	48.33	55.95	61.63	65.90
145.5	-0.8132	42.1906	0.2021	30.30	31.44	33.35	37.07	42.19	48.75	56.43	62.16	66.48
146.5	-0.8194	42.5511	0.2018	30.58	31.72	33.65	37.40	42.55	49.16	56.90	62.69	67.04
147.5	-0.8262	42.9091	0.2015	30.86	32.01	33.95	37.72	42.91	49.56	57.37	63.21	67.61
148.5	-0.8336	43.2644	0.2012	31.14	32.30	34.25	38.05	43.26	49.97	57.84	63.72	68.16
149.5	-0.8416	43.6168	0.2008	31.42	32.59	34.55	38.37	43.62	50.36	58.29	64.23	68.72
150.5	-0.8503	43.9661	0.2004	31.70	32.88	34.85	38.69	43.97	50.76	58.75	64.73	69.26
151.5	-0.8596	44.3120	0.2000	31.99	33.17	35.15	39.00	44.31	51.14	59.19	65.23	69.80
152.5	-0.8695	44.6544	0.1995	32.27	33.46	35.45	39.32	44.65	51.53	59.63	65.72	70.33
153.5	-0.8801	44.9929	0.1990	32.56	33.74	35.74	39.63	44.99	51.90	60.06	66.20	70.85
154.5	-0.8913	45.3274	0.1985	32.84	34.03	36.04	39.94	45.33	52.27	60.49	66.67	71.37
155.5	-0.9031	45.6578	0.1979	33.12	34.32	36.33	40.25	45.66	52.64	60.90	67.14	71.88
156.5	-0.9155	45.9837	0.1974	33.41	34.61	36.63	40.56	45.98	53.00	61.31	67.59	72.38
157.5	-0.9286	46.3050	0.1968	33.69	34.89	36.92	40.86	46.31	53.35	61.71	68.04	72.87
158.5	-0.9422	46.6216	0.1961	33.97	35.18	37.21	41.16	46.62	53.70	62.11	68.48	73.35
159.5	-0.9565	46.9331	0.1955	34.25	35.46	37.49	41.45	46.93	54.04	62.49	68.92	73.83
160.5	-0.9714	47.2396	0.1948	34.53	35.74	37.78	41.75	47.24	54.37	62.87	69.34	74.29
161.5	-0.9869	47.5408	0.1941	34.81	36.02	38.06	42.03	47.54	54.69	63.24	69.75	74.75
162.5	-1.0031	47.8366	0.1933	35.09	36.30	38.34	42.32	47.84	55.01	63.60	70.16	75.20
163.5	-1.0197	48.1269	0.1926	35.36	36.57	38.62	42.60	48.13	55.32	63.95	70.56	75.64
164.5	-1.0370	48.4114	0.1918	35.63	36.85	38.89	42.88	48.41	55.63	64.30	70.94	76.06
165.5	-1.0548	48.6902	0.1910	35.90	37.12	39.16	43.15	48.69	55.92	64.63	71.32	76.48
166.5	-1.0732	48.9630	0.1902	36.17	37.39	39.43	43.42	48.96	56.21	64.95	71.69	76.90
167.5	-1.0922	49.2299	0.1894	36.44	37.65	39.69	43.68	49.23	56.49	65.27	72.04	77.30
168.5	-1.1116	49.4908	0.1886	36.70	37.91	39.95	43.94	49.49	56.76	65.58	72.39	77.69
169.5	-1.1316	49.7454	0.1877	36.96	38.17	40.21	44.19	49.75	57.03	65.87	72.73	78.07

CDC Growth Standards

Table V.7c.
LMS parameters and smoothed percentiles of weight (kg)-for-age in months for girls from 2 to 20 years

Age Group (months)	L	M	S	3rd	5th	10th	25th	50th	75th	90th	95th	97th
170.5	-1.1520	49.9939	0.1869	37.22	38.43	40.46	44.44	49.99	57.29	66.16	73.06	78.44
171.5	-1.1729	50.2362	0.1860	37.47	38.68	40.71	44.69	50.24	57.54	66.44	73.38	78.81
172.5	-1.1942	50.4722	0.1851	37.72	38.93	40.96	44.93	50.47	57.78	66.71	73.69	79.16
173.5	-1.2159	50.7020	0.1842	37.97	39.17	41.20	45.16	50.70	58.01	66.97	73.99	79.50
174.5	-1.2380	50.9254	0.1833	38.21	39.41	41.44	45.39	50.93	58.24	67.22	74.28	79.84
175.5	-1.2604	51.1426	0.1824	38.45	39.65	41.67	45.61	51.14	58.46	67.46	74.56	80.16
176.5	-1.2832	51.3535	0.1815	38.69	39.88	41.89	45.83	51.35	58.67	67.70	74.83	80.48
177.5	-1.3062	51.5582	0.1806	38.92	40.11	42.12	46.05	51.56	58.87	67.92	75.09	80.78
178.5	-1.3295	51.7568	0.1797	39.15	40.33	42.33	46.25	51.76	59.07	68.14	75.35	81.08
179.5	-1.3529	51.9493	0.1788	39.37	40.55	42.55	46.46	51.95	59.26	68.35	75.59	81.37
180.5	-1.3765	52.1357	0.1779	39.59	40.77	42.76	46.65	52.14	59.44	68.55	75.83	81.65
181.5	-1.4002	52.3162	0.1771	39.80	40.98	42.96	46.85	52.32	59.62	68.74	76.06	81.92
182.5	-1.4239	52.4908	0.1762	40.01	41.18	43.16	47.03	52.49	59.79	68.93	76.27	82.18
183.5	-1.4476	52.6597	0.1753	40.22	41.38	43.35	47.21	52.66	59.95	69.10	76.48	82.43
184.5	-1.4712	52.8230	0.1744	40.42	41.58	43.54	47.39	52.82	60.11	69.27	76.69	82.68
185.5	-1.4948	52.9808	0.1736	40.61	41.77	43.72	47.56	52.98	60.26	69.44	76.88	82.92
186.5	-1.5182	53.1333	0.1728	40.80	41.95	43.90	47.73	53.13	60.40	69.59	77.07	83.15
187.5	-1.5413	53.2806	0.1719	40.98	42.13	44.07	47.89	53.28	60.54	69.74	77.25	83.37
188.5	-1.5641	53.4228	0.1711	41.16	42.31	44.24	48.04	53.42	60.68	69.88	77.42	83.58
189.5	-1.5866	53.5603	0.1704	41.34	42.48	44.40	48.20	53.56	60.80	70.02	77.59	83.79
190.5	-1.6087	53.6931	0.1696	41.51	42.64	44.56	48.34	53.69	60.93	70.16	77.75	83.99
191.5	-1.6302	53.8214	0.1688	41.67	42.80	44.72	48.48	53.82	61.05	70.28	77.90	84.18
192.5	-1.6512	53.9454	0.1681	41.83	42.96	44.86	48.62	53.95	61.16	70.40	78.05	84.37
193.5	-1.6717	54.0654	0.1674	41.98	43.11	45.01	48.75	54.07	61.27	70.52	78.20	84.55
194.5	-1.6914	54.1816	0.1668	42.13	43.25	45.15	48.88	54.18	61.38	70.64	78.33	84.72
195.5	-1.7104	54.2941	0.1661	42.27	43.39	45.28	49.00	54.29	61.49	70.75	78.47	84.89
196.5	-1.7285	54.4032	0.1655	42.41	43.52	45.41	49.12	54.40	61.59	70.85	78.60	85.05
197.5	-1.7459	54.5092	0.1649	42.54	43.65	45.53	49.24	54.51	61.69	70.96	78.72	85.21
198.5	-1.7622	54.6122	0.1644	42.67	43.78	45.66	49.35	54.61	61.78	71.06	78.84	85.36
199.5	-1.7776	54.7126	0.1638	42.79	43.90	45.77	49.46	54.71	61.88	71.16	78.96	85.50
200.5	-1.7920	54.8104	0.1634	42.91	44.02	45.88	49.57	54.81	61.97	71.26	79.08	85.64
201.5	-1.8053	54.9061	0.1629	43.02	44.13	45.99	49.67	54.91	62.06	71.35	79.19	85.78
202.5	-1.8174	54.9998	0.1625	43.13	44.23	46.10	49.77	55.00	62.15	71.45	79.30	85.91
203.5	-1.8284	55.0917	0.1621	43.24	44.34	46.20	49.87	55.09	62.24	71.54	79.41	86.04
204.5	-1.8381	55.1822	0.1618	43.34	44.44	46.29	49.96	55.18	62.33	71.64	79.52	86.17
205.5	-1.8466	55.2714	0.1614	43.43	44.53	46.39	50.05	55.27	62.42	71.73	79.62	86.29
206.5	-1.8537	55.3595	0.1612	43.52	44.62	46.48	50.14	55.36	62.50	71.82	79.72	86.41
207.5	-1.8596	55.4469	0.1609	43.61	44.71	46.57	50.23	55.45	62.59	71.92	79.83	86.52
208.5	-1.8641	55.5336	0.1607	43.70	44.79	46.65	50.31	55.53	62.68	72.01	79.93	86.63
209.5	-1.8672	55.6200	0.1606	43.78	44.87	46.73	50.40	55.62	62.77	72.11	80.03	86.74
210.5	-1.8690	55.7062	0.1604	43.85	44.95	46.81	50.48	55.71	62.86	72.21	80.13	86.85
211.5	-1.8694	55.7925	0.1603	43.93	45.03	46.89	50.56	55.79	62.96	72.31	80.24	86.95
212.5	-1.8684	55.8789	0.1603	44.00	45.10	46.96	50.64	55.88	63.05	72.41	80.34	87.05
213.5	-1.8660	55.9657	0.1602	44.06	45.17	47.03	50.72	55.97	63.15	72.51	80.44	87.15
214.5	-1.8623	56.0530	0.1603	44.13	45.23	47.11	50.80	56.05	63.24	72.61	80.54	87.25
215.5	-1.8573	56.1410	0.1603	44.19	45.30	47.17	50.87	56.14	63.34	72.72	80.65	87.34
216.5	-1.8509	56.2297	0.1604	44.25	45.36	47.24	50.95	56.23	63.44	72.83	80.75	87.43
217.5	-1.8433	56.3192	0.1605	44.30	45.42	47.31	51.03	56.32	63.55	72.94	80.86	87.53
218.5	-1.8345	56.4096	0.1606	44.36	45.48	47.37	51.10	56.41	63.65	73.05	80.96	87.62
219.5	-1.8245	56.5010	0.1608	44.41	45.53	47.43	51.18	56.50	63.76	73.16	81.07	87.70
220.5	-1.8133	56.5932	0.1610	44.46	45.59	47.50	51.25	56.59	63.87	73.28	81.17	87.79
221.5	-1.8012	56.6863	0.1612	44.51	45.64	47.56	51.33	56.69	63.98	73.39	81.28	87.87
222.5	-1.7880	56.7803	0.1614	44.55	45.69	47.62	51.40	56.78	64.09	73.51	81.39	87.96
223.5	-1.7739	56.8749	0.1617	44.60	45.74	47.68	51.48	56.87	64.20	73.63	81.49	88.04
224.5	-1.7590	56.9701	0.1619	44.64	45.79	47.73	51.55	56.97	64.32	73.75	81.60	88.12
225.5	-1.7434	57.0656	0.1622	44.68	45.84	47.79	51.63	57.07	64.43	73.87	81.71	88.20
226.5	-1.7272	57.1613	0.1625	44.72	45.88	47.85	51.70	57.16	64.55	74.00	81.81	88.27
227.5	-1.7104	57.2568	0.1628	44.76	45.93	47.90	51.77	57.26	64.66	74.12	81.92	88.35
228.5	-1.6933	57.3518	0.1631	44.80	45.97	47.95	51.85	57.35	64.78	74.24	82.02	88.42
229.5	-1.6759	57.4458	0.1635	44.83	46.01	48.00	51.92	57.45	64.89	74.36	82.12	88.49
230.5	-1.6583	57.5384	0.1638	44.86	46.05	48.05	51.99	57.54	65.01	74.47	82.22	88.56
231.5	-1.6407	57.6291	0.1641	44.89	46.09	48.10	52.06	57.63	65.12	74.59	82.32	88.62
232.5	-1.6233	57.7173	0.1644	44.92	46.12	48.15	52.12	57.72	65.23	74.70	82.41	88.69
233.5	-1.6062	57.8023	0.1648	44.95	46.16	48.19	52.18	57.80	65.33	74.81	82.50	88.75
234.5	-1.5895	57.8833	0.1651	44.97	46.19	48.23	52.24	57.88	65.43	74.91	82.59	88.80
235.5	-1.5735	57.9597	0.1654	44.99	46.21	48.27	52.30	57.96	65.52	75.01	82.67	88.86
236.5	-1.5582	58.0304	0.1657	45.01	46.24	48.30	52.35	58.03	65.61	75.10	82.74	88.91
237.5	-1.5438	58.0945	0.1660	45.03	46.26	48.33	52.39	58.09	65.69	75.18	82.81	88.95
238.5	-1.5306	58.1510	0.1663	45.04	46.27	48.36	52.43	58.15	65.76	75.26	82.88	88.99
239.5	-1.5188	58.1988	0.1665	45.05	46.29	48.38	52.47	58.20	65.83	75.32	82.93	89.03
240.0	-1.5134	58.2190	0.1666	45.05	46.29	48.38	52.48	58.22	65.85	75.35	82.95	89.04

Table V.8a.

LMS parameters and smoothed percentiles of stature (cm)-for-age in months for boys from 2 to 20 years

Age Group (months)	L	M	S	Percentiles								
				3rd	5th	10th	25th	50th	75th	90th	95th	97th
24.0	0.94152	86.4522	0.04032	79.9	80.7	82.0	84.1	86.5	88.8	90.9	92.2	93.0
24.5	1.00721	86.8616	0.04040	80.3	81.1	82.4	84.5	86.9	89.2	91.4	92.6	93.5
25.5	0.83725	87.6525	0.04058	81.0	81.8	83.1	85.3	87.7	90.1	92.2	93.5	94.4
26.5	0.68149	88.4233	0.04072	81.7	82.6	83.8	86.0	88.4	90.9	93.1	94.4	95.3
27.5	0.53878	89.1755	0.04083	82.4	83.3	84.6	86.7	89.2	91.6	93.9	95.3	96.1
28.5	0.40770	89.9104	0.04091	83.1	84.0	85.3	87.4	89.9	92.4	94.7	96.1	97.0
29.5	0.28676	90.6291	0.04095	83.8	84.7	86.0	88.2	90.6	93.2	95.5	96.9	97.8
30.5	0.17449	91.3324	0.04097	84.5	85.3	86.6	88.8	91.3	93.9	96.2	97.7	98.6
31.5	0.06944	92.0213	0.04095	85.2	86.0	87.3	89.5	92.0	94.6	97.0	98.4	99.4
32.5	-0.02972	92.6964	0.04091	85.8	86.7	88.0	90.2	92.7	95.3	97.7	99.2	100.1
33.5	-0.12425	93.3585	0.04084	86.5	87.3	88.6	90.8	93.4	96.0	98.4	99.9	100.9
34.5	-0.21529	94.0082	0.04076	87.1	88.0	89.2	91.5	94.0	96.6	99.1	100.6	101.6
35.5	-0.30385	94.6464	0.04065	87.8	88.6	89.9	92.1	94.6	97.3	99.7	101.3	102.3
36.5	-0.39092	95.2736	0.04053	88.4	89.2	90.5	92.7	95.3	97.9	100.4	101.9	102.9
37.5	-0.25480	95.9147	0.04057	88.9	89.8	91.1	93.3	95.9	98.6	101.1	102.6	103.6
38.5	-0.12565	96.5473	0.04062	89.5	90.3	91.7	93.9	96.5	99.2	101.7	103.2	104.3
39.5	-0.00317	97.1719	0.04067	90.0	90.9	92.2	94.5	97.2	99.9	102.4	103.9	104.9
40.5	0.11291	97.7890	0.04072	90.5	91.4	92.8	95.1	97.8	100.5	103.0	104.5	105.5
41.5	0.22275	98.3990	0.04078	91.1	92.0	93.4	95.7	98.4	101.1	103.6	105.2	106.2
42.5	0.32653	99.0025	0.04085	91.6	92.5	93.9	96.3	99.0	101.8	104.3	105.8	106.8
43.5	0.42436	99.6000	0.04092	92.1	93.0	94.5	96.9	99.6	102.4	104.9	106.4	107.4
44.5	0.51635	100.1918	0.04100	92.6	93.5	95.0	97.4	100.2	103.0	105.5	107.1	108.1
45.5	0.60260	100.7783	0.04108	93.1	94.1	95.5	98.0	100.8	103.6	106.1	107.7	108.7
46.5	0.68317	101.3600	0.04116	93.6	94.6	96.1	98.6	101.4	104.2	106.8	108.3	109.3
47.5	0.75816	101.9373	0.04125	94.1	95.1	96.6	99.1	101.9	104.8	107.4	108.9	109.9
48.5	0.82764	102.5105	0.04134	94.6	95.6	97.1	99.7	102.5	105.4	108.0	109.5	110.5
49.5	0.89169	103.0799	0.04144	95.1	96.1	97.6	100.2	103.1	106.0	108.6	110.1	111.1
50.5	0.95039	103.6459	0.04154	95.6	96.6	98.1	100.7	103.6	106.6	109.2	110.7	111.8
51.5	1.00383	104.2087	0.04164	96.0	97.1	98.6	101.3	104.2	107.1	109.8	111.3	112.4
52.5	1.05214	104.7687	0.04174	96.5	97.6	99.2	101.8	104.8	107.7	110.4	111.9	113.0
53.5	1.09537	105.3262	0.04185	97.0	98.1	99.7	102.3	105.3	108.3	111.0	112.6	113.6
54.5	1.13365	105.8813	0.04196	97.5	98.5	100.2	102.9	105.9	108.9	111.6	113.2	114.2
55.5	1.16710	106.4343	0.04206	98.0	99.0	100.7	103.4	106.4	109.4	112.1	113.8	114.8
56.5	1.19585	106.9855	0.04217	98.4	99.5	101.2	103.9	107.0	110.0	112.7	114.4	115.4
57.5	1.22000	107.5350	0.04228	98.9	100.0	101.7	104.5	107.5	110.6	113.3	115.0	116.0
58.5	1.23972	108.0830	0.04238	99.4	100.5	102.2	105.0	108.1	111.2	113.9	115.6	116.6
59.5	1.25512	108.6296	0.04249	99.9	101.0	102.7	105.5	108.6	111.7	114.5	116.2	117.2
60.5	1.26637	109.1751	0.04259	100.3	101.5	103.2	106.0	109.2	112.3	115.1	116.8	117.8
61.5	1.27361	109.7196	0.04270	100.8	101.9	103.7	106.5	109.7	112.9	115.7	117.4	118.4
62.5	1.27700	110.2631	0.04280	101.3	102.4	104.2	107.1	110.3	113.4	116.3	118.0	119.0
63.5	1.27670	110.8058	0.04290	101.8	102.9	104.7	107.6	110.8	114.0	116.9	118.6	119.6
64.5	1.27289	111.3477	0.04299	102.2	103.4	105.2	108.1	111.3	114.6	117.4	119.1	120.3
65.5	1.26573	111.8890	0.04309	102.7	103.9	105.7	108.6	111.9	115.1	118.0	119.7	120.9
66.5	1.25540	112.4296	0.04318	103.2	104.4	106.2	109.1	112.4	115.7	118.6	120.3	121.5
67.5	1.24209	112.9696	0.04327	103.7	104.9	106.7	109.7	113.0	116.3	119.2	120.9	122.1
68.5	1.22598	113.5090	0.04336	104.2	105.3	107.2	110.2	113.5	116.8	119.8	121.5	122.7
69.5	1.20726	114.0479	0.04344	104.6	105.8	107.7	110.7	114.0	117.4	120.4	122.1	123.3
70.5	1.18614	114.5861	0.04352	105.1	106.3	108.2	111.2	114.6	117.9	120.9	122.7	123.9
71.5	1.16280	115.1238	0.04360	105.6	106.8	108.7	111.7	115.1	118.5	121.5	123.3	124.5
72.5	1.13744	115.6609	0.04367	106.1	107.3	109.2	112.2	115.7	119.1	122.1	123.9	125.1
73.5	1.11029	116.1973	0.04375	106.6	107.8	109.7	112.8	116.2	119.6	122.7	124.5	125.7
74.5	1.08154	116.7329	0.04382	107.1	108.3	110.2	113.3	116.7	120.2	123.3	125.1	126.3
75.5	1.05140	117.2678	0.04388	107.6	108.8	110.7	113.8	117.3	120.7	123.9	125.7	126.9
76.5	1.02010	117.8018	0.04395	108.1	109.3	111.2	114.3	117.8	121.3	124.4	126.3	127.5
77.5	0.98785	118.3348	0.04401	108.5	109.8	111.7	114.8	118.3	121.8	125.0	126.9	128.1
78.5	0.95485	118.8668	0.04407	109.0	110.3	112.2	115.3	118.9	122.4	125.6	127.5	128.7
79.5	0.92133	119.3977	0.04413	109.5	110.8	112.7	115.8	119.4	123.0	126.2	128.1	129.3
80.5	0.88751	119.9272	0.04418	110.0	111.2	113.2	116.4	119.9	123.5	126.7	128.7	129.9
81.5	0.85358	120.4554	0.04424	110.5	111.7	113.7	116.9	120.5	124.1	127.3	129.3	130.5
82.5	0.81976	120.9821	0.04430	111.0	112.2	114.1	117.4	121.0	124.6	127.9	129.9	131.1
83.5	0.78625	121.5072	0.04435	111.5	112.7	114.6	117.9	121.5	125.2	128.5	130.4	131.7
84.5	0.75324	122.0305	0.04440	111.9	113.2	115.1	118.4	122.0	125.7	129.0	131.0	132.3
85.5	0.72094	122.5520	0.04446	112.4	113.7	115.6	118.9	122.6	126.2	129.6	131.6	132.9
86.5	0.68952	123.0714	0.04451	112.9	114.2	116.1	119.4	123.1	126.8	130.2	132.2	133.5
87.5	0.65914	123.5886	0.04457	113.4	114.6	116.6	119.9	123.6	127.3	130.7	132.8	134.1
88.5	0.63000	124.1035	0.04462	113.9	115.1	117.1	120.4	124.1	127.9	131.3	133.3	134.7
89.5	0.60220	124.6160	0.04468	114.3	115.6	117.6	120.9	124.6	128.4	131.8	133.9	135.3
90.5	0.57591	125.1259	0.04474	114.8	116.1	118.0	121.4	125.1	128.9	132.4	134.5	135.8
91.5	0.55123	125.6331	0.04480	115.2	116.5	118.5	121.9	125.6	129.5	132.9	135.0	136.4
92.5	0.52828	126.1374	0.04486	115.7	117.0	119.0	122.3	126.1	130.0	133.5	135.6	137.0
93.5	0.50714	126.6388	0.04492	116.2	117.5	119.5	122.8	126.6	130.5	134.0	136.2	137.6
94.5	0.48790	127.1370	0.04499	116.6	117.9	119.9	123.3	127.1	131.0	134.6	136.7	138.1
95.5	0.47059	127.6320	0.04506	117.1	118.4	120.4	123.8	127.6	131.5	135.1	137.3	138.7

Table V.8b.

LMS parameters and smoothed percentiles of stature (cm)-for-age in months for boys from 2 to 20 years

Age Group (months)	L	M	S	Percentiles 3rd	5th	10th	25th	50th	75th	90th	95th	97th
96.5	0.45527	128.1237	0.04513	117.5	118.8	120.8	124.3	128.1	132.1	135.7	137.8	139.3
97.5	0.44195	128.6119	0.04520	117.9	119.2	121.3	124.7	128.6	132.6	136.2	138.4	139.8
98.5	0.43063	129.0966	0.04528	118.4	119.7	121.7	125.2	129.1	133.1	136.7	138.9	140.4
99.5	0.42129	129.5777	0.04536	118.8	120.1	122.2	125.6	129.6	133.6	137.2	139.5	140.9
100.5	0.41391	130.0550	0.04544	119.2	120.5	122.6	126.1	130.1	134.1	137.8	140.0	141.5
101.5	0.40843	130.5286	0.04553	119.6	121.0	123.0	126.6	130.5	134.6	138.3	140.5	142.0
102.5	0.40478	130.9983	0.04562	120.0	121.4	123.5	127.0	131.0	135.1	138.8	141.0	142.5
103.5	0.40288	131.4641	0.04571	120.5	121.8	123.9	127.4	131.5	135.6	139.3	141.6	143.1
104.5	0.40263	131.9260	0.04581	120.9	122.2	124.3	127.9	131.9	136.0	139.8	142.1	143.6
105.5	0.40391	132.3840	0.04591	121.2	122.6	124.7	128.3	132.4	136.5	140.3	142.6	144.1
106.5	0.40661	132.8381	0.04601	121.6	123.0	125.1	128.8	132.8	137.0	140.8	143.1	144.6
107.5	0.41058	133.2882	0.04611	122.0	123.4	125.5	129.2	133.3	137.5	141.3	143.6	145.1
108.5	0.41569	133.7345	0.04622	122.4	123.8	126.0	129.6	133.7	137.9	141.8	144.1	145.7
109.5	0.42177	134.1769	0.04633	122.8	124.2	126.3	130.0	134.2	138.4	142.3	144.6	146.2
110.5	0.42866	134.6155	0.04644	123.2	124.6	126.7	130.4	134.6	138.9	142.8	145.1	146.7
111.5	0.43621	135.0504	0.04655	123.5	124.9	127.1	130.8	135.1	139.3	143.2	145.6	147.2
112.5	0.44423	135.4818	0.04666	123.9	125.3	127.5	131.3	135.5	139.8	143.7	146.1	147.7
113.5	0.45256	135.9097	0.04678	124.2	125.7	127.9	131.7	135.9	140.2	144.2	146.6	148.2
114.5	0.46103	136.3343	0.04690	124.6	126.0	128.3	132.1	136.3	140.7	144.7	147.1	148.6
115.5	0.46947	136.7557	0.04701	124.9	126.4	128.6	132.5	136.8	141.1	145.1	147.5	149.1
116.5	0.47770	137.1742	0.04713	125.3	126.8	129.0	132.8	137.2	141.6	145.6	148.0	149.6
117.5	0.48558	137.5899	0.04725	125.6	127.1	129.4	133.2	137.6	142.0	146.1	148.5	150.1
118.5	0.49295	138.0032	0.04737	126.0	127.5	129.8	133.6	138.0	142.4	146.5	149.0	150.6
119.5	0.49965	138.4143	0.04749	126.3	127.8	130.1	134.0	138.4	142.9	147.0	149.4	151.1
120.5	0.50556	138.8234	0.04761	126.7	128.2	130.5	134.4	138.8	143.3	147.4	149.9	151.5
121.5	0.51056	139.2310	0.04773	127.0	128.5	130.8	134.8	139.2	143.7	147.9	150.4	152.0
122.5	0.51453	139.6373	0.04785	127.3	128.9	131.2	135.2	139.6	144.2	148.3	150.8	152.5
123.5	0.51738	140.0427	0.04796	127.7	129.2	131.6	135.5	140.0	144.6	148.8	151.3	153.0
124.5	0.51904	140.4477	0.04808	128.0	129.6	131.9	135.9	140.4	145.0	149.2	151.8	153.4
125.5	0.51945	140.8527	0.04819	128.4	129.9	132.3	136.3	140.9	145.5	149.7	152.2	153.9
126.5	0.51859	141.2582	0.04830	128.7	130.2	132.6	136.7	141.3	145.9	150.1	152.7	154.4
127.5	0.51643	141.6646	0.04841	129.0	130.6	133.0	137.1	141.7	146.3	150.6	153.2	154.8
128.5	0.51301	142.0725	0.04852	129.4	131.0	133.4	137.5	142.1	146.8	151.0	153.6	155.3
129.5	0.50835	142.4824	0.04863	129.7	131.3	133.7	137.8	142.5	147.2	151.5	154.1	155.8
130.5	0.50255	142.8949	0.04874	130.1	131.7	134.1	138.2	142.9	147.6	152.0	154.6	156.3
131.5	0.49570	143.3107	0.04884	130.5	132.0	134.5	138.6	143.3	148.1	152.4	155.1	156.8
132.5	0.48794	143.7304	0.04894	130.8	132.4	134.9	139.0	143.7	148.5	152.9	155.5	157.3
133.5	0.47945	144.1545	0.04904	131.2	132.8	135.2	139.4	144.2	149.0	153.4	156.0	157.8
134.5	0.47044	144.5838	0.04913	131.5	133.1	135.6	139.8	144.6	149.4	153.8	156.5	158.3
135.5	0.46115	145.0190	0.04922	131.9	133.5	136.0	140.2	145.0	149.9	154.3	157.0	158.8
136.5	0.45186	145.4607	0.04931	132.3	133.9	136.4	140.7	145.5	150.3	154.8	157.5	159.3
137.5	0.44289	145.9097	0.04940	132.7	134.3	136.8	141.1	145.9	150.8	155.3	158.0	159.8
138.5	0.43458	146.3665	0.04949	133.1	134.7	137.2	141.5	146.4	151.3	155.8	158.6	160.4
139.5	0.42730	146.8320	0.04957	133.5	135.1	137.7	142.0	146.8	151.8	156.3	159.1	160.9
140.5	0.42146	147.3066	0.04965	133.9	135.6	138.1	142.4	147.3	152.3	156.9	159.6	161.4
141.5	0.41748	147.7911	0.04973	134.3	136.0	138.5	142.9	147.8	152.8	157.4	160.2	162.0
142.5	0.41577	148.2859	0.04981	134.8	136.4	139.0	143.4	148.3	153.3	157.9	160.7	162.6
143.5	0.41678	148.7917	0.04988	135.2	136.9	139.5	143.8	148.8	153.8	158.5	161.3	163.1
144.5	0.42092	149.3088	0.04995	135.7	137.3	139.9	144.3	149.3	154.4	159.0	161.9	163.7
145.5	0.42861	149.8376	0.05001	136.1	137.8	140.4	144.8	149.8	154.9	159.6	162.5	164.3
146.5	0.44022	150.3784	0.05008	136.6	138.3	140.9	145.3	150.4	155.5	160.2	163.1	164.9
147.5	0.45610	150.9313	0.05013	137.1	138.8	141.4	145.9	150.9	156.1	160.8	163.7	165.5
148.5	0.47654	151.4964	0.05019	137.5	139.3	141.9	146.4	151.5	156.7	161.4	164.3	166.1
149.5	0.50177	152.0735	0.05023	138.0	139.8	142.4	147.0	152.1	157.3	162.0	164.9	166.8
150.5	0.53195	152.6624	0.05027	138.5	140.3	143.0	147.5	152.7	157.9	162.6	165.5	167.4
151.5	0.56718	153.2627	0.05031	139.1	140.8	143.5	148.1	153.3	158.5	163.3	166.2	168.1
152.5	0.60746	153.8738	0.05033	139.6	141.3	144.1	148.7	153.9	159.1	163.9	166.8	168.7
153.5	0.65270	154.4951	0.05035	140.1	141.9	144.6	149.3	154.5	159.8	164.6	167.5	169.4
154.5	0.70276	155.1255	0.05036	140.6	142.4	145.2	149.9	155.1	160.4	165.2	168.1	170.0
155.5	0.75738	155.7642	0.05035	141.2	143.0	145.8	150.5	155.8	161.1	165.9	168.8	170.7
156.5	0.81624	156.4099	0.05033	141.7	143.6	146.4	151.1	156.4	161.7	166.6	169.5	171.3
157.5	0.87895	157.0612	0.05030	142.3	144.1	147.0	151.7	157.1	162.4	167.2	170.1	172.0
158.5	0.94505	157.7168	0.05026	142.8	144.7	147.6	152.4	157.7	163.1	167.9	170.8	172.7
159.5	1.01405	158.3751	0.05020	143.4	145.3	148.2	153.0	158.4	163.7	168.6	171.4	173.3
160.5	1.08538	159.0344	0.05013	144.0	145.9	148.8	153.6	159.0	164.4	169.2	172.1	174.0
161.5	1.15849	159.6931	0.05003	144.5	146.5	149.4	154.3	159.7	165.1	169.9	172.8	174.6
162.5	1.23277	160.3493	0.04993	145.1	147.0	150.0	154.9	160.3	165.7	170.5	173.4	175.2
163.5	1.30763	161.0015	0.04980	145.7	147.6	150.6	155.6	161.0	166.4	171.2	174.0	175.9
164.5	1.38247	161.6478	0.04966	146.3	148.2	151.2	156.2	161.6	167.0	171.8	174.7	176.5
165.5	1.45672	162.2865	0.04951	146.8	148.8	151.8	156.8	162.3	167.7	172.4	175.3	177.1
166.5	1.52981	162.9161	0.04933	147.4	149.4	152.4	157.4	162.9	168.3	173.1	175.9	177.7
167.5	1.60122	163.5350	0.04915	148.0	150.0	153.0	158.1	163.5	168.9	173.6	176.5	178.3
168.5	1.67043	164.1418	0.04895	148.5	150.5	153.6	158.7	164.1	169.5	174.2	177.0	178.8
169.5	1.73700	164.7352	0.04873	149.1	151.1	154.2	159.3	164.7	170.1	174.8	177.6	179.4

221

Table V.8c.
LMS parameters and smoothed percentiles of stature (cm)-for-age in months for boys from 2 to 20 years

Age Group (months)	L	M	S	Percentiles								
				3rd	5th	10th	25th	50th	75th	90th	95th	97th
170.5	1.80048	165.3140	0.04850	149.6	151.7	154.8	159.8	165.3	170.7	175.3	178.1	179.9
171.5	1.86052	165.8771	0.04827	150.2	152.2	155.3	160.4	165.9	171.2	175.9	178.6	180.4
172.5	1.91677	166.4236	0.04802	150.7	152.8	155.9	161.0	166.4	171.7	176.4	179.1	180.9
173.5	1.96893	166.9528	0.04777	151.2	153.3	156.4	161.5	167.0	172.3	176.9	179.6	181.4
174.5	2.01678	167.4641	0.04751	151.8	153.8	156.9	162.0	167.5	172.7	177.4	180.1	181.8
175.5	2.0601	167.9571	0.0472	152.3	154.3	157.4	162.5	168.0	173.2	177.8	180.5	182.2
176.5	2.0988	168.4313	0.0470	152.8	154.8	157.9	163.0	168.4	173.7	178.3	180.9	182.7
177.5	2.1326	168.8867	0.0467	153.2	155.3	158.4	163.5	168.9	174.1	178.7	181.3	183.0
178.5	2.1617	169.3231	0.0464	153.7	155.8	158.9	163.9	169.3	174.5	179.1	181.7	183.4
179.5	2.1858	169.7405	0.0462	154.2	156.2	159.3	164.4	169.7	174.9	179.5	182.1	183.8
180.5	2.2052	170.1393	0.0459	154.6	156.7	159.8	164.8	170.1	175.3	179.8	182.4	184.1
181.5	2.2197	170.5195	0.0456	155.0	157.1	160.2	165.2	170.5	175.7	180.2	182.8	184.5
182.5	2.22959	170.8815	0.04536	155.5	157.5	160.6	165.6	170.9	176.0	180.5	183.1	184.8
183.5	2.23491	171.2257	0.04510	155.9	157.9	160.9	165.9	171.2	176.3	180.8	183.4	185.1
184.5	2.23583	171.5525	0.04485	156.2	158.3	161.3	166.3	171.6	176.6	181.1	183.7	185.3
185.5	2.23257	171.8626	0.04460	156.6	158.6	161.7	166.6	171.9	176.9	181.4	183.9	185.6
186.5	2.22533	172.1563	0.04436	157.0	159.0	162.0	166.9	172.2	177.2	181.6	184.2	185.8
187.5	2.21435	172.4343	0.04413	157.3	159.3	162.3	167.2	172.4	177.5	181.9	184.4	186.1
188.5	2.19991	172.6972	0.04390	157.7	159.6	162.6	167.5	172.7	177.7	182.1	184.7	186.3
189.5	2.18226	172.9456	0.04369	158.0	159.9	162.9	167.8	172.9	178.0	182.3	184.9	186.5
190.5	2.16170	173.1801	0.04348	158.3	160.2	163.2	168.0	173.2	178.2	182.5	185.1	186.7
191.5	2.13852	173.4014	0.04328	158.6	160.5	163.5	168.3	173.4	178.4	182.7	185.3	186.9
192.5	2.11302	173.6101	0.04309	158.8	160.8	163.7	168.5	173.6	178.6	182.9	185.5	187.1
193.5	2.08549	173.8067	0.04290	159.1	161.0	163.9	168.7	173.8	178.8	183.1	185.6	187.3
194.5	2.05622	173.9920	0.04273	159.4	161.3	164.2	168.9	174.0	178.9	183.3	185.8	187.4
195.5	2.02550	174.1665	0.04256	159.6	161.5	164.4	169.1	174.2	179.1	183.4	185.9	187.6
196.5	1.99360	174.3308	0.04240	159.8	161.7	164.6	169.3	174.3	179.2	183.6	186.1	187.7
197.5	1.96079	174.4854	0.04225	160.0	161.9	164.8	169.4	174.5	179.4	183.7	186.2	187.9
198.5	1.92732	174.6310	0.04211	160.3	162.1	165.0	169.6	174.6	179.5	183.8	186.4	188.0
199.5	1.89343	174.7680	0.04197	160.4	162.3	165.1	169.8	174.8	179.7	184.0	186.5	188.1
200.5	1.85934	174.8969	0.04185	160.6	162.5	165.3	169.9	174.9	179.8	184.1	186.6	188.2
201.5	1.82525	175.0182	0.04173	160.8	162.6	165.4	170.0	175.0	179.9	184.2	186.7	188.3
202.5	1.79134	175.1323	0.04161	161.0	162.8	165.6	170.2	175.1	180.0	184.3	186.8	188.4
203.5	1.75779	175.2398	0.04151	161.1	162.9	165.7	170.3	175.2	180.1	184.4	186.9	188.5
204.5	1.72474	175.3410	0.04141	161.3	163.1	165.8	170.4	175.3	180.2	184.5	187.0	188.6
205.5	1.69232	175.4362	0.04132	161.4	163.2	166.0	170.5	175.4	180.3	184.6	187.1	188.7
206.5	1.66066	175.5259	0.04123	161.5	163.3	166.1	170.6	175.5	180.4	184.6	187.2	188.8
207.5	1.62985	175.6104	0.04115	161.7	163.5	166.2	170.7	175.6	180.4	184.7	187.3	188.9
208.5	1.59996	175.6901	0.04107	161.8	163.6	166.3	170.8	175.7	180.5	184.8	187.3	189.0
209.5	1.57108	175.7652	0.04100	161.9	163.7	166.4	170.9	175.8	180.6	184.9	187.4	189.0
210.5	1.54325	175.8360	0.04094	162.0	163.8	166.5	170.9	175.8	180.7	184.9	187.5	189.1
211.5	1.51652	175.9028	0.04088	162.1	163.9	166.6	171.0	175.9	180.7	185.0	187.5	189.2
212.5	1.49091	175.9658	0.04082	162.2	163.9	166.6	171.1	176.0	180.8	185.1	187.6	189.2
213.5	1.46645	176.0254	0.04077	162.3	164.0	166.7	171.2	176.0	180.8	185.1	187.7	189.3
214.5	1.44315	176.0816	0.04073	162.4	164.1	166.8	171.2	176.1	180.9	185.2	187.7	189.4
215.5	1.42100	176.1348	0.04068	162.4	164.2	166.8	171.3	176.1	180.9	185.2	187.8	189.4
216.5	1.40000	176.1850	0.04064	162.5	164.2	166.9	171.3	176.2	181.0	185.3	187.8	189.5
217.5	1.38014	176.2326	0.04061	162.6	164.3	167.0	171.4	176.2	181.0	185.3	187.9	189.5
218.5	1.36140	176.2776	0.04058	162.6	164.4	167.0	171.4	176.3	181.1	185.4	187.9	189.6
219.5	1.34376	176.3202	0.04055	162.7	164.4	167.1	171.5	176.3	181.1	185.4	187.9	189.6
220.5	1.32720	176.3606	0.04052	162.7	164.5	167.1	171.5	176.4	181.2	185.4	188.0	189.6
221.5	1.31167	176.3989	0.04050	162.8	164.5	167.2	171.6	176.4	181.2	185.5	188.0	189.7
222.5	1.29715	176.4352	0.04047	162.8	164.6	167.2	171.6	176.4	181.2	185.5	188.1	189.7
223.5	1.28360	176.4697	0.04046	162.9	164.6	167.3	171.6	176.5	181.3	185.6	188.1	189.8
224.5	1.27099	176.5024	0.04044	162.9	164.7	167.3	171.7	176.5	181.3	185.6	188.1	189.8
225.5	1.25928	176.5335	0.04042	163.0	164.7	167.3	171.7	176.5	181.3	185.6	188.2	189.8
226.5	1.24844	176.5630	0.04041	163.0	164.7	167.4	171.7	176.6	181.4	185.6	188.2	189.9
227.5	1.23841	176.5911	0.04040	163.0	164.8	167.4	171.8	176.6	181.4	185.7	188.2	189.9
228.5	1.22916	176.6179	0.04039	163.1	164.8	167.4	171.8	176.6	181.4	185.7	188.3	189.9
229.5	1.22066	176.6433	0.04038	163.1	164.8	167.4	171.8	176.6	181.4	185.7	188.3	190.0
230.5	1.21287	176.6676	0.04038	163.1	164.8	167.5	171.8	176.7	181.5	185.8	188.3	190.0
231.5	1.20574	176.6907	0.04037	163.2	164.9	167.5	171.9	176.7	181.5	185.8	188.3	190.0
232.5	1.19925	176.7127	0.04037	163.2	164.9	167.5	171.9	176.7	181.5	185.8	188.4	190.0
233.5	1.19335	176.7337	0.04037	163.2	164.9	167.5	171.9	176.7	181.5	185.8	188.4	190.1
234.5	1.18802	176.7538	0.04036	163.2	164.9	167.6	171.9	176.8	181.6	185.9	188.4	190.1
235.5	1.18321	176.7730	0.04036	163.3	165.0	167.6	171.9	176.8	181.6	185.9	188.4	190.1
236.5	1.17890	176.7913	0.04036	163.3	165.0	167.6	172.0	176.8	181.6	185.9	188.5	190.1
237.5	1.17506	176.8088	0.04036	163.3	165.0	167.6	172.0	176.8	181.6	185.9	188.5	190.1
238.5	1.17164	176.8255	0.04037	163.3	165.0	167.6	172.0	176.8	181.6	185.9	188.5	190.2
239.5	1.16864	176.8415	0.04037	163.3	165.0	167.7	172.0	176.8	181.6	186.0	188.5	190.2
240.0	1.16728	176.8492	0.04037	163.3	165.0	167.7	172.0	176.8	181.7	186.0	188.5	190.2
240.0	1.16728	176.8492	0.04037	163.3	165.0	167.7	172.0	176.8	181.7	186.0	188.5	190.2

Table V.9a.

LMS parameters and smoothed percentiles of stature (cm)-for-age in months for girls from 2 to 20 years

Age Group (months)	L	M	S	3rd	5th	10th	25th	50th	75th	90th	95th	97th
24.0	1.0724	84.9756	0.0408	78.4	79.3	80.5	82.6	85.0	87.3	89.4	90.7	91.5
24.5	1.0513	85.3973	0.0409	78.8	79.6	80.9	83.0	85.4	87.7	89.9	91.1	91.9
25.5	1.0420	86.2903	0.0411	79.6	80.4	81.7	83.9	86.3	88.7	90.8	92.1	93.0
26.5	1.0126	87.1571	0.0413	80.4	81.2	82.5	84.7	87.2	89.6	91.8	93.1	93.9
27.5	0.9705	87.9960	0.0415	81.1	82.0	83.3	85.5	88.0	90.5	92.7	94.0	94.9
28.5	0.9211	88.8055	0.0416	81.9	82.7	84.1	86.3	88.8	91.3	93.6	94.9	95.8
29.5	0.8682	89.5848	0.0417	82.6	83.5	84.8	87.1	89.6	92.1	94.4	95.8	96.6
30.5	0.8145	90.3334	0.0418	83.3	84.2	85.5	87.8	90.3	92.9	95.2	96.6	97.5
31.5	0.7620	91.0515	0.0418	84.0	84.8	86.2	88.5	91.1	93.6	96.0	97.4	98.3
32.5	0.7117	91.7396	0.0418	84.6	85.5	86.9	89.2	91.7	94.3	96.7	98.1	99.0
33.5	0.6643	92.3985	0.0419	85.2	86.1	87.5	89.8	92.4	95.0	97.4	98.8	99.8
34.5	0.6203	93.0295	0.0419	85.8	86.7	88.1	90.4	93.0	95.7	98.1	99.5	100.5
35.5	0.5796	93.6338	0.0420	86.4	87.3	88.7	91.0	93.6	96.3	98.7	100.2	101.1
36.5	0.5420	94.2134	0.0420	86.9	87.8	89.2	91.6	94.2	96.9	99.3	100.8	101.8
37.5	0.5114	94.7964	0.0421	87.4	88.3	89.7	92.1	94.8	97.5	100.0	101.5	102.4
38.5	0.4828	95.3739	0.0422	88.0	88.9	90.3	92.7	95.4	98.1	100.6	102.1	103.1
39.5	0.4555	95.9469	0.0423	88.5	89.4	90.8	93.2	95.9	98.7	101.2	102.7	103.7
40.5	0.4292	96.5164	0.0424	89.0	89.9	91.4	93.8	96.5	99.3	101.8	103.4	104.4
41.5	0.4034	97.0834	0.0425	89.5	90.4	91.9	94.3	97.1	99.9	102.5	104.0	105.0
42.5	0.3779	97.6485	0.0426	90.0	91.0	92.4	94.9	97.6	100.5	103.1	104.6	105.7
43.5	0.3526	98.2125	0.0427	90.5	91.5	92.9	95.4	98.2	101.1	103.7	105.3	106.3
44.5	0.3273	98.7759	0.0428	91.0	92.0	93.5	95.9	98.8	101.7	104.3	105.9	107.0
45.5	0.3020	99.3394	0.0429	91.5	92.5	94.0	96.5	99.3	102.2	104.9	106.5	107.6
46.5	0.2766	99.9033	0.0431	92.0	93.0	94.5	97.0	99.9	102.8	105.5	107.2	108.2
47.5	0.2512	100.4681	0.0432	92.6	93.5	95.0	97.6	100.5	103.4	106.1	107.8	108.9
48.5	0.2257	101.0339	0.0433	93.1	94.0	95.6	98.1	101.0	104.0	106.8	108.4	109.5
49.5	0.2003	101.6012	0.0434	93.6	94.6	96.1	98.7	101.6	104.6	107.4	109.1	110.2
50.5	0.1749	102.1700	0.0435	94.1	95.1	96.6	99.2	102.2	105.2	108.0	109.7	110.8
51.5	0.1497	102.7406	0.0436	94.6	95.6	97.1	99.8	102.7	105.8	108.6	110.3	111.5
52.5	0.1247	103.3130	0.0436	95.1	96.1	97.7	100.3	103.3	106.4	109.2	111.0	112.1
53.5	0.1000	103.8873	0.0437	95.7	96.7	98.2	100.9	103.9	107.0	109.9	111.6	112.8
54.5	0.0757	104.4635	0.0438	96.2	97.2	98.7	101.4	104.5	107.6	110.5	112.2	113.4
55.5	0.0518	105.0415	0.0439	96.7	97.7	99.3	102.0	105.0	108.2	111.1	112.9	114.1
56.5	0.0285	105.6213	0.0440	97.2	98.2	99.8	102.5	105.6	108.8	111.7	113.5	114.7
57.5	0.0059	106.2029	0.0441	97.8	98.8	100.4	103.1	106.2	109.4	112.4	114.2	115.4
58.5	-0.0161	106.7861	0.0441	98.3	99.3	100.9	103.7	106.8	110.0	113.0	114.8	116.0
59.5	-0.0374	107.3707	0.0442	98.8	99.9	101.5	104.2	107.4	110.6	113.6	115.5	116.7
60.5	-0.0577	107.9566	0.0443	99.4	100.4	102.0	104.8	108.0	111.2	114.3	116.1	117.4
61.5	-0.0772	108.5436	0.0443	99.9	100.9	102.6	105.3	108.5	111.8	114.9	116.8	118.0
62.5	-0.0957	109.1316	0.0444	100.4	101.5	103.1	105.9	109.1	112.5	115.5	117.4	118.7
63.5	-0.1132	109.7202	0.0445	101.0	102.0	103.7	106.5	109.7	113.1	116.2	118.1	119.3
64.5	-0.1297	110.3092	0.0445	101.5	102.6	104.2	107.1	110.3	113.7	116.8	118.7	120.0
65.5	-0.1450	110.8984	0.0446	102.0	103.1	104.8	107.6	110.9	114.3	117.4	119.4	120.7
66.5	-0.1592	111.4876	0.0447	102.6	103.6	105.3	108.2	111.5	114.9	118.1	120.0	121.3
67.5	-0.1722	112.0764	0.0447	103.1	104.2	105.9	108.8	112.1	115.5	118.7	120.7	122.0
68.5	-0.1840	112.6646	0.0448	103.6	104.7	106.4	109.3	112.7	116.1	119.4	121.3	122.6
69.5	-0.1947	113.2519	0.0448	104.2	105.3	107.0	109.9	113.3	116.7	120.0	122.0	123.3
70.5	-0.2040	113.8380	0.0449	104.7	105.8	107.5	110.5	113.8	117.3	120.6	122.6	124.0
71.5	-0.2122	114.4226	0.0449	105.2	106.3	108.1	111.0	114.4	118.0	121.2	123.3	124.6
72.5	-0.2191	115.0055	0.0450	105.8	106.9	108.6	111.6	115.0	118.6	121.9	123.9	125.3
73.5	-0.2247	115.5863	0.0450	106.3	107.4	109.1	112.1	115.6	119.2	122.5	124.5	125.9
74.5	-0.2291	116.1648	0.0451	106.8	107.9	109.7	112.7	116.2	119.8	123.1	125.2	126.5
75.5	-0.2323	116.7406	0.0451	107.3	108.5	110.2	113.3	116.7	120.4	123.7	125.8	127.2
76.5	-0.2343	117.3136	0.0451	107.9	109.0	110.8	113.8	117.3	121.0	124.3	126.4	127.8
77.5	-0.2351	117.8833	0.0452	108.4	109.5	111.3	114.4	117.9	121.5	125.0	127.1	128.4
78.5	-0.2348	118.4496	0.0452	108.9	110.0	111.8	114.9	118.4	122.1	125.6	127.7	129.1
79.5	-0.2333	119.0123	0.0453	109.4	110.5	112.3	115.4	119.0	122.7	126.2	128.3	129.7
80.5	-0.2307	119.5710	0.0453	109.9	111.1	112.9	116.0	119.6	123.3	126.8	128.9	130.3
81.5	-0.2271	120.1254	0.0453	110.4	111.6	113.4	116.5	120.1	123.9	127.4	129.5	130.9
82.5	-0.2224	120.6755	0.0454	110.9	112.1	113.9	117.0	120.7	124.4	128.0	130.1	131.5
83.5	-0.2168	121.2210	0.0454	111.4	112.6	114.4	117.6	121.2	125.0	128.5	130.7	132.1
84.5	-0.2102	121.7617	0.0455	111.9	113.1	114.9	118.1	121.8	125.6	129.1	131.3	132.7
85.5	-0.2028	122.2974	0.0455	112.3	113.5	115.4	118.6	122.3	126.1	129.7	131.9	133.3
86.5	-0.1945	122.8279	0.0455	112.8	114.0	115.9	119.1	122.8	126.7	130.3	132.5	133.9
87.5	-0.1855	123.3531	0.0456	113.3	114.5	116.4	119.6	123.4	127.2	130.8	133.0	134.5
88.5	-0.1757	123.8728	0.0456	113.8	115.0	116.9	120.1	123.9	127.8	131.4	133.6	135.1
89.5	-0.1653	124.3870	0.0457	114.2	115.4	117.4	120.6	124.4	128.3	131.9	134.2	135.6
90.5	-0.1544	124.8956	0.0457	114.7	115.9	117.8	121.1	124.9	128.8	132.5	134.7	136.2
91.5	-0.1428	125.3985	0.0457	115.1	116.4	118.3	121.6	125.4	129.3	133.0	135.3	136.7
92.5	-0.1308	125.8956	0.0458	115.6	116.8	118.7	122.1	125.9	129.9	133.5	135.8	137.3
93.5	-0.1184	126.3869	0.0458	116.0	117.3	119.2	122.5	126.4	130.4	134.1	136.3	137.8
94.5	-0.1056	126.8724	0.0459	116.4	117.7	119.7	123.0	126.9	130.9	134.6	136.9	138.4
95.5	-0.0926	127.3522	0.0459	116.9	118.1	120.1	123.5	127.4	131.4	135.1	137.4	138.9

Table V.9b.
LMS parameters and smoothed percentiles of stature (cm)-for-age in months for girls from 2 to 20 years

Age Group (months)	L	M	S	Percentiles 3rd	5th	10th	25th	50th	75th	90th	95th	97th
96.5	-0.0793	127.8263	0.0460	117.3	118.5	120.5	123.9	127.8	131.9	135.6	137.9	139.4
97.5	-0.0658	128.2947	0.0460	117.7	119.0	121.0	124.4	128.3	132.3	136.1	138.4	139.9
98.5	-0.0522	128.7576	0.0461	118.1	119.4	121.4	124.8	128.8	132.8	136.6	138.9	140.4
99.5	-0.0385	129.2152	0.0461	118.5	119.8	121.8	125.3	129.2	133.3	137.1	139.4	140.9
100.5	-0.0247	129.6675	0.0462	118.9	120.2	122.2	125.7	129.7	133.8	137.6	139.9	141.5
101.5	-0.0110	130.1148	0.0463	119.3	120.6	122.6	126.1	130.1	134.2	138.1	140.4	142.0
102.5	0.0027	130.5574	0.0463	119.7	121.0	123.0	126.5	130.6	134.7	138.5	140.9	142.4
103.5	0.0164	130.9954	0.0464	120.0	121.4	123.4	127.0	131.0	135.2	139.0	141.4	142.9
104.5	0.0301	131.4293	0.0465	120.4	121.7	123.8	127.4	131.4	135.6	139.5	141.9	143.4
105.5	0.0436	131.8593	0.0466	120.8	122.1	124.2	127.8	131.9	136.1	140.0	142.3	143.9
106.5	0.0571	132.2859	0.0467	121.1	122.5	124.6	128.2	132.3	136.5	140.4	142.8	144.4
107.5	0.0706	132.7094	0.0468	121.5	122.9	125.0	128.6	132.7	137.0	140.9	143.3	144.9
108.5	0.0841	133.1304	0.0469	121.9	123.2	125.3	129.0	133.1	137.4	141.4	143.8	145.4
109.5	0.0977	133.5493	0.0470	122.2	123.6	125.7	129.4	133.5	137.8	141.8	144.2	145.8
110.5	0.1115	133.9667	0.0471	122.6	123.9	126.1	129.8	134.0	138.3	142.3	144.7	146.3
111.5	0.1254	134.3832	0.0472	122.9	124.3	126.5	130.2	134.4	138.7	142.7	145.2	146.8
112.5	0.1397	134.7995	0.0474	123.2	124.6	126.8	130.6	134.8	139.2	143.2	145.7	147.3
113.5	0.1544	135.2163	0.0475	123.6	125.0	127.2	130.9	135.2	139.6	143.7	146.1	147.8
114.5	0.1698	135.6342	0.0477	123.9	125.3	127.6	131.3	135.6	140.1	144.1	146.6	148.3
115.5	0.1859	136.0540	0.0478	124.3	125.7	127.9	131.7	136.1	140.5	144.6	147.1	148.7
116.5	0.2030	136.4766	0.0480	124.6	126.0	128.3	132.1	136.5	141.0	145.1	147.6	149.2
117.5	0.2212	136.9027	0.0482	124.9	126.4	128.7	132.5	136.9	141.4	145.6	148.1	149.7
118.5	0.2408	137.3333	0.0483	125.3	126.7	129.0	132.9	137.3	141.9	146.0	148.6	150.3
119.5	0.2619	137.7691	0.0485	125.6	127.1	129.4	133.3	137.8	142.3	146.5	149.1	150.8
120.5	0.2847	138.2112	0.0487	126.0	127.5	129.8	133.7	138.2	142.8	147.0	149.6	151.3
121.5	0.3096	138.6602	0.0489	126.3	127.8	130.2	134.1	138.7	143.3	147.5	150.1	151.8
122.5	0.3366	139.1172	0.0491	126.7	128.2	130.5	134.6	139.1	143.8	148.1	150.7	152.4
123.5	0.3659	139.5829	0.0493	127.0	128.6	130.9	135.0	139.6	144.3	148.6	151.2	152.9
124.5	0.3977	140.0581	0.0495	127.4	128.9	131.3	135.4	140.1	144.8	149.1	151.7	153.5
125.5	0.4321	140.5435	0.0496	127.8	129.3	131.8	135.9	140.5	145.3	149.6	152.3	154.0
126.5	0.4692	141.0397	0.0498	128.2	129.7	132.2	136.3	141.0	145.8	150.2	152.8	154.6
127.5	0.5089	141.5472	0.0500	128.5	130.1	132.6	136.8	141.5	146.4	150.8	153.4	155.2
128.5	0.5514	142.0664	0.0501	129.0	130.6	133.1	137.3	142.1	146.9	151.3	154.0	155.7
129.5	0.5963	142.5974	0.0503	129.4	131.0	133.5	137.8	142.6	147.5	151.9	154.6	156.3
130.5	0.6436	143.1404	0.0504	129.8	131.5	134.0	138.3	143.1	148.0	152.5	155.2	156.9
131.5	0.6931	143.6950	0.0505	130.3	131.9	134.5	138.8	143.7	148.6	153.1	155.8	157.5
132.5	0.7443	144.2609	0.0505	130.7	132.4	135.0	139.4	144.3	149.2	153.7	156.4	158.1
133.5	0.7969	144.8376	0.0506	131.2	132.9	135.5	139.9	144.8	149.8	154.3	157.0	158.7
134.5	0.8505	145.4240	0.0506	131.7	133.4	136.0	140.5	145.4	150.4	154.9	157.6	159.3
135.5	0.9044	146.0192	0.0505	132.2	133.9	136.6	141.1	146.0	151.0	155.5	158.2	160.0
136.5	0.9581	146.6217	0.0505	132.7	134.5	137.2	141.6	146.6	151.6	156.1	158.8	160.6
137.5	1.0111	147.2300	0.0504	133.3	135.0	137.7	142.2	147.2	152.2	156.7	159.4	161.2
138.5	1.0625	147.8424	0.0502	133.8	135.6	138.3	142.8	147.8	152.8	157.3	160.0	161.8
139.5	1.1117	148.4569	0.0500	134.4	136.2	138.9	143.4	148.5	153.5	157.9	160.6	162.4
140.5	1.1581	149.0714	0.0498	135.0	136.8	139.5	144.1	149.1	154.1	158.5	161.2	162.9
141.5	1.2011	149.6839	0.0496	135.6	137.4	140.1	144.7	149.7	154.7	159.1	161.8	163.5
142.5	1.2399	150.2920	0.0493	136.2	138.0	140.7	145.3	150.3	155.3	159.7	162.4	164.1
143.5	1.2740	150.8936	0.0489	136.8	138.6	141.3	145.9	150.9	155.9	160.3	162.9	164.6
144.5	1.3030	151.4866	0.0486	137.4	139.2	142.0	146.5	151.5	156.4	160.8	163.5	165.2
145.5	1.3266	152.0687	0.0482	138.1	139.8	142.6	147.1	152.1	157.0	161.4	164.0	165.7
146.5	1.3444	152.6381	0.0478	138.7	140.5	143.2	147.7	152.6	157.5	161.9	164.5	166.2
147.5	1.3564	153.1930	0.0474	139.3	141.1	143.8	148.3	153.2	158.1	162.4	165.0	166.7
148.5	1.3626	153.7317	0.0470	139.9	141.7	144.4	148.8	153.7	158.6	162.9	165.5	167.1
149.5	1.3631	154.2529	0.0466	140.5	142.3	144.9	149.4	154.3	159.1	163.4	165.9	167.6
150.5	1.3582	154.7555	0.0462	141.1	142.8	145.5	149.9	154.8	159.6	163.8	166.4	168.0
151.5	1.3482	155.2385	0.0458	141.7	143.4	146.0	150.4	155.2	160.0	164.3	166.8	168.4
152.5	1.3338	155.7012	0.0454	142.2	143.9	146.6	150.9	155.7	160.4	164.7	167.2	168.8
153.5	1.3154	156.1432	0.0450	142.8	144.5	147.1	151.4	156.1	160.9	165.1	167.6	169.2
154.5	1.2937	156.5643	0.0446	143.3	145.0	147.5	151.8	156.6	161.3	165.4	167.9	169.5
155.5	1.2693	156.9644	0.0442	143.8	145.4	148.0	152.3	157.0	161.6	165.8	168.3	169.9
156.5	1.2430	157.3437	0.0439	144.2	145.9	148.4	152.7	157.3	162.0	166.1	168.6	170.2
157.5	1.2153	157.7025	0.0435	144.7	146.3	148.9	153.1	157.7	162.3	166.4	168.9	170.5
158.5	1.1870	158.0411	0.0432	145.1	146.7	149.2	153.4	158.0	162.6	166.7	169.2	170.8
159.5	1.1585	158.3603	0.0429	145.5	147.1	149.6	153.8	158.4	162.9	167.0	169.5	171.1
160.5	1.1304	158.6606	0.0426	145.9	147.5	150.0	154.1	158.7	163.2	167.3	169.7	171.3
161.5	1.1031	158.9427	0.0424	146.2	147.8	150.3	154.4	158.9	163.5	167.5	170.0	171.6
162.5	1.0770	159.2075	0.0421	146.6	148.1	150.6	154.7	159.2	163.7	167.8	170.2	171.8
163.5	1.0523	159.4557	0.0419	146.9	148.4	150.9	154.9	159.5	164.0	168.0	170.4	172.0
164.5	1.0294	159.6882	0.0417	147.2	148.7	151.2	155.2	159.7	164.2	168.2	170.6	172.2
165.5	1.0083	159.9058	0.0415	147.4	149.0	151.4	155.4	159.9	164.4	168.4	170.8	172.4
166.5	0.9891	160.1094	0.0413	147.7	149.2	151.6	155.6	160.1	164.6	168.6	171.0	172.6
167.5	0.9718	160.2997	0.0412	147.9	149.5	151.8	155.9	160.3	164.8	168.8	171.2	172.7
168.5	0.9566	160.4777	0.0410	148.1	149.7	152.1	156.0	160.5	164.9	168.9	171.3	172.9
169.5	0.9432	160.6441	0.0409	148.3	149.9	152.2	156.2	160.6	165.1	169.1	171.5	173.0

224

CDC Growth Standards

Table V.9c.

LMS parameters and smoothed percentiles of stature (cm)-for-age in months for girls from 2 to 20 years

Age Group (months)	L	M	S	3rd	5th	10th	25th	50th	75th	90th	95th	97th
170.5	0.9318	160.7995	0.0408	148.5	150.0	152.4	156.4	160.8	165.2	169.2	171.6	173.2
171.5	0.9221	160.9449	0.0407	148.7	150.2	152.6	156.5	160.9	165.4	169.4	171.7	173.3
172.5	0.9140	161.0808	0.0406	148.8	150.4	152.7	156.7	161.1	165.5	169.5	171.9	173.4
173.5	0.9075	161.2079	0.0405	149.0	150.5	152.9	156.8	161.2	165.6	169.6	172.0	173.5
174.5	0.9025	161.3268	0.0404	149.1	150.6	153.0	156.9	161.3	165.7	169.7	172.1	173.6
175.5	0.8987	161.4381	0.0403	149.2	150.8	153.1	157.1	161.4	165.8	169.8	172.2	173.7
176.5	0.8961	161.5423	0.0403	149.4	150.9	153.2	157.2	161.5	165.9	169.9	172.3	173.8
177.5	0.8947	161.6399	0.0402	149.5	151.0	153.3	157.3	161.6	166.0	170.0	172.4	173.9
178.5	0.8941	161.7315	0.0402	149.6	151.1	153.4	157.4	161.7	166.1	170.1	172.5	174.0
179.5	0.8945	161.8174	0.0401	149.7	151.2	153.5	157.4	161.8	166.2	170.2	172.5	174.1
180.5	0.8956	161.8980	0.0401	149.7	151.3	153.6	157.5	161.9	166.3	170.2	172.6	174.2
181.5	0.8973	161.9738	0.0400	149.8	151.3	153.7	157.6	162.0	166.4	170.3	172.7	174.2
182.5	0.8997	162.0450	0.0400	149.9	151.4	153.8	157.7	162.0	166.4	170.4	172.7	174.3
183.5	0.9025	162.1120	0.0400	150.0	151.5	153.8	157.7	162.1	166.5	170.4	172.8	174.3
184.5	0.9058	162.1752	0.0400	150.0	151.5	153.9	157.8	162.2	166.6	170.5	172.9	174.4
185.5	0.9094	162.2347	0.0399	150.1	151.6	154.0	157.9	162.2	166.6	170.6	172.9	174.5
186.5	0.9134	162.2908	0.0399	150.1	151.7	154.0	157.9	162.3	166.7	170.6	173.0	174.5
187.5	0.9176	162.3439	0.0399	150.2	151.7	154.1	158.0	162.3	166.7	170.7	173.0	174.6
188.5	0.9220	162.3940	0.0399	150.3	151.8	154.1	158.0	162.4	166.8	170.7	173.1	174.6
189.5	0.9266	162.4414	0.0399	150.3	151.8	154.2	158.1	162.4	166.8	170.8	173.1	174.7
190.5	0.9314	162.4862	0.0398	150.3	151.9	154.2	158.1	162.5	166.9	170.8	173.2	174.7
191.5	0.9362	162.5287	0.0398	150.4	151.9	154.2	158.2	162.5	166.9	170.8	173.2	174.7
192.5	0.9411	162.5690	0.0398	150.4	151.9	154.3	158.2	162.6	166.9	170.9	173.2	174.8
193.5	0.9461	162.6072	0.0398	150.5	152.0	154.3	158.2	162.6	167.0	170.9	173.3	174.8
194.5	0.9511	162.6435	0.0398	150.5	152.0	154.4	158.3	162.6	167.0	170.9	173.3	174.8
195.5	0.9561	162.6781	0.0398	150.5	152.0	154.4	158.3	162.7	167.0	171.0	173.3	174.9
196.5	0.9611	162.7109	0.0398	150.6	152.1	154.4	158.3	162.7	167.1	171.0	173.4	174.9
197.5	0.9661	162.7421	0.0398	150.6	152.1	154.5	158.4	162.7	167.1	171.0	173.4	174.9
198.5	0.9710	162.7719	0.0398	150.6	152.1	154.5	158.4	162.8	167.1	171.1	173.4	175.0
199.5	0.9759	162.8002	0.0398	150.6	152.2	154.5	158.4	162.8	167.2	171.1	173.5	175.0
200.5	0.9808	162.8273	0.0398	150.7	152.2	154.5	158.5	162.8	167.2	171.1	173.5	175.0
201.5	0.9856	162.8531	0.0397	150.7	152.2	154.6	158.5	162.9	167.2	171.2	173.5	175.0
202.5	0.9903	162.8778	0.0397	150.7	152.2	154.6	158.5	162.9	167.2	171.2	173.5	175.1
203.5	0.9949	162.9013	0.0397	150.7	152.3	154.6	158.5	162.9	167.3	171.2	173.6	175.1
204.5	0.9995	162.9238	0.0397	150.7	152.3	154.6	158.6	162.9	167.3	171.2	173.6	175.1
205.5	1.0040	162.9454	0.0397	150.8	152.3	154.6	158.6	162.9	167.3	171.2	173.6	175.1
206.5	1.0084	162.9660	0.0397	150.8	152.3	154.7	158.6	163.0	167.3	171.3	173.6	175.1
207.5	1.0127	162.9858	0.0397	150.8	152.3	154.7	158.6	163.0	167.4	171.3	173.6	175.2
208.5	1.0169	163.0047	0.0397	150.8	152.4	154.7	158.6	163.0	167.4	171.3	173.6	175.2
209.5	1.0211	163.0228	0.0397	150.8	152.4	154.7	158.7	163.0	167.4	171.3	173.7	175.2
210.5	1.0251	163.0402	0.0397	150.9	152.4	154.7	158.7	163.0	167.4	171.3	173.7	175.2
211.5	1.0291	163.0569	0.0397	150.9	152.4	154.8	158.7	163.1	167.4	171.3	173.7	175.2
212.5	1.0330	163.0729	0.0397	150.9	152.4	154.8	158.7	163.1	167.4	171.4	173.7	175.2
213.5	1.0368	163.0882	0.0397	150.9	152.4	154.8	158.7	163.1	167.5	171.4	173.7	175.2
214.5	1.0405	163.1030	0.0397	150.9	152.4	154.8	158.7	163.1	167.5	171.4	173.7	175.3
215.5	1.0441	163.1172	0.0397	150.9	152.5	154.8	158.7	163.1	167.5	171.4	173.8	175.3
216.5	1.0476	163.1308	0.0397	150.9	152.5	154.8	158.8	163.1	167.5	171.4	173.8	175.3
217.5	1.0510	163.1439	0.0397	150.9	152.5	154.8	158.8	163.1	167.5	171.4	173.8	175.3
218.5	1.0543	163.1565	0.0397	151.0	152.5	154.8	158.8	163.2	167.5	171.5	173.8	175.3
219.5	1.0576	163.1686	0.0397	151.0	152.5	154.9	158.8	163.2	167.5	171.5	173.8	175.3
220.5	1.0608	163.1802	0.0397	151.0	152.5	154.9	158.8	163.2	167.5	171.5	173.8	175.3
221.5	1.0639	163.1914	0.0397	151.0	152.5	154.9	158.8	163.2	167.6	171.5	173.8	175.3
222.5	1.0669	163.2022	0.0397	151.0	152.5	154.9	158.8	163.2	167.6	171.5	173.8	175.3
223.5	1.0698	163.2126	0.0397	151.0	152.5	154.9	158.8	163.2	167.6	171.5	173.8	175.4
224.5	1.0727	163.2226	0.0397	151.0	152.5	154.9	158.9	163.2	167.6	171.5	173.8	175.4
225.5	1.0754	163.2322	0.0397	151.0	152.6	154.9	158.9	163.2	167.6	171.5	173.9	175.4
226.5	1.0781	163.2415	0.0397	151.0	152.6	154.9	158.9	163.2	167.6	171.5	173.9	175.4
227.5	1.0808	163.2504	0.0397	151.0	152.6	154.9	158.9	163.3	167.6	171.5	173.9	175.4
228.5	1.0833	163.2590	0.0397	151.0	152.6	154.9	158.9	163.3	167.6	171.5	173.9	175.4
229.5	1.0858	163.2673	0.0397	151.1	152.6	155.0	158.9	163.3	167.6	171.5	173.9	175.4
230.5	1.0882	163.2753	0.0397	151.1	152.6	155.0	158.9	163.3	167.6	171.6	173.9	175.4
231.5	1.0906	163.2830	0.0397	151.1	152.6	155.0	158.9	163.3	167.6	171.6	173.9	175.4
232.5	1.0929	163.2904	0.0396	151.1	152.6	155.0	158.9	163.3	167.7	171.6	173.9	175.4
233.5	1.0951	163.2976	0.0396	151.1	152.6	155.0	158.9	163.3	167.7	171.6	173.9	175.4
234.5	1.0972	163.3045	0.0396	151.1	152.6	155.0	158.9	163.3	167.7	171.6	173.9	175.4
235.5	1.0993	163.3111	0.0396	151.1	152.6	155.0	158.9	163.3	167.7	171.6	173.9	175.4
236.5	1.1014	163.3175	0.0396	151.1	152.6	155.0	158.9	163.3	167.7	171.6	173.9	175.4
237.5	1.1033	163.3237	0.0396	151.1	152.6	155.0	159.0	163.3	167.7	171.6	173.9	175.5
238.5	1.1053	163.3297	0.0396	151.1	152.6	155.0	159.0	163.3	167.7	171.6	173.9	175.5
239.5	1.1071	163.3354	0.0396	151.1	152.6	155.0	159.0	163.3	167.7	171.6	173.9	175.5
240.0	1.1080	163.3383	0.0396	151.1	152.7	155.0	159.0	163.3	167.7	171.6	174.0	175.5

Table V.10a.

LMS parameters and smoothed percentiles of body mass index (kg/m^2)-for-age in months for boys from 2 to 20 years

Age Group (months)	L	M	S	Percentiles									
				3rd	5th	10th	25th	50th	75th	85th	90th	95th	97th
24.0	-2.0112	16.5750	0.0806	14.52	14.74	15.09	15.74	16.58	17.56	18.16	18.61	19.34	19.86
24.5	-1.9824	16.5478	0.0801	14.50	14.72	15.07	15.72	16.55	17.52	18.12	18.56	19.28	19.79
25.5	-1.9241	16.4944	0.0792	14.47	14.68	15.03	15.68	16.49	17.45	18.04	18.47	19.16	19.66
26.5	-1.8655	16.4426	0.0784	14.43	14.65	15.00	15.63	16.44	17.38	17.96	18.38	19.06	19.54
27.5	-1.8073	16.3922	0.0776	14.40	14.61	14.96	15.59	16.39	17.32	17.88	18.29	18.95	19.42
28.5	-1.7501	16.3433	0.0768	14.37	14.58	14.92	15.55	16.34	17.26	17.81	18.21	18.85	19.31
29.5	-1.6948	16.2958	0.0761	14.33	14.55	14.89	15.51	16.30	17.20	17.74	18.13	18.76	19.20
30.5	-1.6421	16.2497	0.0755	14.30	14.51	14.85	15.47	16.25	17.14	17.67	18.06	18.67	19.10
31.5	-1.5927	16.2050	0.0749	14.27	14.48	14.82	15.44	16.20	17.08	17.60	17.98	18.59	19.01
32.5	-1.5474	16.1615	0.0743	14.24	14.45	14.79	15.40	16.16	17.03	17.54	17.92	18.51	18.92
33.5	-1.5069	16.1193	0.0738	14.21	14.42	14.75	15.36	16.12	16.98	17.48	17.85	18.43	18.84
34.5	-1.4718	16.0784	0.0734	14.18	14.39	14.72	15.33	16.08	16.93	17.43	17.79	18.36	18.76
35.5	-1.4426	16.0388	0.0730	14.15	14.36	14.69	15.29	16.04	16.88	17.38	17.73	18.30	18.69
36.5	-1.4200	16.0003	0.0726	14.12	14.33	14.66	15.26	16.00	16.83	17.33	17.68	18.24	18.62
37.5	-1.4043	15.9630	0.0723	14.09	14.30	14.63	15.23	15.96	16.79	17.28	17.63	18.18	18.56
38.5	-1.3959	15.9270	0.0721	14.07	14.27	14.60	15.20	15.93	16.75	17.23	17.58	18.13	18.51
39.5	-1.3949	15.8920	0.0719	14.04	14.25	14.57	15.16	15.89	16.71	17.19	17.54	18.08	18.46
40.5	-1.4017	15.8582	0.0717	14.02	14.22	14.55	15.13	15.86	16.67	17.15	17.50	18.04	18.41
41.5	-1.4161	15.8256	0.0716	13.99	14.19	14.52	15.10	15.83	16.64	17.12	17.46	18.00	18.37
42.5	-1.4382	15.7941	0.0715	13.97	14.17	14.49	15.07	15.79	16.60	17.08	17.42	17.97	18.34
43.5	-1.4677	15.7636	0.0715	13.94	14.14	14.47	15.05	15.76	16.57	17.05	17.39	17.93	18.31
44.5	-1.5044	15.7343	0.0715	13.92	14.12	14.44	15.02	15.73	16.54	17.02	17.36	17.91	18.28
45.5	-1.5479	15.7061	0.0715	13.90	14.10	14.42	14.99	15.71	16.51	16.99	17.34	17.88	18.26
46.5	-1.5979	15.6790	0.0716	13.88	14.08	14.39	14.97	15.68	16.49	16.97	17.31	17.86	18.25
47.5	-1.6537	15.6531	0.0717	13.86	14.05	14.37	14.94	15.65	16.46	16.95	17.29	17.85	18.23
48.5	-1.7149	15.6282	0.0719	13.84	14.03	14.35	14.92	15.63	16.44	16.93	17.28	17.84	18.23
49.5	-1.7807	15.6044	0.0721	13.82	14.01	14.33	14.89	15.60	16.42	16.91	17.26	17.83	18.22
50.5	-1.8505	15.5818	0.0723	13.80	13.99	14.30	14.87	15.58	16.40	16.89	17.25	17.82	18.22
51.5	-1.9236	15.5603	0.0726	13.78	13.98	14.28	14.85	15.56	16.38	16.88	17.24	17.82	18.23
52.5	-1.9992	15.5399	0.0728	13.77	13.96	14.27	14.83	15.54	16.36	16.87	17.23	17.82	18.24
53.5	-2.0767	15.5206	0.0732	13.75	13.94	14.25	14.81	15.52	16.35	16.86	17.23	17.83	18.25
54.5	-2.1553	15.5026	0.0735	13.74	13.92	14.23	14.79	15.50	16.34	16.85	17.22	17.83	18.27
55.5	-2.2344	15.4857	0.0739	13.72	13.91	14.21	14.77	15.49	16.33	16.84	17.22	17.84	18.29
56.5	-2.3133	15.4700	0.0742	13.71	13.89	14.20	14.75	15.47	16.32	16.84	17.22	17.86	18.31
57.5	-2.3914	15.4555	0.0746	13.69	13.88	14.18	14.74	15.46	16.31	16.84	17.23	17.87	18.34
58.5	-2.4680	15.4421	0.0751	13.68	13.86	14.17	14.72	15.44	16.30	16.84	17.23	17.89	18.37
59.5	-2.5428	15.4300	0.0755	13.67	13.85	14.15	14.71	15.43	16.30	16.84	17.24	17.91	18.40
60.5	-2.6152	15.4191	0.0760	13.66	13.84	14.14	14.70	15.42	16.29	16.84	17.25	17.94	18.44
61.5	-2.6848	15.4095	0.0765	13.64	13.83	14.13	14.68	15.41	16.29	16.85	17.27	17.97	18.48
62.5	-2.7513	15.4010	0.0770	13.63	13.82	14.11	14.67	15.40	16.29	16.85	17.28	18.00	18.53
63.5	-2.8145	15.3938	0.0775	13.62	13.80	14.10	14.66	15.39	16.29	16.86	17.30	18.03	18.57
64.5	-2.8740	15.3878	0.0781	13.61	13.79	14.09	14.65	15.39	16.29	16.87	17.31	18.06	18.62
65.5	-2.9298	15.3831	0.0786	13.60	13.79	14.08	14.64	15.38	16.30	16.88	17.33	18.10	18.67
66.5	-2.9818	15.3795	0.0792	13.60	13.78	14.07	14.64	15.38	16.30	16.90	17.36	18.14	18.73
67.5	-3.0298	15.3772	0.0798	13.59	13.77	14.07	14.63	15.38	16.31	16.91	17.38	18.18	18.79
68.5	-3.0739	15.3761	0.0804	13.58	13.76	14.06	14.62	15.38	16.32	16.93	17.41	18.22	18.85
69.5	-3.1141	15.3762	0.0811	13.57	13.75	14.05	14.62	15.38	16.33	16.95	17.43	18.27	18.91
70.5	-3.1504	15.3775	0.0817	13.57	13.75	14.05	14.62	15.38	16.34	16.97	17.46	18.31	18.97
71.5	-3.1829	15.3799	0.0824	13.56	13.74	14.04	14.61	15.38	16.35	16.99	17.49	18.36	19.04
72.5	-3.2117	15.3835	0.0830	13.55	13.74	14.04	14.61	15.38	16.36	17.01	17.52	18.41	19.11
73.5	-3.2369	15.3883	0.0837	13.55	13.73	14.03	14.61	15.39	16.38	17.04	17.56	18.47	19.18
74.5	-3.2588	15.3942	0.0844	13.54	13.73	14.03	14.61	15.39	16.40	17.07	17.59	18.52	19.25
75.5	-3.2773	15.4013	0.0852	13.54	13.72	14.03	14.61	15.40	16.41	17.09	17.63	18.58	19.33
76.5	-3.2927	15.4094	0.0859	13.54	13.72	14.03	14.61	15.41	16.43	17.12	17.67	18.64	19.41
77.5	-3.3051	15.4187	0.0866	13.53	13.72	14.03	14.62	15.42	16.45	17.15	17.71	18.70	19.48
78.5	-3.3148	15.4290	0.0874	13.53	13.72	14.03	14.62	15.43	16.47	17.18	17.75	18.76	19.56
79.5	-3.3218	15.4404	0.0882	13.53	13.72	14.03	14.62	15.44	16.50	17.22	17.79	18.82	19.65
80.5	-3.3263	15.4529	0.0889	13.53	13.72	14.03	14.63	15.45	16.52	17.25	17.83	18.88	19.73
81.5	-3.3286	15.4664	0.0897	13.53	13.72	14.03	14.64	15.47	16.55	17.29	17.88	18.95	19.82
82.5	-3.3287	15.4809	0.0905	13.53	13.72	14.03	14.64	15.48	16.57	17.32	17.93	19.01	19.90
83.5	-3.3269	15.4964	0.0913	13.53	13.72	14.04	14.65	15.50	16.60	17.36	17.97	19.08	19.99
84.5	-3.3232	15.5129	0.0921	13.53	13.72	14.04	14.66	15.51	16.63	17.40	18.02	19.15	20.08
85.5	-3.3178	15.5303	0.0929	13.53	13.72	14.05	14.67	15.53	16.66	17.44	18.07	19.22	20.17
86.5	-3.3109	15.5488	0.0938	13.53	13.73	14.05	14.68	15.55	16.69	17.48	18.12	19.29	20.26
87.5	-3.3026	15.5681	0.0946	13.54	13.73	14.06	14.69	15.57	16.72	17.53	18.18	19.37	20.36
88.5	-3.2930	15.5884	0.0954	13.54	13.74	14.07	14.70	15.59	16.76	17.57	18.23	19.44	20.45
89.5	-3.2823	15.6096	0.0962	13.54	13.74	14.07	14.72	15.61	16.79	17.61	18.28	19.52	20.55
90.5	-3.2705	15.6317	0.0971	13.55	13.75	14.08	14.73	15.63	16.83	17.66	18.34	19.59	20.64
91.5	-3.2577	15.6547	0.0979	13.55	13.75	14.09	14.75	15.65	16.86	17.71	18.40	19.67	20.74
92.5	-3.2441	15.6785	0.0988	13.56	13.76	14.10	14.76	15.68	16.90	17.76	18.45	19.75	20.84
93.5	-3.2298	15.7032	0.0996	13.56	13.77	14.11	14.78	15.70	16.94	17.80	18.51	19.83	20.94
94.5	-3.2148	15.7288	0.1004	13.57	13.78	14.12	14.79	15.73	16.98	17.85	18.57	19.91	21.03
95.5	-3.1992	15.7551	0.1013	13.58	13.79	14.13	14.81	15.76	17.02	17.90	18.63	19.99	21.13

Table V.10b.

LMS parameters and smoothed percentiles of body mass index (kg/m^2)-for-age in months for boys from 2 to 20 years

Age Group (months)	L	M	S	3rd	5th	10th	25th	50th	75th	85th	90th	95th	97th
96.50	-3.1831	15.7823	0.1021	13.59	13.80	14.15	14.83	15.78	17.06	17.96	18.69	20.07	21.24
97.50	-3.1665	15.8103	0.1029	13.59	13.81	14.16	14.85	15.81	17.10	18.01	18.75	20.15	21.34
98.50	-3.1496	15.8390	0.1037	13.60	13.82	14.17	14.87	15.84	17.14	18.06	18.82	20.23	21.44
99.50	-3.1324	15.8686	0.1046	13.61	13.83	14.19	14.89	15.87	17.19	18.12	18.88	20.32	21.54
100.50	-3.1149	15.8989	0.1054	13.62	13.84	14.20	14.91	15.90	17.23	18.17	18.94	20.40	21.64
101.50	-3.0972	15.9299	0.1062	13.64	13.85	14.22	14.93	15.93	17.27	18.23	19.01	20.48	21.75
102.50	-3.0794	15.9617	0.1070	13.65	13.87	14.24	14.95	15.96	17.32	18.28	19.08	20.57	21.85
103.50	-3.0614	15.9942	0.1078	13.66	13.88	14.25	14.98	15.99	17.37	18.34	19.14	20.65	21.95
104.50	-3.0434	16.0274	0.1086	13.67	13.90	14.27	15.00	16.03	17.41	18.40	19.21	20.74	22.06
105.50	-3.0253	16.0613	0.1094	13.69	13.91	14.29	15.03	16.06	17.46	18.45	19.28	20.83	22.16
106.50	-3.0072	16.0959	0.1102	13.70	13.93	14.31	15.05	16.10	17.51	18.51	19.34	20.91	22.27
107.50	-2.9892	16.1312	0.1110	13.72	13.94	14.33	15.08	16.13	17.56	18.57	19.41	21.00	22.37
108.50	-2.9711	16.1671	0.1117	13.73	13.96	14.35	15.10	16.17	17.61	18.63	19.48	21.09	22.48
109.50	-2.9532	16.2037	0.1125	13.75	13.98	14.37	15.13	16.20	17.66	18.69	19.55	21.18	22.58
110.50	-2.9354	16.2409	0.1132	13.76	14.00	14.39	15.16	16.24	17.71	18.75	19.62	21.26	22.69
111.50	-2.9176	16.2788	0.1140	13.78	14.02	14.41	15.19	16.28	17.76	18.82	19.69	21.35	22.79
112.50	-2.9000	16.3173	0.1147	13.80	14.04	14.44	15.22	16.32	17.81	18.88	19.76	21.44	22.90
113.50	-2.8826	16.3564	0.1154	13.82	14.06	14.46	15.25	16.36	17.86	18.94	19.83	21.53	23.00
114.50	-2.8653	16.3961	0.1161	13.84	14.08	14.48	15.28	16.40	17.92	19.00	19.91	21.62	23.10
115.50	-2.8482	16.4363	0.1168	13.86	14.10	14.51	15.31	16.44	17.97	19.07	19.98	21.71	23.21
116.50	-2.8313	16.4772	0.1175	13.88	14.12	14.53	15.34	16.48	18.02	19.13	20.05	21.80	23.31
117.50	-2.8146	16.5186	0.1182	13.90	14.15	14.56	15.37	16.52	18.08	19.20	20.12	21.89	23.42
118.50	-2.7980	16.5606	0.1188	13.92	14.17	14.59	15.41	16.56	18.13	19.26	20.20	21.98	23.52
119.50	-2.7817	16.6031	0.1195	13.94	14.19	14.61	15.44	16.60	18.19	19.32	20.27	22.06	23.62
120.50	-2.7656	16.6461	0.1201	13.97	14.22	14.64	15.47	16.65	18.25	19.39	20.34	22.15	23.73
121.50	-2.7498	16.6897	0.1207	13.99	14.24	14.67	15.51	16.69	18.30	19.46	20.42	22.24	23.83
122.50	-2.7341	16.7338	0.1213	14.01	14.27	14.70	15.54	16.73	18.36	19.52	20.49	22.33	23.93
123.50	-2.7187	16.7784	0.1219	14.04	14.30	14.73	15.58	16.78	18.42	19.59	20.56	22.42	24.03
124.50	-2.7036	16.8235	0.1225	14.06	14.32	14.76	15.61	16.82	18.47	19.66	20.64	22.51	24.13
125.50	-2.6886	16.8691	0.1231	14.09	14.35	14.79	15.65	16.87	18.53	19.72	20.71	22.60	24.24
126.50	-2.6739	16.9151	0.1237	14.12	14.38	14.82	15.69	16.92	18.59	19.79	20.79	22.69	24.34
127.50	-2.6594	16.9616	0.1242	14.14	14.41	14.85	15.73	16.96	18.65	19.86	20.86	22.78	24.44
128.50	-2.6452	17.0086	0.1247	14.17	14.44	14.89	15.76	17.01	18.71	19.92	20.94	22.86	24.54
129.50	-2.6312	17.0560	0.1253	14.20	14.47	14.92	15.80	17.06	18.77	19.99	21.01	22.95	24.63
130.50	-2.6174	17.1039	0.1258	14.23	14.50	14.95	15.84	17.10	18.83	20.06	21.09	23.04	24.73
131.50	-2.6039	17.1522	0.1263	14.26	14.53	14.99	15.88	17.15	18.89	20.13	21.16	23.13	24.83
132.50	-2.5906	17.2009	0.1267	14.29	14.56	15.02	15.92	17.20	18.95	20.20	21.24	23.21	24.93
133.50	-2.5775	17.2500	0.1272	14.32	14.59	15.06	15.96	17.25	19.01	20.27	21.31	23.30	25.02
134.50	-2.5646	17.2995	0.1276	14.35	14.62	15.09	16.00	17.30	19.07	20.33	21.39	23.39	25.12
135.50	-2.5520	17.3494	0.1281	14.38	14.66	15.13	16.05	17.35	19.13	20.40	21.46	23.47	25.21
136.50	-2.5395	17.3997	0.1285	14.41	14.69	15.16	16.09	17.40	19.19	20.47	21.54	23.56	25.31
137.50	-2.5273	17.4504	0.1289	14.44	14.73	15.20	16.13	17.45	19.25	20.54	21.61	23.64	25.40
138.50	-2.5153	17.5014	0.1293	14.48	14.76	15.24	16.17	17.50	19.31	20.61	21.69	23.73	25.49
139.50	-2.5035	17.5528	0.1297	14.51	14.79	15.28	16.22	17.55	19.37	20.68	21.76	23.81	25.58
140.50	-2.4919	17.6045	0.1301	14.54	14.83	15.31	16.26	17.60	19.44	20.75	21.84	23.90	25.68
141.50	-2.4805	17.6565	0.1304	14.58	14.87	15.35	16.31	17.66	19.50	20.82	21.91	23.98	25.77
142.50	-2.4693	17.7089	0.1307	14.61	14.90	15.39	16.35	17.71	19.56	20.89	21.98	24.06	25.86
143.50	-2.4583	17.7616	0.1311	14.65	14.94	15.43	16.40	17.76	19.62	20.95	22.06	24.15	25.94
144.50	-2.4474	17.8146	0.1314	14.68	14.98	15.47	16.44	17.81	19.69	21.02	22.13	24.23	26.03
145.50	-2.4368	17.8679	0.1317	14.72	15.02	15.51	16.49	17.87	19.75	21.09	22.21	24.31	26.12
146.50	-2.4263	17.9216	0.1320	14.76	15.05	15.55	16.53	17.92	19.81	21.16	22.28	24.39	26.21
147.50	-2.4159	17.9754	0.1322	14.79	15.09	15.59	16.58	17.98	19.88	21.23	22.35	24.47	26.29
148.50	-2.4057	18.0296	0.1325	14.83	15.13	15.64	16.63	18.03	19.94	21.30	22.43	24.55	26.38
149.50	-2.3957	18.0840	0.1328	14.87	15.17	15.68	16.67	18.08	20.00	21.37	22.50	24.63	26.46
150.50	-2.3859	18.1387	0.1330	14.91	15.21	15.72	16.72	18.14	20.07	21.44	22.57	24.71	26.54
151.50	-2.3761	18.1937	0.1332	14.95	15.25	15.76	16.77	18.19	20.13	21.51	22.65	24.79	26.62
152.50	-2.3665	18.2488	0.1334	14.99	15.29	15.81	16.82	18.25	20.19	21.58	22.72	24.87	26.71
153.50	-2.3571	18.3043	0.1336	15.03	15.33	15.85	16.87	18.30	20.26	21.65	22.79	24.95	26.79
154.50	-2.3478	18.3599	0.1338	15.07	15.38	15.90	16.92	18.36	20.32	21.71	22.86	25.03	26.86
155.50	-2.3385	18.4157	0.1340	15.11	15.42	15.94	16.97	18.42	20.38	21.78	22.94	25.10	26.94
156.50	-2.3295	18.4718	0.1341	15.15	15.46	15.99	17.02	18.47	20.45	21.85	23.01	25.18	27.02
157.50	-2.3205	18.5281	0.1343	15.19	15.50	16.03	17.07	18.53	20.51	21.92	23.08	25.25	27.10
158.50	-2.3116	18.5845	0.1344	15.23	15.54	16.08	17.12	18.58	20.58	21.99	23.15	25.33	27.17
159.50	-2.3028	18.6411	0.1346	15.27	15.59	16.12	17.17	18.64	20.64	22.06	23.22	25.40	27.25
160.50	-2.2941	18.6979	0.1347	15.31	15.63	16.17	17.22	18.70	20.70	22.12	23.29	25.48	27.32
161.50	-2.2855	18.7549	0.1348	15.36	15.68	16.21	17.27	18.75	20.77	22.19	23.36	25.55	27.40
162.50	-2.2770	18.8120	0.1349	15.40	15.72	16.26	17.32	18.81	20.83	22.26	23.43	25.62	27.47
163.50	-2.2686	18.8693	0.1350	15.44	15.76	16.31	17.37	18.87	20.89	22.33	23.50	25.69	27.54
164.50	-2.2602	18.9267	0.1350	15.48	15.81	16.35	17.42	18.93	20.96	22.39	23.57	25.77	27.61
165.50	-2.2519	18.9842	0.1351	15.53	15.85	16.40	17.47	18.98	21.02	22.46	23.64	25.84	27.68
166.50	-2.2437	19.0419	0.1352	15.57	15.90	16.45	17.53	19.04	21.09	22.53	23.71	25.91	27.75
167.50	-2.2355	19.0997	0.1352	15.62	15.94	16.50	17.58	19.10	21.15	22.60	23.78	25.98	27.82
168.50	-2.2274	19.1576	0.1353	15.66	15.99	16.55	17.63	19.16	21.21	22.66	23.85	26.05	27.88
169.50	-2.2193	19.2156	0.1353	15.71	16.04	16.59	17.68	19.22	21.28	22.73	23.92	26.12	27.95

Table V.10c.

LMS parameters and smoothed percentiles of body mass index (kg/m^2)-for-age in months for boys from 2 to 20 years

Age Group (months)	L	M	S	Percentiles 3rd	5th	10th	25th	50th	75th	85th	90th	95th	97th
170.5	-2.21124	19.2737	0.1353	15.75	16.08	16.64	17.74	19.27	21.34	22.80	23.98	26.18	28.02
171.5	-2.20324	19.3318	0.13532	15.80	16.13	16.69	17.79	19.33	21.41	22.86	24.05	26.25	28.08
172.5	-2.19527	19.3901	0.13532	15.84	16.18	16.74	17.84	19.39	21.47	22.93	24.12	26.32	28.15
173.5	-2.18734	19.4484	0.13532	15.89	16.22	16.79	17.90	19.45	21.53	22.99	24.19	26.38	28.21
174.5	-2.17943	19.5067	0.13531	15.93	16.27	16.84	17.95	19.51	21.60	23.06	24.25	26.45	28.27
175.5	-2.17154	19.5651	0.13529	15.98	16.32	16.89	18.00	19.57	21.66	23.13	24.32	26.52	28.33
176.5	-2.16367	19.6236	0.13527	16.02	16.36	16.94	18.06	19.62	21.72	23.19	24.39	26.58	28.40
177.5	-2.15582	19.6821	0.13524	16.07	16.41	16.99	18.11	19.68	21.79	23.26	24.45	26.65	28.46
178.5	-2.14799	19.7406	0.1352	16.12	16.46	17.04	18.16	19.74	21.85	23.32	24.52	26.71	28.52
179.5	-2.14016	19.7991	0.13516	16.16	16.51	17.09	18.22	19.80	21.91	23.39	24.58	26.77	28.58
180.5	-2.13234	19.8577	0.13511	16.21	16.55	17.14	18.27	19.86	21.98	23.45	24.65	26.84	28.64
181.5	-2.12454	19.9162	0.13506	16.26	16.60	17.19	18.32	19.92	22.04	23.52	24.71	26.90	28.69
182.5	-2.11674	19.9747	0.135	16.30	16.65	17.24	18.38	19.97	22.10	23.58	24.78	26.96	28.75
183.5	-2.10894	20.0332	0.13493	16.35	16.70	17.29	18.43	20.03	22.16	23.64	24.84	27.02	28.81
184.5	-2.10115	20.0917	0.13487	16.40	16.75	17.34	18.49	20.09	22.23	23.71	24.90	27.09	28.87
185.5	-2.09336	20.1502	0.13479	16.44	16.80	17.39	18.54	20.15	22.29	23.77	24.97	27.15	28.92
186.5	-2.08557	20.2086	0.13472	16.49	16.84	17.44	18.60	20.21	22.35	23.83	25.03	27.21	28.98
187.5	-2.07779	20.2669	0.13464	16.54	16.89	17.49	18.65	20.27	22.41	23.90	25.09	27.27	29.03
188.5	-2.07002	20.3252	0.13456	16.58	16.94	17.54	18.70	20.33	22.47	23.96	25.16	27.33	29.09
189.5	-2.06225	20.3835	0.13447	16.63	16.99	17.59	18.76	20.38	22.54	24.02	25.22	27.39	29.14
190.5	-2.0545	20.4416	0.13438	16.68	17.04	17.64	18.81	20.44	22.60	24.09	25.28	27.45	29.20
191.5	-2.04675	20.4997	0.13429	16.72	17.08	17.69	18.87	20.50	22.66	24.15	25.34	27.51	29.25
192.5	-2.03902	20.5576	0.1342	16.77	17.13	17.74	18.92	20.56	22.72	24.21	25.41	27.56	29.30
193.5	-2.0313	20.6155	0.1341	16.82	17.18	17.79	18.97	20.62	22.78	24.27	25.47	27.62	29.36
194.5	-2.02361	20.6733	0.13401	16.86	17.23	17.84	19.03	20.67	22.84	24.33	25.53	27.68	29.41
195.5	-2.01594	20.7309	0.13391	16.91	17.28	17.89	19.08	20.73	22.90	24.40	25.59	27.74	29.46
196.5	-2.00831	20.7884	0.13381	16.96	17.32	17.94	19.13	20.79	22.97	24.46	25.65	27.80	29.52
197.5	-2.00071	20.8457	0.13372	17.00	17.37	17.99	19.19	20.85	23.03	24.52	25.71	27.85	29.57
198.5	-1.99315	20.9029	0.13362	17.05	17.42	18.04	19.24	20.90	23.09	24.58	25.77	27.91	29.62
199.5	-1.98564	20.96	0.13352	17.10	17.47	18.09	19.29	20.96	23.15	24.64	25.83	27.97	29.68
200.5	-1.97819	21.0169	0.13343	17.14	17.51	18.14	19.35	21.02	23.21	24.70	25.89	28.03	29.73
201.5	-1.97081	21.0736	0.13333	17.19	17.56	18.19	19.40	21.07	23.27	24.76	25.96	28.08	29.78
202.5	-1.9635	21.1301	0.13324	17.23	17.61	18.24	19.45	21.13	23.33	24.82	26.02	28.14	29.83
203.5	-1.95627	21.1864	0.13315	17.28	17.66	18.29	19.50	21.19	23.39	24.88	26.08	28.20	29.89
204.5	-1.94913	21.2425	0.13306	17.33	17.70	18.33	19.56	21.24	23.44	24.94	26.14	28.26	29.94
205.5	-1.9421	21.2984	0.13297	17.37	17.75	18.38	19.61	21.30	23.50	25.00	26.19	28.31	29.99
206.5	-1.93518	21.354	0.13289	17.42	17.80	18.43	19.66	21.35	23.56	25.06	26.25	28.37	30.05
207.5	-1.92838	21.4094	0.1328	17.46	17.84	18.48	19.71	21.41	23.62	25.12	26.31	28.43	30.10
208.5	-1.92171	21.4646	0.13273	17.51	17.89	18.53	19.76	21.46	23.68	25.18	26.37	28.49	30.16
209.5	-1.91519	21.5195	0.13265	17.55	17.93	18.57	19.81	21.52	23.74	25.24	26.43	28.55	30.21
210.5	-1.90883	21.5742	0.13258	17.59	17.98	18.62	19.86	21.57	23.80	25.30	26.49	28.60	30.27
211.5	-1.90264	21.6285	0.13252	17.64	18.02	18.67	19.91	21.63	23.85	25.36	26.55	28.66	30.32
212.5	-1.89663	21.6826	0.13246	17.68	18.07	18.72	19.96	21.68	23.91	25.42	26.61	28.72	30.38
213.5	-1.89082	21.7364	0.13241	17.72	18.11	18.76	20.01	21.74	23.97	25.48	26.67	28.78	30.44
214.5	-1.88521	21.7899	0.13236	17.77	18.16	18.81	20.06	21.79	24.03	25.54	26.73	28.84	30.49
215.5	-1.87982	21.843	0.13232	17.81	18.20	18.85	20.11	21.84	24.08	25.60	26.79	28.90	30.55
216.5	-1.87467	21.8959	0.13229	17.85	18.24	18.90	20.16	21.90	24.14	25.66	26.85	28.96	30.61
217.5	-1.86976	21.9484	0.13226	17.89	18.29	18.94	20.21	21.95	24.20	25.71	26.91	29.02	30.67
218.5	-1.86511	22.0005	0.13224	17.93	18.33	18.99	20.26	22.00	24.25	25.77	26.97	29.08	30.73
219.5	-1.86073	22.0523	0.13223	17.98	18.37	19.03	20.31	22.05	24.31	25.83	27.03	29.14	30.79
220.5	-1.85663	22.1037	0.13223	18.02	18.41	19.08	20.35	22.10	24.37	25.89	27.09	29.20	30.86
221.5	-1.85283	22.1548	0.13223	18.06	18.45	19.12	20.40	22.15	24.42	25.95	27.15	29.27	30.92
222.5	-1.84932	22.2054	0.13225	18.10	18.50	19.16	20.45	22.21	24.48	26.01	27.21	29.33	30.99
223.5	-1.84613	22.2557	0.13227	18.14	18.54	19.20	20.49	22.26	24.53	26.07	27.27	29.39	31.05
224.5	-1.84326	22.3055	0.13231	18.17	18.58	19.25	20.54	22.31	24.59	26.13	27.33	29.46	31.12
225.5	-1.84072	22.355	0.13236	18.21	18.62	19.29	20.58	22.35	24.65	26.18	27.40	29.52	31.19
226.5	-1.83852	22.404	0.13242	18.25	18.65	19.33	20.63	22.40	24.70	26.24	27.46	29.59	31.26
227.5	-1.83666	22.4526	0.13248	18.29	18.69	19.37	20.67	22.45	24.75	26.30	27.52	29.66	31.33
228.5	-1.83514	22.5007	0.13257	18.32	18.73	19.41	20.71	22.50	24.81	26.36	27.58	29.73	31.40
229.5	-1.83397	22.5484	0.13266	18.36	18.77	19.45	20.76	22.55	24.86	26.42	27.64	29.80	31.48
230.5	-1.83316	22.5957	0.13277	18.40	18.80	19.49	20.80	22.60	24.92	26.48	27.71	29.87	31.55
231.5	-1.8327	22.6424	0.13289	18.43	18.84	19.52	20.84	22.64	24.97	26.54	27.77	29.94	31.63
232.5	-1.83258	22.6887	0.13302	18.47	18.88	19.56	20.88	22.69	25.03	26.60	27.83	30.01	31.71
233.5	-1.83282	22.7346	0.13317	18.50	18.91	19.60	20.92	22.73	25.08	26.66	27.90	30.08	31.79
234.5	-1.8334	22.7799	0.13334	18.53	18.94	19.63	20.96	22.78	25.13	26.72	27.96	30.16	31.87
235.5	-1.83432	22.8247	0.13352	18.57	18.98	19.67	21.00	22.82	25.19	26.78	28.03	30.23	31.96
236.5	-1.83556	22.8691	0.13372	18.60	19.01	19.70	21.04	22.87	25.24	26.84	28.09	30.31	32.04
237.5	-1.83712	22.9129	0.13393	18.63	19.04	19.74	21.08	22.91	25.29	26.90	28.16	30.39	32.13
238.5	-1.83899	22.9563	0.13416	18.66	19.07	19.77	21.11	22.96	25.34	26.96	28.23	30.47	32.22
239.5	-1.84115	22.9991	0.13441	18.69	19.11	19.80	21.15	23.00	25.40	27.02	28.29	30.55	32.32
240.0	-1.84233	23.0203	0.13454	18.70	19.12	19.82	21.17	23.02	25.42	27.05	28.33	30.59	32.37

Table V.11a.
LMS parameters and smoothed percentiles of body mass index (kg/m^2)-for-age in months for girls from 2 to 20 years

Age Group (months)	L	M	S	Percentiles									
				3rd	5th	10th	25th	50th	75th	85th	90th	95th	97th
24.0	-0.9866	16.4234	0.0855	14.15	14.40	14.80	15.53	16.42	17.43	18.02	18.44	19.11	19.56
24.5	-1.0245	16.3880	0.0850	14.13	14.38	14.78	15.50	16.39	17.39	17.97	18.40	19.06	19.52
25.5	-1.1027	16.3190	0.0842	14.10	14.35	14.74	15.44	16.32	17.30	17.89	18.31	18.97	19.42
26.5	-1.1840	16.2521	0.0835	14.07	14.31	14.70	15.39	16.25	17.23	17.80	18.22	18.88	19.33
27.5	-1.2681	16.1873	0.0827	14.04	14.28	14.65	15.34	16.19	17.15	17.73	18.14	18.80	19.25
28.5	-1.3548	16.1248	0.0821	14.02	14.24	14.61	15.29	16.12	17.08	17.65	18.06	18.72	19.17
29.5	-1.4437	16.0643	0.0815	13.99	14.21	14.58	15.24	16.06	17.01	17.58	17.99	18.64	19.10
30.5	-1.5345	16.0059	0.0809	13.96	14.18	14.54	15.19	16.01	16.94	17.51	17.92	18.58	19.04
31.5	-1.6269	15.9497	0.0804	13.93	14.15	14.50	15.14	15.95	16.88	17.44	17.85	18.51	18.97
32.5	1.7204	15.8955	0.0800	13.91	14.12	14.46	15.10	15.90	16.82	17.38	17.79	18.45	18.92
33.5	-1.8146	15.8434	0.0796	13.88	14.09	14.43	15.05	15.84	16.76	17.32	17.73	18.40	18.87
34.5	-1.9091	15.7933	0.0792	13.85	14.06	14.39	15.01	15.79	16.71	17.27	17.68	18.35	18.82
35.5	-2.0033	15.7453	0.0789	13.83	14.03	14.36	14.97	15.75	16.66	17.22	17.63	18.30	18.78
36.5	-2.0968	15.6992	0.0786	13.80	14.00	14.33	14.93	15.70	16.61	17.17	17.58	18.25	18.74
37.5	-2.1892	15.6552	0.0784	13.78	13.97	14.30	14.89	15.66	16.56	17.12	17.54	18.22	18.71
38.5	-2.2800	15.6132	0.0782	13.75	13.95	14.27	14.85	15.61	16.52	17.08	17.49	18.18	18.68
39.5	-2.3687	15.5732	0.0781	13.73	13.92	14.24	14.82	15.57	16.47	17.04	17.46	18.15	18.65
40.5	-2.4550	15.5351	0.0780	13.71	13.90	14.21	14.79	15.54	16.43	17.00	17.42	18.12	18.63
41.5	-2.5385	15.4989	0.0779	13.68	13.87	14.18	14.75	15.50	16.40	16.96	17.39	18.10	18.62
42.5	-2.6187	15.4647	0.0779	13.66	13.85	14.15	14.72	15.46	16.36	16.93	17.36	18.08	18.60
43.5	-2.6955	15.4324	0.0779	13.64	13.82	14.13	14.69	15.43	16.33	16.90	17.34	18.06	18.60
44.5	-2.7685	15.4019	0.0780	13.62	13.80	14.10	14.66	15.40	16.30	16.88	17.31	18.05	18.59
45.5	-2.8374	15.3734	0.0781	13.60	13.78	14.08	14.64	15.37	16.28	16.85	17.30	18.04	18.59
46.5	-2.9022	15.3466	0.0783	13.58	13.76	14.05	14.61	15.35	16.25	16.83	17.28	18.03	18.60
47.5	-2.9626	15.3217	0.0785	13.56	13.74	14.03	14.59	15.32	16.23	16.82	17.26	18.03	18.60
48.5	-3.0185	15.2985	0.0787	13.54	13.71	14.01	14.56	15.30	16.21	16.80	17.25	18.03	18.61
49.5	-3.0699	15.2772	0.0790	13.52	13.69	13.99	14.54	15.28	16.19	16.79	17.25	18.03	18.63
50.5	-3.1168	15.2576	0.0793	13.50	13.68	13.97	14.52	15.26	16.18	16.78	17.24	18.04	18.65
51.5	-3.1591	15.2397	0.0796	13.48	13.66	13.95	14.50	15.24	16.16	16.77	17.24	18.05	18.67
52.5	-3.1969	15.2235	0.0800	13.46	13.64	13.93	14.48	15.22	16.15	16.76	17.24	18.06	18.69
53.5	-3.2303	15.2089	0.0805	13.45	13.62	13.91	14.47	15.21	16.14	16.76	17.24	18.07	18.72
54.5	-3.2593	15.1961	0.0809	13.43	13.61	13.90	14.45	15.20	16.14	16.76	17.25	18.09	18.75
55.5	-3.2841	15.1848	0.0814	13.41	13.59	13.88	14.44	15.18	16.13	16.76	17.25	18.11	18.78
56.5	-3.3048	15.1751	0.0819	13.40	13.57	13.87	14.42	15.18	16.13	16.77	17.26	18.14	18.82
57.5	-3.3216	15.1670	0.0825	13.38	13.56	13.85	14.41	15.17	16.13	16.77	17.28	18.16	18.86
58.5	-3.3346	15.1605	0.0830	13.37	13.55	13.84	14.40	15.16	16.13	16.78	17.29	18.19	18.90
59.5	-3.3440	15.1554	0.0837	13.36	13.53	13.83	14.39	15.16	16.13	16.79	17.31	18.22	18.95
60.5	-3.3501	15.1519	0.0843	13.34	13.52	13.82	14.38	15.15	16.14	16.80	17.33	18.26	19.00
61.5	-3.3529	15.1498	0.0850	13.33	13.51	13.81	14.38	15.15	16.15	16.82	17.35	18.29	19.05
62.5	-3.3527	15.1492	0.0857	13.32	13.50	13.80	14.37	15.15	16.15	16.83	17.37	18.33	19.10
63.5	-3.3497	15.1499	0.0864	13.31	13.49	13.79	14.36	15.15	16.16	16.85	17.40	18.37	19.16
64.5	-3.3440	15.1521	0.0871	13.30	13.48	13.78	14.36	15.15	16.18	16.87	17.43	18.42	19.21
65.5	-3.3359	15.1557	0.0879	13.29	13.47	13.77	14.36	15.16	16.19	16.89	17.46	18.46	19.27
66.5	-3.3255	15.1606	0.0887	13.28	13.46	13.77	14.36	15.16	16.21	16.92	17.49	18.51	19.34
67.5	-3.3131	15.1668	0.0895	13.27	13.45	13.76	14.35	15.17	16.22	16.94	17.52	18.56	19.40
68.5	-3.2987	15.1743	0.0903	13.26	13.45	13.76	14.35	15.17	16.24	16.97	17.56	18.61	19.47
69.5	-3.2827	15.1831	0.0912	13.25	13.44	13.75	14.36	15.18	16.26	17.00	17.59	18.66	19.54
70.5	-3.2650	15.1931	0.0920	13.25	13.43	13.75	14.36	15.19	16.28	17.03	17.63	18.72	19.61
71.5	-3.2459	15.2044	0.0929	13.24	13.43	13.75	14.36	15.20	16.31	17.07	17.67	18.78	19.68
72.5	-3.2256	15.2169	0.0938	13.23	13.43	13.75	14.37	15.22	16.33	17.10	17.72	18.84	19.75
73.5	-3.2041	15.2306	0.0947	13.23	13.42	13.75	14.37	15.23	16.36	17.14	17.76	18.90	19.83
74.5	-3.1817	15.2454	0.0956	13.22	13.42	13.75	14.38	15.25	16.39	17.17	17.81	18.96	19.91
75.5	-3.1584	15.2614	0.0966	13.22	13.42	13.75	14.38	15.26	16.42	17.21	17.85	19.03	19.99
76.5	-3.1343	15.2785	0.0975	13.22	13.42	13.75	14.39	15.28	16.45	17.25	17.90	19.09	20.07
77.5	-3.1096	15.2968	0.0985	13.22	13.42	13.75	14.40	15.30	16 48	17.29	17.95	19.16	20.16
78.5	-3.0843	15.3161	0.0994	13.21	13.42	13.76	14.41	15.32	16.51	17.34	18.01	19.23	20.24
79.5	-3.0586	15.3364	0.1004	13.21	13.42	13.76	14.42	15.34	16.55	17.38	18.06	19.30	20.33
80.5	-3.0325	15.3579	0.1014	13.21	13.42	13.76	14.43	15.36	16.58	17.43	18.12	19.37	20.42
81.5	-3.0062	15.3803	0.1024	13.21	13.42	13.77	14.45	15.38	16.62	17.48	18.17	19.45	20.50
82.5	-2.9796	15.4037	0.1033	13.21	13.42	13.78	14.46	15.40	16.66	17.52	18.23	19.52	20.60
83.5	-2.9529	15.4282	0.1043	13.22	13.43	13.78	14.47	15.43	16.69	17.57	18.29	19.60	20.69
84.5	-2.9262	15.4536	0.1053	13.22	13.43	13.79	14.49	15.45	16.73	17.63	18.35	19.68	20.78
85.5	-2.8994	15.4799	0.1063	13.22	13.44	13.80	14.50	15.48	16.78	17.68	18.41	19.76	20.88
86.5	-2.8727	15.5072	0.1073	13.23	13.44	13.81	14.52	15.51	16.82	17.73	18.47	19.84	20.97
87.5	-2.8461	15.5354	0.1083	13.23	13.45	13.82	14.54	15.54	16.86	17.79	18.54	19.92	21.07
88.5	-2.8197	15.5644	0.1093	13.23	13.46	13.83	14.56	15.56	16.91	17.84	18.60	20.00	21.17
89.5	-2.7934	15.5944	0.1103	13.24	13.47	13.84	14.58	15.59	16.95	17.90	18.67	20.08	21.26
90.5	-2.7673	15.6252	0.1113	13.25	13.47	13.86	14.60	15.63	17.00	17.95	18.73	20.17	21.36
91.5	-2.7415	15.6568	0.1123	13.25	13.48	13.87	14.62	15.66	17.04	18.01	18.80	20.25	21.47
92.5	-2.7160	15.6893	0.1133	13.26	13.49	13.88	14.64	15.69	17.09	18.07	18.87	20.34	21.57
93.5	-2.6908	15.7226	0.1142	13.27	13.50	13.90	14.66	15.72	17.14	18.13	18.94	20.43	21.67
94.5	-2.6659	15.7566	0.1152	13.28	13.52	13.91	14.68	15.76	17.19	18.19	19.01	20.52	21.77
95.5	-2.6413	15.7914	0.1162	13.29	13.53	13.93	14.71	15.79	17.24	18.25	19.08	20.61	21.88

CDC Growth Standards

Table V.11b.

LMS parameters and smoothed percentiles of body mass index (kg/m^2)-for-age in months for girls from 2 to 20 years

Age Group (months)	L	M	S	3rd	5th	10th	25th	50th	75th	85th	90th	95th	97th
96.5	-2.6172	15.8270	0.1172	13.30	13.54	13.94	14.73	15.83	17.29	18.32	19.15	20.70	21.98
97.5	-2.5934	15.8633	0.1181	13.31	13.55	13.96	14.76	15.86	17.34	18.38	19.23	20.79	22.09
98.5	-2.5701	15.9003	0.1191	13.32	13.57	13.98	14.78	15.90	17.40	18.44	19.30	20.88	22.19
99.5	-2.5471	15.9380	0.1200	13.34	13.58	14.00	14.81	15.94	17.45	18.51	19.37	20.97	22.30
100.5	-2.5246	15.9764	0.1209	13.35	13.60	14.02	14.83	15.98	17.50	18.57	19.45	21.06	22.41
101.5	-2.5026	16.0155	0.1219	13.36	13.61	14.04	14.86	16.02	17.56	18.64	19.52	21.15	22.51
102.5	-2.4810	16.0552	0.1228	13.38	13.63	14.06	14.89	16.06	17.61	18.71	19.60	21.25	22.62
103.5	-2.4598	16.0955	0.1237	13.39	13.65	14.08	14.92	16.10	17.67	18.77	19.68	21.34	22.73
104.5	-2.4391	16.1365	0.1246	13.41	13.67	14.10	14.95	16.14	17.73	18.84	19.75	21.44	22.84
105.5	-2.4188	16.1780	0.1254	13.42	13.68	14.12	14.98	16.18	17.78	18.91	19.83	21.53	22.95
106.5	-2.3991	16.2201	0.1263	13.44	13.70	14.15	15.01	16.22	17.84	18.98	19.91	21.63	23.06
107.5	-2.3798	16.2628	0.1272	13.46	13.72	14.17	15.04	16.26	17.90	19.05	19.99	21.72	23.17
108.5	-2.3609	16.3061	0.1280	13.48	13.74	14.19	15.07	16.31	17.96	19.12	20.07	21.82	23.28
109.5	-2.3426	16.3499	0.1288	13.49	13.77	14.22	15.11	16.35	18.02	19.19	20.15	21.91	23.39
110.5	-2.3247	16.3942	0.1297	13.51	13.79	14.25	15.14	16.39	18.08	19.26	20.23	22.01	23.50
111.5	-2.3072	16.4390	0.1305	13.53	13.81	14.27	15.17	16.44	18.14	19.33	20.31	22.11	23.61
112.5	-2.2903	16.4843	0.1313	13.55	13.83	14.30	15.21	16.48	18.20	19.40	20.39	22.20	23.72
113.5	-2.2738	16.5300	0.1320	13.58	13.86	14.33	15.24	16.53	18.26	19.47	20.47	22.30	23.83
114.5	-2.2578	16.5763	0.1328	13.60	13.88	14.35	15.28	16.58	18.32	19.55	20.55	22.40	23.94
115.5	-2.2422	16.6229	0.1335	13.62	13.90	14.38	15.31	16.62	18.38	19.62	20.63	22.50	24.05
116.5	-2.2271	16.6700	0.1343	13.64	13.93	14.41	15.35	16.67	18.44	19.69	20.71	22.59	24.16
117.5	-2.2125	16.7175	0.1350	13.67	13.95	14.44	15.39	16.72	18.51	19.76	20.79	22.69	24.27
118.5	-2.1983	16.7654	0.1357	13.69	13.98	14.47	15.42	16.77	18.57	19.84	20.87	22.79	24.38
119.5	-2.1846	16.8137	0.1364	13.72	14.01	14.50	15.46	16.81	18.63	19.91	20.95	22.89	24.49
120.5	-2.1713	16.8623	0.1371	13.74	14.04	14.53	15.50	16.86	18.70	19.98	21.04	22.98	24.60
121.5	-2.1585	16.9113	0.1377	13.77	14.06	14.56	15.54	16.91	18.76	20.06	21.12	23.08	24.71
122.5	-2.1461	16.9606	0.1384	13.79	14.09	14.59	15.58	16.96	18.82	20.13	21.20	23.18	24.82
123.5	-2.1341	17.0103	0.1390	13.82	14.12	14.63	15.62	17.01	18.89	20.20	21.28	23.27	24.93
124.5	-2.1225	17.0602	0.1396	13.85	14.15	14.66	15.66	17.06	18.95	20.28	21.36	23.37	25.04
125.5	-2.1114	17.1105	0.1402	13.88	14.18	14.69	15.70	17.11	19.01	20.35	21.45	23.47	25.15
126.5	-2.1007	17.1610	0.1408	13.90	14.21	14.73	15.74	17.16	19.08	20.43	21.53	23.57	25.26
127.5	-2.0905	17.2117	0.1413	13.93	14.24	14.76	15.78	17.21	19.14	20.50	21.61	23.66	25.37
128.5	-2.0806	17.2628	0.1419	13.96	14.27	14.80	15.82	17.26	19.21	20.57	21.69	23.76	25.48
129.5	-2.0712	17.3140	0.1424	13.99	14.30	14.83	15.86	17.31	19.27	20.65	21.77	23.85	25.59
130.5	-2.0621	17.3655	0.1429	14.02	14.34	14.87	15.90	17.37	19.34	20.72	21.86	23.95	25.69
131.5	-2.0535	17.4172	0.1434	14.05	14.37	14.90	15.95	17.42	19.40	20.80	21.94	24.05	25.80
132.5	-2.0452	17.4691	0.1439	14.08	14.40	14.94	15.99	17.47	19.46	20.87	22.02	24.14	25.91
133.5	-2.0374	17.5211	0.1443	14.12	14.44	14.98	16.03	17.52	19.53	20.94	22.10	24.24	26.02
134.5	-2.0299	17.5733	0.1448	14.15	14.47	15.01	16.08	17.57	19.59	21.02	22.18	24.33	26.12
135.5	-2.0228	17.6257	0.1452	14.18	14.51	15.05	16.12	17.63	19.66	21.09	22.26	24.43	26.23
136.5	-2.0161	17.6782	0.1456	14.21	14.54	15.09	16.16	17.68	19.72	21.16	22.34	24.52	26.33
137.5	-2.0098	17.7308	0.1460	14.25	14.58	15.13	16.21	17.73	19.79	21.24	22.42	24.61	26.44
138.5	-2.0038	17.7836	0.1464	14.28	14.61	15.17	16.25	17.78	19.85	21.31	22.50	24.71	26.54
139.5	-1.9982	17.8364	0.1468	14.32	14.65	15.20	16.30	17.84	19.92	21.38	22.58	24.80	26.65
140.5	-1.9930	17.8893	0.1471	14.35	14.68	15.24	16.34	17.89	19.98	21.45	22.66	24.89	26.75
141.5	-1.9881	17.9423	0.1474	14.39	14.72	15.28	16.39	17.94	20.04	21.53	22.74	24.98	26.85
142.5	-1.9835	17.9953	0.1478	14.42	14.76	15.32	16.43	18.00	20.11	21.60	22.82	25.07	26.95
143.5	-1.9794	18.0484	0.1481	14.46	14.79	15.36	16.48	18.05	20.17	21.67	22.90	25.17	27.05
144.5	-1.9755	18.1015	0.1484	14.49	14.83	15.40	16.52	18.10	20.24	21.74	22.97	25.26	27.16
145.5	-1.9720	18.1546	0.1486	14.53	14.87	15.44	16.57	18.15	20.30	21.81	23.05	25.35	27.26
146.5	-1.9689	18.2077	0.1489	14.57	14.91	15.48	16.61	18.21	20.36	21.88	23.13	25.43	27.36
147.5	-1.9660	18.2609	0.1491	14.61	14.95	15.53	16.66	18.26	20.43	21.96	23.21	25.52	27.46
148.5	-1.9635	18.3139	0.1494	14.64	14.99	15.57	16.71	18.31	20.49	22.03	23.28	25.61	27.55
149.5	-1.9614	18.3670	0.1496	14.68	15.03	15.61	16.75	18.37	20.55	22.10	23.36	25.70	27.65
150.5	-1.9595	18.4200	0.1498	14.72	15.07	15.65	16.80	18.42	20.61	22.17	23.43	25.79	27.75
151.5	-1.9580	18.4730	0.1500	14.76	15.11	15.69	16.84	18.47	20.68	22.23	23.51	25.87	27.85
152.5	-1.9568	18.5259	0.1501	14.80	15.15	15.73	16.89	18.53	20.74	22.30	23.58	25.96	27.94
153.5	-1.9559	18.5787	0.1503	14.83	15.19	15.78	16.94	18.58	20.80	22.37	23.66	26.05	28.04
154.5	-1.9553	18.6314	0.1505	14.87	15.23	15.82	16.98	18.63	20.86	22.44	23.73	26.13	28.13
155.5	-1.9550	18.6840	0.1506	14.91	15.27	15.86	17.03	18.68	20.92	22.51	23.81	26.22	28.23
156.5	-1.9550	18.7364	0.1507	14.95	15.31	15.90	17.08	18.74	20.98	22.58	23.88	26.30	28.32
157.5	-1.9553	18.7888	0.1508	14.99	15.35	15.95	17.12	18.79	21.05	22.64	23.95	26.38	28.41
158.5	-1.9559	18.8410	0.1509	15.03	15.39	15.99	17.17	18.84	21.11	22.71	24.02	26.46	28.51
159.5	-1.9568	18.8930	0.1510	15.07	15.43	16.03	17.22	18.89	21.17	22.77	24.09	26.55	28.60
160.5	-1.9579	18.9449	0.1511	15.11	15.47	16.08	17.26	18.94	21.23	22.84	24.17	26.63	28.69
161.5	-1.9594	18.9966	0.1511	15.15	15.51	16.12	17.31	19.00	21.28	22.90	24.24	26.71	28.78
162.5	-1.9611	19.0481	0.1512	15.20	15.56	16.16	17.36	19.05	21.34	22.97	24.30	26.79	28.87
163.5	-1.9631	19.0994	0.1512	15.24	15.60	16.21	17.40	19.10	21.40	23.03	24.37	26.87	28.96
164.5	-1.9654	19.1505	0.1512	15.28	15.64	16.25	17.45	19.15	21.46	23.10	24.44	26.95	29.05
165.5	-1.9679	19.2014	0.1513	15.32	15.68	16.29	17.50	19.20	21.52	23.16	24.51	27.03	29.14
166.5	-1.9707	19.2520	0.1513	15.36	15.72	16.34	17.54	19.25	21.57	23.22	24.58	27.10	29.22
167.5	-1.9738	19.3024	0.1513	15.40	15.77	16.38	17.59	19.30	21.63	23.29	24.65	27.18	29.31
168.5	-1.9771	19.3526	0.1513	15.44	15.81	16.42	17.64	19.35	21.69	23.35	24.71	27.26	29.40

230

CDC Growth Standards

Table V.11c.

LMS parameters and smoothed percentiles of body mass index (kg/m^2)-for-age in months for girls from 2 to 20 years

Age Group (months)	L	M	S	3rd	5th	10th	25th	50th	75th	85th	90th	95th	97th
169.5	-1.9806	19.4024	0.1512	15.48	15.85	16.47	17.68	19.40	21.74	23.41	24.78	27.33	29.48
170.5	-1.9844	19.4520	0.1512	15.53	15.89	16.51	17.73	19.45	21.80	23.47	24.84	27.41	29.57
171.5	-1.9885	19.5014	0.1512	15.57	15.93	16.55	17.77	19.50	21.86	23.53	24.91	27.48	29.65
172.5	-1.9928	19.5504	0.1511	15.61	15.98	16.60	17.82	19.55	21.91	23.59	24.97	27.55	29.74
173.5	-1.9973	19.5991	0.1511	15.65	16.02	16.64	17.86	19.60	21.96	23.65	25.03	27.63	29.82
174.5	-2.0020	19.6475	0.1510	15.69	16.06	16.68	17.91	19.65	22.02	23.71	25.10	27.70	29.90
175.5	-2.0070	19.6955	0.1509	15.73	16.10	16.73	17.95	19.70	22.07	23.76	25.16	27.77	29.98
176.5	-2.0121	19.7432	0.1509	15.77	16.14	16.77	18.00	19.74	22.12	23.82	25.22	27.84	30.06
177.5	-2.0175	19.7906	0.1508	15.81	16.19	16.81	18.04	19.79	22.18	23.88	25.28	27.91	30.15
178.5	-2.0231	19.8376	0.1507	15.86	16.23	16.85	18.09	19.84	22.23	23.93	25.34	27.99	30.23
179.5	-2.0289	19.8843	0.1506	15.90	16.27	16.90	18.13	19.88	22.28	23.99	25.40	28.05	30.31
180.5	-2.0349	19.9306	0.1505	15.94	16.31	16.94	18.17	19.93	22.33	24.05	25.46	28.12	30.39
181.5	-2.0411	19.9765	0.1504	15.98	16.35	16.98	18.22	19.98	22.38	24.10	25.52	28.19	30.46
182.5	-2.0474	20.0220	0.1503	16.02	16.39	17.02	18.26	20.02	22.43	24.15	25.58	28.26	30.54
183.5	-2.0539	20.0670	0.1502	16.06	16.43	17.06	18.30	20.07	22.48	24.21	25.64	28.33	30.62
184.5	-2.0606	20.1117	0.1501	16.10	16.47	17.10	18.35	20.11	22.53	24.26	25.69	28.39	30.70
185.5	-2.0675	20.1560	0.1500	16.14	16.51	17.14	18.39	20.16	22.58	24.31	25.75	28.46	30.78
186.5	-2.0745	20.1998	0.1498	16.18	16.55	17.19	18.43	20.20	22.63	24.36	25.81	28.53	30.85
187.5	-2.0816	20.2432	0.1497	16.22	16.59	17.23	18.47	20.24	22.67	24.42	25.86	28.59	30.93
188.5	-2.0889	20.2861	0.1496	16.26	16.63	17.27	18.51	20.29	22.72	24.47	25.92	28.66	31.00
189.5	-2.0963	20.3286	0.1495	16.30	16.67	17.30	18.55	20.33	22.77	24.52	25.97	28.72	31.08
190.5	-2.1038	20.3706	0.1493	16.34	16.71	17.34	18.59	20.37	22.81	24.57	26.02	28.78	31.16
191.5	-2.1114	20.4122	0.1492	16.37	16.75	17.38	18.63	20.41	22.86	24.62	26.08	28.85	31.23
192.5	-2.1192	20.4533	0.1491	16.41	16.79	17.42	18.67	20.45	22.90	24.66	26.13	28.91	31.30
193.5	-2.1270	20.4938	0.1490	16.45	16.83	17.46	18.71	20.49	22.95	24.71	26.18	28.97	31.38
194.5	-2.1349	20.5339	0.1488	16.49	16.86	17.50	18.75	20.53	22.99	24.76	26.23	29.03	31.45
195.5	-2.1428	20.5735	0.1487	16.52	16.90	17.53	18.79	20.57	23.03	24.81	26.28	29.10	31.53
196.5	-2.1509	20.6126	0.1486	16.56	16.94	17.57	18.82	20.61	23.08	24.85	26.33	29.16	31.60
197.5	-2.1589	20.6511	0.1485	16.60	16.97	17.61	18.86	20.65	23.12	24.90	26.38	29.22	31.67
198.5	-2.1670	20.6891	0.1483	16.63	17.01	17.64	18.90	20.69	23.16	24.94	26.43	29.28	31.75
199.5	-2.1752	20.7266	0.1482	16.67	17.04	17.68	18.93	20.73	23.20	24.99	26.48	29.34	31.82
200.5	-2.1833	20.7636	0.1481	16.70	17.08	17.71	18.97	20.76	23.24	25.03	26.53	29.40	31.89
201.5	-2.1915	20.7999	0.1480	16.74	17.11	17.75	19.00	20.80	23.28	25.08	26.58	29.46	31.97
202.5	-2.1996	20.8358	0.1479	16.77	17.15	17.78	19.04	20.84	23.32	25.12	26.63	29.52	32.04
203.5	-2.2077	20.8711	0.1478	16.80	17.18	17.82	19.07	20.87	23.36	25.16	26.67	29.57	32.11
204.5	-2.2157	20.9058	0.1477	16.84	17.21	17.85	19.11	20.91	23.40	25.20	26.72	29.63	32.19
205.5	-2.2237	20.9399	0.1476	16.87	17.24	17.88	19.14	20.94	23.43	25.25	26.77	29.69	32.26
206.5	-2.2317	20.9734	0.1476	16.90	17.28	17.91	19.17	20.97	23.47	25.29	26.81	29.75	32.33
207.5	-2.2395	21.0064	0.1475	16.93	17.31	17.94	19.20	21.01	23.51	25.33	26.86	29.81	32.41
208.5	-2.2473	21.0387	0.1474	16.96	17.34	17.97	19.23	21.04	23.54	25.37	26.90	29.87	32.48
209.5	-2.2549	21.0705	0.1474	16.99	17.37	18.00	19.26	21.07	23.58	25.41	26.95	29.92	32.55
210.5	-2.2624	21.1016	0.1473	17.02	17.39	18.03	19.29	21.10	23.62	25.45	26.99	29.98	32.63
211.5	-2.2697	21.1322	0.1473	17.05	17.42	18.06	19.32	21.13	23.65	25.49	27.04	30.04	32.70
212.5	-2.2769	21.1621	0.1473	17.07	17.45	18.09	19.35	21.16	23.68	25.53	27.08	30.10	32.77
213.5	-2.2839	21.1913	0.1472	17.10	17.48	18.11	19.38	21.19	23.72	25.57	27.13	30.15	32.85
214.5	-2.2907	21.2200	0.1472	17.12	17.50	18.14	19.40	21.22	23.75	25.60	27.17	30.21	32.92
215.5	-2.2973	21.2480	0.1472	17.15	17.53	18.17	19.43	21.25	23.78	25.64	27.21	30.27	33.00
216.5	-2.3037	21.2753	0.1473	17.17	17.55	18.19	19.45	21.28	23.82	25.68	27.25	30.33	33.07
217.5	-2.3098	21.3020	0.1473	17.20	17.57	18.21	19.48	21.30	23.85	25.71	27.30	30.38	33.15
218.5	-2.3157	21.3281	0.1473	17.22	17.60	18.24	19.50	21.33	23.88	25.75	27.34	30.44	33.23
219.5	-2.3212	21.3534	0.1474	17.24	17.62	18.26	19.53	21.35	23.91	25.79	27.38	30.50	33.30
220.5	-2.3265	21.3781	0.1475	17.26	17.64	18.28	19.55	21.38	23.94	25.82	27.42	30.56	33.38
221.5	-2.3314	21.4021	0.1476	17.28	17.66	18.30	19.57	21.40	23.97	25.86	27.47	30.61	33.46
222.5	-2.3360	21.4255	0.1477	17.30	17.68	18.32	19.59	21.43	24.00	25.89	27.51	30.67	33.54
223.5	-2.3403	21.4481	0.1478	17.31	17.69	18.34	19.61	21.45	24.03	25.93	27.55	30.73	33.62
224.5	-2.3442	21.4701	0.1480	17.33	17.71	18.35	19.63	21.47	24.06	25.96	27.59	30.79	33.70
225.5	-2.3477	21.4913	0.1481	17.35	17.72	18.37	19.65	21.49	24.08	26.00	27.63	30.85	33.78
226.5	-2.3508	21.5119	0.1483	17.36	17.74	18.38	19.66	21.51	24.11	26.03	27.67	30.91	33.86
227.5	-2.3534	21.5317	0.1485	17.37	17.75	18.40	19.68	21.53	24.14	26.07	27.71	30.97	33.94
228.5	-2.3557	21.5508	0.1487	17.38	17.77	18.41	19.70	21.55	24.16	26.10	27.76	31.03	34.02
229.5	-2.3575	21.5692	0.1490	17.39	17.78	18.42	19.71	21.57	24.19	26.13	27.80	31.09	34.11
230.5	-2.3588	21.5869	0.1492	17.40	17.79	18.43	19.72	21.59	24.22	26.17	27.84	31.15	34.19
231.5	-2.3596	21.6038	0.1495	17.41	17.80	18.44	19.74	21.60	24.24	26.20	27.88	31.21	34.28
232.5	-2.3599	21.6200	0.1498	17.42	17.80	18.45	19.75	21.62	24.27	26.23	27.92	31.27	34.37
233.5	-2.3597	21.6354	0.1502	17.43	17.81	18.46	19.76	21.64	24.29	26.27	27.96	31.34	34.45
234.5	-2.3590	21.6501	0.1505	17.43	17.81	18.47	19.77	21.65	24.31	26.30	28.00	31.40	34.54
235.5	-2.3577	21.6640	0.1509	17.43	17.82	18.47	19.78	21.66	24.34	26.33	28.05	31.47	34.63
236.5	-2.3559	21.6771	0.1513	17.43	17.82	18.48	19.78	21.68	24.36	26.36	28.09	31.53	34.73
237.5	-2.3535	21.6895	0.1518	17.44	17.82	18.48	19.79	21.69	24.38	26.40	28.13	31.60	34.82
238.5	-2.3505	21.7011	0.1522	17.43	17.82	18.48	19.79	21.70	24.41	26.43	28.17	31.66	34.91
239.5	-2.3470	21.7119	0.1527	17.43	17.82	18.48	19.80	21.71	24.43	26.46	28.22	31.73	35.01
240.0	-2.3450	21.7170	0.1530	17.43	17.82	18.48	19.80	21.72	24.44	26.48	28.24	31.76	35.06

LIST OF FIGURES: CDC GROWTH CHARTS

Source: http://www.cdc.gov/growthcharts/ May 30, 2000.

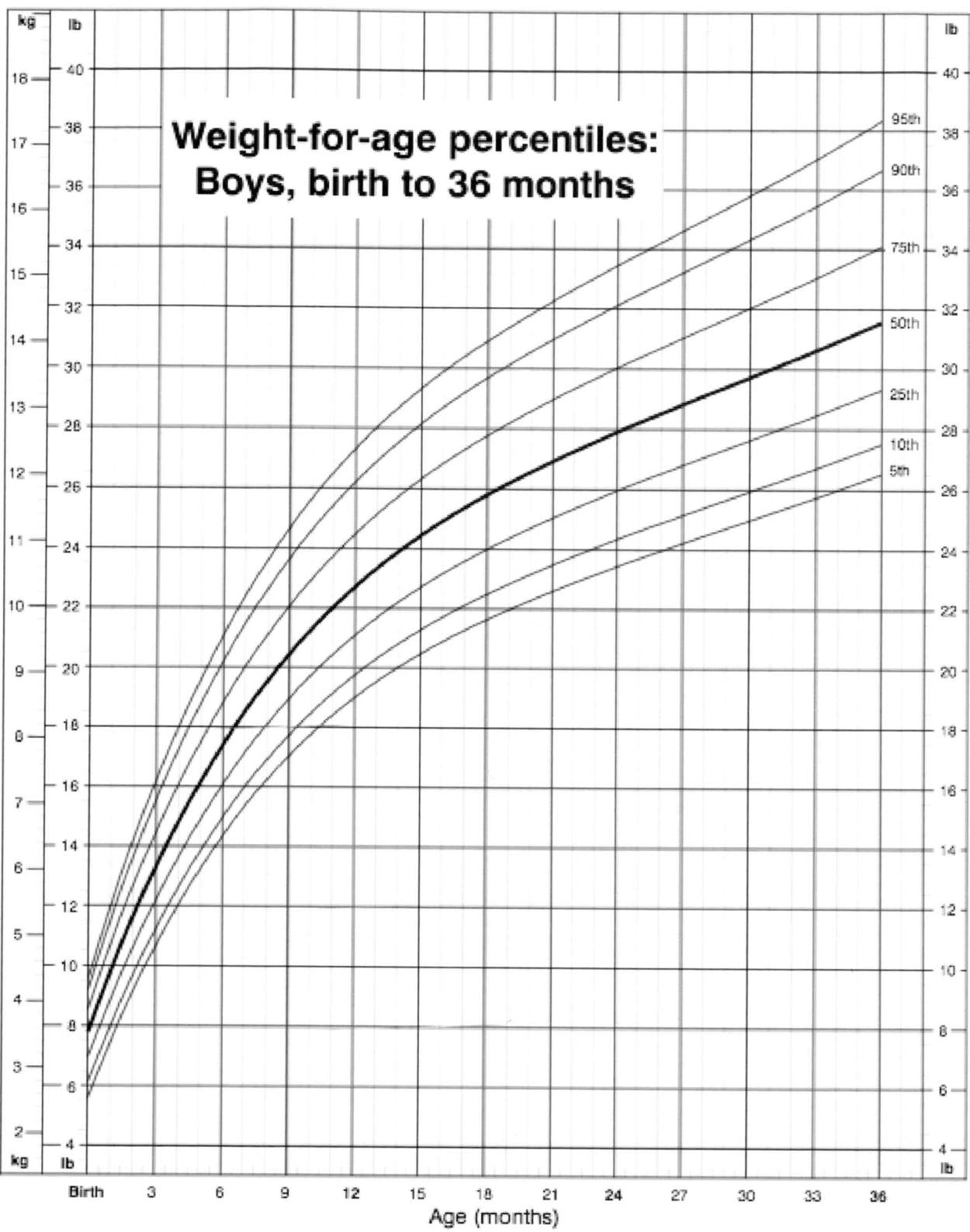

Figure V.1. Percentiles of Weight (kg) and Pounds (lb.) by Age for Boys from Birth to 36 Months.

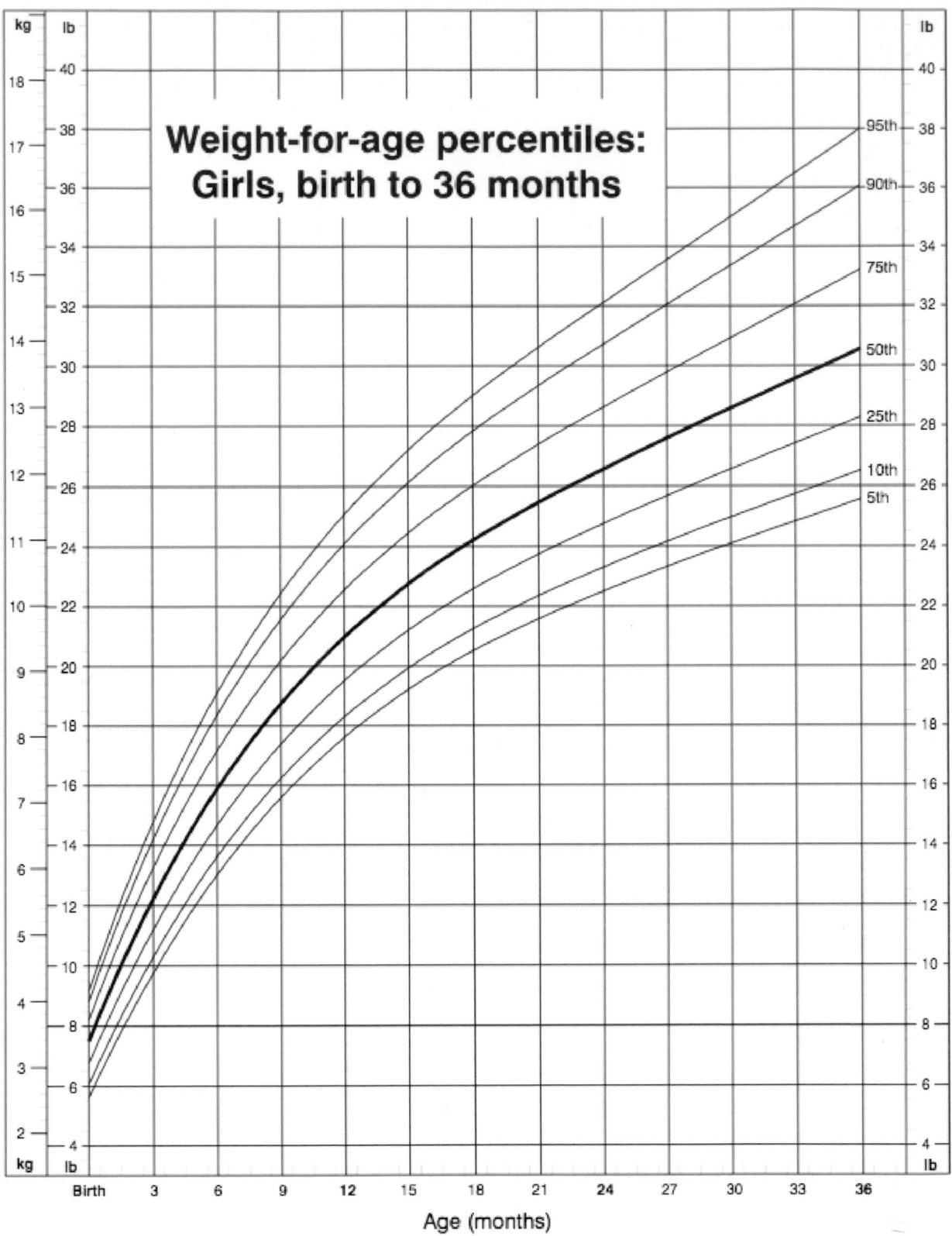

Figure V.2. Percentiles of Weight (kg) and Pounds (lb.) by Age for Girls from Birth to 36 Months.

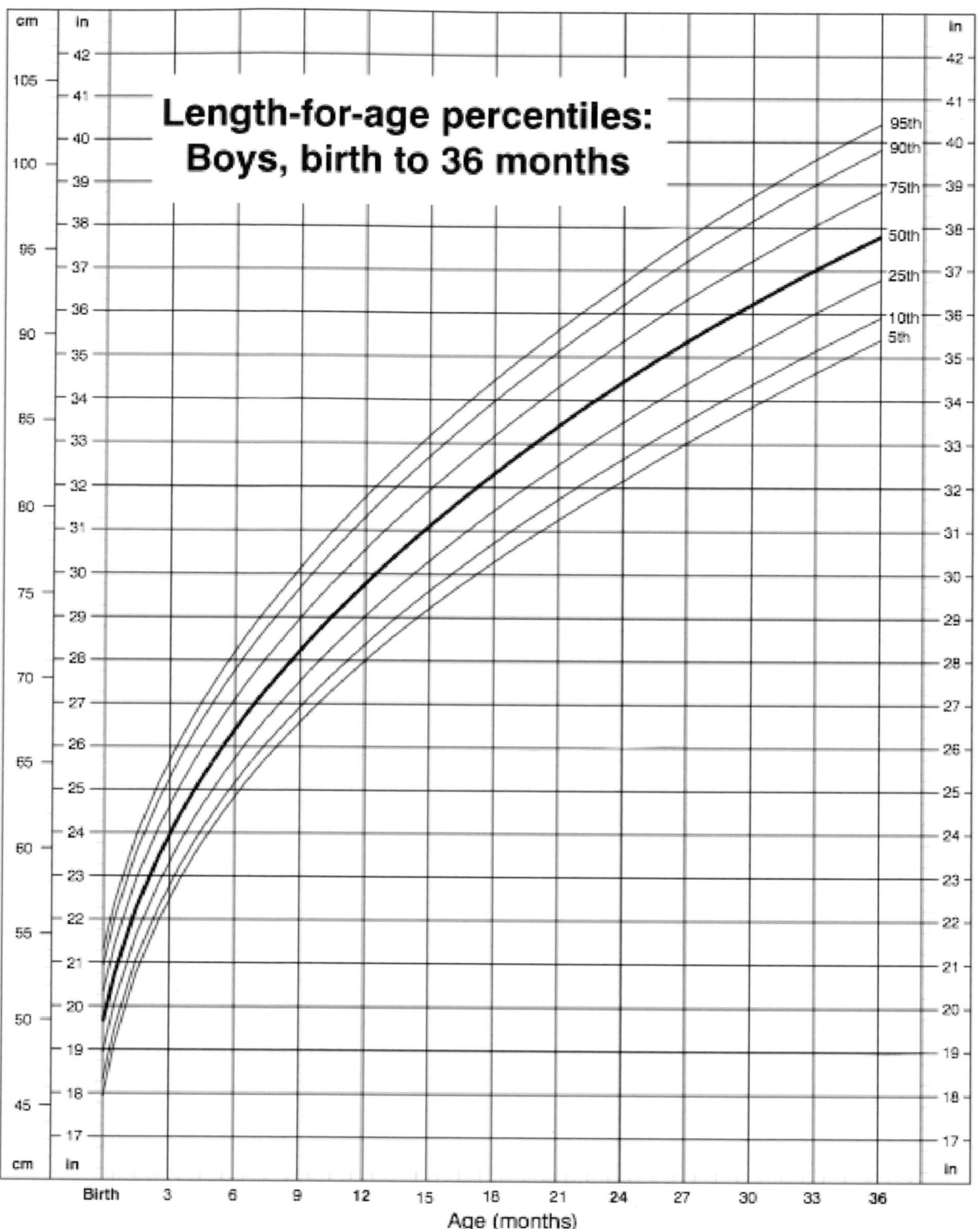

Figure V.3. Percentiles of Recumbent Length in Centimeters (cm) and Inches (in.) by Age for Boys from Birth to 36 Months.

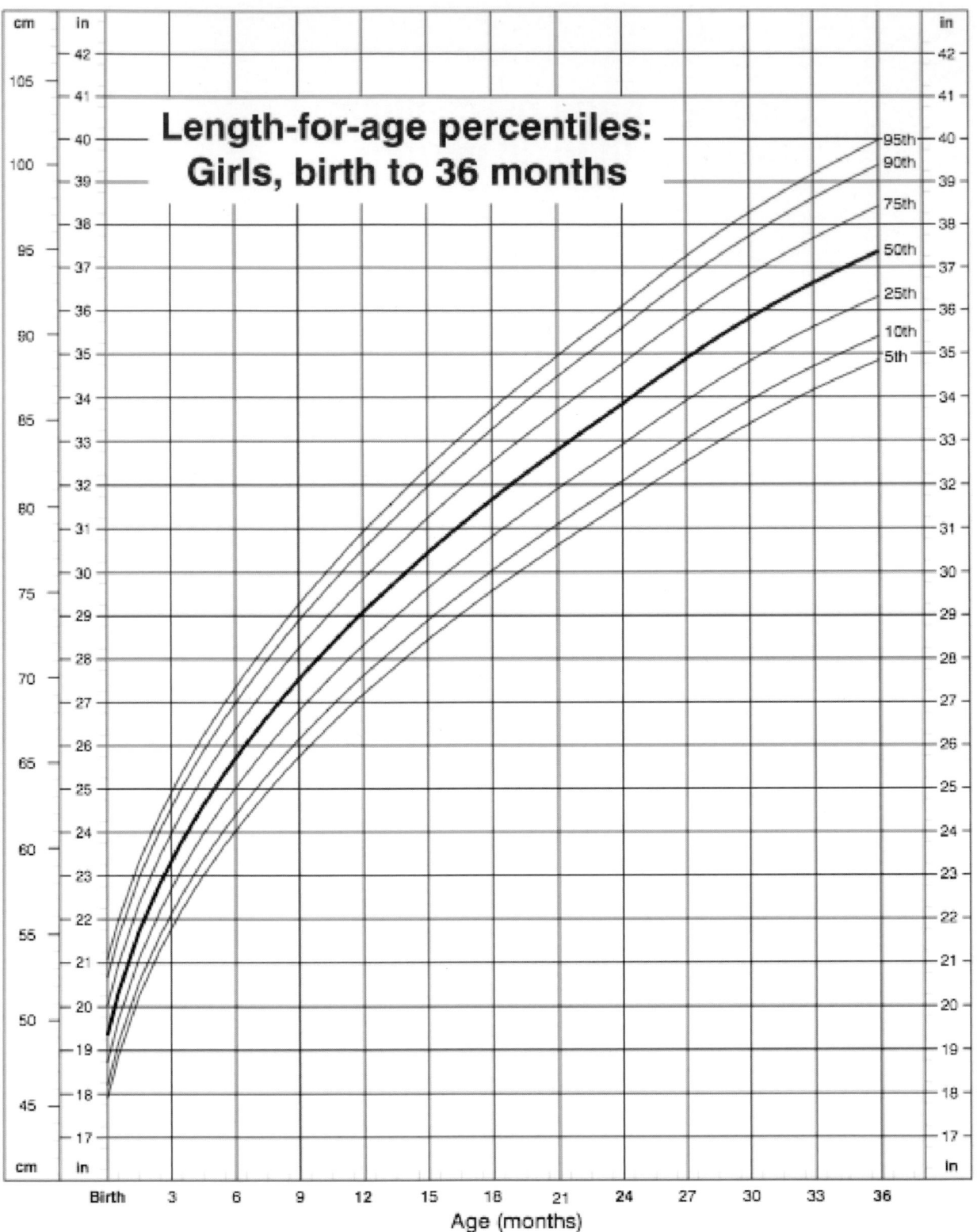

Figure V.4. Percentiles of Recumbent Length in Centimeters (cm) and Inches (in.) by Age for Girls from Birth to 36 Months.

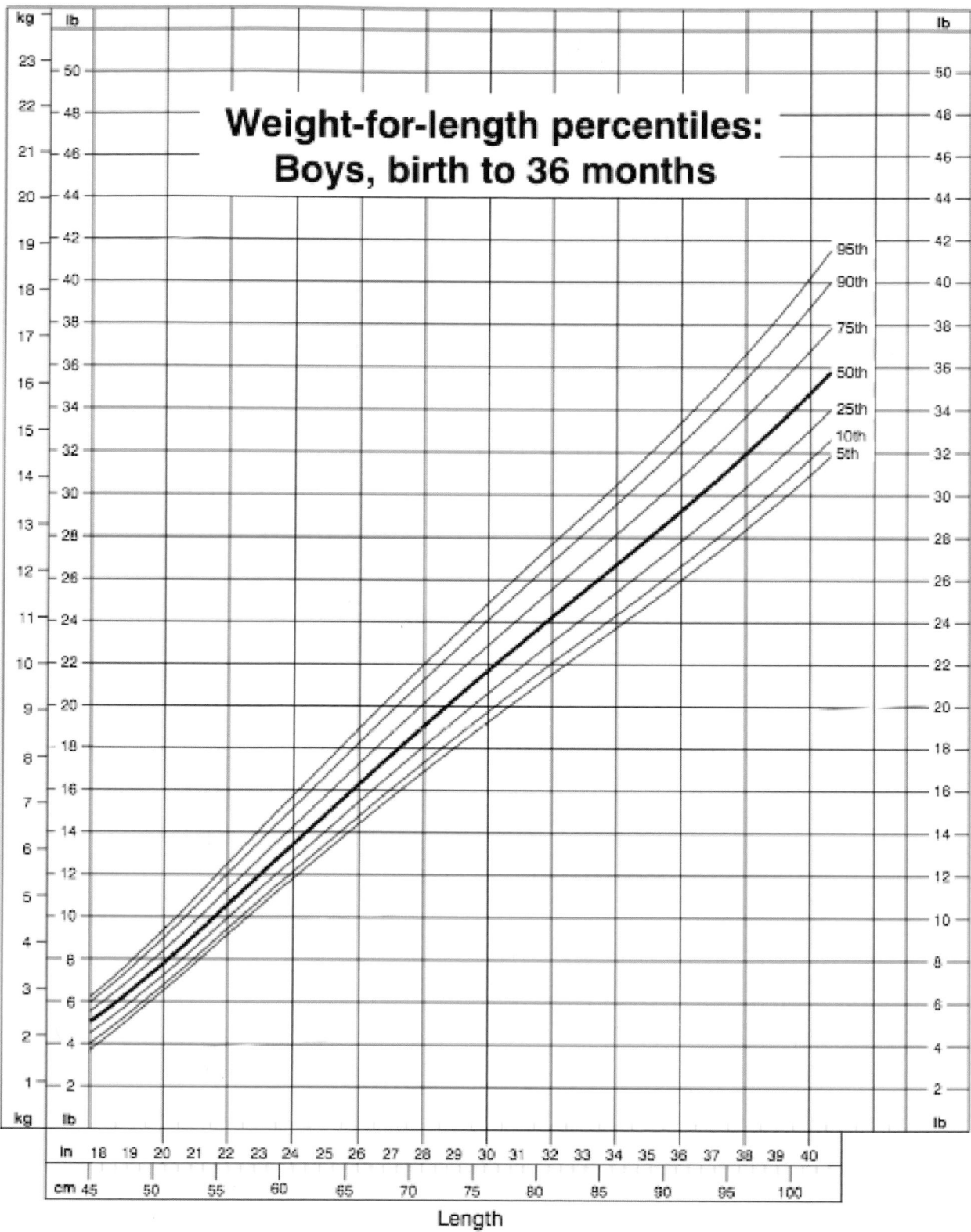

Figure V.5. Percentiles of Recumbent Length in Centimeters (cm) and Inches (in.) and Weight in Kilograms (kg) and Pounds (lb.) by Age for Boys from Birth to 36 Months.

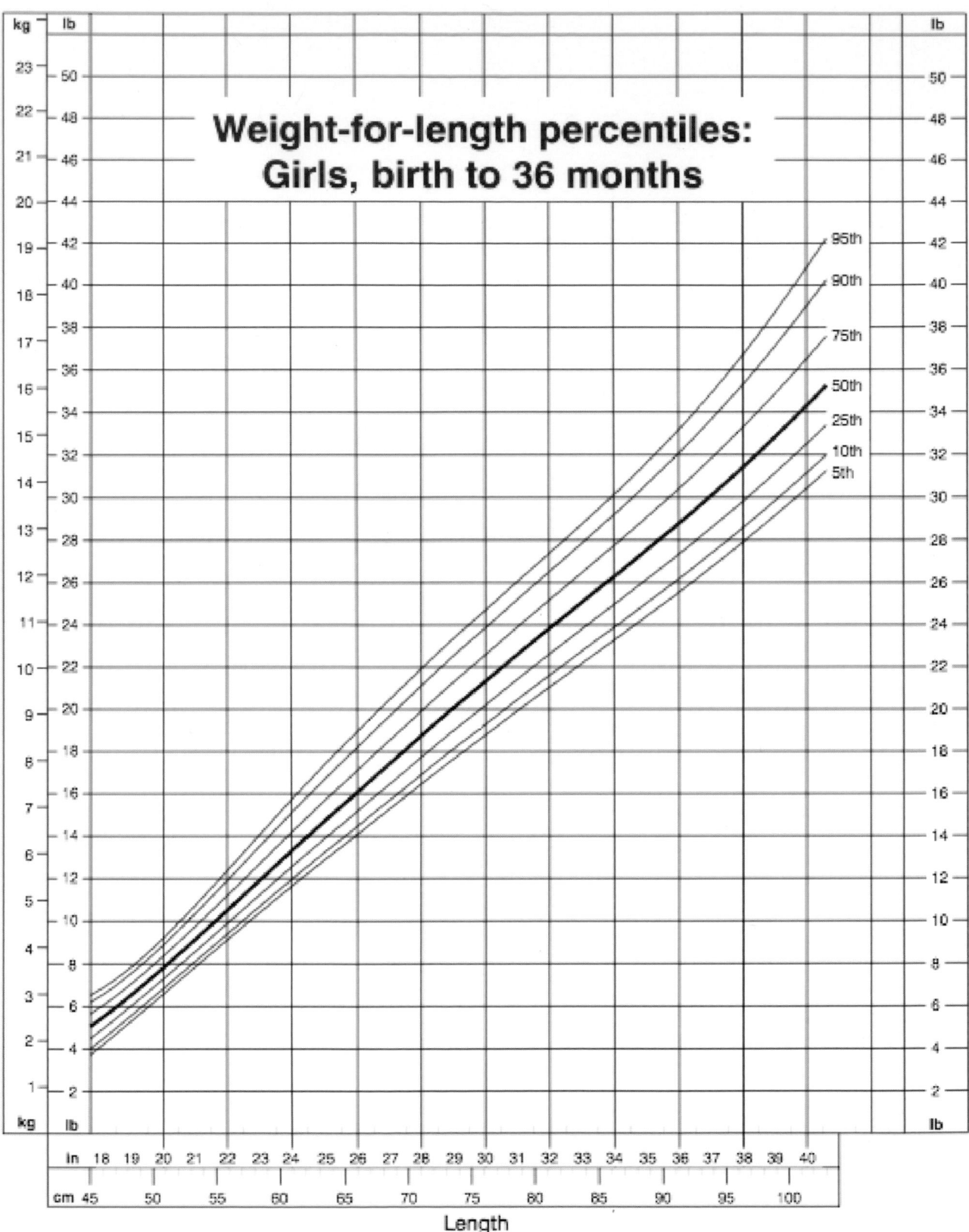

Figure V.6. Percentiles of Recumbent Length in Centimeters (cm) and Inches (in.) and Weight in Kilograms (kg) and Pounds (lb.) by Age for Girls from Birth to 36 Months.

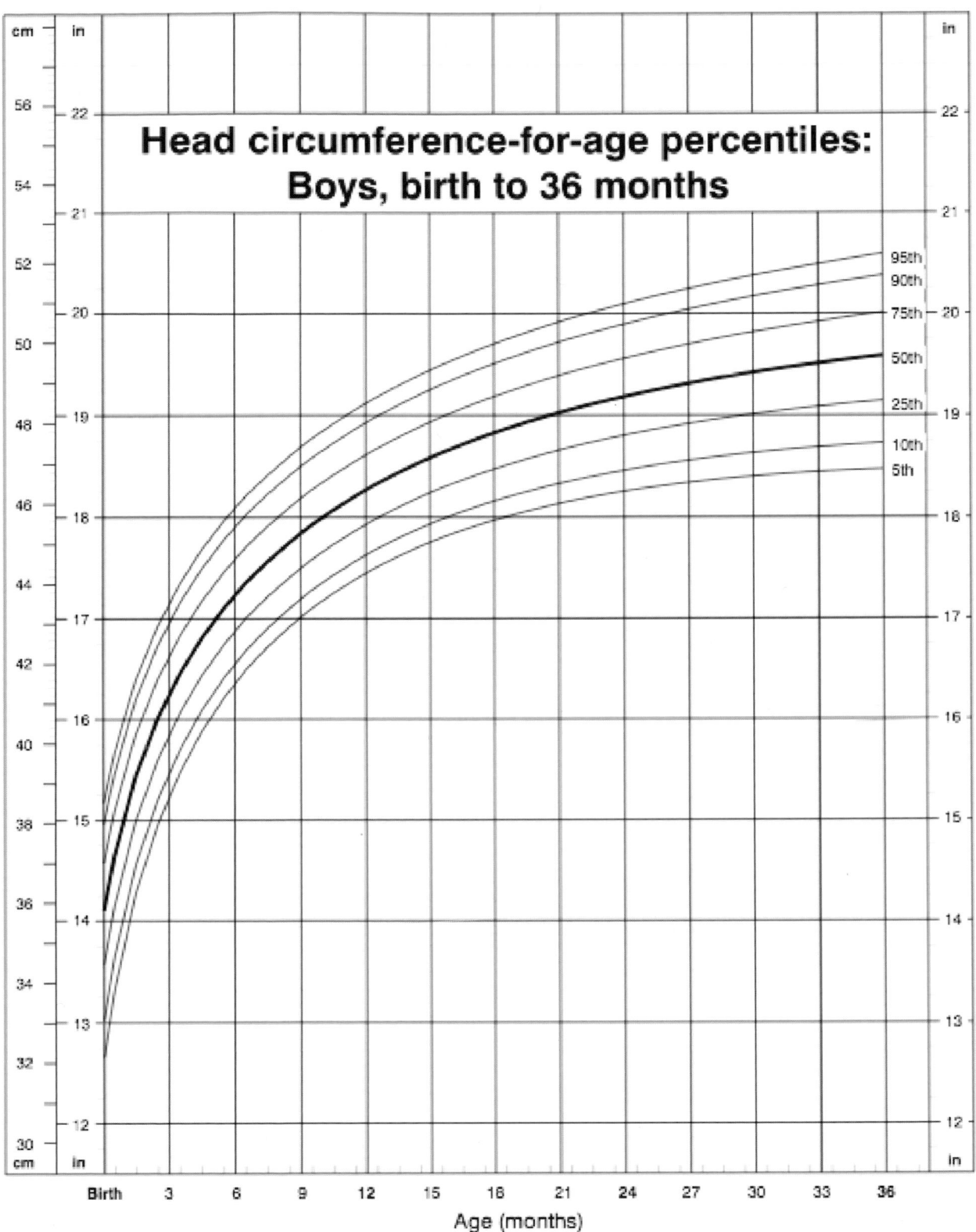

Figure V.7. Percentiles of Head Circumference in Centimeters (cm) and Inches (in.) by Age for Boys from Birth to 36 Months.

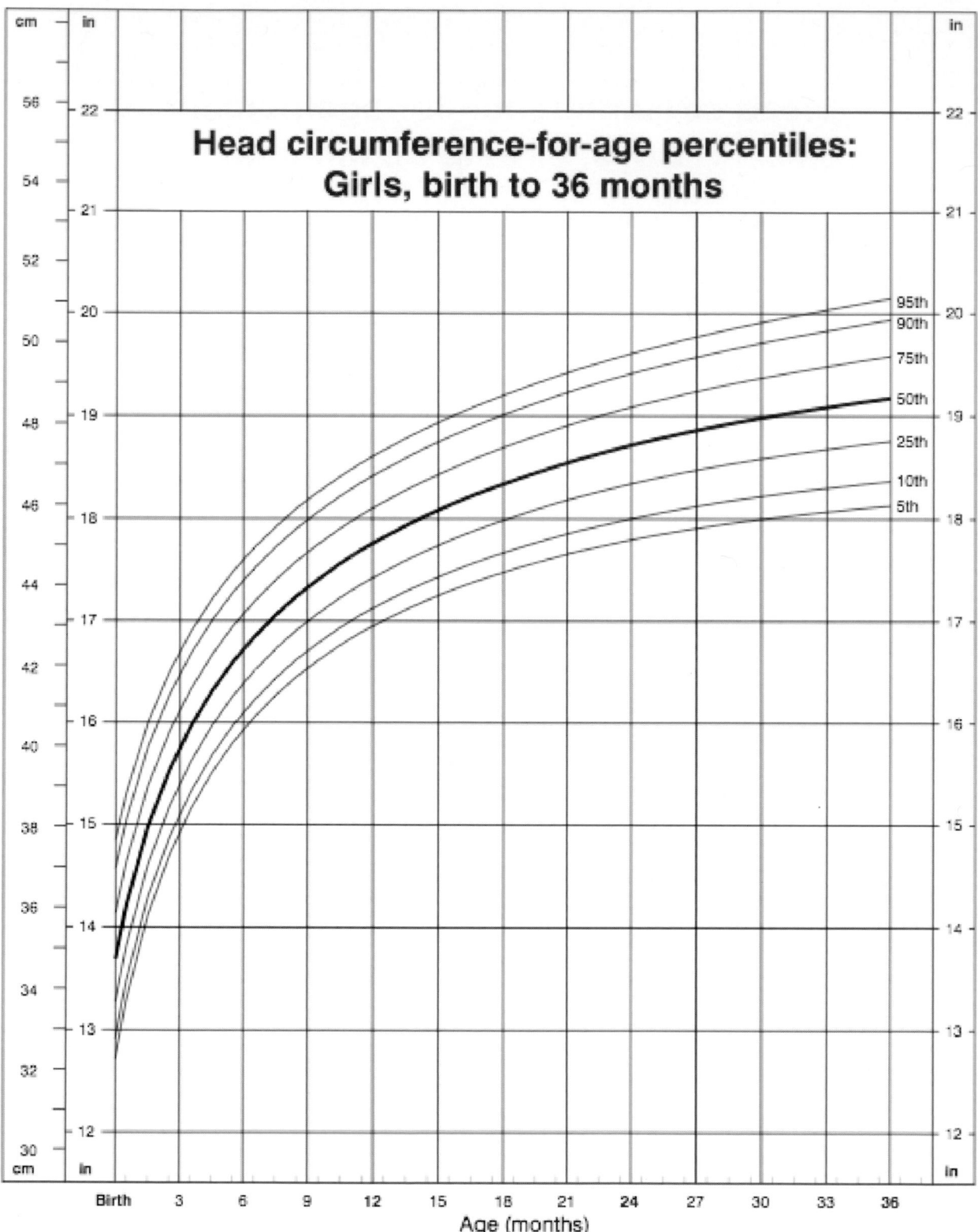

Figure V.8. Percentiles of Head Circumference in Centimeters (cm) and Inches (in.) by Age for Girls from Birth to 36 Months.

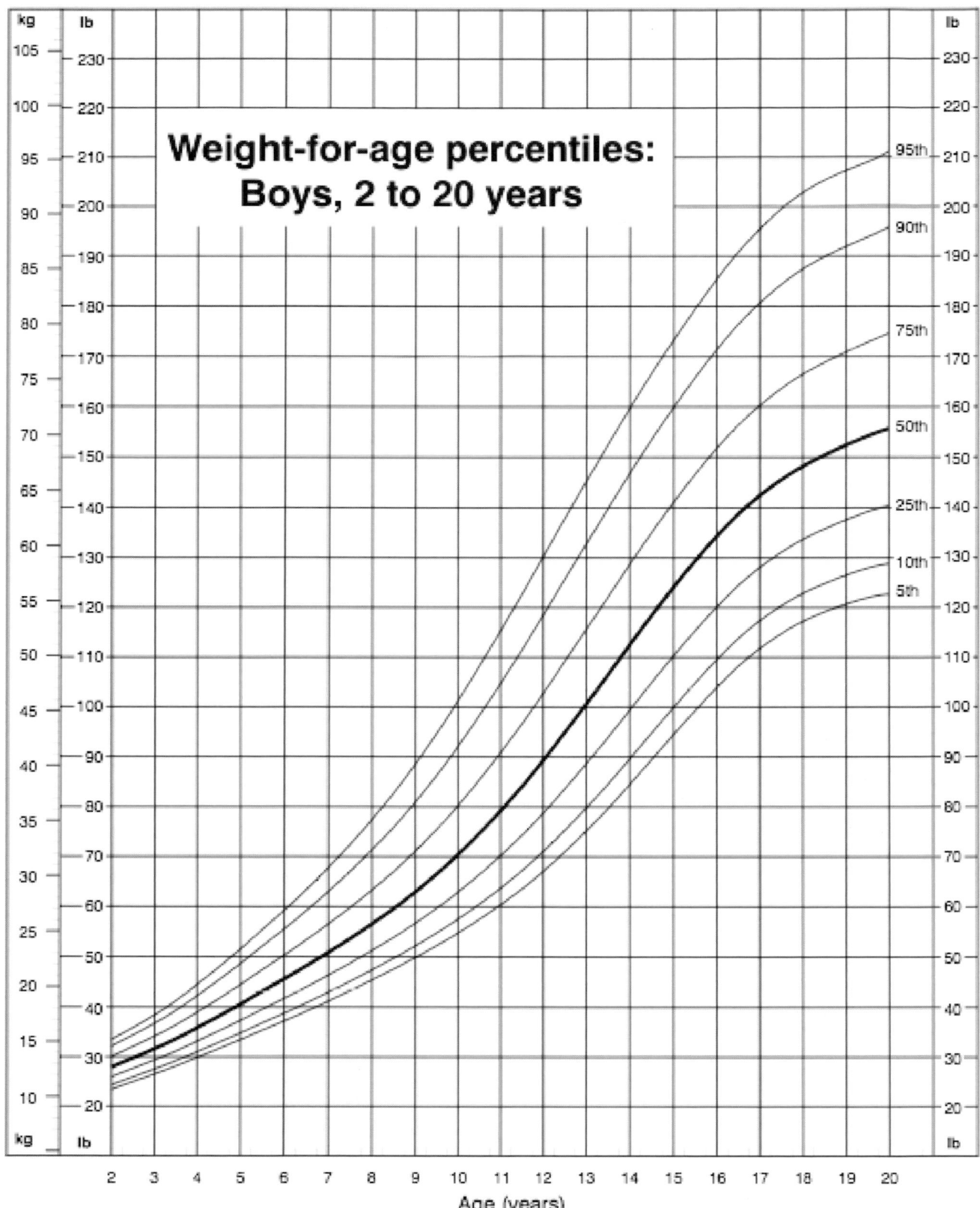

Figure V.9. Percentiles of Weight in Kilograms (kg) and Pounds (lb.) for Males Ranging in Age from 2 to 20 Years.

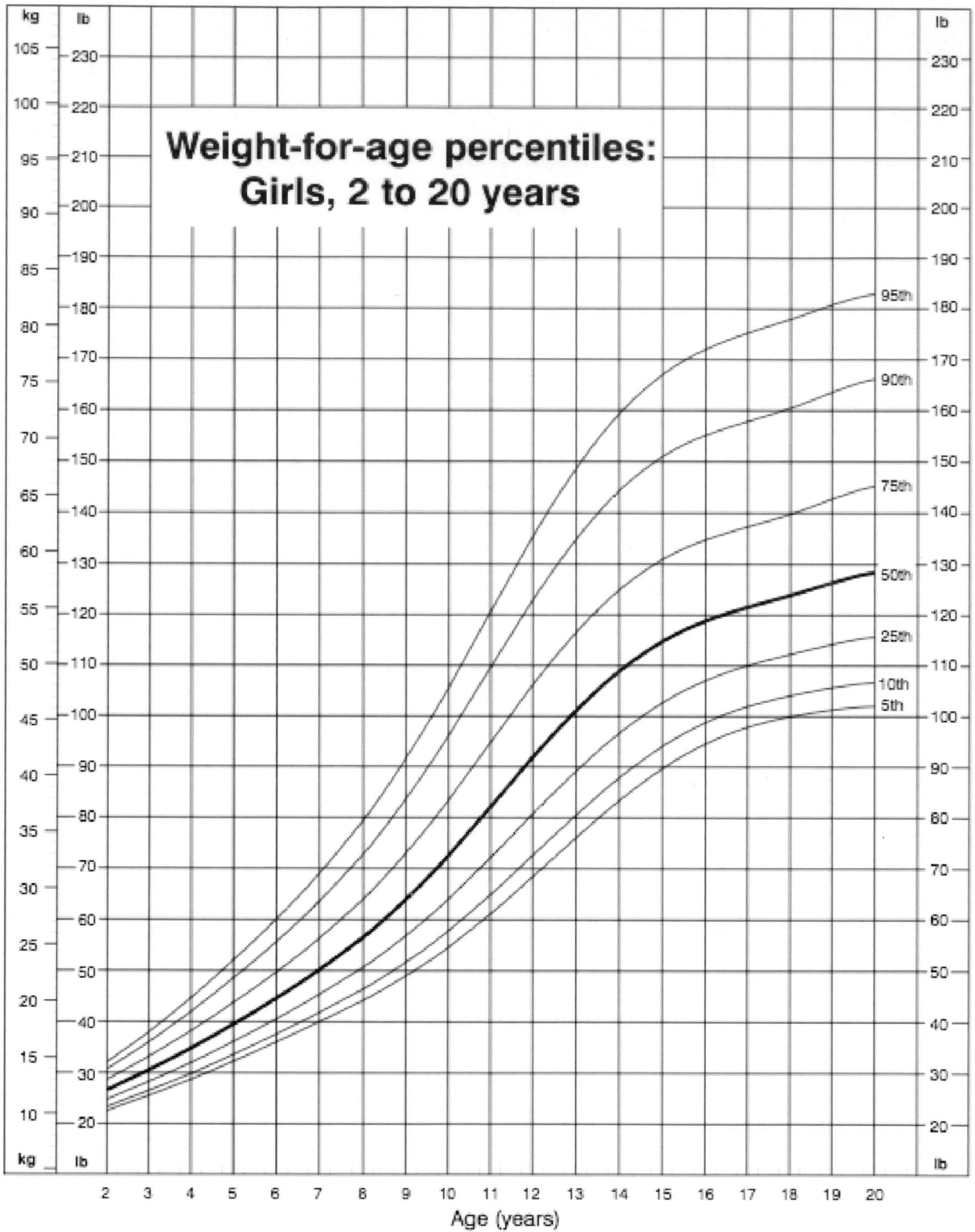

Figure V.10. Percentiles of Weight in Kilograms (kg) and Pounds (lb.) for Females Ranging in Age from 2 to 20 Years.

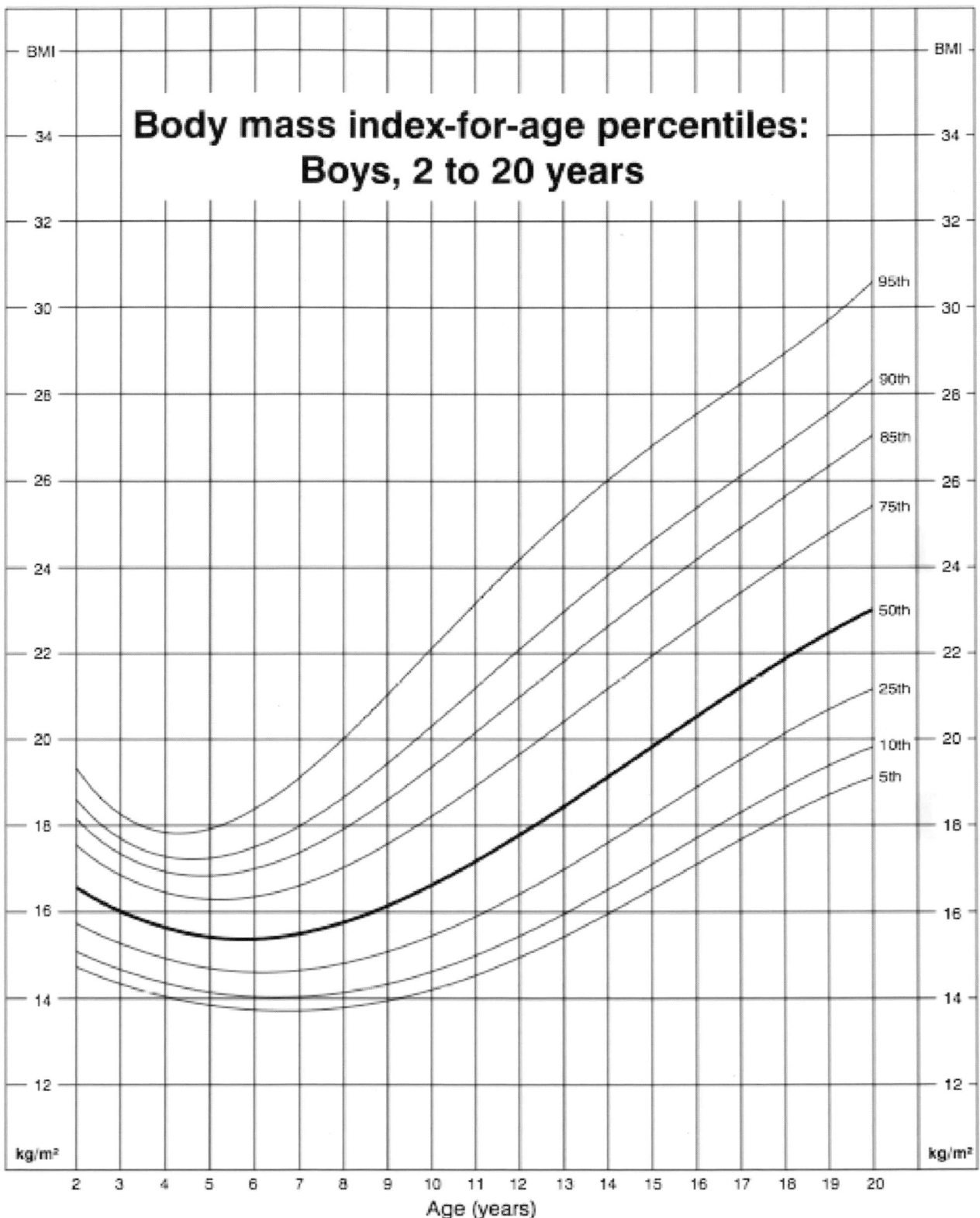

Figure V.11. Percentiles of Body Mass Index (kg/m^2) for Males Ranging in Age from 2 to 20 Years.

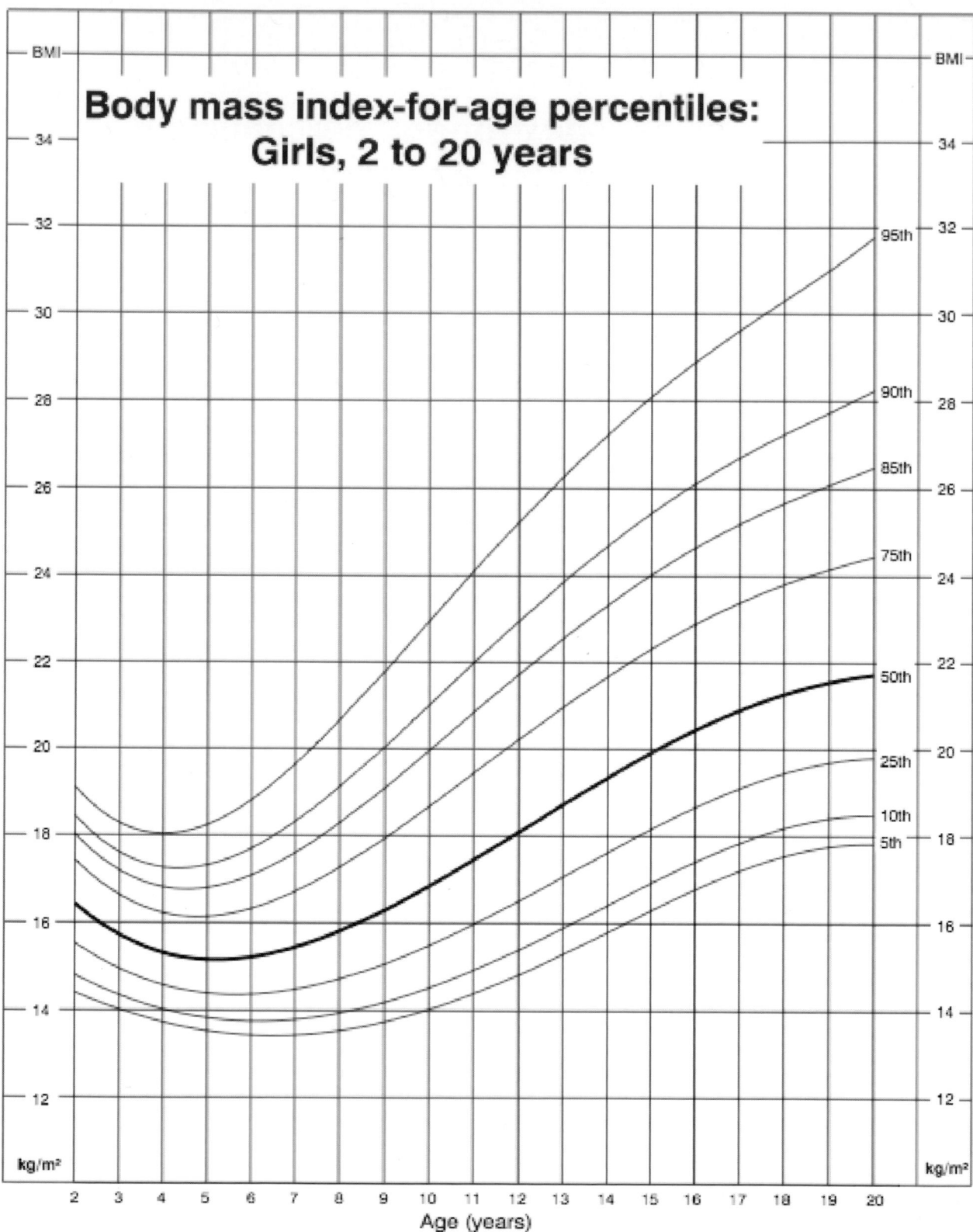

Figure V.12. Percentiles of Body Mass Index (kg/m^2) for Females Ranging in Age from 2 to 20 Years.

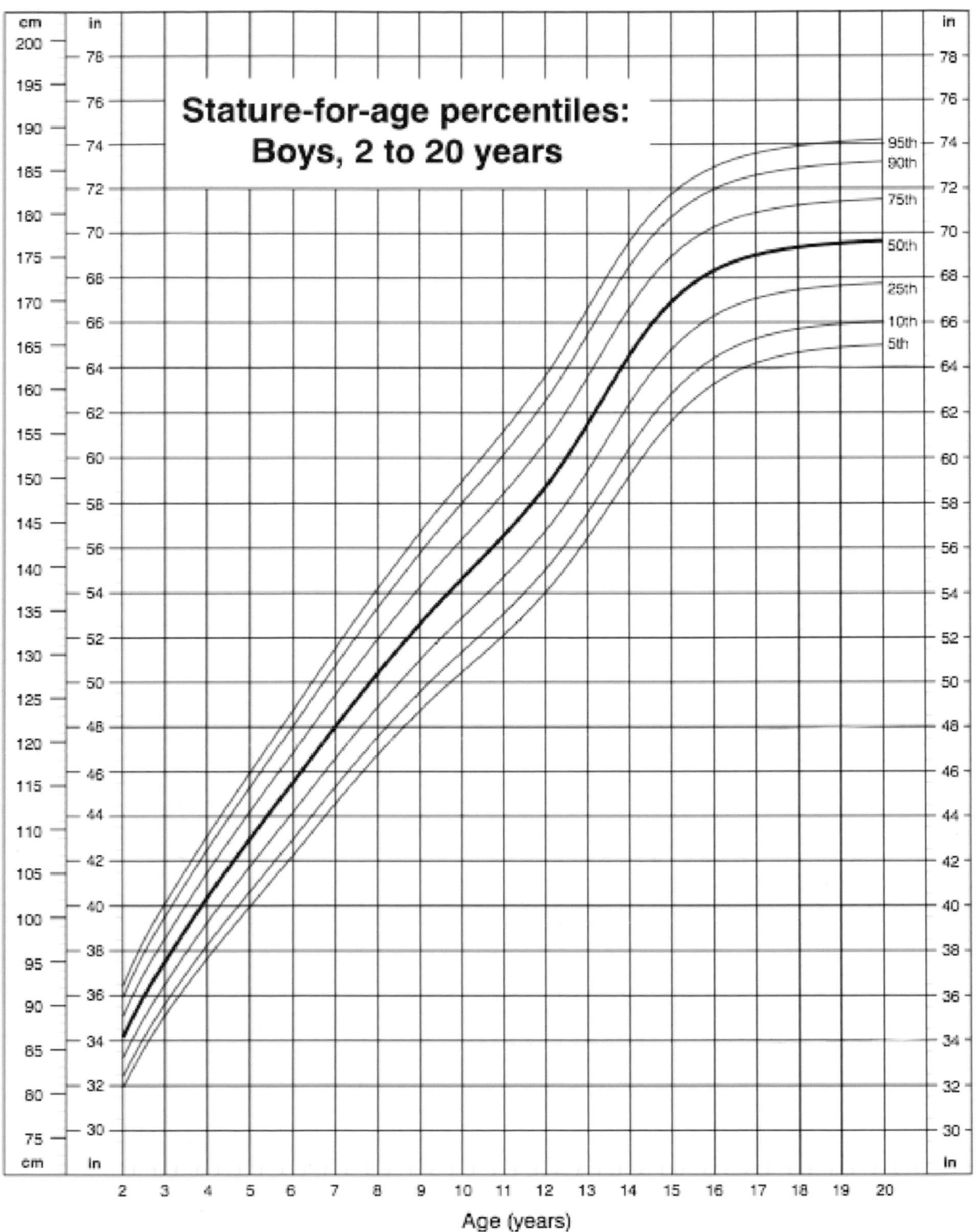

Figure V.13. Percentiles of Stature in Centimeters (cm) and Inches (in.) for Males Ranging in Age from 2 to 20 Years.

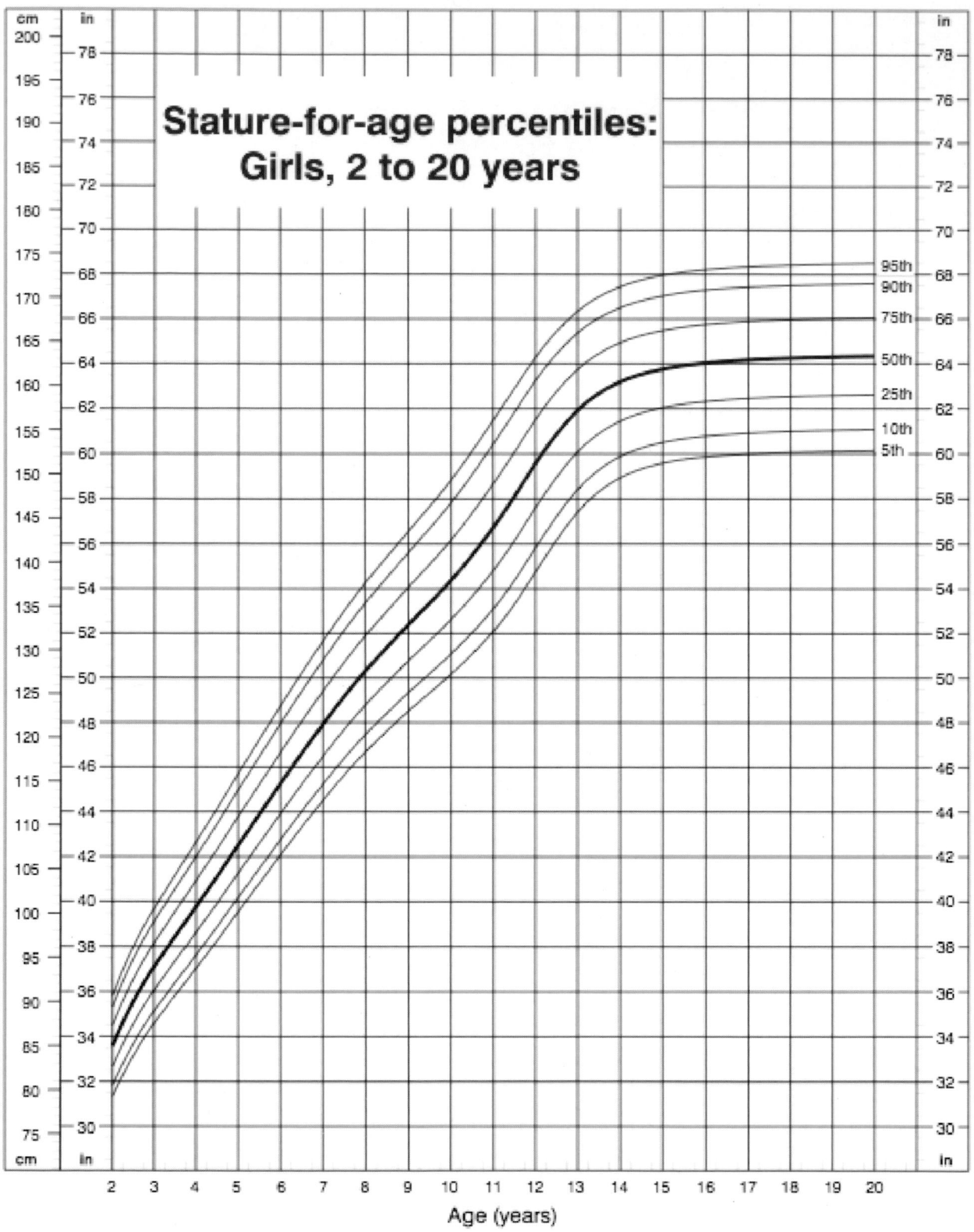

Figure V.14. Percentiles of Stature in Centimeters (cm) and Inches (in.) for Females Ranging in Age from 2 to 20 Years.

THE WHO CHILD GROWTH STANDARDS FROM BIRTH TO 5 YEARS

The World Health Organization (WHO) released a new international child growth standard for infants and children ranging in age from birth to 5 years (2). This new reference is based upon the WHO Multi-centre Growth Reference Study (MGRS), which was initiated in 1986 to collect, standardize, and disseminate child anthropometric data in a uniform format (3, 4). The MGRS was a population-based study conducted between 1997 and 2003 in Brazil, Ghana, India, Norway, Oman, and the United States. The MGRS combined a longitudinal follow-up from birth to 24 months with a cross-sectional component of children aged 18–71 months.

In the longitudinal component, mothers and newborns were enrolled at birth and visited at home a total of 21 times at weeks 1, 2, 4 and 6; monthly from 2–12 months; and bimonthly in the 2nd year. The criteria for inclusion in the study were: no known health or environmental constraints to growth, mothers willing to follow MGRS feeding recommendations (i.e., exclusive or predominant breast-feeding for at least 4 mo, introduction of complementary foods by 6 mo of age, and continued breast-feeding to at least 12 mo of age), no maternal smoking before and after delivery, single term birth, and absence of significant morbidity. Full-term low birth-weight infants were not excluded.

Eligibility criteria for the cross-sectional component were the same as those for the longitudinal component with the exception of infant feeding practices. A minimum of 3 mo of any breast-feeding was required for participants in the study's cross-sectional component. The database includes population-based surveys that fulfill common inclusion criteria related to sampling frame and procedure, sample size, and standard measurement techniques. The data was checked for validity and consistency and raw data sets were analyzed following a standard procedure to obtain comparable results (4).

A major premise of these standards is that the breast-fed infant is the biological norm for growth and that environmental differences—not genetic endowment—are the principal determinants of disparities in child growth. Since many countries such as Canada, the United Kingdom, the United States, and others are becoming multiethnic in composition, the use of reference based upon diverse ethnic samples is quite appropriate. Field tests conducted in two relatively affluent settings, Argentina and Italy, and two more economically stressed populations, the Maldives and Pakistan, found an overall concordance between clinical assessments and the new standard-based indicators (6). Furthermore, the means and percentiles of the new standard are lower than those of the CDC (7).

The WHO standards include information of weight, recumbent length, and body mass index, head circumference, mid-upper arm circumference, and triceps and subscapular skinfold thickness by age in weeks and months from birth to 5 years of age. The percentiles for weight, length, height, body mass index (BMI), head circumference, arm circumference, triceps skinfold and subscapular skinfolds are presented in **Tables V.12** to **V.27** according to the following format:

Weight-for-age: Birth to 13 weeks

Weight-for-age: Birth to 5 years

Weight-for-length: Birth to 2 years

Weight-for-height: 2 to 5 years

Length-for-age: Birth to 13 weeks

Length-for-age: Birth to 2 years

Height-for-age: 2 to 5 years

BMI-for-age: Birth to 13 weeks

BMI-for-age: Birth to 2 years

BMI-for-age: 2 to 5 years

Head circumference-for-age: Birth to 5 years

Arm circumference-for-age: 3 months to 5 years

Triceps skinfold-for-age: 3 months to 5 years

Subscapular skinfold-for-age: 3 months to 5 years

These references provide the skew factor (L), means (M), coefficients of variation (S), and standard deviations (SD) referred to as LMS parameters and the smoothed percentiles. **Figures V.15** to **V.30** present the growth charts for weight, length, body mass index, head circumference, mid-upper arm circumference and skinfold thickness at the triceps and subscapular sites developed using the WHO anthropometric reference (2).

LIST OF TABLES: WHO CHILD GROWTH STANDARDS

from 2 to 5 years.

Table V.20b. LMS parameters and smoothed percentiles of weight (kg)-for-height (cm) for girls from 2 to 5 years.

Table V.21. LMS parameters and smoothed percentiles of body mass index (kg/cm^2)-for-age (month) for boys and girls from birth to 13 weeks.

Table V.22. LMS parameters and smoothed percentiles of body mass index (kg/cm^2)-for-age (month) for boys and girls from birth to 2 years.

Table V.23. LMS parameters and smoothed percentiles of body mass index (kg/cm^2)-for-age (month) for boys and girls from 2 to 5 years.

Table V.24a. LMS parameters and smoothed percentiles of head circumference (cm)-for-age (month) for boys from birth to 5 years.

Table V.24b. LMS parameters and smoothed percentiles of head circumference (cm)-for-age (month) for girls from birth to 5 years.

Table V.25a. LMS parameters and smoothed percentiles of mid-upper arm circumference (cm)-for-age (month) for boys from 3 months to 5 years.

Table V.25b. LMS parameters and smoothed percentiles of mid-upper arm circumference (cm)-for-age (month) for girls from 3 months to 5 years.

Table V.26a. LMS parameters and smoothed percentiles of triceps skinfold thickness (mm)-for-age (month) for boys from 3 months to 5 years.

Table V.26b. LMS parameters and smoothed percentiles of triceps skinfold thickness (mm)-for-age (month) for girls from 3 months to 5 years.

Table V.27a. LMS parameters and smoothed percentiles of subscapular skinfold thickness (mm)-for-age (month) for boys from 3 months to 5 years.

Table V.27b. LMS parameters and smoothed percentiles of subscapular skinfold thickness (mm)-for-age (month) for girls from 3 months to 5 years.

Table V.12.

LMS parameters and smoothed percentiles of weight (kg)-for-age (week) for boys and girls from birth to 13 weeks

Age Group (weeks)	L	M	S	Percentiles										
				1st	3rd	5th	15th	25th	50th	75th	85th	95th	97th	99th
Boys														
0.0	0.3487	3.3464	0.1460	2.5	2.6	2.9	3.0	3.3	3.7	3.9	4.2	4.3	4.6	54.3
1.0	0.2776	3.4879	0.1448	2.6	2.7	3.0	3.2	3.5	3.8	4.0	4.4	4.5	4.8	59.3
2.0	0.2581	3.7529	0.1414	2.8	3.0	3.2	3.4	3.8	4.1	4.3	4.7	4.9	5.1	63.1
3.0	0.2442	4.0603	0.1381	3.1	3.2	3.5	3.7	4.1	4.5	4.7	5.1	5.2	5.5	66.2
4.0	0.2331	4.3671	0.1350	3.4	3.5	3.8	4.0	4.4	4.8	5.0	5.4	5.6	5.9	68.7
5.0	0.2237	4.6590	0.1322	3.6	3.7	4.1	4.3	4.7	5.1	5.3	5.8	5.9	6.3	70.8
6.0	0.2155	4.9303	0.1296	3.8	4.0	4.3	4.5	4.9	5.4	5.6	6.1	6.3	6.6	72.6
7.0	0.2081	5.1817	0.1273	4.1	4.2	4.5	4.8	5.2	5.6	5.9	6.4	6.5	6.9	74.2
8.0	0.2014	5.4149	0.1252	4.3	4.4	4.7	5.0	5.4	5.9	6.2	6.6	6.8	7.2	75.7
9.0	0.1952	5.6319	0.1233	4.4	4.6	4.9	5.2	5.6	6.1	6.4	6.9	7.1	7.4	77.2
10.0	0.1894	5.8346	0.1216	4.6	4.8	5.1	5.4	5.8	6.3	6.6	7.1	7.3	7.7	78.6
11.0	0.1840	6.0242	0.1200	4.8	4.9	5.3	5.6	6.0	6.5	6.8	7.3	7.5	7.9	80.0
12.0	0.1789	6.2019	0.1186	4.9	5.1	5.5	5.7	6.2	6.7	7.0	7.5	7.7	8.1	81.3
13.0	0.1740	6.3690	0.1173	5.1	5.2	5.6	5.9	6.4	6.9	7.2	7.7	7.9	8.3	82.6
Girls														
0.0	0.3809	3.2322	0.1417	2.4	2.5	2.8	2.9	3.2	3.6	3.7	4.0	4.2	4.4	53.5
1.0	0.2671	3.3388	0.1460	2.5	2.6	2.9	3.0	3.3	3.7	3.9	4.2	4.4	4.6	58.2
2.0	0.2304	3.5693	0.1434	2.7	2.8	3.1	3.2	3.6	3.9	4.1	4.5	4.6	4.9	61.8
3.0	0.2024	3.8352	0.1406	2.9	3.0	3.3	3.5	3.8	4.2	4.4	4.8	5.0	5.3	64.7
4.0	0.1789	4.0987	0.1381	3.1	3.3	3.5	3.7	4.1	4.5	4.7	5.1	5.3	5.6	67.1
5.0	0.1582	4.3476	0.1358	3.3	3.5	3.8	4.0	4.3	4.8	5.0	5.4	5.6	5.9	69.2
6.0	0.1395	4.5793	0.1339	3.5	3.7	4.0	4.2	4.6	5.0	5.3	5.7	5.9	6.2	71.0
7.0	0.1224	4.7950	0.1323	3.7	3.8	4.2	4.4	4.8	5.2	5.5	5.9	6.1	6.5	72.7
8.0	0.1065	4.9959	0.1309	3.9	4.0	4.4	4.6	5.0	5.5	5.7	6.2	6.4	6.7	74.3
9.0	0.0918	5.1842	0.1297	4.1	4.2	4.5	4.7	5.2	5.7	5.9	6.4	6.6	7.0	75.8
10.0	0.0779	5.3618	0.1286	4.2	4.3	4.7	4.9	5.4	5.8	6.1	6.6	6.8	7.2	77.2
11.0	0.0648	5.5295	0.1277	4.3	4.5	4.8	5.1	5.5	6.0	6.3	6.8	7.0	7.4	78.6
12.0	0.0525	5.6883	0.1269	4.5	4.6	5.0	5.2	5.7	6.2	6.5	7.0	7.2	7.6	80.0
13.0	0.0407	5.8393	0.1262	4.6	4.7	5.1	5.4	5.8	6.4	6.7	7.2	7.4	7.8	81.3

Table V.13a.

LMS parameters and smoothed percentiles of weight (kg)-for-age (month) for boys from birth to 5 years

Age Group (months)	L	M	S	Percentiles										
				1st	3rd	5th	15th	25th	50th	75th	85th	95th	97th	99th
0.0	0.3487	3.3464	0.1460	2.3	2.5	2.6	2.9	3.0	3.3	3.7	3.9	4.2	4.3	4.6
1.0	0.2297	4.4709	0.1340	3.2	3.4	3.6	3.9	4.1	4.5	4.9	5.1	5.5	5.7	6
2.0	0.1970	5.5675	0.1239	4.1	4.4	4.5	4.9	5.1	5.6	6.0	6.3	6.8	7.0	7.4
3.0	0.1738	6.3762	0.1173	4.8	5.1	5.2	5.6	5.9	6.4	6.9	7.2	7.7	7.9	8.3
4.0	0.1553	7.0023	0.1132	5.4	5.6	5.8	6.2	6.5	7.0	7.6	7.9	8.4	8.6	9.1
5.0	0.1395	7.5105	0.1108	5.8	6.1	6.2	6.7	7.0	7.5	8.1	8.4	9.0	9.2	9.7
6.0	0.1257	7.9340	0.1096	6.1	6.4	6.6	7.1	7.4	7.9	8.5	8.9	9.5	9.7	10.2
7.0	0.1134	8.2970	0.1090	6.4	6.7	6.9	7.4	7.7	8.3	8.9	9.3	9.9	10.2	10.7
8.0	0.1021	8.6151	0.1088	6.7	7.0	7.2	7.7	8.0	8.6	9.3	9.6	10.3	10.5	11.1
9.0	0.0917	8.9014	0.1088	6.9	7.2	7.4	7.9	8.3	8.9	9.6	10.0	10.6	10.9	11.4
10.0	0.0820	9.1649	0.1089	7.1	7.5	7.7	8.2	8.5	9.2	9.9	10.3	10.9	11.2	11.8
11.0	0.0730	9.4122	0.1091	7.3	7.7	7.9	8.4	8.7	9.4	10.1	10.5	11.2	11.5	12.1
12.0	0.0644	9.6479	0.1093	7.5	7.8	8.1	8.6	9.0	9.6	10.4	10.8	11.5	11.8	12.4
13.0	0.0563	9.8749	0.1095	7.6	8.0	8.2	8.8	9.2	9.9	10.6	11.1	11.8	12.1	12.7
14.0	0.0487	10.0953	0.1098	7.8	8.2	8.4	9.0	9.4	10.1	10.9	11.3	12.1	12.4	13
15.0	0.0413	10.3108	0.1101	8.0	8.4	8.6	9.2	9.6	10.3	11.1	11.6	12.3	12.7	13.3
0.4	3.2322	10.5228	0.1104	8.1	8.5	8.8	9.4	9.8	10.5	11.3	11.8	12.6	12.9	13.6
17.0	0.0275	10.7319	0.1108	8.3	8.7	8.9	9.6	10.0	10.7	11.6	12.0	12.9	13.2	13.9
18.0	0.0211	10.9385	0.1112	8.4	8.9	9.1	9.7	10.1	10.9	11.8	12.3	13.1	13.5	14.2
19.0	0.0148	11.1430	0.1116	8.6	9.0	9.3	9.9	10.3	11.1	12.0	12.5	13.4	13.7	14.4
20.0	0.0087	11.3462	0.1121	8.7	9.2	9.4	10.1	10.5	11.3	12.2	12.7	13.6	14.0	14.7
21.0	0.0029	11.5486	0.1126	8.9	9.3	9.6	10.3	10.7	11.5	12.5	13.0	13.9	14.3	15
22.0	-0.0028	11.7504	0.1131	9.0	9.5	9.8	10.5	10.9	11.8	12.7	13.2	14.2	14.5	15.3
23.0	-0.0083	11.9514	0.1137	9.2	9.7	9.9	10.6	11.1	12.0	12.9	13.4	14.4	14.8	15.6
24.0	-0.0137	12.1515	0.1143	9.3	9.8	10.1	10.8	11.3	12.2	13.1	13.7	14.7	15.1	15.9
25.0	-0.0189	12.3502	0.1149	9.5	10.0	10.2	11.0	11.4	12.4	13.3	13.9	14.9	15.3	16.1
26.0	-0.0240	12.5466	0.1154	9.6	10.1	10.4	11.1	11.6	12.5	13.6	14.1	15.2	15.6	16.4
27.0	-0.0289	12.7401	0.1160	9.7	10.2	10.5	11.3	11.8	12.7	13.8	14.4	15.4	15.9	16.7
28.0	-0.0337	12.9303	0.1166	9.9	10.4	10.7	11.5	12.0	12.9	14.0	14.6	15.7	16.1	17
29.0	-0.0385	13.1169	0.1172	10.0	10.5	10.8	11.6	12.1	13.1	14.2	14.8	15.9	16.4	17.3
30.0	-0.0431	13.3000	0.1178	10.1	10.7	11.0	11.8	12.3	13.3	14.4	15.0	16.2	16.6	17.5
31.0	-0.0476	13.4798	0.1184	10.3	10.8	11.1	11.9	12.4	13.5	14.6	15.2	16.4	16.9	17.8
32.0	-0.0520	13.6567	0.1190	10.4	10.9	11.2	12.1	12.6	13.7	14.8	15.5	16.6	17.1	18
33.0	-0.0564	13.8309	0.1195	10.5	11.1	11.4	12.2	12.8	13.8	15.0	15.7	16.9	17.3	18.3
34.0	-0.0606	14.0031	0.1201	10.6	11.2	11.5	12.4	12.9	14.0	15.2	15.9	17.1	17.6	18.6
35.0	-0.0648	14.1736	0.1206	10.7	11.3	11.6	12.5	13.1	14.2	15.4	16.1	17.3	17.8	18.8
36.0	-0.0689	14.3429	0.1212	10.8	11.4	11.8	12.7	13.2	14.3	15.6	16.3	17.5	18.0	19.1
37.0	-0.0729	14.5113	0.1217	11.0	11.6	11.9	12.8	13.4	14.5	15.8	16.5	17.8	18.3	19.3
38.0	-0.0769	14.6791	0.1222	11.1	11.7	12.0	12.9	13.5	14.7	15.9	16.7	18.0	18.5	19.6
39.0	-0.0808	14.8466	0.1227	11.2	11.8	12.2	13.1	13.7	14.8	16.1	16.9	18.2	18.7	19.8
40.0	-0.0846	15.0140	0.1232	11.3	11.9	12.3	13.2	13.8	15.0	16.3	17.1	18.4	19.0	20.1
41.0	-0.0883	15.1813	0.1237	11.4	12.1	12.4	13.4	14.0	15.2	16.5	17.3	18.6	19.2	20.3
42.0	-0.0920	15.3486	0.1243	11.5	12.2	12.5	13.5	14.1	15.3	16.7	17.5	18.9	19.4	20.6
43.0	-0.0957	15.5158	0.1248	11.7	12.3	12.7	13.6	14.3	15.5	16.9	17.7	19.1	19.7	20.8
44.0	-0.0993	15.6828	0.1253	11.8	12.4	12.8	13.8	14.4	15.7	17.1	17.9	19.3	19.9	21.1
45.0	-0.1028	15.8497	0.1259	11.9	12.5	12.9	13.9	14.6	15.8	17.3	18.1	19.5	20.1	21.3
46.0	-0.1063	16.0163	0.1264	12.0	12.7	13.0	14.1	14.7	16.0	17.4	18.3	19.8	20.4	21.6
47.0	-0.1097	16.1827	0.1270	12.1	12.8	13.2	14.2	14.9	16.2	17.6	18.5	20.0	20.6	21.9
48.0	-0.1131	16.3489	0.1276	12.2	12.9	13.3	14.3	15.0	16.3	17.8	18.7	20.2	20.9	22.1
49.0	-0.1165	16.5150	0.1282	12.3	13.0	13.4	14.5	15.2	16.5	18.0	18.9	20.4	21.1	22.4
50.0	-0.1198	16.6811	0.1288	12.4	13.1	13.5	14.6	15.3	16.7	18.2	19.1	20.7	21.3	22.6
51.0	-0.1230	16.8471	0.1294	12.5	13.3	13.7	14.7	15.4	16.8	18.4	19.3	20.9	21.6	22.9
52.0	-0.1262	17.0132	0.1301	12.6	13.4	13.8	14.9	15.6	17.0	18.6	19.5	21.1	21.8	23.2
53.0	-0.1294	17.1792	0.1307	12.7	13.5	13.9	15.0	15.7	17.2	18.8	19.7	21.4	22.1	23.4
54.0	-0.1325	17.3452	0.1313	12.9	13.6	14.0	15.2	15.9	17.3	19.0	19.9	21.6	22.3	23.7
55.0	-0.1356	17.5111	0.1320	13.0	13.7	14.1	15.3	16.0	17.5	19.2	20.1	21.8	22.5	24
56.0	-0.1387	17.6768	0.1326	13.1	13.8	14.3	15.4	16.2	17.7	19.3	20.3	22.1	22.8	24.2
57.0	-0.1417	17.8422	0.1333	13.2	13.9	14.4	15.6	16.3	17.8	19.5	20.5	22.3	23.0	24.5
58.0	-0.1447	18.0073	0.1339	13.3	14.1	14.5	15.7	16.5	18.0	19.7	20.7	22.5	23.3	24.8
59.0	-0.1477	18.1722	0.1345	13.4	14.2	14.6	15.8	16.6	18.2	19.9	20.9	22.8	23.5	25
60.0	-0.1506	18.3366	0.1352	13.5	14.3	14.7	16.0	16.7	18.3	20.1	21.1	23.0	23.8	25.3

WHO Growth Standards

Table V.13b.

LMS parameters and smoothed percentiles of weight (kg)-for-age (month) for girls from birth to 5 years

Age Group (months)	L	M	S	Percentiles										
				1st	3rd	5th	15th	25th	50th	75th	85th	95th	97th	99th
0.0	0.3809	3.2322	0.1417	2.3	2.4	2.5	2.8	2.9	3.2	3.6	3.7	4.0	4.2	4.4
1.0	0.1714	4.1873	0.1372	3.0	3.2	3.3	3.6	3.8	4.2	4.6	4.8	5.2	5.4	5.7
2.0	0.0962	5.1282	0.1300	3.8	4.0	4.1	4.5	4.7	5.1	5.6	5.9	6.4	6.5	6.9
3.0	0.0402	5.8458	0.1262	4.4	4.6	4.7	5.1	5.4	5.8	6.4	6.7	7.2	7.4	7.8
4.0	-0.0050	6.4237	0.1240	4.8	5.1	5.2	5.6	5.9	6.4	7.0	7.3	7.9	8.1	8.6
5.0	-0.0430	6.8985	0.1227	5.2	5.5	5.6	6.1	6.4	6.9	7.5	7.8	8.4	8.7	9.2
6.0	-0.0756	7.2970	0.1220	5.5	5.8	6.0	6.4	6.7	7.3	7.9	8.3	8.9	9.2	9.7
7.0	-0.1039	7.6422	0.1218	5.8	6.1	6.3	6.7	7.0	7.6	8.3	8.7	9.4	9.6	10.2
8.0	-0.1288	7.9487	0.1218	6.0	6.3	6.5	7.0	7.3	7.9	8.6	9.0	9.7	10.0	10.6
9.0	-0.1507	8.2254	0.1220	6.2	6.6	6.8	7.3	7.6	8.2	8.9	9.3	10.1	10.4	11
10.0	-0.1700	8.4800	0.1222	6.4	6.8	7.0	7.5	7.8	8.5	9.2	9.6	10.4	10.7	11.3
11.0	-0.1872	8.7192	0.1225	6.6	7.0	7.2	7.7	8.0	8.7	9.5	9.9	10.7	11.0	11.7
12.0	-0.2024	8.9481	0.1227	6.8	7.1	7.3	7.9	8.2	8.9	9.7	10.2	11.0	11.3	12
13.0	-0.2158	9.1699	0.1228	6.9	7.3	7.5	8.1	8.4	9.2	10.0	10.4	11.3	11.6	12.3
14.0	-0.2278	9.3870	0.1229	7.1	7.5	7.7	8.3	8.6	9.4	10.2	10.7	11.5	11.9	12.6
15.0	-0.2384	9.6008	0.1230	7.3	7.7	7.9	8.5	8.8	9.6	10.4	10.9	11.8	12.2	12.9
0.4	3.2322	9.8124	0.1230	7.4	7.8	8.1	8.7	9.0	9.8	10.7	11.2	12.1	12.5	13.2
17.0	-0.2562	10.0226	0.1231	7.6	8.0	8.2	8.8	9.2	10.0	10.9	11.4	12.3	12.7	13.5
18.0	-0.2637	10.2315	0.1231	7.8	8.2	8.4	9.0	9.4	10.2	11.1	11.6	12.6	13.0	13.8
19.0	-0.2703	10.4393	0.1232	7.9	8.3	8.6	9.2	9.6	10.4	11.4	11.9	12.9	13.3	14.1
20.0	-0.2762	10.6464	0.1232	8.1	8.5	8.7	9.4	9.8	10.6	11.6	12.1	13.1	13.5	14.4
21.0	-0.2815	10.8534	0.1234	8.2	8.7	8.9	9.6	10.0	10.9	11.8	12.4	13.4	13.8	14.6
22.0	-0.2862	11.0608	0.1235	8.4	8.8	9.1	9.8	10.2	11.1	12.0	12.6	13.6	14.1	14.9
23.0	-0.2903	11.2688	0.1237	8.5	9.0	9.2	9.9	10.4	11.3	12.3	12.8	13.9	14.3	15.2
24.0	-0.2941	11.4775	0.1239	8.7	9.2	9.4	10.1	10.6	11.5	12.5	13.1	14.2	14.6	15.5
25.0	-0.2975	11.6864	0.1241	8.9	9.3	9.6	10.3	10.8	11.7	12.7	13.3	14.4	14.9	15.8
26.0	-0.3005	11.8947	0.1244	9.0	9.5	9.8	10.5	10.9	11.9	12.9	13.6	14.7	15.2	16.1
27.0	-0.3032	12.1015	0.1247	9.2	9.6	9.9	10.7	11.1	12.1	13.2	13.8	15.0	15.4	16.4
28.0	-0.3057	12.3059	0.1251	9.3	9.8	10.1	10.8	11.3	12.3	13.4	14.0	15.2	15.7	16.7
29.0	-0.3080	12.5073	0.1255	9.5	10.0	10.2	11.0	11.5	12.5	13.6	14.3	15.5	16.0	17
30.0	-0.3101	12.7055	0.1259	9.6	10.1	10.4	11.2	11.7	12.7	13.8	14.5	15.7	16.2	17.3
31.0	-0.3120	12.9006	0.1263	9.7	10.3	10.5	11.3	11.9	12.9	14.1	14.7	16.0	16.5	17.6
32.0	-0.3138	13.0930	0.1268	9.9	10.4	10.7	11.5	12.0	13.1	14.3	15.0	16.2	16.8	17.8
33.0	-0.3155	13.2837	0.1274	10.0	10.5	10.8	11.7	12.2	13.3	14.5	15.2	16.5	17.0	18.1
34.0	-0.3171	13.4731	0.1279	10.1	10.7	11.0	11.8	12.4	13.5	14.7	15.4	16.8	17.3	18.4
35.0	-0.3186	13.6618	0.1286	10.3	10.8	11.1	12.0	12.5	13.7	14.9	15.7	17.0	17.6	18.7
36.0	-0.3201	13.8503	0.1292	10.4	11.0	11.3	12.1	12.7	13.9	15.1	15.9	17.3	17.8	19
37.0	-0.3216	14.0385	0.1299	10.5	11.1	11.4	12.3	12.9	14.0	15.3	16.1	17.5	18.1	19.3
38.0	-0.3230	14.2265	0.1306	10.6	11.2	11.6	12.5	13.0	14.2	15.6	16.3	17.8	18.4	19.6
39.0	-0.3243	14.4140	0.1314	10.8	11.4	11.7	12.6	13.2	14.4	15.8	16.6	18.0	18.6	19.9
40.0	-0.3257	14.6010	0.1321	10.9	11.5	11.8	12.8	13.4	14.6	16.0	16.8	18.3	18.9	20.2
41.0	-0.3270	14.7873	0.1329	11.0	11.6	12.0	12.9	13.5	14.8	16.2	17.0	18.6	19.2	20.5
42.0	-0.3283	14.9727	0.1338	11.1	11.8	12.1	13.1	13.7	15.0	16.4	17.3	18.8	19.5	20.8
43.0	-0.3296	15.1573	0.1346	11.3	11.9	12.2	13.2	13.9	15.2	16.6	17.5	19.1	19.7	21.1
44.0	-0.3309	15.3410	0.1355	11.4	12.0	12.4	13.4	14.0	15.3	16.8	17.7	19.3	20.0	21.4
45.0	-0.3322	15.5240	0.1363	11.5	12.1	12.5	13.5	14.2	15.5	17.0	17.9	19.6	20.3	21.7
46.0	-0.3335	15.7064	0.1372	11.6	12.3	12.6	13.7	14.3	15.7	17.3	18.2	19.9	20.6	22
47.0	-0.3348	15.8882	0.1380	11.7	12.4	12.8	13.8	14.5	15.9	17.5	18.4	20.1	20.8	22.3
48.0	-0.3361	16.0697	0.1388	11.8	12.5	12.9	14.0	14.7	16.1	17.7	18.6	20.4	21.1	22.6
49.0	-0.3374	16.2511	0.1397	11.9	12.6	13.0	14.1	14.8	16.3	17.9	18.9	20.6	21.4	22.9
50.0	-0.3387	16.4322	0.1405	12.1	12.8	13.2	14.3	15.0	16.4	18.1	19.1	20.9	21.7	23.2
51.0	-0.3400	16.6133	0.1413	12.2	12.9	13.3	14.4	15.1	16.6	18.3	19.3	21.2	22.0	23.5
52.0	-0.3414	16.7942	0.1421	12.3	13.0	13.4	14.5	15.3	16.8	18.5	19.5	21.4	22.2	23.9
53.0	-0.3427	16.9748	0.1429	12.4	13.1	13.5	14.7	15.4	17.0	18.7	19.8	21.7	22.5	24.2
54.0	-0.3440	17.1551	0.1437	12.5	13.2	13.7	14.8	15.6	17.2	18.9	20.0	22.0	22.8	24.5
55.0	-0.3453	17.3347	0.1445	12.6	13.4	13.8	15.0	15.8	17.3	19.1	20.2	22.2	23.1	24.8
56.0	-0.3466	17.5136	0.1453	12.7	13.5	13.9	15.1	15.9	17.5	19.3	20.4	22.5	23.3	25.1
57.0	-0.3479	17.6916	0.1460	12.8	13.6	14.0	15.3	16.1	17.7	19.6	20.7	22.7	23.6	25.4
58.0	-0.3492	17.8686	0.1468	12.9	13.7	14.2	15.4	16.2	17.9	19.8	20.9	23.0	23.9	25.7
59.0	-0.3505	18.0445	0.1475	13.1	13.8	14.3	15.5	16.4	18.0	20.0	21.1	23.3	24.2	26
60.0	-0.3518	18.2193	0.1482	13.2	14.0	14.4	15.7	16.5	18.2	20.2	21.3	23.5	24.4	26.3

Table V.14.

LMS parameters and smoothed percentiles of length (cm)-for-age (week) for boys and girls from birth to 13 weeks

Age Group (weeks)	L	M	S	Percentiles										
				1st	3rd	5th	15th	25th	50th	75th	85th	95th	97th	99th
Boys														
0.0	1.0	49.8842	0.0380	45.5	46.3	46.8	47.9	48.6	49.9	51.2	51.8	53.0	53.4	54.3
1.0	1.0	51.1152	0.0372	46.7	47.5	48.0	49.1	49.8	51.1	52.4	53.1	54.2	54.7	55.5
2.0	1.0	52.3461	0.0365	47.9	48.8	49.2	50.4	51.1	52.3	53.6	54.3	55.5	55.9	56.8
3.0	1.0	53.3905	0.0361	48.9	49.8	50.2	51.4	52.1	53.4	54.7	55.4	56.6	57.0	57.9
4.0	1.0	54.3881	0.0357	49.9	50.7	51.2	52.4	53.1	54.4	55.7	56.4	57.6	58.0	58.9
5.0	1.0	55.3374	0.0353	50.8	51.7	52.1	53.3	54.0	55.3	56.7	57.4	58.6	59.0	59.9
6.0	1.0	56.2357	0.0350	51.7	52.5	53.0	54.2	54.9	56.2	57.6	58.3	59.5	59.9	60.8
7.0	1.0	57.0851	0.0347	52.5	53.4	53.8	55.0	55.7	57.1	58.4	59.1	60.3	60.8	61.7
8.0	1.0	57.8889	0.0344	53.3	54.1	54.6	55.8	56.5	57.9	59.2	60.0	61.2	61.6	62.5
9.0	1.0	58.6536	0.0342	54.0	54.9	55.4	56.6	57.3	58.7	60.0	60.7	61.9	62.4	63.3
10.0	1.0	59.3872	0.0339	54.7	55.6	56.1	57.3	58.0	59.4	60.7	61.5	62.7	63.2	64.1
11.0	1.0	60.0894	0.0337	55.4	56.3	56.8	58.0	58.7	60.1	61.5	62.2	63.4	63.9	64.8
12.0	1.0	60.7605	0.0335	56.0	56.9	57.4	58.7	59.4	60.8	62.1	62.9	64.1	64.6	65.5
13.0	1.0	61.4013	0.0333	56.6	57.6	58.0	59.3	60.0	61.4	62.8	63.5	64.8	65.2	66.2
Girls														
0.0	0.4	3.2322	0.0379	44.8	45.6	46.1	47.2	47.9	49.1	50.4	51.1	52.2	52.7	53.5
1.0	1.0	50.3298	0.0374	45.9	46.8	47.2	48.4	49.1	50.3	51.6	52.3	53.4	53.9	54.7
2.0	1.0	51.5120	0.0369	47.1	47.9	48.4	49.5	50.2	51.5	52.8	53.5	54.6	55.1	55.9
3.0	1.0	52.4695	0.0367	48.0	48.8	49.3	50.5	51.2	52.5	53.8	54.5	55.6	56.1	56.9
4.0	1.0	53.3809	0.0365	48.9	49.7	50.2	51.4	52.1	53.4	54.7	55.4	56.6	57.0	57.9
5.0	1.0	54.2454	0.0363	49.7	50.5	51.0	52.2	52.9	54.2	55.6	56.3	57.5	57.9	58.8
6.0	1.0	55.0642	0.0361	50.4	51.3	51.8	53.0	53.7	55.1	56.4	57.1	58.3	58.8	59.7
7.0	1.0	55.8406	0.0359	51.2	52.1	52.5	53.8	54.5	55.8	57.2	57.9	59.1	59.6	60.5
8.0	1.0	56.5767	0.0358	51.9	52.8	53.2	54.5	55.2	56.6	57.9	58.7	59.9	60.4	61.3
9.0	1.0	57.2761	0.0356	52.5	53.4	53.9	55.2	55.9	57.3	58.7	59.4	60.6	61.1	62.0
10.0	1.0	57.9436	0.0355	53.2	54.1	54.6	55.8	56.6	57.9	59.3	60.1	61.3	61.8	62.7
11.0	1.0	58.5816	0.0354	53.8	54.7	55.2	56.4	57.2	58.6	60.0	60.7	62.0	62.5	63.4
12.0	1.0	59.1922	0.0353	54.3	55.3	55.8	57.0	57.8	59.2	60.6	61.4	62.6	63.1	64.1
13.0	1.0	59.7773	0.0352	54.9	55.8	56.3	57.6	58.4	59.8	61.2	62.0	63.2	63.7	64.7

Table V.15.
LMS parameters and smoothed percentiles of length (cm)-for-age (month) for boys and girls from birth to 2 years

Age Group (months)	L	M	S	Percentiles										
				1st	3rd	5th	15th	25th	50th	75th	85th	95th	97th	99th
Boys														
0.0	1.0	49.8842	0.0380	45.5	46.3	46.8	47.9	48.6	49.9	51.2	51.8	53.0	53.4	54.3
1.0	1.0	54.7244	0.0356	50.2	51.1	51.5	52.7	53.4	54.7	56.0	56.7	57.9	58.4	59.3
2.0	1.0	58.4249	0.0342	53.8	54.7	55.1	56.4	57.1	58.4	59.8	60.5	61.7	62.2	63.1
3.0	1.0	61.4292	0.0333	56.7	57.6	58.1	59.3	60.1	61.4	62.8	63.5	64.8	65.3	66.2
4.0	1.0	63.8860	0.0326	59.0	60.0	60.5	61.7	62.5	63.9	65.3	66.0	67.3	67.8	68.7
5.0	1.0	65.9026	0.0320	61.0	61.9	62.4	63.7	64.5	65.9	67.3	68.1	69.4	69.9	70.8
6.0	1.0	67.6236	0.0317	62.6	63.6	64.1	65.4	66.2	67.6	69.1	69.8	71.1	71.6	72.6
7.0	1.0	69.1645	0.0314	64.1	65.1	65.6	66.9	67.7	69.2	70.6	71.4	72.7	73.2	74.2
8.0	1.0	70.5994	0.0312	65.5	66.5	67.0	68.3	69.1	70.6	72.1	72.9	74.2	74.7	75.7
9.0	1.0	71.9687	0.0312	66.8	67.7	68.3	69.6	70.5	72.0	73.5	74.3	75.7	76.2	77.2
10.0	1.0	73.2812	0.0312	68.0	69.0	69.5	70.9	71.7	73.3	74.8	75.6	77.0	77.6	78.6
11.0	1.0	74.5388	0.0313	69.1	70.2	70.7	72.1	73.0	74.5	76.1	77.0	78.4	78.9	80.0
12.0	1.0	75.7488	0.0314	70.2	71.3	71.8	73.3	74.1	75.7	77.4	78.2	79.7	80.2	81.3
13.0	1.0	76.9186	0.0315	71.3	72.4	**72.9**	74.4	75.3	76.9	78.6	79.4	80.9	81.5	82.6
14.0	1.0	78.0497	0.0317	72.3	73.4	74.0	75.5	76.4	78.0	79.7	80.6	82.1	82.7	83.8
15.0	0.4	3.2322	0.0320	73.3	74.4	75.0	76.5	77.4	79.1	80.9	81.8	83.3	83.9	85.0
16.0	1.0	80.2113	0.0322	74.2	75.4	76.0	77.5	78.5	80.2	82.0	82.9	84.5	85.1	86.2
17.0	1.0	81.2487	0.0325	75.1	76.3	76.9	78.5	79.5	81.2	83.0	84.0	85.6	86.2	87.4
18.0	1.0	82.2587	0.0328	76.0	77.2	77.8	79.5	80.4	82.3	84.1	85.1	86.7	87.3	88.5
19.0	1.0	83.2418	0.0331	76.8	78.1	78.7	80.4	81.4	83.2	85.1	86.1	87.8	88.4	89.7
20.0	1.0	84.1996	0.0334	77.7	78.9	79.6	81.3	82.3	84.2	86.1	87.1	88.8	89.5	90.7
21.0	1.0	85.1348	0.0338	78.4	79.7	80.4	82.2	83.2	85.1	87.1	88.1	89.9	90.5	91.8
22.0	1.0	86.0477	0.0341	79.2	80.5	81.2	83.0	84.1	86.0	88.0	89.1	90.9	91.6	92.9
23.0	1.0	86.9410	0.0345	80.0	81.3	82.0	83.8	84.9	86.9	89.0	90.0	91.9	92.6	93.9
24.0	1.0	87.8161	0.0348	80.7	82.1	82.8	84.6	85.8	87.8	89.9	91.0	92.8	93.6	94.9
Girls														
0.0	1.0	49.1477	0.0379	44.8	45.6	46.1	47.2	47.9	49.1	50.4	51.1	52.2	52.7	53.5
1.0	1.0	53.6872	0.0364	49.1	50.0	50.5	51.7	52.4	53.7	55.0	55.7	56.9	57.4	58.2
2.0	1.0	57.0673	0.0357	52.3	53.2	53.7	55.0	55.7	57.1	58.4	59.2	60.4	60.9	61.8
3.0	1.0	59.8029	0.0352	54.9	55.8	56.3	57.6	58.4	59.8	61.2	62.0	63.3	63.8	64.7
4.0	1.0	62.0899	0.0349	57.1	58.0	58.5	59.8	60.6	62.1	63.5	64.3	65.7	66.2	67.1
5.0	1.0	64.0301	0.0346	58.9	59.9	60.4	61.7	62.5	64.0	65.5	66.3	67.7	68.2	69.2
6.0	1.0	65.7311	0.0345	60.5	61.5	62.0	63.4	64.2	65.7	67.3	68.1	69.5	70.0	71.0
7.0	1.0	67.2873	0.0344	61.9	62.9	63.5	64.9	65.7	67.3	68.8	69.7	71.1	71.6	72.7
8.0	1.0	68.7498	0.0344	63.2	64.3	64.9	66.3	67.2	68.7	70.3	71.2	72.6	73.2	74.3
9.0	1.0	70.1435	0.0344	64.5	65.6	66.2	67.6	68.5	70.1	71.8	72.6	74.1	74.7	75.8
10.0	1.0	71.4818	0.0345	65.7	66.8	67.4	68.9	69.8	71.5	73.1	74.0	75.5	76.1	77.2
11.0	1.0	72.7710	0.0346	66.9	68.0	68.6	70.2	71.1	72.8	74.5	75.4	76.9	77.5	78.6
12.0	1.0	74.0150	0.0348	68.0	69.2	69.8	71.3	72.3	74.0	75.8	76.7	78.3	78.9	80.0
13.0	1.0	75.2176	0.0350	69.1	70.3	**70.9**	72.5	73.4	75.2	77.0	77.9	79.5	80.2	81.3
14.0	1.0	76.3817	0.0351	70.1	71.3	72.0	73.6	74.6	76.4	78.2	79.2	80.8	81.4	82.6
15.0	1.0	77.5099	0.0353	71.1	72.4	73.0	74.7	75.7	77.5	79.4	80.3	82.0	82.7	83.9
16.0	1.0	78.6055	0.0356	72.1	73.3	74.0	75.7	76.7	78.6	80.5	81.5	83.2	83.9	85.1
17.0	1.0	79.6710	0.0358	73.0	74.3	75.0	76.7	77.7	79.7	81.6	82.6	84.4	85.0	86.3
18.0	1.0	80.7079	0.0360	74.0	75.2	75.9	77.7	78.7	80.7	82.7	83.7	85.5	86.2	87.5
19.0	1.0	81.7182	0.0362	74.8	76.2	76.9	78.7	79.7	81.7	83.7	84.8	86.6	87.3	88.6
20.0	1.0	82.7036	0.0364	75.7	77.0	77.7	79.6	80.7	82.7	84.7	85.8	87.7	88.4	89.7
21.0	1.0	83.6654	0.0367	76.5	77.9	78.6	80.5	81.6	83.7	85.7	86.8	88.7	89.4	90.8
22.0	1.0	84.6040	0.0369	77.3	78.7	79.5	81.4	82.5	84.6	86.7	87.8	89.7	90.5	91.9
23.0	1.0	85.5202	0.0371	78.1	79.6	80.3	82.2	83.4	85.5	87.7	88.8	90.7	91.5	92.9
24.0	1.0	86.4153	0.0373	78.9	80.3	81.1	83.1	84.2	86.4	88.6	89.8	91.7	92.5	93.9

Table V.16.
LMS parameters and smoothed percentiles of length (cm)-for-age (month) for boys and girls from 2 to 5 years

Age Group (months)	L	M	S	1st	3rd	5th	15th	25th	50th	75th	85th	95th	97th	99th
Boys														
24.0	1.0	87.1161	0.0351	80.0	81.4	82.1	83.9	85.1	87.1	89.2	90.3	92.1	92.9	94.2
25.0	1.0	87.9720	0.0354	80.7	82.1	82.8	84.7	85.9	88.0	90.1	91.2	93.1	93.8	95.2
26.0	1.0	88.8065	0.0358	81.4	82.8	83.6	85.5	86.7	88.8	90.9	92.1	94.0	94.8	96.2
27.0	1.0	89.6197	0.0361	82.1	83.5	84.3	86.3	87.4	89.6	91.8	93.0	94.9	95.7	97.1
28.0	1.0	90.4120	0.0364	82.8	84.2	85.0	87.0	88.2	90.4	92.6	93.8	95.8	96.6	98.1
29.0	1.0	91.1828	0.0367	83.4	84.9	85.7	87.7	88.9	91.2	93.4	94.7	96.7	97.5	99.0
30.0	1.0	91.9327	0.0370	84.0	85.5	86.3	88.4	89.6	91.9	94.2	95.5	97.5	98.3	99.9
31.0	1.0	92.6631	0.0373	84.6	86.2	87.0	89.1	90.3	92.7	95.0	96.2	98.4	99.2	100.7
32.0	1.0	93.3753	0.0376	85.2	86.8	87.6	89.7	91.0	93.4	95.7	97.0	99.2	100.0	101.5
33.0	1.0	94.0711	0.0379	85.8	87.4	88.2	90.4	91.7	94.1	96.5	97.8	99.9	100.8	102.4
34.0	1.0	94.7532	0.0381	86.4	88.0	88.8	91.0	92.3	94.8	97.2	98.5	100.7	101.5	103.2
35.0	1.0	95.4236	0.0384	86.9	88.5	89.4	91.6	93.0	95.4	97.9	99.2	101.4	102.3	103.9
36.0	1.0	96.0835	0.0386	87.5	89.1	90.0	92.2	93.6	96.1	98.6	99.9	102.2	103.1	104.7
37.0	1.0	96.7337	0.0388	88.0	89.7	90.6	92.8	94.2	96.7	99.3	100.6	102.9	103.8	105.5
38.0	1.0	97.3749	0.0390	88.5	90.2	91.1	93.4	94.8	97.4	99.9	101.3	103.6	104.5	106.2
39.0	0.4	3.2322	0.0392	89.1	90.8	91.7	94.0	95.4	98.0	100.6	102.0	104.3	105.2	106.9
40.0	1.0	98.6310	0.0394	89.6	91.3	92.2	94.6	96.0	98.6	101.3	102.7	105.0	105.9	107.7
41.0	1.0	99.2459	0.0395	90.1	91.9	92.8	95.2	96.6	99.2	101.9	103.3	105.7	106.6	108.4
42.0	1.0	99.8515	0.0397	90.6	92.4	93.3	95.7	97.2	99.9	102.5	104.0	106.4	107.3	109.1
43.0	1.0	100.4485	0.0399	91.1	92.9	93.9	96.3	97.7	100.4	103.1	104.6	107.0	108.0	109.8
44.0	1.0	101.0374	0.0400	91.6	93.4	94.4	96.8	98.3	101.0	103.8	105.2	107.7	108.6	110.4
45.0	1.0	101.6186	0.0402	92.1	93.9	94.9	97.4	98.9	101.6	104.4	105.8	108.3	109.3	111.1
46.0	1.0	102.1933	0.0403	92.6	94.4	95.4	97.9	99.4	102.2	105.0	106.5	109.0	109.9	111.8
47.0	1.0	102.7625	0.0405	93.1	94.9	95.9	98.5	100.0	102.8	105.6	107.1	109.6	110.6	112.4
48.0	1.0	103.3273	0.0406	93.6	95.4	96.4	99.0	100.5	103.3	106.2	107.7	110.2	111.2	113.1
49.0	1.0	103.8886	0.0407	94.0	95.9	96.9	99.5	101.0	103.9	106.7	108.3	110.8	111.8	113.7
50.0	1.0	104.4473	0.0409	94.5	96.4	97.4	100.0	101.6	104.4	107.3	108.9	111.5	112.5	114.4
51.0	1.0	105.0041	0.0410	95.0	96.9	97.9	100.5	102.1	105.0	107.9	109.5	112.1	113.1	115.0
52.0	1.0	105.5596	0.0411	95.5	97.4	98.4	101.1	102.6	105.6	108.5	110.1	112.7	113.7	115.7
53.0	1.0	106.1138	0.0413	95.9	97.9	98.9	101.6	103.2	106.1	109.1	110.7	113.3	114.3	116.3
54.0	1.0	106.6668	0.0414	96.4	98.4	99.4	102.1	103.7	106.7	109.6	111.2	113.9	115.0	116.9
55.0	1.0	107.2188	0.0415	96.9	98.8	99.9	102.6	104.2	107.2	110.2	111.8	114.5	115.6	117.6
56.0	1.0	107.7697	0.0417	97.3	99.3	100.4	103.1	104.7	107.8	110.8	112.4	115.2	116.2	118.2
57.0	1.0	108.3198	0.0418	97.8	99.8	100.9	103.6	105.3	108.3	111.4	113.0	115.8	116.8	118.8
58.0	1.0	108.8689	0.0419	98.3	100.3	101.4	104.1	105.8	108.9	111.9	113.6	116.4	117.4	119.5
59.0	1.0	109.4170	0.0420	98.7	100.8	101.9	104.7	106.3	109.4	112.5	114.2	117.0	118.1	120.1
60.0	1.0	109.9638	0.0421	99.2	101.2	102.3	105.2	106.8	110.0	113.1	114.8	117.6	118.7	120.7
Girls														
24.0	1.0	85.7153	0.0376	78.2	79.6	80.4	82.4	83.5	85.7	87.9	89.1	91.0	91.8	93.2
25.0	1.0	86.5904	0.0379	79.0	80.4	81.2	83.2	84.4	86.6	88.8	90.0	92.0	92.8	94.2
26.0	1.0	87.4462	0.0381	79.7	81.2	82.0	84.0	85.2	87.4	89.7	90.9	92.9	93.7	95.2
27.0	1.0	88.2830	0.0383	80.4	81.9	82.7	84.8	86.0	88.3	90.6	91.8	93.8	94.6	96.1
28.0	1.0	89.1004	0.0385	81.1	82.6	83.5	85.5	86.8	89.1	91.4	92.7	94.7	95.6	97.1
29.0	1.0	89.8991	0.0387	81.8	83.4	84.2	86.3	87.6	89.9	92.2	93.5	95.6	96.4	98.0
30.0	1.0	90.6797	0.0389	82.5	84.0	84.9	87.0	88.3	90.7	93.1	94.3	96.5	97.3	98.9
31.0	1.0	91.4430	0.0391	83.1	84.7	85.6	87.7	89.0	91.4	93.9	95.2	97.3	98.2	99.8
32.0	1.0	92.1906	0.0393	83.8	85.4	86.2	88.4	89.7	92.2	94.6	95.9	98.2	99.0	100.6
33.0	1.0	92.9239	0.0395	84.4	86.0	86.9	89.1	90.4	92.9	95.4	96.7	99.0	99.8	101.5
34.0	1.0	93.6444	0.0397	85.0	86.7	87.5	89.8	91.1	93.6	96.2	97.5	99.8	100.6	102.3
35.0	1.0	94.3533	0.0399	85.6	87.3	88.2	90.5	91.8	94.4	96.9	98.3	100.5	101.4	103.1
36.0	1.0	95.0515	0.0401	86.2	87.9	88.8	91.1	92.5	95.1	97.6	99.0	101.3	102.2	103.9
37.0	1.0	95.7399	0.0402	86.8	88.5	89.4	91.7	93.1	95.7	98.3	99.7	102.1	103.0	104.7
38.0	1.0	96.4187	0.0404	87.4	89.1	90.0	92.4	93.8	96.4	99.0	100.5	102.8	103.7	105.5
39.0	1.0	97.0885	0.0406	87.9	89.7	90.6	93.0	94.4	97.1	99.7	101.2	103.6	104.5	106.3
40.0	0.4	3.2322	0.0407	88.5	90.3	91.2	93.6	95.1	97.7	100.4	101.9	104.3	105.2	107.0
41.0	1.0	98.4015	0.0409	89.0	90.8	91.8	94.2	95.7	98.4	101.1	102.6	105.0	106.0	107.8
42.0	1.0	99.0448	0.0411	89.6	91.4	92.4	94.8	96.3	99.0	101.8	103.3	105.7	106.7	108.5
43.0	1.0	99.6795	0.0412	90.1	92.0	92.9	95.4	96.9	99.7	102.4	103.9	106.4	107.4	109.2
44.0	1.0	100.3058	0.0414	90.7	92.5	93.5	96.0	97.5	100.3	103.1	104.6	107.1	108.1	110.0
45.0	1.0	100.9238	0.0415	91.2	93.0	94.0	96.6	98.1	100.9	103.7	105.3	107.8	108.8	110.7
46.0	1.0	101.5337	0.0416	91.7	93.6	94.6	97.2	98.7	101.5	104.4	105.9	108.5	109.5	111.4
47.0	1.0	102.1360	0.0418	92.2	94.1	95.1	97.7	99.3	102.1	105.0	106.6	109.2	110.2	112.1
48.0	1.0	102.7312	0.0419	92.7	94.6	95.6	98.3	99.8	102.7	105.6	107.2	109.8	110.8	112.8
49.0	1.0	103.3197	0.0421	93.2	95.1	96.2	98.8	100.4	103.3	106.3	107.8	110.5	111.5	113.4
50.0	1.0	103.9021	0.0422	93.7	95.7	96.7	99.4	100.9	103.9	106.9	108.4	111.1	112.1	114.1
51.0	1.0	104.4786	0.0423	94.2	96.2	97.2	99.9	101.5	104.5	107.5	109.1	111.8	112.8	114.8
52.0	1.0	105.0494	0.0425	94.7	96.7	97.7	100.4	102.0	105.0	108.1	109.7	112.4	113.4	115.4
53.0	1.0	105.6148	0.0426	95.2	97.2	98.2	101.0	102.6	105.6	108.6	110.3	113.0	114.1	116.1
54.0	1.0	106.1748	0.0427	95.6	97.6	98.7	101.5	103.1	106.2	109.2	110.9	113.6	114.7	116.7
55.0	1.0	106.7295	0.0429	96.1	98.1	99.2	102.0	103.6	106.7	109.8	111.5	114.3	115.3	117.4
56.0	1.0	107.2788	0.0430	96.6	98.6	99.7	102.5	104.2	107.3	110.4	112.1	114.9	116.0	118.0
57.0	1.0	107.8227	0.0431	97.0	99.1	100.2	103.0	104.7	107.8	111.0	112.6	115.5	116.6	118.6
58.0	1.0	108.3613	0.0432	97.5	99.6	100.7	103.5	105.2	108.4	111.5	113.2	116.1	117.2	119.3
59.0	1.0	108.8948	0.0433	97.9	100.0	101.1	104.0	105.7	108.9	112.1	113.8	116.7	117.8	119.9
60.0	1.0	109.4233	0.0435	98.4	100.5	101.6	104.5	106.2	109.4	112.6	114.4	117.2	118.4	120.5

Table V.17a.

LMS parameters and smoothed percentiles of weight (kg)-for-length (cm) for boys from birth to 2 years

Length (cm)	L	M	S	1st	3rd	5th	15th	25th	50th	75th	85th	95th	97th	99th
45.0	-0.3521	2.4410	0.0918	2.0	2.1	2.1	2.2	2.3	2.4	2.6	2.7	2.9	2.9	3.0
45.5	-0.3521	2.5244	0.0915	2.1	2.1	2.2	2.3	2.4	2.5	2.7	2.8	2.9	3.0	3.1
46.0	-0.3521	2.6077	0.0912	2.1	2.2	2.3	2.4	2.5	2.6	2.8	2.9	3.0	3.1	3.3
46.5	-0.3521	2.6913	0.0909	2.2	2.3	2.3	2.5	2.5	2.7	2.9	3.0	3.1	3.2	3.4
47.0	-0.3521	2.7755	0.0907	2.3	2.4	2.4	2.5	2.6	2.8	3.0	3.1	3.2	3.3	3.5
47.5	-0.3521	2.8609	0.0904	2.3	2.4	2.5	2.6	2.7	2.9	3.0	3.1	3.3	3.4	3.6
48.0	-0.3521	2.9480	0.0901	2.4	2.5	2.6	2.7	2.8	2.9	3.1	3.2	3.4	3.5	3.7
48.5	-0.3521	3.0377	0.0898	2.5	2.6	2.6	2.8	2.9	3.0	3.2	3.3	3.5	3.6	3.8
49.0	-0.3521	3.1308	0.0895	2.6	2.7	2.7	2.9	2.9	3.1	3.3	3.4	3.6	3.7	3.9
49.5	-0.3521	3.2276	0.0892	2.6	2.7	2.8	2.9	3.0	3.2	3.4	3.5	3.8	3.8	4.0
50.0	-0.3521	3.3278	0.0889	2.7	2.8	2.9	3.0	3.1	3.3	3.5	3.7	3.9	4.0	4.1
50.5	-0.3521	3.4311	0.0886	2.8	2.9	3.0	3.1	3.2	3.4	3.6	3.8	4.0	4.1	4.2
51.0	-0.3521	3.5376	0.0883	2.9	3.0	3.1	3.2	3.3	3.5	3.8	3.9	4.1	4.2	4.4
51.5	-0.3521	3.6477	0.0880	3.0	3.1	3.2	3.3	3.4	3.6	3.9	4.0	4.2	4.3	4.5
52.0	-0.3521	3.7620	0.0877	3.1	3.2	3.3	3.4	3.5	3.8	4.0	4.1	4.4	4.5	4.6
52.5	-0.3521	3.8814	0.0874	3.2	3.3	3.4	3.6	3.7	3.9	4.1	4.3	4.5	4.6	4.8
53.0	0.3809	3.2322	0.0871	3.3	3.4	3.5	3.7	3.8	4.0	4.3	4.4	4.6	4.7	4.9
53.5	-0.3521	4.1354	0.0868	3.4	3.5	3.6	3.8	3.9	4.1	4.4	4.5	4.8	4.9	5.1
54.0	-0.3521	4.2693	0.0865	3.5	3.6	3.7	3.9	4.0	4.3	4.5	4.7	4.9	5.0	5.3
54.5	-0.3521	4.4066	0.0862	3.6	3.8	3.8	4.0	4.2	4.4	4.7	4.8	5.1	5.2	5.4
55.0	-0.3521	4.5467	0.0859	3.7	3.9	4.0	4.2	4.3	4.5	4.8	5.0	5.3	5.4	5.6
55.5	-0.3521	4.6892	0.0856	3.9	4.0	4.1	4.3	4.4	4.7	5.0	5.1	5.4	5.5	5.8
56.0	-0.3521	4.8338	0.0854	4.0	4.1	4.2	4.4	4.6	4.8	5.1	5.3	5.6	5.7	5.9
56.5	-0.3521	4.9796	0.0851	4.1	4.3	4.3	4.6	4.7	5.0	5.3	5.4	5.7	5.9	6.1
57.0	-0.3521	5.1259	0.0848	4.2	4.4	4.5	4.7	4.8	5.1	5.4	5.6	5.9	6.0	6.3
57.5	-0.3521	5.2721	0.0846	4.4	4.5	4.6	4.8	5.0	5.3	5.6	5.8	6.1	6.2	6.5
58.0	-0.3521	5.4180	0.0843	4.5	4.6	4.7	5.0	5.1	5.4	5.7	5.9	6.2	6.4	6.6
58.5	-0.3521	5.5632	0.0841	4.6	4.8	4.9	5.1	5.3	5.6	5.9	6.1	6.4	6.5	6.8
59.0	-0.3521	5.7074	0.0838	4.7	4.9	5.0	5.2	5.4	5.7	6.0	6.2	6.6	6.7	7.0
59.5	-0.3521	5.8501	0.0836	4.8	5.0	5.1	5.4	5.5	5.9	6.2	6.4	6.7	6.9	7.2
60.0	-0.3521	5.9907	0.0834	5.0	5.1	5.2	5.5	5.7	6.0	6.3	6.5	6.9	7.0	7.3
60.5	-0.3521	6.1284	0.0832	5.1	5.3	5.4	5.6	5.8	6.1	6.5	6.7	7.1	7.2	7.5
61.0	-0.3521	6.2632	0.0831	5.2	5.4	5.5	5.8	5.9	6.3	6.6	6.8	7.2	7.4	7.7
61.5	-0.3521	6.3954	0.0829	5.3	5.5	5.6	5.9	6.1	6.4	6.8	7.0	7.4	7.5	7.8
62.0	-0.3521	6.5251	0.0828	5.4	5.6	5.7	6.0	6.2	6.5	6.9	7.1	7.5	7.7	8.0
62.5	-0.3521	6.6527	0.0827	5.5	5.7	5.8	6.1	6.3	6.7	7.0	7.3	7.6	7.8	8.1
63.0	-0.3521	6.7786	0.0826	5.6	5.8	5.9	6.2	6.4	6.8	7.2	7.4	7.8	8.0	8.3
63.5	-0.3521	6.9028	0.0825	5.7	5.9	6.0	6.3	6.5	6.9	7.3	7.5	7.9	8.1	8.4
64.0	-0.3521	7.0255	0.0824	5.8	6.0	6.2	6.5	6.6	7.0	7.4	7.7	8.1	8.2	8.6
64.5	-0.3521	7.1467	0.0823	5.9	6.1	6.3	6.6	6.8	7.1	7.6	7.8	8.2	8.4	8.7
65.0	-0.3521	7.2666	0.0822	6.0	6.3	6.4	6.7	6.9	7.3	7.7	7.9	8.3	8.5	8.9
65.5	-0.3521	7.3854	0.0822	6.1	6.4	6.5	6.8	7.0	7.4	7.8	8.1	8.5	8.7	9.0
66.0	-0.3521	7.5034	0.0822	6.2	6.5	6.6	6.9	7.1	7.5	7.9	8.2	8.6	8.8	9.1
66.5	-0.3521	7.6206	0.0821	6.3	6.6	6.7	7.0	7.2	7.6	8.1	8.3	8.8	8.9	9.3
67.0	-0.3521	7.7370	0.0821	6.4	6.7	6.8	7.1	7.3	7.7	8.2	8.4	8.9	9.1	9.4
67.5	-0.3521	7.8526	0.0821	6.5	6.8	6.9	7.2	7.4	7.9	8.3	8.6	9.0	9.2	9.6
68.0	-0.3521	7.9674	0.0821	6.6	6.9	7.0	7.3	7.5	8.0	8.4	8.7	9.2	9.3	9.7
68.5	-0.3521	8.0816	0.0822	6.7	7.0	7.1	7.4	7.7	8.1	8.5	8.8	9.3	9.5	9.8
69.0	-0.3521	8.1955	0.0822	6.8	7.1	7.2	7.5	7.8	8.2	8.7	8.9	9.4	9.6	10.0
69.5	-0.3521	8.3092	0.0822	6.9	7.1	7.3	7.6	7.9	8.3	8.8	9.1	9.5	9.7	10.1
70.0	-0.3521	8.4227	0.0823	7.0	7.2	7.4	7.7	8.0	8.4	8.9	9.2	9.7	9.9	10.3
70.5	-0.3521	8.5358	0.0824	7.1	7.3	7.5	7.8	8.1	8.5	9.0	9.3	9.8	10.0	10.4
71.0	-0.3521	8.6480	0.0824	7.2	7.4	7.6	8.0	8.2	8.6	9.1	9.4	9.9	10.1	10.5
71.5	-0.3521	8.7594	0.0825	7.3	7.5	7.7	8.1	8.3	8.8	9.3	9.6	10.1	10.3	10.7
72.0	-0.3521	8.8697	0.0825	7.4	7.6	7.8	8.2	8.4	8.9	9.4	9.7	10.2	10.4	10.8
72.5	-0.3521	8.9788	0.0826	7.5	7.7	7.9	8.3	8.5	9.0	9.5	9.8	10.3	10.5	11.0
73.0	-0.3521	9.0865	0.0827	7.5	7.8	8.0	8.4	8.6	9.1	9.6	9.9	10.4	10.7	11.1
73.5	-0.3521	9.1927	0.0828	7.6	7.9	8.0	8.4	8.7	9.2	9.7	10.0	10.6	10.8	11.2
74.0	-0.3521	9.2974	0.0828	7.7	8.0	8.1	8.5	8.8	9.3	9.8	10.1	10.7	10.9	11.4
74.5	-0.3521	9.4010	0.0829	7.8	8.1	8.2	8.6	8.9	9.4	9.9	10.3	10.8	11.0	11.5
75.0	-0.3521	9.5032	0.0830	7.9	8.2	8.3	8.7	9.0	9.5	10.1	10.4	10.9	11.2	11.6
75.5	-0.3521	9.6041	0.0830	8.0	8.2	8.4	8.8	9.1	9.6	10.2	10.5	11.0	11.3	11.7
76.0	-0.3521	9.7033	0.0831	8.0	8.3	8.5	8.9	9.2	9.7	10.3	10.6	11.2	11.4	11.9
76.5	-0.3521	9.8007	0.0831	8.1	8.4	8.6	9.0	9.3	9.8	10.4	10.7	11.3	11.5	12.0
77.0	-0.3521	9.8963	0.0831	8.2	8.5	8.7	9.1	9.4	9.9	10.5	10.8	11.4	11.6	12.1
77.5	-0.3521	9.9902	0.0832	8.3	8.6	8.7	9.2	9.5	10.0	10.6	10.9	11.5	11.7	12.2
78.0	-0.3521	10.0827	0.0832	8.4	8.7	8.8	9.3	9.5	10.1	10.7	11.0	11.6	11.8	12.3
78.5	-0.3521	10.1741	0.0832	8.4	8.7	8.9	9.3	9.6	10.2	10.8	11.1	11.7	12.0	12.4
79.0	-0.3521	10.2649	0.0832	8.5	8.8	9.0	9.4	9.7	10.3	10.9	11.2	11.8	12.1	12.5
79.5	-0.3521	10.3558	0.0831	8.6	8.9	9.1	9.5	9.8	10.4	11.0	11.3	11.9	12.2	12.7
80.0	-0.3521	10.4475	0.0831	8.7	9.0	9.1	9.6	9.9	10.4	11.1	11.4	12.0	12.3	12.8

257

Table V.17b.
LMS parameters and smoothed percentiles of weight (kg)-for-length (cm) for boys from birth to 2 years

Length (cm)	L	M	S	1st	3rd	5th	15th	25th	50th	75th	85th	95th	97th	99th
80.5	-0.3521	10.5405	0.0830	8.7	9.1	9.2	9.7	10.0	10.5	11.2	11.5	12.1	12.4	12.9
81.0	-0.3521	10.6352	0.0829	8.8	9.1	9.3	9.8	10.1	10.6	11.3	11.6	12.2	12.5	13.0
81.5	-0.3521	10.7322	0.0828	8.9	9.2	9.4	9.9	10.2	10.7	11.4	11.7	12.3	12.6	13.1
82.0	-0.3521	10.8321	0.0827	9.0	9.3	9.5	10.0	10.2	10.8	11.5	11.8	12.5	12.7	13.2
82.5	-0.3521	10.9350	0.0826	9.1	9.4	9.6	10.1	10.3	10.9	11.6	11.9	12.6	12.8	13.3
83.0	-0.3521	11.0415	0.0825	9.2	9.5	9.7	10.1	10.4	11.0	11.7	12.0	12.7	13.0	13.5
83.5	-0.3521	11.1516	0.0823	9.3	9.6	9.8	10.3	10.6	11.2	11.8	12.2	12.8	13.1	13.6
84.0	-0.3521	11.2651	0.0822	9.4	9.7	9.9	10.4	10.7	11.3	11.9	12.3	12.9	13.2	13.7
84.5	-0.3521	11.3817	0.0820	9.5	9.8	10.0	10.5	10.8	11.4	12.0	12.4	13.1	13.3	13.9
85.0	-0.3521	11.5007	0.0818	9.6	9.9	10.1	10.6	10.9	11.5	12.2	12.5	13.2	13.5	14.0
85.5	-0.3521	11.6218	0.0816	9.7	10.0	10.2	10.7	11.0	11.6	12.3	12.7	13.3	13.6	14.1
86.0	-0.3521	11.7444	0.0815	9.8	10.1	10.3	10.8	11.1	11.7	12.4	12.8	13.5	13.7	14.3
86.5	-0.3521	11.8678	0.0813	9.9	10.2	10.4	10.9	11.2	11.9	12.5	12.9	13.6	13.9	14.4
87.0	-0.3521	11.9916	0.0811	10.0	10.3	10.5	11.0	11.4	12.0	12.7	13.1	13.7	14.0	14.6
87.5	-0.3521	12.1152	0.0810	10.1	10.4	10.6	11.2	11.5	12.1	12.8	13.2	13.9	14.2	14.7
88.0	-0.3521	12.2382	0.0808	10.2	10.6	10.7	11.3	11.6	12.2	12.9	13.3	14.0	14.3	14.9
88.5	0.3809	3.2322	0.0807	10.3	10.7	10.9	11.4	11.7	12.4	13.1	13.5	14.2	14.4	15.0
89.0	-0.3521	12.4815	0.0806	10.4	10.8	11.0	11.5	11.8	12.5	13.2	13.6	14.3	14.6	15.2
89.5	-0.3521	12.6017	0.0805	10.5	10.9	11.1	11.6	11.9	12.6	13.3	13.7	14.4	14.7	15.3
90.0	-0.3521	12.7209	0.0804	10.6	11.0	11.2	11.7	12.1	12.7	13.4	13.8	14.6	14.9	15.4
90.5	-0.3521	12.8392	0.0803	10.7	11.1	11.3	11.8	12.2	12.8	13.6	14.0	14.7	15.0	15.6
91.0	-0.3521	12.9569	0.0803	10.8	11.2	11.4	11.9	12.3	13.0	13.7	14.1	14.8	15.1	15.7
91.5	-0.3521	13.0742	0.0803	10.9	11.3	11.5	12.0	12.4	13.1	13.8	14.2	15.0	15.3	15.9
92.0	-0.3521	13.1910	0.0803	11.0	11.4	11.6	12.2	12.5	13.2	13.9	14.4	15.1	15.4	16.0
92.5	-0.3521	13.3075	0.0803	11.1	11.5	11.7	12.3	12.6	13.3	14.1	14.5	15.2	15.5	16.1
93.0	-0.3521	13.4239	0.0803	11.2	11.6	11.8	12.4	12.7	13.4	14.2	14.6	15.4	15.7	16.3
93.5	-0.3521	13.5404	0.0803	11.3	11.7	11.9	12.5	12.8	13.5	14.3	14.7	15.5	15.8	16.4
94.0	-0.3521	13.6572	0.0803	11.4	11.8	12.0	12.6	12.9	13.7	14.4	14.9	15.6	16.0	16.6
94.5	-0.3521	13.7746	0.0804	11.5	11.9	12.1	12.7	13.1	13.8	14.5	15.0	15.8	16.1	16.7
95.0	-0.3521	13.8928	0.0805	11.6	12.0	12.2	12.8	13.2	13.9	14.7	15.1	15.9	16.2	16.9
95.5	-0.3521	14.0120	0.0806	11.7	12.1	12.3	12.9	13.3	14.0	14.8	15.3	16.0	16.4	17.0
96.0	-0.3521	14.1325	0.0807	11.8	12.2	12.4	13.0	13.4	14.1	14.9	15.4	16.2	16.5	17.2
96.5	-0.3521	14.2544	0.0808	11.9	12.3	12.5	13.1	13.5	14.3	15.1	15.5	16.3	16.7	17.3
97.0	-0.3521	14.3782	0.0809	12.0	12.4	12.6	13.2	13.6	14.4	15.2	15.7	16.5	16.8	17.5
97.5	-0.3521	14.5038	0.0811	12.1	12.5	12.7	13.4	13.7	14.5	15.3	15.8	16.6	17.0	17.6
98.0	-0.3521	14.6316	0.0812	12.2	12.6	12.8	13.5	13.9	14.6	15.5	15.9	16.8	17.1	17.8
98.5	-0.3521	14.7614	0.0814	12.3	12.7	13.0	13.6	14.0	14.8	15.6	16.1	16.9	17.3	18.0
99.0	-0.3521	14.8934	0.0816	12.4	12.8	13.1	13.7	14.1	14.9	15.7	16.2	17.1	17.4	18.1
99.5	-0.3521	15.0275	0.0818	12.5	12.9	13.2	13.8	14.2	15.0	15.9	16.4	17.2	17.6	18.3
100.0	-0.3521	15.1637	0.0820	12.6	13.0	13.3	13.9	14.4	15.2	16.0	16.5	17.4	17.8	18.5
100.5	-0.3521	15.3018	0.0822	12.7	13.2	13.4	14.1	14.5	15.3	16.2	16.7	17.6	17.9	18.7
101.0	-0.3521	15.4419	0.0824	12.8	13.3	13.5	14.2	14.6	15.4	16.3	16.8	17.7	18.1	18.8
101.5	-0.3521	15.5838	0.0827	12.9	13.4	13.6	14.3	14.7	15.6	16.5	17.0	17.9	18.3	19.0
102.0	-0.3521	15.7276	0.0829	13.0	13.5	13.8	14.5	14.9	15.7	16.6	17.2	18.1	18.5	19.2
102.5	-0.3521	15.8732	0.0832	13.2	13.6	13.9	14.6	15.0	15.9	16.8	17.3	18.3	18.6	19.4
103.0	-0.3521	16.0206	0.0834	13.3	13.8	14.0	14.7	15.2	16.0	17.0	17.5	18.4	18.8	19.6
103.5	-0.3521	16.1697	0.0837	13.4	13.9	14.1	14.8	15.3	16.2	17.1	17.7	18.6	19.0	19.8
104.0	-0.3521	16.3204	0.0840	13.5	14.0	14.3	15.0	15.4	16.3	17.3	17.8	18.8	19.2	20.0
104.5	-0.3521	16.4728	0.0843	13.6	14.1	14.4	15.1	15.6	16.5	17.4	18.0	19.0	19.4	20.2
105.0	-0.3521	16.6268	0.0845	13.7	14.2	14.5	15.3	15.7	16.6	17.6	18.2	19.2	19.6	20.4
105.5	-0.3521	16.7826	0.0848	13.9	14.4	14.6	15.4	15.9	16.8	17.8	18.4	19.4	19.8	20.6
106.0	-0.3521	16.9401	0.0851	14.0	14.5	14.8	15.5	16.0	16.9	18.0	18.5	19.6	20.0	20.8
106.5	-0.3521	17.0995	0.0854	14.1	14.6	14.9	15.7	16.2	17.1	18.1	18.7	19.7	20.2	21.0
107.0	-0.3521	17.2607	0.0857	14.2	14.8	15.0	15.8	16.3	17.3	18.3	18.9	19.9	20.4	21.2
107.5	-0.3521	17.4237	0.0860	14.4	14.9	15.2	16.0	16.5	17.4	18.5	19.1	20.1	20.6	21.4
108.0	-0.3521	17.5885	0.0863	14.5	15.0	15.3	16.1	16.6	17.6	18.7	19.3	20.3	20.8	21.7
108.5	-0.3521	17.7553	0.0866	14.6	15.2	15.5	16.3	16.8	17.8	18.8	19.5	20.5	21.0	21.9
109.0	-0.3521	17.9242	0.0869	14.7	15.3	15.6	16.4	16.9	17.9	19.0	19.6	20.8	21.2	22.1
109.5	-0.3521	18.0954	0.0872	14.9	15.4	15.7	16.6	17.1	18.1	19.2	19.8	21.0	21.4	22.3
110.0	-0.3521	18.2689	0.0876	15.0	15.6	15.9	16.7	17.2	18.3	19.4	20.0	21.2	21.6	22.6

WHO Growth Standards

Table V.18a.
LMS parameters and smoothed percentiles of weight (kg)-for-length (cm) for girls from birth to 2 years

Length (cm)	L	M	S	1st	3rd	5th	15th	25th	50th	75th	85th	95th	97th	99th
45.0	-0.3833	2.4607	0.0903	2.0	2.1	2.1	2.2	2.3	2.5	2.6	2.7	2.9	2.9	3.1
45.5	-0.3833	2.5457	0.0903	2.1	2.2	2.2	2.3	2.4	2.5	2.7	2.8	3.0	3.0	3.2
46.0	-0.3833	2.6306	0.0904	2.1	2.2	2.3	2.4	2.5	2.6	2.8	2.9	3.1	3.1	3.3
46.5	-0.3833	2.7155	0.0904	2.2	2.3	2.3	2.5	2.6	2.7	2.9	3.0	3.2	3.2	3.4
47.0	-0.3833	2.8007	0.0904	2.3	2.4	2.4	2.6	2.6	2.8	3.0	3.1	3.3	3.3	3.5
47.5	-0.3833	2.8867	0.0905	2.4	2.4	2.5	2.6	2.7	2.9	3.1	3.2	3.4	3.4	3.6
48.0	-0.3833	2.9741	0.0905	2.4	2.5	2.6	2.7	2.8	3.0	3.2	3.3	3.5	3.5	3.7
48.5	-0.3833	3.0636	0.0906	2.5	2.6	2.7	2.8	2.9	3.1	3.3	3.4	3.6	3.7	3.8
49.0	-0.3833	3.1560	0.0906	2.6	2.7	2.7	2.9	3.0	3.2	3.4	3.5	3.7	3.8	3.9
49.5	-0.3833	3.2520	0.0906	2.7	2.8	2.8	3.0	3.1	3.3	3.5	3.6	3.8	3.9	4.1
50.0	-0.3833	3.3518	0.0907	2.7	2.8	2.9	3.1	3.2	3.4	3.6	3.7	3.9	4.0	4.2
50.5	-0.3833	3.4557	0.0907	2.8	2.9	3.0	3.2	3.3	3.5	3.7	3.8	4.0	4.1	4.3
51.0	-0.3833	3.5636	0.0908	2.9	3.0	3.1	3.2	3.4	3.6	3.8	3.9	4.2	4.3	4.4
51.5	-0.3833	3.6754	0.0908	3.0	3.1	3.2	3.4	3.5	3.7	3.9	4.0	4.3	4.4	4.6
52.0	-0.3833	3.7911	0.0909	3.1	3.2	3.3	3.5	3.6	3.8	4.0	4.2	4.4	4.5	4.7
52.5	-0.3833	3.9105	0.0909	3.2	3.3	3.4	3.6	3.7	3.9	4.2	4.3	4.6	4.7	4.9
53.0	0.3809	3.2322	0.0909	3.3	3.4	3.5	3.7	3.8	4.0	4.3	4.4	4.7	4.8	5.0
53.5	-0.3833	4.1591	0.0910	3.4	3.5	3.6	3.8	3.9	4.2	4.4	4.6	4.9	5.0	5.2
54.0	-0.3833	4.2875	0.0910	3.5	3.6	3.7	3.9	4.0	4.3	4.6	4.7	5.0	5.1	5.3
54.5	-0.3833	4.4179	0.0911	3.6	3.7	3.8	4.0	4.2	4.4	4.7	4.9	5.2	5.3	5.5
55.0	-0.3833	4.5498	0.0911	3.7	3.9	3.9	4.1	4.3	4.5	4.8	5.0	5.3	5.4	5.7
55.5	-0.3833	4.6827	0.0911	3.8	4.0	4.0	4.3	4.4	4.7	5.0	5.2	5.5	5.6	5.8
56.0	-0.3833	4.8162	0.0912	3.9	4.1	4.2	4.4	4.5	4.8	5.1	5.3	5.6	5.8	6.0
56.5	-0.3833	4.9500	0.0912	4.0	4.2	4.3	4.5	4.7	5.0	5.3	5.5	5.8	5.9	6.2
57.0	-0.3833	5.0837	0.0913	4.1	4.3	4.4	4.6	4.8	5.1	5.4	5.6	5.9	6.1	6.3
57.5	-0.3833	5.2173	0.0913	4.3	4.4	4.5	4.8	4.9	5.2	5.6	5.7	6.1	6.2	6.5
58.0	-0.3833	5.3507	0.0913	4.4	4.5	4.6	4.9	5.0	5.4	5.7	5.9	6.2	6.4	6.7
58.5	-0.3833	5.4834	0.0913	4.5	4.6	4.7	5.0	5.2	5.5	5.8	6.0	6.4	6.5	6.8
59.0	-0.3833	5.6151	0.0913	4.6	4.8	4.9	5.1	5.3	5.6	6.0	6.2	6.6	6.7	7.0
59.5	-0.3833	5.7454	0.0914	4.7	4.9	5.0	5.2	5.4	5.7	6.1	6.3	6.7	6.9	7.2
60.0	-0.3833	5.8742	0.0914	4.8	5.0	5.1	5.4	5.5	5.9	6.3	6.5	6.9	7.0	7.3
60.5	-0.3833	6.0014	0.0914	4.9	5.1	5.2	5.5	5.6	6.0	6.4	6.6	7.0	7.2	7.5
61.0	-0.3833	6.1270	0.0914	5.0	5.2	5.3	5.6	5.8	6.1	6.5	6.7	7.2	7.3	7.6
61.5	0.3833	6.2511	0.0914	5.1	5.3	5.4	5.7	5.9	6.3	6.7	6.9	7.3	7.5	7.8
62.0	-0.3833	6.3738	0.0914	5.2	5.4	5.5	5.8	6.0	6.4	6.8	7.0	7.4	7.6	8.0
62.5	-0.3833	6.4948	0.0913	5.3	5.5	5.6	5.9	6.1	6.5	6.9	7.2	7.6	7.8	8.1
63.0	-0.3833	6.6144	0.0913	5.4	5.6	5.7	6.0	6.2	6.6	7.0	7.3	7.7	7.9	8.3
63.5	-0.3833	6.7328	0.0913	5.5	5.7	5.8	6.1	6.3	6.7	7.2	7.4	7.9	8.0	8.4
64.0	-0.3833	6.8501	0.0913	5.6	5.8	5.9	6.2	6.4	6.9	7.3	7.5	8.0	8.2	8.5
64.5	-0.3833	6.9662	0.0912	5.7	5.9	6.0	6.3	6.6	7.0	7.4	7.7	8.1	8.3	8.7
65.0	-0.3833	7.0812	0.0912	5.8	6.0	6.1	6.5	6.7	7.1	7.5	7.8	8.3	8.5	8.8
65.5	-0.3833	7.1950	0.0912	5.9	6.1	6.2	6.6	6.8	7.2	7.7	7.9	8.4	8.6	9.0
66.0	-0.3833	7.3076	0.0911	6.0	6.2	6.3	6.7	6.9	7.3	7.8	8.0	8.5	8.7	9.1
66.5	-0.3833	7.4189	0.0911	6.1	6.3	6.4	6.8	7.0	7.4	7.9	8.2	8.7	8.9	9.3
67.0	-0.3833	7.5288	0.0910	6.1	6.4	6.5	6.9	7.1	7.5	8.0	8.3	8.8	9.0	9.4
67.5	-0.3833	7.6375	0.0910	6.2	6.5	6.6	7.0	7.2	7.6	8.1	8.4	8.9	9.1	9.5
68.0	-0.3833	7.7448	0.0909	6.3	6.6	6.7	7.1	7.3	7.7	8.2	8.5	9.0	9.2	9.7
68.5	-0.3833	7.8509	0.0909	6.4	6.7	6.8	7.2	7.4	7.9	8.4	8.6	9.2	9.4	9.8
69.0	-0.3833	7.9559	0.0908	6.5	6.7	6.9	7.3	7.5	8.0	8.5	8.8	9.3	9.5	9.9
69.5	-0.3833	8.0599	0.0907	6.6	6.8	7.0	7.3	7.6	8.1	8.6	8.9	9.4	9.6	10.0
70.0	-0.3833	8.1630	0.0907	6.7	6.9	7.1	7.4	7.7	8.2	8.7	9.0	9.5	9.7	10.2
70.5	-0.3833	8.2651	0.0906	6.7	7.0	7.1	7.5	7.8	8.3	8.8	9.1	9.6	9.9	10.3
71.0	-0.3833	8.3666	0.0906	6.8	7.1	7.2	7.6	7.9	8.4	8.9	9.2	9.8	10.0	10.4
71.5	-0.3833	8.4676	0.0905	6.9	7.2	7.3	7.7	8.0	8.5	9.0	9.3	9.9	10.1	10.5
72.0	-0.3833	8.5679	0.0904	7.0	7.3	7.4	7.8	8.1	8.6	9.1	9.4	10.0	10.2	10.7
72.5	-0.3833	8.6674	0.0904	7.1	7.4	7.5	7.9	8.2	8.7	9.2	9.5	10.1	10.3	10.8
73.0	-0.3833	8.7661	0.0903	7.2	7.4	7.6	8.0	8.3	8.8	9.3	9.6	10.2	10.4	10.9
73.5	-0.3833	8.8638	0.0903	7.2	7.5	7.7	8.1	8.3	8.9	9.4	9.7	10.3	10.6	11.0
74.0	-0.3833	8.9601	0.0902	7.3	7.6	7.8	8.2	8.4	9.0	9.5	9.9	10.4	10.7	11.2
74.5	-0.3833	9.0552	0.0901	7.4	7.7	7.8	8.3	8.5	9.1	9.6	10.0	10.5	10.8	11.3
75.0	-0.3833	9.1490	0.0901	7.5	7.8	7.9	8.3	8.6	9.1	9.7	10.1	10.7	10.9	11.4
75.5	-0.3833	9.2418	0.0900	7.6	7.8	8.0	8.4	8.7	9.2	9.8	10.2	10.8	11.0	11.5
76.0	-0.3833	9.3337	0.0899	7.6	7.9	8.1	8.5	8.8	9.3	9.9	10.3	10.9	11.1	11.6
76.5	-0.3833	9.4252	0.0899	7.7	8.0	8.2	8.6	8.9	9.4	10.0	10.4	11.0	11.2	11.7
77.0	-0.3833	9.5166	0.0898	7.8	8.1	8.2	8.7	9.0	9.5	10.1	10.5	11.1	11.3	11.8
77.5	-0.3833	9.6086	0.0897	7.9	8.2	8.3	8.8	9.1	9.6	10.2	10.6	11.2	11.4	11.9
78.0	-0.3833	9.7015	0.0897	7.9	8.2	8.4	8.9	9.1	9.7	10.3	10.7	11.3	11.5	12.1
78.5	-0.3833	9.7957	0.0896	8.0	8.3	8.5	8.9	9.2	9.8	10.4	10.8	11.4	11.7	12.2
79.0	0.3833	9.8915	0.0895	8.1	8.4	8.6	9.0	9.3	9.9	10.5	10.9	11.5	11.8	12.3
79.5	-0.3833	9.9892	0.0895	8.2	8.5	8.7	9.1	9.4	10.0	10.6	11.0	11.6	11.9	12.4
80.0	-0.3833	10.0891	0.0894	8.3	8.6	8.7	9.2	9.5	10.1	10.7	11.1	11.7	12.0	12.5

Table V.18b.

LMS parameters and smoothed percentiles of weight (kg)-for-length (cm) for girls from birth to 2 years

Length (cm)	L	M	S	1st	3rd	5th	15th	25th	50th	75th	85th	95th	97th	99th
80.5	-0.3833	10.1916	0.0893	8.3	8.7	8.8	9.3	9.6	10.2	10.8	11.2	11.9	12.1	12.7
81.0	-0.3833	10.2965	0.0893	8.4	8.8	8.9	9.4	9.7	10.3	10.9	11.3	12.0	12.2	12.8
81.5	-0.3833	10.4041	0.0892	8.5	8.8	9.0	9.5	9.8	10.4	11.1	11.4	12.1	12.4	12.9
82.0	-0.3833	10.5140	0.0892	8.6	8.9	9.1	9.6	9.9	10.5	11.2	11.6	12.2	12.5	13.1
82.5	-0.3833	10.6263	0.0891	8.7	9.0	9.2	9.7	10.0	10.6	11.3	11.7	12.4	12.6	13.2
83.0	-0.3833	10.7410	0.0891	8.8	9.1	9.3	9.8	10.1	10.7	11.4	11.8	12.5	12.8	13.3
83.5	-0.3833	10.8578	0.0891	8.9	9.2	9.4	9.9	10.2	10.9	11.5	11.9	12.6	12.9	13.5
84.0	-0.3833	10.9767	0.0890	9.0	9.3	9.5	10.0	10.3	11.0	11.7	12.1	12.8	13.1	13.6
84.5	-0.3833	11.0974	0.0890	9.1	9.4	9.6	10.1	10.5	11.1	11.8	12.2	12.9	13.2	13.8
85.0	-0.3833	11.2198	0.0890	9.2	9.5	9.7	10.2	10.6	11.2	11.9	12.3	13.0	13.3	13.9
85.5	-0.3833	11.3435	0.0890	9.3	9.6	9.8	10.4	10.7	11.3	12.1	12.5	13.2	13.5	14.1
86.0	-0.3833	11.4684	0.0890	9.4	9.8	9.9	10.5	10.8	11.5	12.2	12.6	13.3	13.6	14.2
86.5	-0.3833	11.5940	0.0890	9.5	9.9	10.1	10.6	10.9	11.6	12.3	12.7	13.5	13.8	14.4
87.0	-0.3833	11.7201	0.0890	9.6	10.0	10.2	10.7	11.0	11.7	12.5	12.9	13.6	13.9	14.5
87.5	-0.3833	11.8461	0.0890	9.7	10.1	10.3	10.8	11.2	11.8	12.6	13.0	13.8	14.1	14.7
88.0	-0.3833	11.9720	0.0890	9.8	10.2	10.4	10.9	11.3	12.0	12.7	13.2	13.9	14.2	14.9
88.5	0.3809	3.2322	0.0890	9.9	10.3	10.5	11.0	11.4	12.1	12.9	13.3	14.1	14.4	15.0
89.0	-0.3833	12.2229	0.0890	10.0	10.4	10.6	11.2	11.5	12.2	13.0	13.4	14.2	14.5	15.2
89.5	-0.3833	12.3477	0.0890	10.1	10.5	10.7	11.3	11.6	12.3	13.1	13.6	14.4	14.7	15.3
90.0	-0.3833	12.4723	0.0891	10.2	10.6	10.8	11.4	11.8	12.5	13.3	13.7	14.5	14.8	15.5
90.5	-0.3833	12.5965	0.0891	10.3	10.7	10.9	11.5	11.9	12.6	13.4	13.8	14.6	15.0	15.6
91.0	-0.3833	12.7205	0.0891	10.4	10.8	11.0	11.6	12.0	12.7	13.5	14.0	14.8	15.1	15.8
91.5	-0.3833	12.8443	0.0892	10.5	10.9	11.1	11.7	12.1	12.8	13.7	14.1	14.9	15.3	15.9
92.0	-0.3833	12.9681	0.0892	10.6	11.0	11.2	11.8	12.2	13.0	13.8	14.2	15.1	15.4	16.1
92.5	-0.3833	13.0920	0.0893	10.7	11.1	11.3	12.0	12.3	13.1	13.9	14.4	15.2	15.6	16.3
93.0	-0.3833	13.2158	0.0893	10.8	11.2	11.5	12.1	12.5	13.2	14.0	14.5	15.4	15.7	16.4
93.5	-0.3833	13.3399	0.0894	10.9	11.3	11.6	12.2	12.6	13.3	14.2	14.7	15.5	15.9	16.6
94.0	-0.3833	13.4643	0.0895	11.0	11.4	11.7	12.3	12.7	13.5	14.3	14.8	15.7	16.0	16.7
94.5	-0.3833	13.5892	0.0896	11.1	11.5	11.8	12.4	12.8	13.6	14.4	14.9	15.8	16.2	16.9
95.0	-0.3833	13.7146	0.0896	11.2	11.6	11.9	12.5	12.9	13.7	14.6	15.1	16.0	16.3	17.0
95.5	-0.3833	13.8408	0.0897	11.3	11.8	12.0	12.6	13.0	13.8	14.7	15.2	16.1	16.5	17.2
96.0	-0.3833	13.9676	0.0898	11.4	11.9	12.1	12.7	13.2	14.0	14.9	15.4	16.3	16.6	17.4
96.5	-0.3833	14.0953	0.0899	11.5	12.0	12.2	12.9	13.3	14.1	15.0	15.5	16.4	16.8	17.5
97.0	-0.3833	14.2239	0.0900	11.6	12.1	12.3	13.0	13.4	14.2	15.1	15.6	16.6	16.9	17.7
97.5	-0.3833	14.3537	0.0901	11.7	12.2	12.4	13.1	13.5	14.4	15.3	15.8	16.7	17.1	17.9
98.0	-0.3833	14.4848	0.0902	11.8	12.3	12.5	13.2	13.6	14.5	15.4	15.9	16.9	17.3	18.0
98.5	-0.3833	14.6174	0.0903	11.9	12.4	12.7	13.3	13.8	14.6	15.5	16.1	17.0	17.4	18.2
99.0	-0.3833	14.7519	0.0904	12.0	12.5	12.8	13.5	13.9	14.8	15.7	16.2	17.2	17.6	18.4
99.5	-0.3833	14.8882	0.0906	12.2	12.6	12.9	13.6	14.0	14.9	15.8	16.4	17.4	17.8	18.5
100.0	-0.3833	15.0267	0.0907	12.3	12.7	13.0	13.7	14.1	15.0	16.0	16.5	17.5	17.9	18.7
100.5	-0.3833	15.1676	0.0908	12.4	12.9	13.1	13.8	14.3	15.2	16.1	16.7	17.7	18.1	18.9
101.0	-0.3833	15.3108	0.0910	12.5	13.0	13.2	14.0	14.4	15.3	16.3	16.9	17.9	18.3	19.1
101.5	-0.3833	15.4564	0.0911	12.6	13.1	13.4	14.1	14.5	15.5	16.4	17.0	18.0	18.5	19.3
102.0	-0.3833	15.6046	0.0913	12.7	13.2	13.5	14.2	14.7	15.6	16.6	17.2	18.2	18.6	19.5
102.5	-0.3833	15.7553	0.0914	12.8	13.3	13.6	14.4	14.8	15.8	16.8	17.4	18.4	18.8	19.7
103.0	-0.3833	15.9087	0.0916	13.0	13.5	13.7	14.5	15.0	15.9	16.9	17.5	18.6	19.0	19.9
103.5	-0.3833	16.0645	0.0917	13.1	13.6	13.9	14.6	15.1	16.1	17.1	17.7	18.8	19.2	20.1
104.0	-0.3833	16.2229	0.0919	13.2	13.7	14.0	14.8	15.3	16.2	17.3	17.9	19.0	19.4	20.3
104.5	-0.3833	16.3837	0.0920	13.3	13.9	14.1	14.9	15.4	16.4	17.4	18.1	19.1	19.6	20.5
105.0	-0.3833	16.5470	0.0922	13.5	14.0	14.3	15.1	15.6	16.5	17.6	18.2	19.3	19.8	20.7
105.5	-0.3833	16.7129	0.0924	13.6	14.1	14.4	15.2	15.7	16.7	17.8	18.4	19.5	20.0	20.9
106.0	-0.3833	16.8814	0.0925	13.7	14.3	14.6	15.4	15.9	16.9	18.0	18.6	19.7	20.2	21.1
106.5	-0.3833	17.0527	0.0927	13.9	14.4	14.7	15.5	16.0	17.1	18.2	18.8	20.0	20.4	21.4
107.0	-0.3833	17.2269	0.0929	14.0	14.5	14.8	15.7	16.2	17.2	18.4	19.0	20.2	20.6	21.6
107.5	-0.3833	17.4039	0.0931	14.1	14.7	15.0	15.8	16.4	17.4	18.5	19.2	20.4	20.9	21.8
108.0	-0.3833	17.5839	0.0933	14.3	14.8	15.1	16.0	16.5	17.6	18.7	19.4	20.6	21.1	22.1
108.5	-0.3833	17.7668	0.0934	14.4	15.0	15.3	16.2	16.7	17.8	18.9	19.6	20.8	21.3	22.3
109.0	-0.3833	17.9526	0.0936	14.6	15.1	15.5	16.3	16.9	18.0	19.1	19.8	21.0	21.5	22.5
109.5	-0.3833	18.1412	0.0938	14.7	15.3	15.6	16.5	17.0	18.1	19.3	20.0	21.3	21.8	22.8
110.0	-0.3833	18.3324	0.0940	14.9	15.4	15.8	16.7	17.2	18.3	19.5	20.2	21.5	22.0	23.0

Table V.19a.

LMS parameters and smoothed percentiles of weight (kg)-for-height (cm) for boys from 2 to 5 years

Height (cm)	L	M	S	1st	3rd	5th	15th	25th	50th	75th	85th	95th	97th	99th
									Percentiles					
65.0	-0.3521	7.4327	0.0822	6.2	6.4	6.5	6.8	7.0	7.4	7.9	8.1	8.5	8.7	9.1
65.5	-0.3521	7.5504	0.0821	6.3	6.5	6.6	6.9	7.1	7.6	8.0	8.2	8.7	8.9	9.2
66.0	-0.3521	7.6673	0.0821	6.4	6.6	6.7	7.1	7.3	7.7	8.1	8.4	8.8	9.0	9.3
66.5	-0.3521	7.7834	0.0821	6.5	6.7	6.8	7.2	7.4	7.8	8.2	8.5	8.9	9.1	9.5
67.0	-0.3521	7.8986	0.0821	6.6	6.8	6.9	7.3	7.5	7.9	8.4	8.6	9.1	9.3	9.6
67.5	-0.3521	8.0132	0.0821	6.7	6.9	7.0	7.4	7.6	8.0	8.5	8.7	9.2	9.4	9.8
68.0	-0.3521	8.1272	0.0822	6.8	7.0	7.1	7.5	7.7	8.1	8.6	8.9	9.3	9.5	9.9
68.5	-0.3521	8.2410	0.0822	6.8	7.1	7.2	7.6	7.8	8.2	8.7	9.0	9.5	9.7	10.0
69.0	-0.3521	8.3547	0.0823	6.9	7.2	7.3	7.7	7.9	8.4	8.8	9.1	9.6	9.8	10.2
69.5	-0.3521	8.4680	0.0823	7.0	7.3	7.4	7.8	8.0	8.5	9.0	9.2	9.7	9.9	10.3
70.0	-0.3521	8.5808	0.0824	7.1	7.4	7.5	7.9	8.1	8.6	9.1	9.4	9.9	10.1	10.5
70.5	-0.3521	8.6927	0.0824	7.2	7.5	7.6	8.0	8.2	8.7	9.2	9.5	10.0	10.2	10.6
71.0	-0.3521	8.8036	0.0825	7.3	7.6	7.7	8.1	8.3	8.8	9.3	9.6	10.1	10.3	10.7
71.5	-0.3521	8.9135	0.0826	7.4	7.7	7.8	8.2	8.4	8.9	9.4	9.7	10.2	10.5	10.9
72.0	-0.3521	9.0221	0.0826	7.5	7.8	7.9	8.3	8.5	9.0	9.5	9.8	10.4	10.6	11.0
72.5	-0.3521	9.1292	0.0827	7.6	7.8	8.0	8.4	8.6	9.1	9.7	10.0	10.5	10.7	11.1
73.0	0.3809	3.2322	0.0828	7.7	7.9	8.1	8.5	8.7	9.2	9.8	10.1	10.6	10.8	11.3
73.5	-0.3521	9.3390	0.0829	7.8	8.0	8.2	8.6	8.8	9.3	9.9	10.2	10.7	11.0	11.4
74.0	-0.3521	9.4420	0.0829	7.8	8.1	8.3	8.7	8.9	9.4	10.0	10.3	10.9	11.1	11.5
74.5	-0.3521	9.5438	0.0830	7.9	8.2	8.4	8.8	9.0	9.5	10.1	10.4	11.0	11.2	11.7
75.0	-0.3521	9.6440	0.0830	8.0	8.3	8.4	8.9	9.1	9.6	10.2	10.5	11.1	11.3	11.8
75.5	-0.3521	9.7425	0.0831	8.1	8.4	8.5	9.0	9.2	9.7	10.3	10.6	11.2	11.4	11.9
76.0	-0.3521	9.8392	0.0831	8.2	8.5	8.6	9.0	9.3	9.8	10.4	10.7	11.3	11.6	12.0
76.5	-0.3521	9.9341	0.0832	8.2	8.5	8.7	9.1	9.4	9.9	10.5	10.8	11.4	11.7	12.1
77.0	-0.3521	10.0274	0.0832	8.3	8.6	8.8	9.2	9.5	10.0	10.6	10.9	11.5	11.8	12.3
77.5	-0.3521	10.1194	0.0832	8.4	8.7	8.9	9.3	9.6	10.1	10.7	11.0	11.6	11.9	12.4
78.0	-0.3521	10.2105	0.0832	8.5	8.8	8.9	9.4	9.7	10.2	10.8	11.1	11.7	12.0	12.5
78.5	-0.3521	10.3012	0.0832	8.5	8.8	9.0	9.5	9.7	10.3	10.9	11.2	11.9	12.1	12.6
79.0	-0.3521	10.3923	0.0831	8.6	8.9	9.1	9.5	9.8	10.4	11.0	11.3	12.0	12.2	12.7
79.5	-0.3521	10.4845	0.0831	8.7	9.0	9.2	9.6	9.9	10.5	11.1	11.4	12.1	12.3	12.8
80.0	-0.3521	10.5781	0.0830	8.8	9.1	9.3	9.7	10.0	10.6	11.2	11.5	12.2	12.4	12.9
80.5	-0.3521	10.6737	0.0829	8.9	9.2	9.3	9.8	10.1	10.7	11.3	11.6	12.3	12.5	13.0
81.0	-0.3521	10.7718	0.0828	8.9	9.3	9.4	9.9	10.2	10.8	11.4	11.8	12.4	12.6	13.1
81.5	-0.3521	10.8728	0.0827	9.0	9.3	9.5	10.0	10.3	10.9	11.5	11.9	12.5	12.8	13.3
82.0	-0.3521	10.9772	0.0826	9.1	9.4	9.6	10.1	10.4	11.0	11.6	12.0	12.6	12.9	13.4
82.5	-0.3521	11.0851	0.0824	9.2	9.5	9.7	10.2	10.5	11.1	11.7	12.1	12.7	13.0	13.5
83.0	-0.3521	11.1966	0.0823	9.3	9.6	9.8	10.3	10.6	11.2	11.8	12.2	12.9	13.1	13.6
83.5	-0.3521	11.3114	0.0821	9.4	9.7	9.9	10.4	10.7	11.3	12.0	12.3	13.0	13.3	13.8
84.0	-0.3521	11.4290	0.0819	9.5	9.8	10.0	10.5	10.8	11.4	12.1	12.5	13.1	13.4	13.9
84.5	-0.3521	11.5490	0.0817	9.6	9.9	10.1	10.6	10.9	11.5	12.2	12.6	13.3	13.5	14.1
85.0	-0.3521	11.6707	0.0816	9.7	10.1	10.2	10.7	11.1	11.7	12.3	12.7	13.4	13.7	14.2
85.5	-0.3521	11.7937	0.0814	9.8	10.2	10.3	10.9	11.2	11.8	12.5	12.8	13.5	13.8	14.3
86.0	-0.3521	11.9173	0.0812	9.9	10.3	10.5	11.0	11.3	11.9	12.6	13.0	13.7	13.9	14.5
86.5	-0.3521	12.0411	0.0811	10.0	10.4	10.6	11.1	11.4	12.0	12.7	13.1	13.8	14.1	14.6
87.0	-0.3521	12.1645	0.0809	10.1	10.5	10.7	11.2	11.5	12.2	12.9	13.2	13.9	14.2	14.8
87.5	-0.3521	12.2871	0.0808	10.2	10.6	10.8	11.3	11.6	12.3	13.0	13.4	14.1	14.4	14.9
88.0	-0.3521	12.4089	0.0806	10.3	10.7	10.9	11.4	11.8	12.4	13.1	13.5	14.2	14.5	15.1
88.5	-0.3521	12.5298	0.0805	10.5	10.8	11.0	11.5	11.9	12.5	13.2	13.6	14.4	14.6	15.2
89.0	-0.3521	12.6495	0.0805	10.6	10.9	11.1	11.7	12.0	12.6	13.4	13.8	14.5	14.8	15.4
89.5	-0.3521	12.7683	0.0804	10.7	11.0	11.2	11.8	12.1	12.8	13.5	13.9	14.6	14.9	15.5
90.0	-0.3521	12.8864	0.0803	10.8	11.1	11.3	11.9	12.2	12.9	13.6	14.0	14.8	15.1	15.6
90.5	-0.3521	13.0038	0.0803	10.9	11.2	11.4	12.0	12.3	13.0	13.7	14.1	14.9	15.2	15.8
91.0	-0.3521	13.1209	0.0803	11.0	11.3	11.5	12.1	12.4	13.1	13.9	14.3	15.0	15.3	15.9
91.5	-0.3521	13.2376	0.0802	11.0	11.4	11.6	12.2	12.5	13.2	14.0	14.4	15.2	15.5	16.1
92.0	-0.3521	13.3541	0.0803	11.1	11.5	11.7	12.3	12.7	13.4	14.1	14.5	15.3	15.6	16.2
92.5	-0.3521	13.4705	0.0803	11.2	11.6	11.8	12.4	12.8	13.5	14.2	14.7	15.4	15.7	16.3
93.0	-0.3521	13.5870	0.0803	11.3	11.7	11.9	12.5	12.9	13.6	14.4	14.8	15.6	15.9	16.5
93.5	-0.3521	13.7041	0.0804	11.4	11.8	12.0	12.6	13.0	13.7	14.5	14.9	15.7	16.0	16.6
94.0	-0.3521	13.8217	0.0804	11.5	11.9	12.1	12.7	13.1	13.8	14.6	15.0	15.8	16.1	16.8
94.5	-0.3521	13.9403	0.0805	11.6	12.0	12.2	12.8	13.2	13.9	14.7	15.2	16.0	16.3	16.9
95.0	-0.3521	14.0600	0.0806	11.7	12.1	12.4	12.9	13.3	14.1	14.9	15.3	16.1	16.4	17.1

Table V.19b.
LMS parameters and smoothed percentiles of weight (kg)-for-height (cm) for boys from 2 to 5 years

Height (cm)	L	M	S	1st	3rd	5th	15th	25th	50th	75th	85th	95th	97th	99th
									Percentiles					
95.5	-0.3521	14.1811	0.0807	11.8	12.2	12.5	13.1	13.4	14.2	15.0	15.4	16.2	16.6	17.2
96.0	-0.3521	14.3037	0.0808	11.9	12.3	12.6	13.2	13.6	14.3	15.1	15.6	16.4	16.7	17.4
96.5	-0.3521	14.4282	0.0810	12.0	12.4	12.7	13.3	13.7	14.4	15.2	15.7	16.5	16.9	17.5
97.0	-0.3521	14.5547	0.0811	12.1	12.5	12.8	13.4	13.8	14.6	15.4	15.9	16.7	17.0	17.7
97.5	-0.3521	14.6832	0.0813	12.2	12.7	12.9	13.5	13.9	14.7	15.5	16.0	16.8	17.2	17.9
98.0	-0.3521	14.8140	0.0815	12.3	12.8	13.0	13.6	14.0	14.8	15.7	16.1	17.0	17.3	18.0
98.5	-0.3521	14.9468	0.0817	12.4	12.9	13.1	13.8	14.2	14.9	15.8	16.3	17.2	17.5	18.2
99.0	-0.3521	15.0818	0.0819	12.5	13.0	13.2	13.9	14.3	15.1	15.9	16.4	17.3	17.7	18.4
99.5	-0.3521	15.2187	0.0821	12.7	13.1	13.3	14.0	14.4	15.2	16.1	16.6	17.5	17.8	18.5
100.0	-0.3521	15.3576	0.0823	12.8	13.2	13.5	14.1	14.5	15.4	16.2	16.7	17.6	18.0	18.7
100.5	-0.3521	15.4985	0.0825	12.9	13.3	13.6	14.2	14.7	15.5	16.4	16.9	17.8	18.2	18.9
101.0	-0.3521	15.6412	0.0828	13.0	13.4	13.7	14.4	14.8	15.6	16.5	17.1	18.0	18.4	19.1
101.5	-0.3521	15.7857	0.0830	13.1	13.6	13.8	14.5	14.9	15.8	16.7	17.2	18.2	18.5	19.3
102.0	-0.3521	15.9320	0.0833	13.2	13.7	13.9	14.6	15.1	15.9	16.9	17.4	18.3	18.7	19.5
102.5	-0.3521	16.0801	0.0835	13.3	13.8	14.1	14.8	15.2	16.1	17.0	17.6	18.5	18.9	19.7
103.0	-0.3521	16.2298	0.0838	13.4	13.9	14.2	14.9	15.3	16.2	17.2	17.7	18.7	19.1	19.9
103.5	0.3809	3.2322	0.0841	13.6	14.0	14.3	15.0	15.5	16.4	17.3	17.9	18.9	19.3	20.1
104.0	-0.3521	16.5342	0.0844	13.7	14.2	14.4	15.2	15.6	16.5	17.5	18.1	19.1	19.5	20.3
104.5	-0.3521	16.6889	0.0846	13.8	14.3	14.6	15.3	15.8	16.7	17.7	18.2	19.2	19.7	20.5
105.0	-0.3521	16.8454	0.0849	13.9	14.4	14.7	15.4	15.9	16.8	17.8	18.4	19.4	19.9	20.7
105.5	-0.3521	17.0036	0.0852	14.0	14.5	14.8	15.6	16.1	17.0	18.0	18.6	19.6	20.1	20.9
106.0	-0.3521	17.1637	0.0855	14.2	14.7	15.0	15.7	16.2	17.2	18.2	18.8	19.8	20.3	21.1
106.5	-0.3521	17.3256	0.0858	14.3	14.8	15.1	15.9	16.4	17.3	18.4	19.0	20.0	20.5	21.3
107.0	-0.3521	17.4894	0.0861	14.4	14.9	15.2	16.0	16.5	17.5	18.5	19.1	20.2	20.7	21.5
107.5	-0.3521	17.6550	0.0864	14.5	15.1	15.4	16.2	16.7	17.7	18.7	19.3	20.4	20.9	21.7
108.0	-0.3521	17.8226	0.0867	14.7	15.2	15.5	16.3	16.8	17.8	18.9	19.5	20.6	21.1	22
108.5	-0.3521	17.9924	0.0870	14.8	15.3	15.6	16.5	17.0	18.0	19.1	19.7	20.8	21.3	22.2
109.0	-0.3521	18.1645	0.0874	14.9	15.5	15.8	16.6	17.1	18.2	19.3	19.9	21.1	21.5	22.4
109.5	-0.3521	18.3390	0.0877	15.1	15.6	15.9	16.8	17.3	18.3	19.5	20.1	21.3	21.7	22.7
110.0	-0.3521	18.5158	0.0880	15.2	15.8	16.1	16.9	17.5	18.5	19.7	20.3	21.5	22.0	22.9
110.5	-0.3521	18.6948	0.0883	15.3	15.9	16.2	17.1	17.6	18.7	19.9	20.5	21.7	22.2	23.1
111.0	-0.3521	18.8759	0.0886	15.5	16.1	16.4	17.2	17.8	18.9	20.1	20.7	21.9	22.4	23.4
111.5	-0.3521	19.0590	0.0890	15.6	16.2	16.5	17.4	18.0	19.1	20.3	20.9	22.1	22.6	23.6
112.0	-0.3521	19.2439	0.0893	15.7	16.3	16.7	17.6	18.1	19.2	20.5	21.1	22.4	22.9	23.9
112.5	-0.3521	19.4304	0.0896	15.9	16.5	16.8	17.7	18.3	19.4	20.7	21.4	22.6	23.1	24.1
113.0	-0.3521	19.6185	0.0899	16.0	16.6	17.0	17.9	18.5	19.6	20.9	21.6	22.8	23.4	24.4
113.5	-0.3521	19.8081	0.0902	16.2	16.8	17.1	18.1	18.7	19.8	21.1	21.8	23.1	23.6	24.6
114.0	-0.3521	19.9990	0.0905	16.3	17.0	17.3	18.2	18.8	20.0	21.3	22.0	23.3	23.8	24.9
114.5	-0.3521	20.1912	0.0909	16.5	17.1	17.5	18.4	19.0	20.2	21.5	22.2	23.5	24.1	25.2
115.0	-0.3521	20.3846	0.0912	16.6	17.3	17.6	18.6	19.2	20.4	21.7	22.4	23.8	24.3	25.4
115.5	-0.3521	20.5789	0.0915	16.8	17.4	17.8	18.7	19.4	20.6	21.9	22.7	24.0	24.6	25.7
116.0	-0.3521	20.7741	0.0918	16.9	17.6	17.9	18.9	19.5	20.8	22.1	22.9	24.3	24.8	25.9
116.5	-0.3521	20.9700	0.0921	17.1	17.7	18.1	19.1	19.7	21.0	22.3	23.1	24.5	25.1	26.2
117.0	-0.3521	21.1666	0.0924	17.2	17.9	18.3	19.3	19.9	21.2	22.5	23.3	24.7	25.3	26.5
117.5	-0.3521	21.3636	0.0927	17.4	18.0	18.4	19.4	20.1	21.4	22.8	23.6	25.0	25.6	26.7
118.0	-0.3521	21.5611	0.0930	17.5	18.2	18.6	19.6	20.3	21.6	23.0	23.8	25.2	25.8	27
118.5	-0.3521	21.7588	0.0933	17.7	18.4	18.7	19.8	20.4	21.8	23.2	24.0	25.5	26.1	27.3
119.0	-0.3521	21.9568	0.0936	17.8	18.5	18.9	20.0	20.6	22.0	23.4	24.2	25.7	26.3	27.5
119.5	-0.3521	22.1549	0.0939	17.9	18.7	19.1	20.1	20.8	22.2	23.6	24.5	26.0	26.6	27.8
120.0	-0.3521	22.3530	0.0942	18.1	18.8	19.2	20.3	21.0	22.4	23.8	24.7	26.2	26.8	28.1

WHO Growth Standards

Table V.20a.

LMS parameters and smoothed percentiles of weight (kg)-for-height (cm) for girls from 2 to 5 years

Height (cm)	L	M	S	1st	3rd	5th	15th	25th	50th	75th	85th	95th	97th	99th
65.0	-0.3833	7.2402	0.0911	5.9	6.1	6.3	6.6	6.8	7.2	7.7	8.0	8.4	8.6	9.0
65.5	-0.3833	7.3523	0.0911	6.0	6.2	6.4	6.7	6.9	7.4	7.8	8.1	8.6	8.8	9.2
66.0	-0.3833	7.4630	0.0910	6.1	6.3	6.5	6.8	7.0	7.5	7.9	8.2	8.7	8.9	9.3
66.5	-0.3833	7.5724	0.0910	6.2	6.4	6.5	6.9	7.1	7.6	8.1	8.3	8.8	9.0	9.4
67.0	-0.3833	7.6806	0.0909	6.3	6.5	6.6	7.0	7.2	7.7	8.2	8.5	9.0	9.2	9.6
67.5	-0.3833	7.7874	0.0909	6.4	6.6	6.7	7.1	7.3	7.8	8.3	8.6	9.1	9.3	9.7
68.0	-0.3833	7.8930	0.0908	6.4	6.7	6.8	7.2	7.4	7.9	8.4	8.7	9.2	9.4	9.8
68.5	-0.3833	7.9976	0.0908	6.5	6.8	6.9	7.3	7.5	8.0	8.5	8.8	9.3	9.5	10.0
69.0	-0.3833	8.1012	0.0907	6.6	6.9	7.0	7.4	7.6	8.1	8.6	8.9	9.4	9.7	10.1
69.5	-0.3833	8.2039	0.0907	6.7	7.0	7.1	7.5	7.7	8.2	8.7	9.0	9.6	9.8	10.2
70.0	-0.3833	8.3058	0.0906	6.8	7.0	7.2	7.6	7.8	8.3	8.8	9.1	9.7	9.9	10.3
70.5	-0.3833	8.4071	0.0905	6.9	7.1	7.3	7.7	7.9	8.4	8.9	9.3	9.8	10.0	10.5
71.0	-0.3833	8.5078	0.0905	6.9	7.2	7.4	7.8	8.0	8.5	9.0	9.4	9.9	10.1	10.6
71.5	-0.3833	8.6078	0.0904	7.0	7.3	7.4	7.9	8.1	8.6	9.2	9.5	10.0	10.3	10.7
72.0	-0.3833	8.7070	0.0904	7.1	7.4	7.5	7.9	8.2	8.7	9.3	9.6	10.1	10.4	10.8
72.5	-0.3833	8.8053	0.0903	7.2	7.5	7.6	8.0	8.3	8.8	9.4	9.7	10.3	10.5	11.0
73.0	0.3809	3.2322	0.0902	7.3	7.6	7.7	8.1	8.4	8.9	9.5	9.8	10.4	10.6	11.1
73.5	-0.3833	8.9983	0.0902	7.4	7.6	7.8	8.2	8.5	9.0	9.6	9.9	10.5	10.7	11.2
74.0	-0.3833	9.0928	0.0901	7.4	7.7	7.9	8.3	8.6	9.1	9.7	10.0	10.6	10.8	11.3
74.5	-0.3833	9.1862	0.0900	7.5	7.8	8.0	8.4	8.7	9.2	9.8	10.1	10.7	10.9	11.4
75.0	-0.3833	9.2786	0.0900	7.6	7.9	8.0	8.5	8.7	9.3	9.9	10.2	10.8	11.1	11.5
75.5	-0.3833	9.3703	0.0899	7.7	8.0	8.1	8.6	8.8	9.4	10.0	10.3	10.9	11.2	11.7
76.0	-0.3833	9.4617	0.0898	7.7	8.0	8.2	8.6	8.9	9.5	10.1	10.4	11.0	11.3	11.8
76.5	-0.3833	9.5533	0.0898	7.8	8.1	8.3	8.7	9.0	9.6	10.2	10.5	11.1	11.4	11.9
77.0	-0.3833	9.6456	0.0897	7.9	8.2	8.4	8.8	9.1	9.6	10.3	10.6	11.2	11.5	12.0
77.5	-0.3833	9.7390	0.0896	8.0	8.3	8.4	8.9	9.2	9.7	10.4	10.7	11.3	11.6	12.1
78.0	-0.3833	9.8338	0.0896	8.0	8.4	8.5	9.0	9.3	9.8	10.5	10.8	11.4	11.7	12.2
78.5	-0.3833	9.9303	0.0895	8.1	8.4	8.6	9.1	9.4	9.9	10.6	10.9	11.6	11.8	12.3
79.0	-0.3833	10.0289	0.0894	8.2	8.5	8.7	9.2	9.4	10.0	10.7	11.0	11.7	11.9	12.5
79.5	-0.3833	10.1298	0.0894	8.3	8.6	8.8	9.2	9.5	10.1	10.8	11.1	11.8	12.1	12.6
80.0	-0.3833	10.2332	0.0893	8.4	8.7	8.9	9.3	9.6	10.2	10.9	11.2	11.9	12.2	12.7
80.5	-0.3833	10.3393	0.0893	8.5	8.8	9.0	9.4	9.7	10.3	11.0	11.4	12.0	12.3	12.8
81.0	-0.3833	10.4477	0.0892	8.6	8.9	9.1	9.5	9.8	10.4	11.1	11.5	12.2	12.4	13.0
81.5	-0.3833	10.5586	0.0892	8.6	9.0	9.2	9.6	9.9	10.6	11.2	11.6	12.3	12.6	13.1
82.0	-0.3833	10.6719	0.0891	8.7	9.1	9.3	9.7	10.1	10.7	11.3	11.7	12.4	12.7	13.2
82.5	-0.3833	10.7874	0.0891	8.8	9.2	9.4	9.9	10.2	10.8	11.5	11.9	12.5	12.8	13.4
83.0	-0.3833	10.9051	0.0891	8.9	9.3	9.5	10.0	10.3	10.9	11.6	12.0	12.7	13.0	13.5
83.5	-0.3833	11.0248	0.0890	9.0	9.4	9.6	10.1	10.4	11.0	11.7	12.1	12.8	13.1	13.7
84.0	-0.3833	11.1462	0.0890	9.1	9.5	9.7	10.2	10.5	11.1	11.8	12.2	13.0	13.3	13.8
84.5	-0.3833	11.2691	0.0890	9.2	9.6	9.8	10.3	10.6	11.3	12.0	12.4	13.1	13.4	14.0
85.0	-0.3833	11.3934	0.0890	9.3	9.7	9.9	10.4	10.7	11.4	12.1	12.5	13.2	13.5	14.1
85.5	-0.3833	11.5186	0.0890	9.4	9.8	10.0	10.5	10.9	11.5	12.2	12.7	13.4	13.7	14.3
86.0	-0.3833	11.6444	0.0890	9.5	9.9	10.1	10.6	11.0	11.6	12.4	12.8	13.5	13.8	14.4
86.5	-0.3833	11.7705	0.0890	9.6	10.0	10.2	10.8	11.1	11.8	12.5	12.9	13.7	14.0	14.6
87.0	-0.3833	11.8965	0.0890	9.7	10.1	10.3	10.9	11.2	11.9	12.6	13.1	13.8	14.1	14.8
87.5	-0.3833	12.0223	0.0890	9.9	10.2	10.4	11.0	11.3	12.0	12.8	13.2	14.0	14.3	14.9
88.0	-0.3833	12.1478	0.0890	10.0	10.3	10.5	11.1	11.4	12.1	12.9	13.3	14.1	14.4	15.1
88.5	-0.3833	12.2729	0.0890	10.1	10.4	10.6	11.2	11.6	12.3	13.0	13.5	14.3	14.6	15.2
89.0	-0.3833	12.3976	0.0890	10.2	10.5	10.8	11.3	11.7	12.4	13.2	13.6	14.4	14.7	15.4
89.5	-0.3833	12.5220	0.0891	10.3	10.6	10.9	11.4	11.8	12.5	13.3	13.8	14.6	14.9	15.5
90.0	-0.3833	12.6461	0.0891	10.4	10.8	11.0	11.5	11.9	12.6	13.4	13.9	14.7	15.0	15.7
90.5	-0.3833	12.7700	0.0892	10.5	10.9	11.1	11.7	12.0	12.8	13.6	14.0	14.9	15.2	15.9
91.0	-0.3833	12.8939	0.0892	10.6	11.0	11.2	11.8	12.1	12.9	13.7	14.2	15.0	15.3	16.0
91.5	-0.3833	13.0177	0.0893	10.7	11.1	11.3	11.9	12.3	13.0	13.8	14.3	15.1	15.5	16.2
92.0	-0.3833	13.1415	0.0893	10.8	11.2	11.4	12.0	12.4	13.1	14.0	14.4	15.3	15.6	16.3
92.5	-0.3833	13.2654	0.0894	10.9	11.3	11.5	12.1	12.5	13.3	14.1	14.6	15.4	15.8	16.5
93.0	-0.3833	13.3896	0.0894	11.0	11.4	11.6	12.2	12.6	13.4	14.2	14.7	15.6	15.9	16.6
93.5	-0.3833	13.5142	0.0895	11.1	11.5	11.7	12.3	12.7	13.5	14.4	14.9	15.7	16.1	16.8
94.0	-0.3833	13.6393	0.0896	11.2	11.6	11.8	12.4	12.8	13.6	14.5	15.0	15.9	16.2	16.9
94.5	-0.3833	13.7650	0.0897	11.3	11.7	11.9	12.6	13.0	13.8	14.6	15.1	16.0	16.4	17.1
95.0	-0.3833	13.8914	0.0898	11.4	11.8	12.0	12.7	13.1	13.9	14.8	15.3	16.2	16.5	17.3
95.5	-0.3833	14.0186	0.0898	11.5	11.9	12.1	12.8	13.2	14.0	14.9	15.4	16.3	16.7	17.4
96.0	-0.3833	14.1466	0.0899	11.6	12.0	12.3	12.9	13.3	14.1	15.0	15.6	16.5	16.9	17.6
96.5	-0.3833	14.2757	0.0900	11.7	12.1	12.4	13.0	13.4	14.3	15.2	15.7	16.6	17.0	17.8
97.0	-0.3833	14.4059	0.0902	11.8	12.2	12.5	13.1	13.6	14.4	15.3	15.8	16.8	17.2	17.9
97.5	-0.3833	14.5376	0.0903	11.9	12.3	12.6	13.3	13.7	14.5	15.5	16.0	16.9	17.3	18.1
98.0	-0.3833	14.6710	0.0904	12.0	12.4	12.7	13.4	13.8	14.7	15.6	16.1	17.1	17.5	18.3
98.5	0.3833	14.8062	0.0905	12.1	12.6	12.8	13.5	13.9	14.8	15.7	16.3	17.3	17.7	18.4
99.0	-0.3833	14.9434	0.0906	12.2	12.7	12.9	13.6	14.1	14.9	15.9	16.4	17.4	17.8	18.6

263

Table V.20b.
LMS parameters and smoothed percentiles of weight (kg)-for-height (cm) for girls from 2 to 5 years

Height (cm)	L	M	S	1st	3rd	5th	15th	25th	50th	75th	85th	95th	97th	99th
99.5	-0.3833	15.0828	0.0908	12.3	12.8	13.0	13.8	14.2	15.1	16.0	16.6	17.6	18.0	18.8
100.0	-0.3833	15.2246	0.0909	12.4	12.9	13.2	13.9	14.3	15.2	16.2	16.8	17.8	18.2	19.0
100.5	-0.3833	15.3687	0.0910	12.5	13.0	13.3	14.0	14.5	15.4	16.4	16.9	17.9	18.3	19.2
101.0	-0.3833	15.5154	0.0912	12.7	13.1	13.4	14.1	14.6	15.5	16.5	17.1	18.1	18.5	19.4
101.5	-0.3833	15.6646	0.0913	12.8	13.3	13.5	14.3	14.7	15.7	16.7	17.2	18.3	18.7	19.5
102.0	-0.3833	15.8164	0.0915	12.9	13.4	13.7	14.4	14.9	15.8	16.8	17.4	18.5	18.9	19.7
102.5	-0.3833	15.9707	0.0916	13.0	13.5	13.8	14.5	15.0	16.0	17.0	17.6	18.7	19.1	19.9
103.0	-0.3833	16.1276	0.0918	13.1	13.6	13.9	14.7	15.2	16.1	17.2	17.8	18.8	19.3	20.2
103.5	-0.3833	16.2870	0.0919	13.3	13.8	14.1	14.8	15.3	16.3	17.3	17.9	19.0	19.5	20.4
104.0	-0.3833	16.4488	0.0921	13.4	13.9	14.2	15.0	15.5	16.4	17.5	18.1	19.2	19.7	20.6
104.5	-0.3833	16.6131	0.0923	13.5	14.0	14.3	15.1	15.6	16.6	17.7	18.3	19.4	19.9	20.8
105.0	-0.3833	16.7800	0.0924	13.6	14.2	14.5	15.3	15.8	16.8	17.9	18.5	19.6	20.1	21.0
105.5	-0.3833	16.9496	0.0926	13.8	14.3	14.6	15.4	15.9	16.9	18.1	18.7	19.8	20.3	21.2
106.0	-0.3833	17.1220	0.0928	13.9	14.5	14.8	15.6	16.1	17.1	18.2	18.9	20.0	20.5	21.4
106.5	-0.3833	17.2973	0.0930	14.1	14.6	14.9	15.7	16.3	17.3	18.4	19.1	20.2	20.7	21.7
107.0	-0.3833	17.4755	0.0932	14.2	14.7	15.1	15.9	16.4	17.5	18.6	19.3	20.5	21.0	21.9
107.5	0.3809	3.2322	0.0933	14.3	14.9	15.2	16.1	16.6	17.7	18.8	19.5	20.7	21.2	22.1
108.0	-0.3833	17.8407	0.0935	14.5	15.0	15.4	16.2	16.8	17.8	19.0	19.7	20.9	21.4	22.4
108.5	-0.3833	18.0277	0.0937	14.6	15.2	15.5	16.4	16.9	18.0	19.2	19.9	21.1	21.6	22.6
109.0	-0.3833	18.2174	0.0939	14.8	15.4	15.7	16.6	17.1	18.2	19.4	20.1	21.4	21.9	22.9
109.5	-0.3833	18.4096	0.0941	14.9	15.5	15.8	16.7	17.3	18.4	19.6	20.3	21.6	22.1	23.1
110.0	-0.3833	18.6043	0.0943	15.1	15.7	16.0	16.9	17.5	18.6	19.8	20.6	21.8	22.4	23.4
110.5	-0.3833	18.8015	0.0945	15.2	15.8	16.2	17.1	17.7	18.8	20.1	20.8	22.1	22.6	23.7
111.0	-0.3833	19.0009	0.0947	15.4	16.0	16.3	17.3	17.8	19.0	20.3	21.0	22.3	22.8	23.9
111.5	-0.3833	19.2024	0.0949	15.5	16.2	16.5	17.4	18.0	19.2	20.5	21.2	22.6	23.1	24.2
112.0	-0.3833	19.4060	0.0951	15.7	16.3	16.7	17.6	18.2	19.4	20.7	21.5	22.8	23.4	24.5
112.5	-0.3833	19.6116	0.0953	15.9	16.5	16.8	17.8	18.4	19.6	20.9	21.7	23.1	23.6	24.7
113.0	-0.3833	19.8190	0.0955	16.0	16.7	17.0	18.0	18.6	19.8	21.2	21.9	23.3	23.9	25.0
113.5	-0.3833	20.0280	0.0957	16.2	16.8	17.2	18.2	18.8	20.0	21.4	22.2	23.6	24.1	25.3
114.0	-0.3833	20.2385	0.0959	16.3	17.0	17.4	18.4	19.0	20.2	21.6	22.4	23.8	24.4	25.6
114.5	-0.3833	20.4502	0.0961	16.5	17.2	17.5	18.5	19.2	20.5	21.8	22.6	24.1	24.7	25.8
115.0	-0.3833	20.6629	0.0963	16.7	17.3	17.7	18.7	19.4	20.7	22.1	22.9	24.3	24.9	26.1
115.5	-0.3833	20.8766	0.0965	16.8	17.5	17.9	18.9	19.6	20.9	22.3	23.1	24.6	25.2	26.4
116.0	-0.3833	21.0909	0.0967	17.0	17.7	18.1	19.1	19.8	21.1	22.5	23.4	24.9	25.5	26.7
116.5	-0.3833	21.3059	0.0969	17.2	17.9	18.3	19.3	20.0	21.3	22.8	23.6	25.1	25.7	27.0
117.0	-0.3833	21.5213	0.0971	17.3	18.0	18.4	19.5	20.2	21.5	23.0	23.8	25.4	26.0	27.3
117.5	-0.3833	21.7370	0.0973	17.5	18.2	18.6	19.7	20.4	21.7	23.2	24.1	25.6	26.3	27.5
118.0	-0.3833	21.9529	0.0975	17.7	18.4	18.8	19.9	20.6	22.0	23.5	24.3	25.9	26.5	27.8
118.5	-0.3833	22.1690	0.0977	17.8	18.6	19.0	20.1	20.8	22.2	23.7	24.6	26.2	26.8	28.1
119.0	-0.3833	22.3851	0.0979	18.0	18.7	19.1	20.3	21.0	22.4	23.9	24.8	26.4	27.1	28.4
119.5	-0.3833	22.6012	0.0981	18.2	18.9	19.3	20.5	21.2	22.6	24.2	25.1	26.7	27.4	28.7
120.0	-0.3833	22.8173	0.0983	18.3	19.1	19.5	20.6	21.4	22.8	24.4	25.3	27.0	27.6	29.0

Table V.21.

LMS parameters and smoothed percentiles of body mass index (kg/cm^2)-for-age (month) for boys and girls from birth to 13 weeks

Age Group (weeks)	L	M	S	Percentiles										
				1st	3rd	5th	15th	25th	50th	75th	85th	95th	97th	99th
Boys														
0.0	-0.3053	13.4069	0.0956	10.8	11.3	11.5	12.2	12.6	13.4	14.3	14.8	15.8	16.1	16.9
1.0	0.5247	13.3421	0.0982	10.5	11.0	11.3	12.0	12.5	13.3	14.2	14.7	15.6	15.9	16.6
2.0	0.4177	13.6377	0.0945	10.8	11.3	11.6	12.3	12.8	13.6	14.5	15.0	15.9	16.2	16.8
3.0	0.3449	14.2241	0.0923	11.4	11.9	12.2	12.9	13.4	14.2	15.1	15.6	16.5	16.8	17.5
4.0	0.2881	14.7714	0.0907	11.9	12.4	12.7	13.4	13.9	14.8	15.7	16.2	17.1	17.4	18.1
5.0	0.2409	15.2355	0.0895	12.3	12.8	13.1	13.9	14.3	15.2	16.2	16.7	17.6	18.0	18.7
6.0	0.2003	15.6107	0.0886	12.6	13.2	13.5	14.2	14.7	15.6	16.6	17.1	18.0	18.4	19.1
7.0	0.1645	15.9169	0.0878	12.9	13.5	13.8	14.5	15.0	15.9	16.9	17.4	18.4	18.7	19.5
8.0	0.1324	16.1698	0.0872	13.2	13.7	14.0	14.8	15.2	16.2	17.1	17.7	18.6	19.0	19.8
9.0	0.1032	16.3787	0.0866	13.4	13.9	14.2	15.0	15.4	16.4	17.4	17.9	18.9	19.3	20.0
10.0	0.0766	16.5494	0.0861	13.5	14.1	14.4	15.1	15.6	16.5	17.5	18.1	19.1	19.4	20.2
11.0	0.0520	16.6882	0.0857	13.7	14.2	14.5	15.3	15.7	16.7	17.7	18.2	19.2	19.6	20.3
12.0	0.0291	16.8016	0.0853	13.8	14.3	14.6	15.4	15.9	16.8	17.8	18.4	19.3	19.7	20.5
13.0	0.0077	16.8950	0.0850	13.9	14.4	14.7	15.5	16.0	16.9	17.9	18.4	19.4	19.8	20.6
Girls														
0.0	0.3809	3.2322	0.0927	10.8	11.2	11.5	12.1	12.5	13.3	14.2	14.7	15.5	15.9	16.6
1.0	0.6319	13.2113	0.0989	10.3	10.8	11.1	11.9	12.3	13.2	14.1	14.6	15.4	15.8	16.4
2.0	0.5082	13.4501	0.0974	10.6	11.1	11.4	12.1	12.6	13.5	14.3	14.8	15.7	16.0	16.7
3.0	0.4263	13.9505	0.0965	11.0	11.5	11.8	12.6	13.1	14.0	14.9	15.4	16.3	16.6	17.3
4.0	0.3637	14.4208	0.0958	11.4	12.0	12.3	13.0	13.5	14.4	15.4	15.9	16.8	17.2	17.9
5.0	0.3124	14.8157	0.0952	11.8	12.3	12.6	13.4	13.9	14.8	15.8	16.3	17.3	17.6	18.4
6.0	0.2688	15.1380	0.0947	12.1	12.6	12.9	13.7	14.2	15.1	16.1	16.7	17.6	18.0	18.8
7.0	0.2306	15.4063	0.0943	12.3	12.9	13.2	14.0	14.4	15.4	16.4	17.0	17.9	18.3	19.1
8.0	0.1966	15.6311	0.0939	12.5	13.1	13.4	14.2	14.7	15.6	16.6	17.2	18.2	18.6	19.4
9.0	0.1658	15.8232	0.0936	12.7	13.2	13.5	14.3	14.9	15.8	16.8	17.4	18.4	18.8	19.6
10.0	0.1377	15.9874	0.0933	12.8	13.4	13.7	14.5	15.0	16.0	17.0	17.6	18.6	19.0	19.8
11.0	0.1118	16.1277	0.0930	13.0	13.5	13.8	14.6	15.1	16.1	17.2	17.8	18.8	19.2	20.0
12.0	0.0877	16.2485	0.0928	13.1	13.6	13.9	14.8	15.3	16.2	17.3	17.9	18.9	19.3	20.1
13.0	0.0652	16.3531	0.0926	13.2	13.7	14.0	14.9	15.4	16.4	17.4	18.0	19.0	19.4	20.3

Table V.22.

LMS parameters and smoothed percentiles of body mass index (kg/cm^2)-for-age (month) for boys and girls from birth to 2 years

Age Group (months)	L	M	S	Percentiles										
				1st	3rd	5th	15th	25th	50th	75th	85th	95th	97th	99th
Boys														
0.0	-0.3053	13.4069	0.0956	10.8	11.3	11.5	12.2	12.6	13.4	14.3	14.8	15.8	16.1	16.9
1.0	0.2708	14.9441	0.0903	12.0	12.6	12.8	13.6	14.1	14.9	15.9	16.4	17.3	17.6	18.3
2.0	0.1118	16.3195	0.0868	13.3	13.8	14.1	14.9	15.4	16.3	17.3	17.8	18.8	19.2	19.9
3.0	0.0068	16.8987	0.0850	13.9	14.4	14.7	15.5	16.0	16.9	17.9	18.5	19.4	19.8	20.6
4.0	-0.0727	17.1579	0.0838	14.1	14.7	15.0	15.7	16.2	17.2	18.2	18.7	19.7	20.1	20.9
5.0	-0.1370	17.2919	0.0830	14.3	14.8	15.1	15.9	16.4	17.3	18.3	18.9	19.8	20.2	21.0
6.0	-0.1913	17.3422	0.0823	14.4	14.9	15.2	15.9	16.4	17.3	18.3	18.9	19.9	20.3	21.1
7.0	-0.2385	17.3288	0.0818	14.4	14.9	15.2	15.9	16.4	17.3	18.3	18.9	19.9	20.3	21.1
8.0	-0.2802	17.2647	0.0814	14.4	14.9	15.1	15.9	16.3	17.3	18.2	18.8	19.8	20.2	21.0
9.0	-0.3176	17.1662	0.0810	14.3	14.8	15.1	15.8	16.3	17.2	18.1	18.7	19.7	20.1	20.8
10.0	-0.3516	17.0488	0.0807	14.2	14.7	15.0	15.7	16.2	17.0	18.0	18.6	19.5	19.9	20.7
11.0	-0.3828	16.9239	0.0804	14.1	14.6	14.9	15.6	16.0	16.9	17.9	18.4	19.4	19.8	20.5
12.0	-0.4115	16.7981	0.0801	14.0	14.5	14.8	15.5	15.9	16.8	17.7	18.3	19.2	19.6	20.4
13.0	-0.4382	16.6743	0.0798	13.9	14.4	14.7	15.4	15.8	16.7	17.6	18.1	19.1	19.5	20.2
14.0	-0.4630	16.5548	0.0796	13.9	14.3	14.6	15.3	15.7	16.6	17.5	18.0	18.9	19.3	20.1
15.0	0.3809	3.2322	0.0794	13.8	14.2	14.5	15.2	15.6	16.4	17.4	17.9	18.8	19.2	19.9
16.0	-0.5082	16.3335	0.0791	13.7	14.2	14.4	15.1	15.5	16.3	17.2	17.8	18.7	19.1	19.8
17.0	-0.5289	16.2329	0.0789	13.6	14.1	14.3	15.0	15.4	16.2	17.1	17.6	18.6	18.9	19.7
18.0	-0.5484	16.1392	0.0787	13.6	14.0	14.2	14.9	15.3	16.1	17.0	17.5	18.5	18.8	19.6
19.0	-0.5669	16.0528	0.0785	13.5	13.9	14.2	14.8	15.2	16.1	16.9	17.4	18.4	18.7	19.5
20.0	-0.5846	15.9743	0.0784	13.4	13.9	14.1	14.8	15.2	16.0	16.9	17.4	18.3	18.6	19.4
21.0	-0.6014	15.9039	0.0782	13.4	13.8	14.1	14.7	15.1	15.9	16.8	17.3	18.2	18.6	19.3
22.0	-0.6174	15.8412	0.0780	13.3	13.8	14.0	14.6	15.0	15.8	16.7	17.2	18.1	18.5	19.2
23.0	-0.6328	15.7852	0.0779	13.3	13.7	14.0	14.6	15.0	15.8	16.7	17.1	18.0	18.4	19.1
24.0	-0.6473	15.7356	0.0777	13.3	13.7	13.9	14.5	14.9	15.7	16.6	17.1	18.0	18.3	19.1
Girls														
0.0	-0.0631	13.3363	0.0927	10.8	11.2	11.5	12.1	12.5	13.3	14.2	14.7	15.5	15.9	16.6
1.0	0.3448	14.5679	0.0956	11.6	12.1	12.4	13.2	13.6	14.6	15.5	16.1	17.0	17.3	18.0
2.0	0.1749	15.7679	0.0937	12.6	13.2	13.5	14.3	14.8	15.8	16.8	17.4	18.4	18.8	19.5
3.0	0.0643	16.3574	0.0925	13.2	13.7	14.0	14.9	15.4	16.4	17.4	18.0	19.0	19.4	20.3
4.0	-0.0191	16.6703	0.0917	13.5	14.0	14.3	15.2	15.7	16.7	17.7	18.3	19.4	19.8	20.6
5.0	-0.0864	16.8386	0.0910	13.7	14.2	14.5	15.3	15.8	16.8	17.9	18.5	19.6	20.0	20.8
6.0	-0.1429	16.9083	0.0904	13.7	14.3	14.6	15.4	15.9	16.9	18.0	18.6	19.6	20.1	20.9
7.0	-0.1916	16.9020	0.0898	13.8	14.3	14.6	15.4	15.9	16.9	18.0	18.6	19.6	20.1	20.9
8.0	-0.2344	16.8404	0.0894	13.7	14.3	14.6	15.4	15.9	16.8	17.9	18.5	19.6	20.0	20.8
9.0	-0.2725	16.7406	0.0890	13.7	14.2	14.5	15.3	15.8	16.7	17.8	18.4	19.4	19.9	20.7
10.0	-0.3068	16.6184	0.0886	13.6	14.1	14.4	15.2	15.7	16.6	17.7	18.2	19.3	19.7	20.6
11.0	-0.3381	16.4875	0.0883	13.5	14.0	14.3	15.1	15.5	16.5	17.5	18.1	19.1	19.6	20.4
12.0	-0.3667	16.3568	0.0880	13.4	13.9	14.2	15.0	15.4	16.4	17.4	17.9	19.0	19.4	20.2
13.0	-0.3932	16.2311	0.0877	13.3	13.8	14.1	14.8	15.3	16.2	17.2	17.8	18.8	19.2	20.1
14.0	-0.4177	16.1128	0.0874	13.3	13.7	14.0	14.7	15.2	16.1	17.1	17.7	18.7	19.1	19.9
15.0	-0.4407	16.0028	0.0872	13.2	13.7	13.9	14.6	15.1	16.0	17.0	17.5	18.6	19.0	19.8
16.0	-0.4623	15.9017	0.0869	13.1	13.6	13.8	14.6	15.0	15.9	16.9	17.4	18.4	18.8	19.7
17.0	-0.4825	15.8096	0.0867	13.0	13.5	13.8	14.5	14.9	15.8	16.8	17.3	18.3	18.7	19.5
18.0	-0.5017	15.7263	0.0865	13.0	13.4	13.7	14.4	14.8	15.7	16.7	17.2	18.2	18.6	19.4
19.0	-0.5199	15.6517	0.0863	12.9	13.4	13.6	14.3	14.8	15.7	16.6	17.2	18.1	18.5	19.3
20.0	-0.5372	15.5855	0.0861	12.9	13.3	13.6	14.3	14.7	15.6	16.5	17.1	18.1	18.5	19.3
21.0	-0.5537	15.5278	0.0859	12.8	13.3	13.6	14.2	14.7	15.5	16.5	17.0	18.0	18.4	19.2
22.0	-0.5695	15.4787	0.0858	12.8	13.3	13.5	14.2	14.6	15.5	16.4	17.0	17.9	18.3	19.1
23.0	-0.5846	15.4380	0.0856	12.8	13.2	13.5	14.2	14.6	15.4	16.4	16.9	17.9	18.3	19.1
24.0	-0.5989	15.4052	0.0855	12.8	13.2	13.5	14.1	14.6	15.4	16.3	16.9	17.8	18.2	19.0

Table V.23.

LMS parameters and smoothed percentiles of body mass index (kg/cm^2)-for-age (month) for boys and girls from 2 to 5 years

Age Group (months)	L	M	S	Percentiles										
				1st	3rd	5th	15th	25th	50th	75th	85th	95th	97th	99th
Boys														
24.0	-0.6187	16.0189	0.0779	13.5	13.9	14.2	14.8	15.2	16.0	16.9	17.4	18.3	18.7	19.4
25.0	-0.5840	15.9800	0.0779	13.5	13.9	14.1	14.8	15.2	16.0	16.9	17.4	18.3	18.6	19.4
26.0	-0.5497	15.9414	0.0780	13.4	13.8	14.1	14.7	15.1	15.9	16.8	17.3	18.2	18.6	19.3
27.0	-0.5166	15.9036	0.0781	13.4	13.8	14.0	14.7	15.1	15.9	16.8	17.3	18.2	18.5	19.2
28.0	-0.4850	15.8667	0.0782	13.3	13.8	14.0	14.7	15.1	15.9	16.7	17.2	18.1	18.5	19.2
29.0	-0.4552	15.8306	0.0783	13.3	13.7	14.0	14.6	15.0	15.8	16.7	17.2	18.1	18.4	19.1
30.0	-0.4274	15.7953	0.0784	13.3	13.7	13.9	14.6	15.0	15.8	16.7	17.2	18.0	18.4	19.1
31.0	-0.4016	15.7606	0.0785	13.2	13.7	13.9	14.5	15.0	15.8	16.6	17.1	18.0	18.4	19.1
32.0	-0.3782	15.7267	0.0787	13.2	13.6	13.9	14.5	14.9	15.7	16.6	17.1	18.0	18.3	19.0
33.0	-0.3572	15.6934	0.0788	13.1	13.6	13.8	14.5	14.9	15.7	16.6	17.0	17.9	18.3	19.0
34.0	-0.3388	15.6610	0.0790	13.1	13.5	13.8	14.4	14.9	15.7	16.5	17.0	17.9	18.2	18.9
35.0	-0.3231	15.6294	0.0791	13.1	13.5	13.8	14.4	14.8	15.6	16.5	17.0	17.9	18.2	18.9
36.0	-0.3101	15.5988	0.0793	13.0	13.5	13.7	14.4	14.8	15.6	16.5	17.0	17.8	18.2	18.9
37.0	-0.3000	15.5693	0.0795	13.0	13.5	13.7	14.4	14.8	15.6	16.4	16.9	17.8	18.1	18.8
38.0	-0.2927	15.5410	0.0797	13.0	13.4	13.7	14.3	14.7	15.5	16.4	16.9	17.8	18.1	18.8
39.0	0.3809	3.2322	0.0799	12.9	13.4	13.6	14.3	14.7	15.5	16.4	16.9	17.7	18.1	18.8
40.0	-0.2869	15.4885	0.0801	12.9	13.4	13.6	14.3	14.7	15.5	16.4	16.8	17.7	18.1	18.8
41.0	-0.2881	15.4645	0.0804	12.9	13.3	13.6	14.2	14.7	15.5	16.3	16.8	17.7	18.0	18.7
42.0	-0.2919	15.4420	0.0806	12.9	13.3	13.6	14.2	14.6	15.4	16.3	16.8	17.7	18.0	18.7
43.0	-0.2981	15.4210	0.0809	12.8	13.3	13.5	14.2	14.6	15.4	16.3	16.8	17.7	18.0	18.7
44.0	-0.3067	15.4013	0.0812	12.8	13.3	13.5	14.2	14.6	15.4	16.3	16.8	17.7	18.0	18.7
45.0	-0.3174	15.3827	0.0814	12.8	13.2	13.5	14.2	14.6	15.4	16.3	16.8	17.6	18.0	18.7
46.0	-0.3303	15.3652	0.0817	12.8	13.2	13.5	14.1	14.5	15.4	16.2	16.7	17.6	18.0	18.7
47.0	-0.3452	15.3485	0.0821	12.8	13.2	13.5	14.1	14.5	15.3	16.2	16.7	17.6	18.0	18.7
48.0	-0.3622	15.3326	0.0824	12.7	13.2	13.4	14.1	14.5	15.3	16.2	16.7	17.6	18.0	18.7
49.0	-0.3811	15.3174	0.0827	12.7	13.2	13.4	14.1	14.5	15.3	16.2	16.7	17.6	18.0	18.7
50.0	-0.4019	15.3029	0.0831	12.7	13.2	13.4	14.1	14.5	15.3	16.2	16.7	17.6	18.0	18.7
51.0	-0.4245	15.2891	0.0834	12.7	13.1	13.4	14.0	14.5	15.3	16.2	16.7	17.6	18.0	18.7
52.0	-0.4488	15.2759	0.0838	12.7	13.1	13.4	14.0	14.4	15.3	16.2	16.7	17.6	18.0	18.7
53.0	-0.4747	15.2633	0.0842	12.7	13.1	13.3	14.0	14.4	15.3	16.2	16.7	17.6	18.0	18.7
54.0	-0.5019	15.2514	0.0846	12.6	13.1	13.3	14.0	14.4	15.3	16.2	16.7	17.6	18.0	18.8
55.0	-0.5303	15.2400	0.0850	12.6	13.1	13.3	14.0	14.4	15.2	16.2	16.7	17.6	18.0	18.8
56.0	-0.5599	15.2291	0.0854	12.6	13.1	13.3	14.0	14.4	15.2	16.1	16.7	17.6	18.0	18.8
57.0	-0.5905	15.2188	0.0858	12.6	13.0	13.3	14.0	14.4	15.2	16.1	16.7	17.6	18.0	18.8
58.0	-0.6223	15.2091	0.0862	12.6	13.0	13.3	13.9	14.4	15.2	16.1	16.7	17.6	18.0	18.8
59.0	-0.6552	15.2000	0.0866	12.6	13.0	13.3	13.9	14.4	15.2	16.1	16.7	17.7	18.1	18.9
60.0	-0.6892	15.1916	0.0870	12.6	13.0	13.3	13.9	14.3	15.2	16.1	16.7	17.7	18.1	18.9
Girls														
24.0	-0.5684	15.6881	0.0845	13.0	13.5	13.7	14.4	14.8	15.7	16.6	17.2	18.1	18.5	19.3
25.0	-0.5684	15.6590	0.0845	13.0	13.4	13.7	14.4	14.8	15.7	16.6	17.1	18.1	18.5	19.3
26.0	-0.5684	15.6308	0.0845	13.0	13.4	13.7	14.4	14.8	15.6	16.6	17.1	18.1	18.5	19.3
27.0	-0.5684	15.6037	0.0845	13.0	13.4	13.7	14.3	14.8	15.6	16.5	17.1	18.0	18.4	19.2
28.0	-0.5684	15.5777	0.0844	12.9	13.4	13.6	14.3	14.7	15.6	16.5	17.0	18.0	18.4	19.2
29.0	-0.5684	15.5523	0.0844	12.9	13.4	13.6	14.3	14.7	15.6	16.5	17.0	18.0	18.4	19.2
30.0	-0.5684	15.5276	0.0844	12.9	13.3	13.6	14.3	14.7	15.5	16.5	17.0	17.9	18.3	19.1
31.0	-0.5684	15.5034	0.0845	12.9	13.3	13.6	14.2	14.7	15.5	16.4	17.0	17.9	18.3	19.1
32.0	-0.5684	15.4798	0.0846	12.8	13.3	13.5	14.2	14.6	15.5	16.4	16.9	17.9	18.3	19.1
33.0	-0.5684	15.4572	0.0847	12.8	13.3	13.5	14.2	14.6	15.5	16.4	16.9	17.9	18.3	19.0
34.0	-0.5684	15.4356	0.0848	12.8	13.2	13.5	14.2	14.6	15.4	16.4	16.9	17.9	18.2	19.0
35.0	-0.5684	15.4155	0.0851	12.8	13.2	13.5	14.1	14.6	15.4	16.3	16.9	17.8	18.2	19.0
36.0	-0.5684	15.3968	0.0854	12.8	13.2	13.5	14.1	14.5	15.4	16.3	16.9	17.8	18.2	19.0
37.0	-0.5684	15.3796	0.0857	12.7	13.2	13.4	14.1	14.5	15.4	16.3	16.8	17.8	18.2	19.0
38.0	-0.5684	15.3638	0.0861	12.7	13.2	13.4	14.1	14.5	15.4	16.3	16.8	17.8	18.2	19.0
39.0	-0.5684	15.3493	0.0865	12.7	13.1	13.4	14.1	14.5	15.3	16.3	16.8	17.8	18.2	19.0
40.0	0.3809	3.2322	0.0870	12.7	13.1	13.4	14.0	14.5	15.3	16.3	16.8	17.8	18.2	19.0
41.0	-0.5684	15.3233	0.0876	12.6	13.1	13.3	14.0	14.5	15.3	16.3	16.8	17.8	18.2	19.0
42.0	-0.5684	15.3116	0.0881	12.6	13.1	13.3	14.0	14.4	15.3	16.3	16.8	17.8	18.2	19.0
43.0	-0.5684	15.3007	0.0887	12.6	13.0	13.3	14.0	14.4	15.3	16.3	16.8	17.8	18.2	19.1
44.0	-0.5684	15.2905	0.0893	12.6	13.0	13.3	14.0	14.4	15.3	16.3	16.8	17.8	18.2	19.1
45.0	-0.5684	15.2814	0.0899	12.5	13.0	13.3	14.0	14.4	15.3	16.3	16.8	17.8	18.3	19.1
46.0	-0.5684	15.2732	0.0905	12.5	13.0	13.2	13.9	14.4	15.3	16.3	16.8	17.8	18.3	19.1
47.0	-0.5684	15.2661	0.0911	12.5	13.0	13.2	13.9	14.4	15.3	16.3	16.8	17.9	18.3	19.1
48.0	-0.5684	15.2602	0.0917	12.5	12.9	13.2	13.9	14.4	15.3	16.3	16.8	17.9	18.3	19.2
49.0	-0.5684	15.2556	0.0923	12.5	12.9	13.2	13.9	14.4	15.3	16.3	16.8	17.9	18.3	19.2
50.0	-0.5684	15.2523	0.0929	12.4	12.9	13.2	13.9	14.3	15.3	16.3	16.8	17.9	18.3	19.2
51.0	-0.5684	15.2503	0.0935	12.4	12.9	13.2	13.9	14.3	15.3	16.3	16.8	17.9	18.4	19.2
52.0	-0.5684	15.2496	0.0940	12.4	12.9	13.1	13.9	14.3	15.2	16.3	16.9	17.9	18.4	19.3
53.0	-0.5684	15.2502	0.0946	12.4	12.9	13.1	13.9	14.3	15.3	16.3	16.9	17.9	18.4	19.3
54.0	-0.5684	15.2519	0.0952	12.4	12.9	13.1	13.9	14.3	15.3	16.3	16.9	18.0	18.4	19.3
55.0	-0.5684	15.2544	0.0957	12.4	12.9	13.1	13.9	14.3	15.3	16.3	16.9	18.0	18.4	19.4
56.0	-0.5684	15.2575	0.0962	12.4	12.8	13.1	13.8	14.3	15.3	16.3	16.9	18.0	18.5	19.4
57.0	-0.5684	15.2612	0.0967	12.4	12.8	13.1	13.8	14.3	15.3	16.3	16.9	18.0	18.5	19.4
58.0	-0.5684	15.2653	0.0971	12.3	12.8	13.1	13.8	14.3	15.3	16.3	16.9	18.0	18.5	19.4
59.0	-0.5684	15.2698	0.0975	12.3	12.8	13.1	13.8	14.3	15.3	16.3	16.9	18.1	18.5	19.5
60.0	-0.5684	15.2747	0.0979	12.3	12.8	13.1	13.8	14.3	15.3	16.3	17.0	18.1	18.6	19.5

Table V.24a.

LMS parameters and smoothed percentiles of head circumference (cm)-for-age (month) for boys from birth to 5 years

Age Group (months)	L	M	S	1st	3rd	5th	15th	25th	50th	75th	85th	95th	97th	99th
0.0	1	34.46180	0.03686	31.5	32.1	32.4	33.1	33.6	34.5	35.3	35.8	36.6	36.9	37.4
1.0	1	37.27590	0.03133	34.6	35.1	35.4	36.1	36.5	37.3	38.1	38.5	39.2	39.5	40.0
2.0	1	39.12850	0.02997	36.4	36.9	37.2	37.9	38.3	39.1	39.9	40.3	41.1	41.3	41.9
3.0	1	40.51350	0.02918	37.8	38.3	38.6	39.3	39.7	40.5	41.3	41.7	42.5	42.7	43.3
4.0	1	41.63170	0.02868	38.9	39.4	39.7	40.4	40.8	41.6	42.4	42.9	43.6	43.9	44.4
5.0	1	42.55760	0.02837	39.7	40.3	40.6	41.3	41.7	42.6	43.4	43.8	44.5	44.8	45.4
6.0	1	43.33060	0.02817	40.5	41.0	41.3	42.1	42.5	43.3	44.2	44.6	45.3	45.6	46.2
7.0	1	43.98030	0.02804	41.1	41.7	42.0	42.7	43.1	44.0	44.8	45.3	46.0	46.3	46.8
8.0	1	44.53000	0.02796	41.6	42.2	42.5	43.2	43.7	44.5	45.4	45.8	46.6	46.9	47.4
9.0	1	44.99980	0.02792	42.1	42.6	42.9	43.7	44.2	45.0	45.8	46.3	47.1	47.4	47.9
10.0	1	45.40510	0.02790	42.5	43.0	43.3	44.1	44.6	45.4	46.3	46.7	47.5	47.8	48.4
11.0	1	45.75730	0.02789	42.8	43.4	43.7	44.4	44.9	45.8	46.6	47.1	47.9	48.2	48.7
12.0	1	46.06610	0.02789	43.1	43.6	44.0	44.7	45.2	46.1	46.9	47.4	48.2	48.5	49.1
13.0	1	46.33950	0.02789	43.3	43.9	44.2	45.0	45.5	46.3	47.2	47.7	48.5	48.8	49.3
14.0	1	46.58440	0.02791	43.6	44.1	44.4	45.2	45.7	46.6	47.5	47.9	48.7	49.0	49.6
15.0	1	46.80600	0.02792	43.8	44.3	44.7	45.5	45.9	46.8	47.7	48.2	49.0	49.3	49.8
16.0	0	3.23220	0.02795	44.0	44.5	44.8	45.6	46.1	47.0	47.9	48.4	49.2	49.5	50.1
17.0	1	47.19620	0.02797	44.1	44.7	45.0	45.8	46.3	47.2	48.1	48.6	49.4	49.7	50.3
18.0	1	47.37110	0.02800	44.3	44.9	45.2	46.0	46.5	47.4	48.3	48.7	49.6	49.9	50.5
19.0	1	47.53570	0.02803	44.4	45.0	45.3	46.2	46.6	47.5	48.4	48.9	49.7	50.0	50.6
20.0	1	47.69190	0.02806	44.6	45.2	45.5	46.3	46.8	47.7	48.6	49.1	49.9	50.2	50.8
21.0	1	47.84080	0.02810	44.7	45.3	45.6	46.4	46.9	47.8	48.7	49.2	50.1	50.4	51.0
22.0	1	47.98330	0.02813	44.8	45.4	45.8	46.6	47.1	48.0	48.9	49.4	50.2	50.5	51.1
23.0	1	48.12010	0.02817	45.0	45.6	45.9	46.7	47.2	48.1	49.0	49.5	50.3	50.7	51.3
24.0	1	48.25150	0.02821	45.1	45.7	46.0	46.8	47.3	48.3	49.2	49.7	50.5	50.8	51.4
25.0	1	48.37770	0.02825	45.2	45.8	46.1	47.0	47.5	48.4	49.3	49.8	50.6	50.9	51.6
26.0	1	48.49890	0.02830	45.3	45.9	46.2	47.1	47.6	48.5	49.4	49.9	50.8	51.1	51.7
27.0	1	48.61510	0.02834	45.4	46.0	46.3	47.2	47.7	48.6	49.5	50.0	50.9	51.2	51.8
28.0	1	48.72640	0.02838	45.5	46.1	46.5	47.3	47.8	48.7	49.7	50.2	51.0	51.3	51.9
29.0	1	48.83310	0.02842	45.6	46.2	46.6	47.4	47.9	48.8	49.8	50.3	51.1	51.4	52.1
30.0	1	48.93510	0.02847	45.7	46.3	46.6	47.5	48.0	48.9	49.9	50.4	51.2	51.6	52.2
31.0	1	49.03270	0.02851	45.8	46.4	46.7	47.6	48.1	49.0	50.0	50.5	51.3	51.7	52.3
32.0	1	49.12600	0.02855	45.9	46.5	46.8	47.7	48.2	49.1	50.1	50.6	51.4	51.8	52.4
33.0	1	49.21530	0.02859	45.9	46.6	46.9	47.8	48.3	49.2	50.2	50.7	51.5	51.9	52.5
34.0	1	49.30070	0.02863	46.0	46.6	47.0	47.8	48.3	49.3	50.3	50.8	51.6	52.0	52.6
35.0	1	49.38260	0.02867	46.1	46.7	47.1	47.9	48.4	49.4	50.3	50.8	51.7	52.0	52.7
36.0	1	49.46120	0.02871	46.2	46.8	47.1	48.0	48.5	49.5	50.4	50.9	51.8	52.1	52.8
37.0	1	49.53670	0.02875	46.2	46.9	47.2	48.1	48.6	49.5	50.5	51.0	51.9	52.2	52.8
38.0	1	49.60930	0.02878	46.3	46.9	47.3	48.1	48.6	49.6	50.6	51.1	52.0	52.3	52.9
39.0	1	49.67910	0.02882	46.3	47.0	47.3	48.2	48.7	49.7	50.6	51.2	52.0	52.4	53.0
40.0	1	49.74650	0.02886	46.4	47.0	47.4	48.3	48.8	49.7	50.7	51.2	52.1	52.4	53.1
41.0	1	49.81160	0.02889	46.5	47.1	47.4	48.3	48.8	49.8	50.8	51.3	52.2	52.5	53.2
42.0	1	49.87450	0.02893	46.5	47.2	47.5	48.4	48.9	49.9	50.8	51.4	52.2	52.6	53.2
43.0	1	49.93540	0.02896	46.6	47.2	47.6	48.4	49.0	49.9	50.9	51.4	52.3	52.7	53.3
44.0	1	49.99420	0.02899	46.6	47.3	47.6	48.5	49.0	50.0	51.0	51.5	52.4	52.7	53.4
45.0	1	50.05120	0.02903	46.7	47.3	47.7	48.5	49.1	50.1	51.0	51.6	52.4	52.8	53.4
46.0	L	50.10640	0.02906	46.7	47.4	47.7	48.6	49.1	50.1	51.1	51.6	52.5	52.8	53.5
47.0	1	50.15980	0.02909	46.8	47.4	47.8	48.6	49.2	50.2	51.1	51.7	52.6	52.9	53.6
48.0	1	50.21150	0.02912	46.8	47.5	47.8	48.7	49.2	50.2	51.2	51.7	52.6	53.0	53.6
49.0	1	50.26170	0.02915	46.9	47.5	47.9	48.7	49.3	50.3	51.2	51.8	52.7	53.0	53.7
50.0	1	50.31050	0.02918	46.9	47.5	47.9	48.8	49.3	50.3	51.3	51.8	52.7	53.1	53.7
51.0	1	50.35780	0.02921	46.9	47.6	47.9	48.8	49.4	50.4	51.3	51.9	52.8	53.1	53.8
52.0	1	50.40390	0.02924	47.0	47.6	48.0	48.9	49.4	50.4	51.4	51.9	52.8	53.2	53.8
53.0	1	50.44880	0.02927	47.0	47.7	48.0	48.9	49.5	50.4	51.4	52.0	52.9	53.2	53.9
54.0	1	50.49260	0.02929	47.1	47.7	48.1	49.0	49.5	50.5	51.5	52.0	52.9	53.3	53.9
55.0	1	50.53540	0.02932	47.1	47.7	48.1	49.0	49.5	50.5	51.5	52.1	53.0	53.3	54.0
56.0	1	50.57720	0.02935	47.1	47.8	48.1	49.0	49.6	50.6	51.6	52.1	53.0	53.4	54.0
57.0	1	50.61830	0.02938	47.2	47.8	48.2	49.1	49.6	50.6	51.6	52.2	53.1	53.4	54.1
58.0	1	50.65870	0.02940	47.2	47.9	48.2	49.1	49.7	50.7	51.7	52.2	53.1	53.5	54.1
59.0	1	50.69840	0.02943	47.2	47.9	48.2	49.2	49.7	50.7	51.7	52.2	53.2	53.5	54.2
60.0	1	50.73750	0.02946	47.3	47.9	48.3	49.2	49.7	50.7	51.7	52.3	53.2	53.5	54.2

Table V.24b.
LMS parameters and smoothed percentiles of head circumference (cm)-for-age (month) for girls from birth to 5 years

Age Group (months)	L	M	S	Percentiles										
				1st	3rd	5th	15th	25th	50th	75th	85th	95th	97th	99th
0.0	1	33.87870	0.03496	31.1	31.7	31.9	32.7	33.1	33.9	34.7	35.1	35.8	36.1	36.6
1.0	1	36.54630	0.03210	33.8	34.3	34.6	35.3	35.8	36.5	37.3	37.8	38.5	38.8	39.3
2.0	1	38.25210	0.03168	35.4	36.0	36.3	37.0	37.4	38.3	39.1	39.5	40.2	40.5	41.1
3.0	1	39.53280	0.03140	36.6	37.2	37.5	38.2	38.7	39.5	40.4	40.8	41.6	41.9	42.4
4.0	1	40.58170	0.03119	37.6	38.2	38.5	39.3	39.7	40.6	41.4	41.9	42.7	43.0	43.5
5.0	1	41.45900	0.03102	38.5	39.0	39.3	40.1	40.6	41.5	42.3	42.8	43.6	43.9	44.5
6.0	1	42.19950	0.03087	39.2	39.7	40.1	40.8	41.3	42.2	43.1	43.5	44.3	44.6	45.2
7.0	1	42.82900	0.03075	39.8	40.4	40.7	41.5	41.9	42.8	43.7	44.2	45.0	45.3	45.9
8.0	1	43.36710	0.03063	40.3	40.9	41.2	42.0	42.5	43.4	44.3	44.7	45.6	45.9	46.5
9.0	1	43.83000	0.03053	40.7	41.3	41.6	42.4	42.9	43.8	44.7	45.2	46.0	46.3	46.9
10.0	1	44.23190	0.03044	41.1	41.7	42.0	42.8	43.3	44.2	45.1	45.6	46.4	46.8	47.4
11.0	1	44.58440	0.03035	41.4	42.0	42.4	43.2	43.7	44.6	45.5	46.0	46.8	47.1	47.7
12.0	1	44.89650	0.03027	41.7	42.3	42.7	43.5	44.0	44.9	45.8	46.3	47.1	47.5	48.1
13.0	1	45.17520	0.03019	42.0	42.6	42.9	43.8	44.3	45.2	46.1	46.6	47.4	47.7	48.3
14.0	1	45.42650	0.03012	42.2	42.9	43.2	44.0	44.5	45.4	46.3	46.8	47.7	48.0	48.6
15.0	1	45.65510	0.03006	42.5	43.1	43.4	44.2	44.7	45.7	46.6	47.1	47.9	48.2	48.8
16.0	0	3.23220	0.02999	42.7	43.3	43.6	44.4	44.9	45.9	46.8	47.3	48.1	48.5	49.1
17.0	1	46.05980	0.02993	42.9	43.5	43.8	44.6	45.1	46.1	47.0	47.5	48.3	48.7	49.3
18.0	1	46.24240	0.02987	43.0	43.6	44.0	44.8	45.3	46.2	47.2	47.7	48.5	48.8	49.5
19.0	1	46.41520	0.02982	43.2	43.8	44.1	45.0	45.5	46.4	47.3	47.8	48.7	49.0	49.6
20.0	1	46.58010	0.02977	43.4	44.0	44.3	45.1	45.6	46.6	47.5	48.0	48.9	49.2	49.8
21.0	1	46.73840	0.02972	43.5	44.1	44.5	45.3	45.8	46.7	47.7	48.2	49.0	49.4	50.0
22.0	1	46.89130	0.02967	43.7	44.3	44.6	45.4	46.0	46.9	47.8	48.3	49.2	49.5	50.1
23.0	1	47.03910	0.02962	43.8	44.4	44.7	45.6	46.1	47.0	48.0	48.5	49.3	49.7	50.3
24.0	1	47.18220	0.02957	43.9	44.6	44.9	45.7	46.2	47.2	48.1	48.6	49.5	49.8	50.4
25.0	1	47.32040	0.02953	44.1	44.7	45.0	45.9	46.4	47.3	48.3	48.8	49.6	49.9	50.6
26.0	1	47.45360	0.02949	44.2	44.8	45.2	46.0	46.5	47.5	48.4	48.9	49.8	50.1	50.7
27.0	1	47.58170	0.02945	44.3	44.9	45.3	46.1	46.6	47.6	48.5	49.0	49.9	50.2	50.8
28.0	1	47.70450	0.02941	44.4	45.1	45.4	46.3	46.8	47.7	48.7	49.2	50.0	50.3	51.0
29.0	1	47.82190	0.02937	44.6	45.2	45.5	46.4	46.9	47.8	48.8	49.3	50.1	50.5	51.1
30.0	1	47.93400	0.02933	44.7	45.3	45.6	46.5	47.0	47.9	48.9	49.4	50.2	50.6	51.2
31.0	1	48.04100	0.02929	44.8	45.4	45.7	46.6	47.1	48.0	49.0	49.5	50.4	50.7	51.3
32.0	1	48.14320	0.02926	44.9	45.5	45.8	46.7	47.2	48.1	49.1	49.6	50.5	50.8	51.4
33.0	1	48.24080	0.02922	45.0	45.6	45.9	46.8	47.3	48.2	49.2	49.7	50.6	50.9	51.5
34.0	1	48.33430	0.02919	45.1	45.7	46.0	46.9	47.4	48.3	49.3	49.8	50.7	51.0	51.6
35.0	1	48.42390	0.02915	45.1	45.8	46.1	47.0	47.5	48.4	49.4	49.9	50.7	51.1	51.7
36.0	1	48.50990	0.02912	45.2	45.9	46.2	47.0	47.6	48.5	49.5	50.0	50.8	51.2	51.8
37.0	1	48.59260	0.02909	45.3	45.9	46.3	47.1	47.6	48.6	49.5	50.1	50.9	51.3	51.9
38.0	1	48.67220	0.02906	45.4	46.0	46.3	47.2	47.7	48.7	49.6	50.1	51.0	51.3	52.0
39.0	1	48.74890	0.02903	45.5	46.1	46.4	47.3	47.8	48.7	49.7	50.2	51.1	51.4	52.0
40.0	1	48.82280	0.02900	45.5	46.2	46.5	47.4	47.9	48.8	49.8	50.3	51.2	51.5	52.1
41.0	1	48.89410	0.02897	45.6	46.2	46.6	47.4	47.9	48.9	49.8	50.4	51.2	51.6	52.2
42.0	1	48.96290	0.02894	45.7	46.3	46.6	47.5	48.0	49.0	49.9	50.4	51.3	51.6	52.3
43.0	1	49.02940	0.02891	45.7	46.4	46.7	47.6	48.1	49.0	50.0	50.5	51.4	51.7	52.3
44.0	1	49.09370	0.02888	45.8	46.4	46.8	47.6	48.1	49.1	50.1	50.6	51.4	51.8	52.4
45.0	1	49.15600	0.02886	45.9	46.5	46.8	47.7	48.2	49.2	50.1	50.6	51.5	51.8	52.5
46.0	1	49.21640	0.02883	45.9	46.5	46.9	47.7	48.3	49.2	50.2	50.7	51.6	51.9	52.5
47.0	1	49.27510	0.02880	46.0	46.6	46.9	47.8	48.3	49.3	50.2	50.7	51.6	51.9	52.6
48.0	1	49.33210	0.02878	46.0	46.7	47.0	47.9	48.4	49.3	50.3	50.8	51.7	52.0	52.6
49.0	1	49.38770	0.02875	46.1	46.7	47.1	47.9	48.4	49.4	50.3	50.9	51.7	52.1	52.7
50.0	1	49.44190	0.02873	46.1	46.8	47.1	48.0	48.5	49.4	50.4	50.9	51.8	52.1	52.7
51.0	1	49.49470	0.02870	46.2	46.8	47.2	48.0	48.5	49.5	50.5	51.0	51.8	52.2	52.8
52.0	1	49.54640	0.02868	46.2	46.9	47.2	48.1	48.6	49.5	50.5	51.0	51.9	52.2	52.9
53.0	1	49.59690	0.02865	46.3	46.9	47.3	48.1	48.6	49.6	50.6	51.1	51.9	52.3	52.9
54.0	1	49.64640	0.02863	46.3	47.0	47.3	48.2	48.7	49.6	50.6	51.1	52.0	52.3	53.0
55.0	1	49.69470	0.02861	46.4	47.0	47.4	48.2	48.7	49.7	50.7	51.2	52.0	52.4	53.0
56.0	1	49.74210	0.02859	46.4	47.1	47.4	48.3	48.8	49.7	50.7	51.2	52.1	52.4	53.1
57.0	1	49.78850	0.02856	46.5	47.1	47.4	48.3	48.8	49.8	50.7	51.3	52.1	52.5	53.1
58.0	1	49.83410	0.02854	46.5	47.2	47.5	48.4	48.9	49.8	50.8	51.3	52.2	52.5	53.1
59.0	1	49.87890	0.02852	46.6	47.2	47.5	48.4	48.9	49.9	50.8	51.4	52.2	52.6	53.2
60.0	1	49.92290	0.02850	46.6	47.2	47.6	48.4	49.0	49.9	50.9	51.4	52.3	52.6	53.0

Table V.25a.

LMS parameters and smoothed percentiles of mid-upper arm circumference (cm)-for-age (month) for boys from 3 months to 5 years

Age Group (months)	L	M	S	Percentiles										
				1st	3rd	5th	15th	25th	50th	75th	85th	95th	97th	99th
3	0.3928	13.4817	0.07475	11.3	11.7	11.9	12.5	12.8	13.5	14.2	14.6	15.2	15.5	16.0
4	0.3475	13.8097	0.07523	11.5	11.9	12.2	12.8	13.1	13.8	14.5	14.9	15.6	15.9	16.4
5	0.3092	14.0585	0.07566	11.7	12.2	12.4	13.0	13.4	14.1	14.8	15.2	15.9	16.2	16.7
6	0.2755	14.2389	0.07601	11.9	12.3	12.5	13.1	13.5	14.2	15.0	15.4	16.1	16.4	16.9
7	0.2453	14.3678	0.07629	12.0	12.4	12.6	13.3	13.6	14.4	15.1	15.5	16.3	16.5	17.1
8	0.2179	14.4591	0.0765	12.1	12.5	12.7	13.3	13.7	14.5	15.2	15.6	16.4	16.7	17.2
9	0.1925	14.5245	0.07665	12.1	12.5	12.8	13.4	13.8	14.5	15.3	15.7	16.5	16.7	17.3
10	0.169	14.5733	0.07676	12.2	12.6	12.8	13.5	13.8	14.6	15.3	15.8	16.5	16.8	17.4
11	0.1469	14.6119	0.07683	12.2	12.6	12.9	13.5	13.9	14.6	15.4	15.8	16.6	16.9	17.4
12	0.1261	14.6449	0.07689	12.2	12.7	12.9	13.5	13.9	14.6	15.4	15.9	16.6	16.9	17.5
13	0.1064	14.6758	0.07694	12.2	12.7	12.9	13.5	13.9	14.7	15.5	15.9	16.6	16.9	17.5
14	0.0876	14.7063	0.07699	12.3	12.7	12.9	13.6	14.0	14.7	15.5	15.9	16.7	17.0	17.6
15	0.0697	14.738	0.07703	12.3	12.7	13.0	13.6	14.0	14.7	15.5	16.0	16.7	17.0	17.6
16	0.0526	14.7723	0.07707	12.3	12.8	13.0	13.6	14.0	14.8	15.6	16.0	16.8	17.1	17.7
17	0.0362	14.8095	0.0771	12.4	12.8	13.0	13.7	14.1	14.8	15.6	16.0	16.8	17.1	17.7
18	0.0204	14.8496	0.07713	12.4	12.8	13.1	13.7	14.1	14.8	15.6	16.1	16.9	17.2	17.8
19	0.3809	3.2322	0.07717	12.4	12.9	13.1	13.7	14.1	14.9	15.7	16.1	16.9	17.2	17.8
20	-0.0097	14.9388	0.07721	12.5	12.9	13.2	13.8	14.2	14.9	15.7	16.2	17.0	17.3	17.9
21	-0.0239	14.9883	0.07725	12.5	13.0	13.2	13.8	14.2	15.0	15.8	16.2	17.0	17.3	17.9
22	-0.0378	15.041	0.07731	12.6	13.0	13.2	13.9	14.3	15.0	15.8	16.3	17.1	17.4	18.0
23	-0.0512	15.0964	0.07738	12.6	13.1	13.3	13.9	14.3	15.1	15.9	16.4	17.2	17.5	18.1
24	-0.0643	15.1536	0.07746	12.7	13.1	13.3	14.0	14.4	15.2	16.0	16.4	17.2	17.5	18.2
25	-0.077	15.2115	0.07755	12.7	13.2	13.4	14.0	14.4	15.2	16.0	16.5	17.3	17.6	18.2
26	-0.0894	15.2693	0.07767	12.8	13.2	13.4	14.1	14.5	15.3	16.1	16.6	17.4	17.7	18.3
27	-0.1014	15.3259	0.0778	12.8	13.3	13.5	14.1	14.5	15.3	16.2	16.6	17.4	17.8	18.4
28	-0.1132	15.3808	0.07794	12.9	13.3	13.5	14.2	14.6	15.4	16.2	16.7	17.5	17.8	18.5
29	-0.1248	15.4336	0.0781	12.9	13.3	13.6	14.2	14.6	15.4	16.3	16.7	17.6	17.9	18.5
30	-0.136	15.4839	0.07827	12.9	13.4	13.6	14.3	14.7	15.5	16.3	16.8	17.6	18.0	18.6
31	-0.147	15.5317	0.07846	13.0	13.4	13.7	14.3	14.7	15.5	16.4	16.9	17.7	18.0	18.7
32	-0.1578	15.5771	0.07866	13.0	13.5	13.7	14.4	14.8	15.6	16.4	16.9	17.8	18.1	18.8
33	-0.1684	15.6201	0.07887	13.0	13.5	13.7	14.4	14.8	15.6	16.5	17.0	17.8	18.2	18.8
34	-0.1788	15.6611	0.07909	13.1	13.5	13.8	14.4	14.9	15.7	16.5	17.0	17.9	18.2	18.9
35	-0.189	15.7003	0.07933	13.1	13.6	13.8	14.5	14.9	15.7	16.6	17.1	17.9	18.3	18.9
36	-0.1989	15.738	0.07956	13.1	13.6	13.8	14.5	14.9	15.7	16.6	17.1	18.0	18.3	19.0
37	-0.2087	15.7745	0.07981	13.1	13.6	13.9	14.5	15.0	15.8	16.7	17.1	18.0	18.4	19.1
38	-0.2184	15.8101	0.08006	13.2	13.6	13.9	14.6	15.0	15.8	16.7	17.2	18.1	18.4	19.1
39	-0.2278	15.845	0.08032	13.2	13.7	13.9	14.6	15.0	15.8	16.7	17.2	18.1	18.5	19.2
40	-0.2372	15.8793	0.08058	13.2	13.7	13.9	14.6	15.0	15.9	16.8	17.3	18.2	18.5	19.2
41	-0.2463	15.9132	0.08085	13.2	13.7	14.0	14.6	15.1	15.9	16.8	17.3	18.2	18.6	19.3
42	-0.2553	15.9467	0.08112	13.3	13.7	14.0	14.7	15.1	15.9	16.9	17.4	18.3	18.6	19.3
43	-0.2642	15.9797	0.08139	13.3	13.8	14.0	14.7	15.1	16.0	16.9	17.4	18.3	18.7	19.4
44	-0.273	16.0124	0.08166	13.3	13.8	14.0	14.7	15.2	16.0	16.9	17.4	18.4	18.7	19.5
45	-0.2816	16.0447	0.08194	13.3	13.8	14.1	14.8	15.2	16.0	17.0	17.5	18.4	18.8	19.5
46	-0.2901	16.0767	0.08222	13.3	13.8	14.1	14.8	15.2	16.1	17.0	17.5	18.5	18.8	19.6
47	-0.2985	16.1085	0.0825	13.4	13.8	14.1	14.8	15.2	16.1	17.0	17.6	18.5	18.9	19.6
48	-0.3067	16.14	0.08278	13.4	13.9	14.1	14.8	15.3	16.1	17.1	17.6	18.5	18.9	19.7
49	-0.3149	16.1714	0.08307	13.4	13.9	14.1	14.9	15.3	16.2	17.1	17.6	18.6	19.0	19.7
50	-0.3229	16.2027	0.08335	13.4	13.9	14.2	14.9	15.3	16.2	17.1	17.7	18.6	19.0	19.8
51	-0.3309	16.234	0.08364	13.4	13.9	14.2	14.9	15.4	16.2	17.2	17.7	18.7	19.1	19.9
52	-0.3387	16.2654	0.08392	13.5	13.9	14.2	14.9	15.4	16.3	17.2	17.8	18.7	19.1	19.9
53	-0.3464	16.2968	0.08421	13.5	14.0	14.2	15.0	15.4	16.3	17.3	17.8	18.8	19.2	20.0
54	-0.3541	16.3283	0.0845	13.5	14.0	14.3	15.0	15.4	16.3	17.3	17.8	18.8	19.2	20.0
55	-0.3616	16.3599	0.08479	13.5	14.0	14.3	15.0	15.5	16.4	17.3	17.9	18.9	19.3	20.1
56	-0.3691	16.3916	0.08508	13.5	14.0	14.3	15.0	15.5	16.4	17.4	17.9	18.9	19.3	20.1
57	-0.3765	16.4233	0.08537	13.6	14.1	14.3	15.1	15.5	16.4	17.4	18.0	19.0	19.4	20.2
58	-0.3838	16.4551	0.08566	13.6	14.1	14.3	15.1	15.5	16.5	17.4	18.0	19.0	19.4	20.2
59	-0.391	16.4871	0.08595	13.6	14.1	14.4	15.1	15.6	16.5	17.5	18.1	19.1	19.5	20.3
60	-0.3981	16.5191	0.08624	13.6	14.1	14.4	15.1	15.6	16.5	17.5	18.1	19.1	19.5	20.4

WHO Growth Standards

Table V.25b.

LMS parameters and smoothed percentiles of mid-upper arm circumference (cm)-for-age (month) for girls from 3 months to 5 years

Age Group (months)	L	M	S	Percentiles										
				1st	3rd	5th	15th	25th	50th	75th	85th	95th	97th	99th
3	-0.1733	13.0284	0.08263	10.8	11.2	11.4	12.0	12.3	13.0	13.8	14.2	14.9	15.3	15.8
4	-0.1733	13.3649	0.08298	11.1	11.5	11.7	12.3	12.6	13.4	14.1	14.6	15.3	15.7	16.3
5	-0.1733	13.6061	0.08325	11.2	11.7	11.9	12.5	12.9	13.6	14.4	14.8	15.6	15.9	16.6
6	-0.1733	13.7771	0.08343	11.4	11.8	12.0	12.6	13.0	13.8	14.6	15.0	15.8	16.2	16.8
7	-0.1733	13.9018	0.08352	11.5	11.9	12.1	12.8	13.1	13.9	14.7	15.2	16.0	16.3	16.9
8	-0.1733	13.9952	0.08351	11.6	12.0	12.2	12.8	13.2	14.0	14.8	15.3	16.1	16.4	17.1
9	-0.1733	14.0665	0.08342	11.6	12.0	12.3	12.9	13.3	14.1	14.9	15.3	16.2	16.5	17.1
10	-0.1733	14.1217	0.08326	11.7	12.1	12.3	13.0	13.4	14.1	14.9	15.4	16.2	16.6	17.2
11	-0.1733	14.1667	0.08305	11.7	12.1	12.4	13.0	13.4	14.2	15.0	15.5	16.3	16.6	17.2
12	-0.1733	14.2065	0.0828	11.8	12.2	12.4	13.0	13.4	14.2	15.0	15.5	16.3	16.6	17.3
13	-0.1733	14.2455	0.08254	11.8	12.2	12.5	13.1	13.5	14.2	15.1	15.5	16.3	16.7	17.3
14	-0.1733	14.2859	0.08227	11.8	12.3	12.5	13.1	13.5	14.3	15.1	15.6	16.4	16.7	17.4
15	-0.1733	14.3289	0.08202	11.9	12.3	12.5	13.2	13.6	14.3	15.1	15.6	16.4	16.8	17.4
16	-0.1733	14.3752	0.08179	11.9	12.4	12.6	13.2	13.6	14.4	15.2	15.7	16.5	16.8	17.4
17	-0.1733	14.4254	0.0816	12.0	12.4	12.6	13.3	13.7	14.4	15.2	15.7	16.5	16.9	17.5
18	-0.1733	14.4795	0.08143	12.0	12.4	12.7	13.3	13.7	14.5	15.3	15.8	16.6	16.9	17.6
19	0.3809	3.2322	0.08131	12.1	12.5	12.7	13.4	13.8	14.5	15.4	15.8	16.6	17.0	17.6
20	-0.1733	14.5987	0.08123	12.1	12.6	12.8	13.4	13.8	14.6	15.4	15.9	16.7	17.0	17.7
21	-0.1733	14.6639	0.08118	12.2	12.6	12.9	13.5	13.9	14.7	15.5	16.0	16.8	17.1	17.8
22	-0.1733	14.7328	0.08118	12.2	12.7	12.9	13.6	14.0	14.7	15.6	16.0	16.9	17.2	17.9
23	-0.1733	14.8049	0.08121	12.3	12.7	13.0	13.6	14.0	14.8	15.6	16.1	16.9	17.3	17.9
24	-0.1733	14.8795	0.08127	12.4	12.8	13.0	13.7	14.1	14.9	15.7	16.2	17.0	17.4	18.0
25	-0.1733	14.9559	0.08136	12.4	12.9	13.1	13.8	14.2	15.0	15.8	16.3	17.1	17.5	18.1
26	-0.1733	15.0327	0.08147	12.5	12.9	13.2	13.8	14.2	15.0	15.9	16.4	17.2	17.6	18.2
27	-0.1733	15.1085	0.08161	12.5	13.0	13.2	13.9	14.3	15.1	16.0	16.5	17.3	17.7	18.3
28	-0.1733	15.1817	0.08178	12.6	13.0	13.3	14.0	14.4	15.2	16.0	16.5	17.4	17.7	18.4
29	-0.1733	15.2514	0.08196	12.6	13.1	13.3	14.0	14.4	15.3	16.1	16.6	17.5	17.8	18.5
30	-0.1733	15.3168	0.08217	12.7	13.2	13.4	14.1	14.5	15.3	16.2	16.7	17.6	17.9	18.6
31	-0.1733	15.3779	0.0824	12.7	13.2	13.4	14.1	14.6	15.4	16.3	16.8	17.6	18.0	18.7
32	-0.1733	15.4351	0.08265	12.8	13.2	13.5	14.2	14.6	15.4	16.3	16.8	17.7	18.1	18.8
33	-0.1733	15.4895	0.08292	12.8	13.3	13.5	14.2	14.7	15.5	16.4	16.9	17.8	18.1	18.8
34	-0.1733	15.5423	0.0832	12.8	13.3	13.6	14.3	14.7	15.5	16.4	17.0	17.9	18.2	18.9
35	-0.1733	15.5941	0.08351	12.9	13.4	13.6	14.3	14.7	15.6	16.5	17.0	17.9	18.3	19.0
36	-0.1733	15.6456	0.08383	12.9	13.4	13.7	14.4	14.8	15.6	16.6	17.1	18.0	18.4	19.1
37	-0.1733	15.6969	0.08416	12.9	13.4	13.7	14.4	14.8	15.7	16.6	17.1	18.1	18.4	19.2
38	-0.1733	15.7483	0.08451	13.0	13.5	13.7	14.4	14.9	15.7	16.7	17.2	18.1	18.5	19.2
39	-0.1733	15.7997	0.08487	13.0	13.5	13.8	14.5	14.9	15.8	16.7	17.3	18.2	18.6	19.3
40	-0.1733	15.8509	0.08525	13.0	13.5	13.8	14.5	15.0	15.9	16.8	17.3	18.3	18.6	19.4
41	-0.1733	15.9016	0.08563	13.1	13.6	13.8	14.6	15.0	15.9	16.9	17.4	18.3	18.7	19.5
42	-0.1733	15.9518	0.08602	13.1	13.6	13.9	14.6	15.1	16.0	16.9	17.5	18.4	18.8	19.6
43	-0.1733	16.0016	0.08642	13.1	13.6	13.9	14.6	15.1	16.0	17.0	17.5	18.5	18.9	19.6
44	-0.1733	16.0509	0.08683	13.2	13.7	13.9	14.7	15.1	16.1	17.0	17.6	18.5	18.9	19.7
45	-0.1733	16.1001	0.08723	13.2	13.7	14.0	14.7	15.2	16.1	17.1	17.6	18.6	19.0	19.8
46	-0.1733	16.1491	0.08765	13.2	13.7	14.0	14.8	15.2	16.1	17.1	17.7	18.7	19.1	19.9
47	-0.1733	16.1983	0.08806	13.2	13.8	14.0	14.8	15.3	16.2	17.2	17.8	18.8	19.2	20.0
48	-0.1733	16.2477	0.08848	13.3	13.8	14.1	14.8	15.3	16.2	17.3	17.8	18.8	19.2	20.0
49	-0.1733	16.2974	0.0889	13.3	13.8	14.1	14.9	15.4	16.3	17.3	17.9	18.9	19.3	20.1
50	-0.1733	16.3475	0.08932	13.3	13.9	14.1	14.9	15.4	16.3	17.4	17.9	19.0	19.4	20.2
51	-0.1733	16.3981	0.08974	13.4	13.9	14.2	15.0	15.4	16.4	17.4	18.0	19.0	19.5	20.3
52	-0.1733	16.449	0.09016	13.4	13.9	14.2	15.0	15.5	16.4	17.5	18.1	19.1	19.5	20.4
53	-0.1733	16.5001	0.09057	13.4	14.0	14.2	15.0	15.5	16.5	17.5	18.1	19.2	19.6	20.5
54	-0.1733	16.5514	0.09099	13.4	14.0	14.3	15.1	15.6	16.6	17.6	18.2	19.3	19.7	20.5
55	-0.1733	16.6026	0.0914	13.5	14.0	14.3	15.1	15.6	16.6	17.7	18.3	19.3	19.8	20.6
56	-0.1733	16.6534	0.09181	13.5	14.0	14.3	15.2	15.7	16.7	17.7	18.3	19.4	19.8	20.7
57	-0.1733	16.7039	0.09221	13.5	14.1	14.4	15.2	15.7	16.7	17.8	18.4	19.5	19.9	20.8
58	-0.1733	16.7539	0.09262	13.6	14.1	14.4	15.2	15.7	16.8	17.8	18.5	19.6	20.0	20.9
59	-0.1733	16.8034	0.09301	13.6	14.1	14.4	15.3	15.8	16.8	17.9	18.5	19.6	20.1	20.9
60	-0.1733	16.8526	0.09341	13.6	14.2	14.5	15.3	15.8	16.9	18.0	18.6	19.7	20.1	21.0

Table V.26a.

LMS parameters and smoothed percentiles of triceps skinfold thickness (mm)-for-age (month) for boys from 3 months to 5 years

Age Group (months)	L	M	S	Percentiles										
				1st	3rd	5th	15th	25th	50th	75th	85th	95th	97th	99th
3	0.0027	9.7639	0.16618	6.6	7.1	7.4	8.2	8.7	9.8	10.9	11.6	12.8	13.3	14.4
4	-0.0165	9.5840	0.17264	6.4	6.9	7.2	8.0	8.5	9.6	10.8	11.5	12.7	13.3	14.3
5	-0.0326	9.3885	0.17824	6.2	6.7	7.0	7.8	8.3	9.4	10.6	11.3	12.6	13.2	14.3
6	-0.0466	9.1729	0.18304	6.0	6.5	6.8	7.6	8.1	9.2	10.4	11.1	12.4	13.0	14.1
7	-0.059	8.9535	0.18685	5.8	6.3	6.6	7.4	7.9	9.0	10.2	10.9	12.2	12.8	13.9
8	-0.0703	8.7435	0.18968	5.7	6.1	6.4	7.2	7.7	8.7	9.9	10.7	12.0	12.5	13.7
9	-0.0806	8.5518	0.19166	5.5	6.0	6.3	7.0	7.5	8.6	9.7	10.4	11.8	12.3	13.5
10	-0.0901	8.3812	0.193	5.4	5.9	6.1	6.9	7.4	8.4	9.6	10.3	11.6	12.1	13.3
11	-0.099	8.2323	0.19389	5.3	5.8	6.0	6.7	7.2	8.2	9.4	10.1	11.4	11.9	13.1
12	-0.1073	8.1041	0.19453	5.2	5.7	5.9	6.6	7.1	8.1	9.2	9.9	11.2	11.8	12.9
13	-0.1152	7.9958	0.19506	5.1	5.6	5.8	6.5	7.0	8.0	9.1	9.8	11.1	11.6	12.7
14	-0.1227	7.9064	0.19558	5.1	5.5	5.8	6.5	6.9	7.9	9.0	9.7	11.0	11.5	12.6
15	-0.1297	7.8345	0.19612	5.0	5.5	5.7	6.4	6.9	7.8	9.0	9.6	10.9	11.4	12.5
16	-0.1365	7.7781	0.19668	5.0	5.4	5.7	6.4	6.8	7.8	8.9	9.6	10.8	11.4	12.5
17	-0.143	7.7351	0.19728	5.0	5.4	5.6	6.3	6.8	7.7	8.8	9.5	10.8	11.3	12.4
18	-0.1492	7.7036	0.19793	4.9	5.4	5.6	6.3	6.7	7.7	8.8	9.5	10.8	11.3	12.4
19	0.3809	3.2322	0.19862	4.9	5.3	5.6	6.3	6.7	7.7	8.8	9.5	10.7	11.3	12.4
20	-0.1609	7.6697	0.19937	4.9	5.3	5.6	6.3	6.7	7.7	8.8	9.5	10.7	11.3	12.4
21	-0.1665	7.6652	0.20018	4.9	5.3	5.6	6.3	6.7	7.7	8.8	9.5	10.8	11.3	12.4
22	-0.1719	7.6675	0.20105	4.9	5.3	5.6	6.2	6.7	7.7	8.8	9.5	10.8	11.3	12.5
23	-0.1771	7.6750	0.20196	4.9	5.3	5.6	6.2	6.7	7.7	8.8	9.5	10.8	11.4	12.5
24	-0.1821	7.6863	0.20293	4.9	5.3	5.6	6.3	6.7	7.7	8.8	9.5	10.8	11.4	12.6
25	-0.187	7.7003	0.20394	4.9	5.3	5.6	6.3	6.7	7.7	8.9	9.6	10.9	11.5	12.7
26	-0.1918	7.7156	0.20497	4.9	5.3	5.6	6.3	6.7	7.7	8.9	9.6	10.9	11.5	12.7
27	-0.1965	7.7312	0.20603	4.9	5.3	5.6	6.3	6.7	7.7	8.9	9.6	11.0	11.6	12.8
28	-0.201	7.7463	0.2071	4.9	5.3	5.6	6.3	6.7	7.7	8.9	9.6	11.0	11.6	12.9
29	-0.2054	7.7602	0.20818	4.9	5.3	5.6	6.3	6.8	7.8	8.9	9.7	11.1	11.7	12.9
30	-0.2097	7.7726	0.20928	4.9	5.3	5.6	6.3	6.8	7.8	9.0	9.7	11.1	11.7	13.0
31	-0.2139	7.7832	0.21039	4.9	5.3	5.6	6.3	6.8	7.8	9.0	9.7	11.2	11.8	13.1
32	-0.218	7.7920	0.21153	4.9	5.3	5.6	6.3	6.8	7.8	9.0	9.8	11.2	11.8	13.1
33	-0.2221	7.7989	0.21269	4.9	5.3	5.6	6.3	6.8	7.8	9.0	9.8	11.2	11.9	13.2
34	-0.226	7.8040	0.21389	4.9	5.3	5.6	6.3	6.8	7.8	9.0	9.8	11.3	11.9	13.2
35	-0.2299	7.8074	0.21513	4.9	5.3	5.6	6.3	6.8	7.8	9.0	9.8	11.3	11.9	13.3
36	-0.2336	7.8094	0.21641	4.9	5.3	5.5	6.3	6.8	7.8	9.1	9.8	11.3	12.0	13.3
37	-0.2374	7.8101	0.21773	4.8	5.3	5.5	6.3	6.8	7.8	9.1	9.8	11.4	12.0	13.4
38	-0.241	7.8096	0.21909	4.8	5.3	5.5	6.3	6.8	7.8	9.1	9.9	11.4	12.1	13.5
39	-0.2446	7.8080	0.22049	4.8	5.3	5.5	6.3	6.7	7.8	9.1	9.9	11.4	12.1	13.5
40	-0.2481	7.8051	0.22194	4.8	5.2	5.5	6.2	6.7	7.8	9.1	9.9	11.4	12.1	13.6
41	-0.2515	7.8009	0.22343	4.8	5.2	5.5	6.2	6.7	7.8	9.1	9.9	11.5	12.2	13.6
42	-0.2549	7.7954	0.22496	4.8	5.2	5.5	6.2	6.7	7.8	9.1	9.9	11.5	12.2	13.7
43	-0.2583	7.7885	0.22653	4.8	5.2	5.5	6.2	6.7	7.8	9.1	9.9	11.5	12.2	13.7
44	-0.2616	7.7804	0.22813	4.7	5.2	5.4	6.2	6.7	7.8	9.1	9.9	11.5	12.3	13.8
45	-0.2648	7.7710	0.22975	4.7	5.2	5.4	6.2	6.7	7.8	9.1	9.9	11.6	12.3	13.8
46	-0.268	7.7605	0.2314	4.7	5.1	5.4	6.2	6.7	7.8	9.1	9.9	11.6	12.3	13.9
47	-0.2711	7.7489	0.23306	4.7	5.1	5.4	6.1	6.6	7.7	9.1	9.9	11.6	12.4	13.9
48	-0.2742	7.7364	0.23473	4.7	5.1	5.4	6.1	6.6	7.7	9.1	10.0	11.6	12.4	14.0
49	-0.2772	7.7233	0.23642	4.6	5.1	5.3	6.1	6.6	7.7	9.1	10.0	11.7	12.4	14.0
50	-0.2802	7.7096	0.23811	4.6	5.1	5.3	6.1	6.6	7.7	9.1	10.0	11.7	12.4	14.1
51	-0.2832	7.6955	0.23981	4.6	5.0	5.3	6.1	6.6	7.7	9.1	10.0	11.7	12.5	14.1
52	-0.2861	7.6812	0.24151	4.6	5.0	5.3	6.0	6.6	7.7	9.1	10.0	11.7	12.5	14.2
53	-0.289	7.6669	0.24322	4.5	5.0	5.3	6.0	6.5	7.7	9.1	10.0	11.7	12.5	14.2
54	-0.2918	7.6525	0.24494	4.5	5.0	5.2	6.0	6.5	7.7	9.1	10.0	11.7	12.6	14.3
55	-0.2946	7.6383	0.24666	4.5	4.9	5.2	6.0	6.5	7.6	9.1	10.0	11.8	12.6	14.3
56	-0.2974	7.6242	0.24839	4.5	4.9	5.2	5.9	6.5	7.6	9.1	10.0	11.8	12.6	14.4
57	-0.3001	7.6104	0.25013	4.5	4.9	5.2	5.9	6.5	7.6	9.0	10.0	11.8	12.6	14.4
58	-0.3028	7.5968	0.25186	4.4	4.9	5.1	5.9	6.4	7.6	9.0	10.0	11.8	12.7	14.5
59	-0.3055	7.5835	0.2536	4.4	4.9	5.1	5.9	6.4	7.6	9.0	10.0	11.8	12.7	14.5
60	-0.3081	7.5706	0.25533	4.4	4.8	5.1	5.9	6.4	7.6	9.0	10.0	11.9	12.7	14.6

Table V.26b.

LMS parameters and smoothed percentiles of triceps skinfold thickness (mm)-for-age (month) for girls from 3 months to 5 years

Age Group (months)	L	M	S	Percentiles										
				1st	3rd	5th	15th	25th	50th	75th	85th	95th	97th	99th
3	0.1875	9.7516	0.17535	6.4	6.9	7.2	8.1	8.7	9.8	11.0	11.7	12.9	13.4	14.4
4	0.1256	9.5866	0.18337	6.2	6.7	7.0	7.9	8.5	9.6	10.8	11.6	12.9	13.4	14.5
5	0.0761	9.3716	0.19007	6.0	6.5	6.8	7.7	8.2	9.4	10.6	11.4	12.8	13.3	14.5
6	0.0349	9.1194	0.1954	5.8	6.3	6.6	7.4	8.0	9.1	10.4	11.2	12.6	13.1	14.3
7	-0.0003	8.8621	0.19934	5.6	6.1	6.4	7.2	7.7	8.9	10.1	10.9	12.3	12.9	14.1
8	-0.0307	8.6228	0.20192	5.4	5.9	6.2	7.0	7.5	8.6	9.9	10.6	12.0	12.6	13.8
9	-0.0572	8.4164	0.20339	5.3	5.8	6.0	6.8	7.3	8.4	9.7	10.4	11.8	12.4	13.6
10	-0.0799	8.2468	0.20413	5.2	5.7	5.9	6.7	7.2	8.2	9.5	10.2	11.6	12.2	13.4
11	-0.0995	8.1114	0.20442	5.1	5.6	5.8	6.6	7.1	8.1	9.3	10.0	11.4	12.0	13.2
12	-0.1161	8.0042	0.20445	5.0	5.5	5.8	6.5	7.0	8.0	9.2	9.9	11.3	11.9	13.1
13	-0.1303	7.9197	0.20432	5.0	5.4	5.7	6.4	6.9	7.9	9.1	9.8	11.2	11.7	12.9
14	-0.1424	7.8538	0.20409	5.0	5.4	5.7	6.4	6.9	7.9	9.0	9.7	11.1	11.7	12.8
15	-0.1527	7.8041	0.20384	4.9	5.4	5.6	6.3	6.8	7.8	9.0	9.7	11.0	11.6	12.8
16	-0.1615	7.7681	0.20363	4.9	5.4	5.6	6.3	6.8	7.8	8.9	9.6	11.0	11.5	12.7
17	-0.169	7.7443	0.2035	4.9	5.3	5.6	6.3	6.8	7.7	8.9	9.6	10.9	11.5	12.7
18	-0.1755	7.7315	0.2035	4.9	5.3	5.6	6.3	6.8	7.7	8.9	9.6	10.9	11.5	12.7
19	0.3809	3.2322	0.20364	4.9	5.3	5.6	6.3	6.7	7.7	8.9	9.6	10.9	11.5	12.7
20	-0.1859	7.7347	0.20393	4.9	5.3	5.6	6.3	6.8	7.7	8.9	9.6	10.9	11.5	12.7
21	-0.1901	7.7484	0.20437	4.9	5.3	5.6	6.3	6.8	7.7	8.9	9.6	11.0	11.5	12.8
22	-0.1939	7.7692	0.20496	4.9	5.4	5.6	6.3	6.8	7.8	8.9	9.7	11.0	11.6	12.8
23	-0.1973	7.7958	0.20568	4.9	5.4	5.6	6.3	6.8	7.8	9.0	9.7	11.1	11.7	12.9
24	-0.2004	7.8273	0.20652	4.9	5.4	5.6	6.3	6.8	7.8	9.0	9.7	11.1	11.7	13.0
25	-0.2032	7.8628	0.20748	5.0	5.4	5.7	6.4	6.8	7.9	9.1	9.8	11.2	11.8	13.1
26	-0.2058	7.9006	0.20855	5.0	5.4	5.7	6.4	6.9	7.9	9.1	9.9	11.3	11.9	13.2
27	-0.2081	7.9396	0.20971	5.0	5.4	5.7	6.4	6.9	7.9	9.2	9.9	11.4	12.0	13.3
28	-0.2103	7.9786	0.21096	5.0	5.5	5.7	6.4	6.9	8.0	9.2	10.0	11.4	12.1	13.4
29	-0.2122	8.0167	0.21228	5.0	5.5	5.7	6.5	7.0	8.0	9.3	10.0	11.5	12.2	13.5
30	-0.214	8.0535	0.21366	5.0	5.5	5.7	6.5	7.0	8.1	9.3	10.1	11.6	12.3	13.6
31	-0.2155	8.0887	0.21509	5.0	5.5	5.8	6.5	7.0	8.1	9.4	10.2	11.7	12.4	13.7
32	-0.217	8.1224	0.21657	5.0	5.5	5.8	6.5	7.0	8.1	9.4	10.2	11.8	12.4	13.8
33	-0.2183	8.1545	0.21809	5.0	5.5	5.8	6.5	7.1	8.2	9.5	10.3	11.8	12.5	14.0
34	-0.2195	8.1855	0.21964	5.0	5.5	5.8	6.6	7.1	8.2	9.5	10.3	11.9	12.6	14.1
35	-0.2207	8.2156	0.22122	5.0	5.5	5.8	6.6	7.1	8.2	9.6	10.4	12.0	12.7	14.2
36	-0.2217	8.245	0.22282	5.0	5.5	5.8	6.6	7.1	8.2	9.6	10.5	12.1	12.8	14.3
37	-0.2227	8.2738	0.22444	5.0	5.5	5.8	6.6	7.1	8.3	9.7	10.5	12.2	12.9	14.4
38	-0.2237	8.3019	0.22608	5.0	5.5	5.8	6.6	7.1	8.3	9.7	10.6	12.2	13.0	14.5
39	-0.2246	8.3294	0.22772	5.0	5.5	5.8	6.6	7.2	8.3	9.7	10.6	12.3	13.1	14.6
40	-0.2254	8.356	0.22937	5.0	5.5	5.8	6.6	7.2	8.4	9.8	10.7	12.4	13.2	14.8
41	-0.2262	8.3818	0.23101	5.0	5.5	5.8	6.6	7.2	8.4	9.8	10.7	12.5	13.2	14.9
42	-0.227	8.4068	0.23264	5.0	5.5	5.8	6.6	7.2	8.4	9.9	10.8	12.5	13.3	15.0
43	-0.2278	8.4311	0.23427	5.0	5.5	5.8	6.7	7.2	8.4	9.9	10.8	12.6	13.4	15.1
44	-0.2285	8.455	0.23587	5.0	5.5	5.8	6.7	7.2	8.5	9.9	10.9	12.7	13.5	15.2
45	-0.2292	8.4786	0.23747	5.0	5.5	5.8	6.7	7.2	8.5	10.0	10.9	12.8	13.6	15.3
46	-0.2298	8.5019	0.23904	5.0	5.5	5.8	6.7	7.3	8.5	10.0	11.0	12.8	13.7	15.4
47	-0.2304	8.525	0.2406	5.0	5.5	5.8	6.7	7.3	8.5	10.1	11.0	12.9	13.7	15.5
48	-0.231	8.5481	0.24215	5.0	5.5	5.8	6.7	7.3	8.5	10.1	11.1	13.0	13.8	15.6
49	-0.2316	8.5711	0.24367	5.0	5.5	5.8	6.7	7.3	8.6	10.1	11.1	13.1	13.9	15.7
50	-0.2321	8.5942	0.24517	5.0	5.5	5.8	6.7	7.3	8.6	10.2	11.2	13.1	14.0	15.8
51	-0.2326	8.6174	0.24665	5.0	5.5	5.8	6.7	7.3	8.6	10.2	11.2	13.2	14.1	16.0
52	-0.2331	8.6406	0.24811	5.0	5.5	5.9	6.7	7.3	8.6	10.2	11.3	13.3	14.2	16.1
53	-0.2336	8.6641	0.24954	5.0	5.6	5.9	6.7	7.3	8.7	10.3	11.3	13.3	14.2	16.2
54	-0.2341	8.6876	0.25095	5.0	5.6	5.9	6.7	7.4	8.7	10.3	11.4	13.4	14.3	16.3
55	-0.2346	8.7112	0.25233	5.0	5.6	5.9	6.8	7.4	8.7	10.4	11.4	13.5	14.4	16.4
56	-0.235	8.7349	0.25369	5.0	5.6	5.9	6.8	7.4	8.7	10.4	11.5	13.6	14.5	16.5
57	-0.2355	8.7586	0.25502	5.0	5.6	5.9	6.8	7.4	8.8	10.4	11.5	13.6	14.6	16.6
58	-0.2359	8.7824	0.25633	5.0	5.6	5.9	6.8	7.4	8.8	10.5	11.6	13.7	14.7	16.7
59	-0.2363	8.8061	0.25761	5.0	5.6	5.9	6.8	7.4	8.8	10.5	11.6	13.8	14.7	16.8
60	-0.2368	8.8298	0.25887	5.0	5.6	5.9	6.8	7.4	8.8	10.6	11.7	13.8	14.8	16.9

Table V.27a.

LMS parameters and smoothed percentiles of subscapular skinfold thickness (mm)-for-age (month) for boys from 3 months to 5 years

Age Group (months)	L	M	S	Percentiles										
				1st	3rd	5th	15th	25th	50th	75th	85th	95th	97th	99th
3	-0.3033	7.6899	0.1702	5.3	5.7	5.9	6.5	6.9	7.7	8.6	9.2	10.3	10.8	11.7
4	-0.3278	7.4968	0.17097	5.2	5.5	5.7	6.3	6.7	7.5	8.4	9.0	10.1	10.5	11.5
5	-0.3503	7.3207	0.17167	5.0	5.4	5.6	6.2	6.5	7.3	8.2	8.8	9.9	10.3	11.3
6	-0.3712	7.1588	0.17232	4.9	5.3	5.5	6.0	6.4	7.2	8.1	8.6	9.7	10.1	11.0
7	-0.3909	7.0104	0.17293	4.8	5.2	5.4	5.9	6.3	7.0	7.9	8.4	9.5	9.9	10.9
8	-0.4097	6.8753	0.17352	4.7	5.1	5.2	5.8	6.1	6.9	7.8	8.3	9.3	9.8	10.7
9	-0.4276	6.753	0.17408	4.6	5.0	5.2	5.7	6.0	6.8	7.6	8.1	9.2	9.6	10.5
10	-0.4449	6.6428	0.17462	4.6	4.9	5.1	5.6	5.9	6.6	7.5	8.0	9.0	9.5	10.4
11	-0.4616	6.5442	0.17514	4.5	4.8	5.0	5.5	5.8	6.5	7.4	7.9	8.9	9.4	10.3
12	-0.4777	6.4562	0.17564	4.4	4.8	4.9	5.4	5.8	6.5	7.3	7.8	8.8	9.2	10.2
13	-0.4934	6.378	0.17613	4.4	4.7	4.9	5.4	5.7	6.4	7.2	7.7	8.7	9.2	10.1
14	-0.5087	6.3085	0.1766	4.3	4.6	4.8	5.3	5.6	6.3	7.1	7.6	8.6	9.1	10.0
15	-0.5236	6.2468	0.17707	4.3	4.6	4.8	5.2	5.6	6.2	7.1	7.6	8.6	9.0	9.9
16	-0.5381	6.1921	0.17752	4.3	4.6	4.7	5.2	5.5	6.2	7.0	7.5	8.5	8.9	9.9
17	-0.5524	6.1435	0.17797	4.2	4.5	4.7	5.2	5.5	6.1	7.0	7.5	8.5	8.9	9.8
18	-0.5663	6.1003	0.1784	4.2	4.5	4.7	5.1	5.4	6.1	6.9	7.4	8.4	8.9	9.8
19	0.3809	3.2322	0.17883	4.2	4.5	4.6	5.1	5.4	6.1	6.9	7.4	8.4	8.8	9.8
20	-0.5934	6.0274	0.17925	4.2	4.4	4.6	5.1	5.4	6.0	6.8	7.3	8.3	8.8	9.7
21	-0.6066	5.9972	0.17966	4.1	4.4	4.6	5.0	5.3	6.0	6.8	7.3	8.3	8.8	9.7
22	-0.6196	5.9706	0.18006	4.1	4.4	4.5	5.0	5.3	6.0	6.8	7.3	8.3	8.7	9.7
23	-0.6324	5.947	0.18046	4.1	4.4	4.5	5.0	5.3	5.9	6.8	7.3	8.3	8.7	9.7
24	-0.6449	5.9258	0.18085	4.1	4.4	4.5	5.0	5.3	5.9	6.7	7.2	8.2	8.7	9.7
25	-0.6573	5.9067	0.18124	4.1	4.3	4.5	4.9	5.3	5.9	6.7	7.2	8.2	8.7	9.7
26	-0.6695	5.8891	0.18162	4.1	4.3	4.5	4.9	5.2	5.9	6.7	7.2	8.2	8.7	9.7
27	-0.6816	5.8729	0.18199	4.0	4.3	4.5	4.9	5.2	5.9	6.7	7.2	8.2	8.7	9.7
28	-0.6935	5.8576	0.18237	4.0	4.3	4.5	4.9	5.2	5.9	6.7	7.2	8.2	8.7	9.7
29	-0.7053	5.8431	0.18273	4.0	4.3	4.4	4.9	5.2	5.8	6.6	7.2	8.2	8.7	9.7
30	-0.7169	5.829	0.18309	4.0	4.3	4.4	4.9	5.2	5.8	6.6	7.1	8.2	8.7	9.7
31	-0.7283	5.815	0.18345	4.0	4.3	4.4	4.9	5.2	5.8	6.6	7.1	8.2	8.7	9.7
32	-0.7397	5.8011	0.18381	4.0	4.3	4.4	4.9	5.2	5.8	6.6	7.1	8.2	8.6	9.7
33	-0.7509	5.787	0.18416	4.0	4.3	4.4	4.8	5.1	5.8	6.6	7.1	8.2	8.6	9.7
34	-0.762	5.7727	0.1845	4.0	4.2	4.4	4.8	5.1	5.8	6.6	7.1	8.2	8.6	9.7
35	-0.773	5.758	0.18485	4.0	4.2	4.4	4.8	5.1	5.8	6.6	7.1	8.1	8.6	9.7
36	-0.7839	5.743	0.18519	4.0	4.2	4.4	4.8	5.1	5.7	6.5	7.1	8.1	8.6	9.7
37	-0.7947	5.7278	0.18552	4.0	4.2	4.4	4.8	5.1	5.7	6.5	7.1	8.1	8.6	9.7
38	-0.8054	5.7125	0.18585	3.9	4.2	4.3	4.8	5.1	5.7	6.5	7.0	8.1	8.6	9.7
39	-0.8159	5.6971	0.18618	3.9	4.2	4.3	4.8	5.1	5.7	6.5	7.0	8.1	8.6	9.7
40	-0.8264	5.6815	0.18651	3.9	4.2	4.3	4.7	5.0	5.7	6.5	7.0	8.1	8.6	9.7
41	-0.8368	5.6658	0.18684	3.9	4.2	4.3	4.7	5.0	5.7	6.5	7.0	8.1	8.6	9.7
42	-0.8471	5.65	0.18716	3.9	4.2	4.3	4.7	5.0	5.6	6.5	7.0	8.1	8.6	9.7
43	-0.8574	5.6339	0.18748	3.9	4.1	4.3	4.7	5.0	5.6	6.4	7.0	8.1	8.6	9.7
44	-0.8675	5.6174	0.18779	3.9	4.1	4.3	4.7	5.0	5.6	6.4	7.0	8.0	8.6	9.7
45	-0.8775	5.6006	0.18811	3.9	4.1	4.3	4.7	5.0	5.6	6.4	6.9	8.0	8.6	9.7
46	-0.8875	5.5834	0.18842	3.9	4.1	4.2	4.7	4.9	5.6	6.4	6.9	8.0	8.5	9.7
47	-0.8974	5.5659	0.18873	3.8	4.1	4.2	4.6	4.9	5.6	6.4	6.9	8.0	8.5	9.7
48	-0.9073	5.5482	0.18903	3.8	4.1	4.2	4.6	4.9	5.5	6.4	6.9	8.0	8.5	9.7
49	-0.917	5.5303	0.18934	3.8	4.1	4.2	4.6	4.9	5.5	6.3	6.9	8.0	8.5	9.7
50	-0.9267	5.5125	0.18964	3.8	4.1	4.2	4.6	4.9	5.5	6.3	6.8	8.0	8.5	9.7
51	-0.9363	5.4948	0.18994	3.8	4.0	4.2	4.6	4.9	5.5	6.3	6.8	8.0	8.5	9.7
52	-0.9459	5.4774	0.19024	3.8	4.0	4.2	4.6	4.9	5.5	6.3	6.8	7.9	8.5	9.7
53	-0.9554	5.4606	0.19053	3.8	4.0	4.2	4.6	4.8	5.5	6.3	6.8	7.9	8.5	9.7
54	-0.9648	5.4443	0.19083	3.8	4.0	4.1	4.5	4.8	5.4	6.2	6.8	7.9	8.5	9.7
55	-0.9742	5.4288	0.19112	3.8	4.0	4.1	4.5	4.8	5.4	6.2	6.8	7.9	8.5	9.7
56	-0.9835	5.414	0.19141	3.7	4.0	4.1	4.5	4.8	5.4	6.2	6.8	7.9	8.4	9.7
57	-0.9928	5.4	0.1917	3.7	4.0	4.1	4.5	4.8	5.4	6.2	6.7	7.9	8.4	9.7
58	-1.002	5.3868	0.19199	3.7	4.0	4.1	4.5	4.8	5.4	6.2	6.7	7.9	8.4	9.7
59	-1.0111	5.3744	0.19227	3.7	3.9	4.1	4.5	4.8	5.4	6.2	6.7	7.9	8.4	9.7
60	-1.0202	5.3628	0.19255	3.7	3.9	4.1	4.5	4.7	5.4	6.2	6.7	7.9	8.4	9.8

Table V.27b.

LMS parameters and smoothed percentiles of subscapular skinfold thickness (mm)-for-age (month) for girls from 3 months to 5 years

Age Group (months)	L	M	S	Percentiles										
				1st	3rd	5th	15th	25th	50th	75th	85th	95th	97th	99th
3	-0.2026	7.7846	0.18428	5.2	5.6	5.8	6.5	6.9	7.8	8.8	9.5	10.6	11.2	12.2
4	-0.2577	7.5405	0.1843	5.0	5.4	5.6	6.3	6.7	7.5	8.6	9.2	10.3	10.8	11.9
5	-0.302	7.3384	0.18428	4.9	5.3	5.5	6.1	6.5	7.3	8.3	8.9	10.1	10.6	11.6
6	-0.3394	7.1637	0.18425	4.8	5.2	5.4	6.0	6.3	7.2	8.1	8.7	9.9	10.4	11.4
7	-0.3718	7.0118	0.18421	4.7	5.1	5.3	5.8	6.2	7.0	8.0	8.5	9.7	10.2	11.2
8	-0.4005	6.8807	0.18412	4.6	5.0	5.2	5.7	6.1	6.9	7.8	8.4	9.5	10.0	11.0
9	-0.4263	6.7679	0.18399	4.6	4.9	5.1	5.6	6.0	6.8	7.7	8.3	9.4	9.8	10.9
10	-0.4498	6.6707	0.18387	4.5	4.8	5.0	5.6	5.9	6.7	7.6	8.1	9.2	9.7	10.7
11	-0.4713	6.5867	0.18381	4.5	4.8	5.0	5.5	5.8	6.6	7.5	8.0	9.1	9.6	10.6
12	-0.4912	6.5138	0.18383	4.4	4.7	4.9	5.4	5.8	6.5	7.4	8.0	9.0	9.5	10.5
13	-0.5098	6.4505	0.18394	4.4	4.7	4.9	5.4	5.7	6.5	7.3	7.9	9.0	9.4	10.5
14	-0.5272	6.3955	0.18415	4.3	4.7	4.8	5.3	5.7	6.4	7.3	7.8	8.9	9.4	10.4
15	-0.5435	6.3474	0.18446	4.3	4.6	4.8	5.3	5.6	6.3	7.2	7.8	8.8	9.3	10.3
16	-0.559	6.3055	0.18487	4.3	4.6	4.8	5.3	5.6	6.3	7.2	7.7	8.8	9.3	10.3
17	-0.5736	6.2689	0.18538	4.3	4.6	4.7	5.2	5.6	6.3	7.1	7.7	8.8	9.2	10.3
18	-0.5876	6.2373	0.18598	4.2	4.5	4.7	5.2	5.5	6.2	7.1	7.7	8.7	9.2	10.3
19	0.3809	3.2322	0.18666	4.2	4.5	4.7	5.2	5.5	6.2	7.1	7.6	8.7	9.2	10.3
20	-0.6136	6.1868	0.18741	4.2	4.5	4.7	5.1	5.5	6.2	7.1	7.6	8.7	9.2	10.3
21	-0.6257	6.1669	0.18823	4.2	4.5	4.6	5.1	5.5	6.2	7.0	7.6	8.7	9.2	10.3
22	-0.6374	6.15	0.18911	4.2	4.5	4.6	5.1	5.4	6.2	7.0	7.6	8.7	9.2	10.3
23	-0.6487	6.1355	0.19005	4.2	4.4	4.6	5.1	5.4	6.1	7.0	7.6	8.7	9.2	10.3
24	-0.6595	6.1232	0.19104	4.1	4.4	4.6	5.1	5.4	6.1	7.0	7.6	8.7	9.2	10.4
25	-0.67	6.1129	0.19207	4.1	4.4	4.6	5.1	5.4	6.1	7.0	7.6	8.7	9.2	10.4
26	-0.6801	6.1041	0.19315	4.1	4.4	4.6	5.1	5.4	6.1	7.0	7.6	8.7	9.3	10.4
27	-0.6899	6.0968	0.19426	4.1	4.4	4.6	5.0	5.4	6.1	7.0	7.6	8.7	9.3	10.5
28	-0.6994	6.0905	0.1954	4.1	4.4	4.6	5.0	5.4	6.1	7.0	7.6	8.8	9.3	10.5
29	-0.7086	6.0851	0.19657	4.1	4.4	4.5	5.0	5.4	6.1	7.0	7.6	8.8	9.3	10.6
30	-0.7175	6.0806	0.19776	4.1	4.4	4.5	5.0	5.4	6.1	7.0	7.6	8.8	9.4	10.6
31	-0.7262	6.0766	0.19898	4.1	4.4	4.5	5.0	5.3	6.1	7.0	7.6	8.8	9.4	10.7
32	-0.7347	6.0733	0.20021	4.1	4.4	4.5	5.0	5.3	6.1	7.0	7.6	8.9	9.4	10.7
33	-0.7429	6.0705	0.20145	4.1	4.3	4.5	5.0	5.3	6.1	7.0	7.6	8.9	9.5	10.8
34	-0.7509	6.0683	0.2027	4.1	4.3	4.5	5.0	5.3	6.1	7.0	7.6	8.9	9.5	10.9
35	-0.7587	6.0665	0.20395	4.0	4.3	4.5	5.0	5.3	6.1	7.0	7.6	8.9	9.5	10.9
36	-0.7664	6.0652	0.20521	4.0	4.3	4.5	5.0	5.3	6.1	7.0	7.7	9.0	9.6	11.0
37	-0.7738	6.0643	0.20647	4.0	4.3	4.5	5.0	5.3	6.1	7.0	7.7	9.0	9.6	11.1
38	-0.7811	6.0637	0.20773	4.0	4.3	4.5	5.0	5.3	6.1	7.0	7.7	9.0	9.7	11.1
39	-0.7882	6.0633	0.20899	4.0	4.3	4.5	5.0	5.3	6.1	7.0	7.7	9.1	9.7	11.2
40	-0.7952	6.0632	0.21024	4.0	4.3	4.5	5.0	5.3	6.1	7.0	7.7	9.1	9.7	11.3
41	-0.802	6.0632	0.21149	4.0	4.3	4.5	5.0	5.3	6.1	7.1	7.7	9.1	9.8	11.3
42	-0.8087	6.0634	0.21273	4.0	4.3	4.5	4.9	5.3	6.1	7.1	7.7	9.1	9.8	11.4
43	-0.8152	6.0637	0.21396	4.0	4.3	4.5	4.9	5.3	6.1	7.1	7.7	9.2	9.9	11.5
44	-0.8217	6.0641	0.21518	4.0	4.3	4.4	4.9	5.3	6.1	7.1	7.8	9.2	9.9	11.6
45	-0.828	6.0647	0.21638	4.0	4.3	4.4	4.9	5.3	6.1	7.1	7.8	9.2	10.0	11.6
46	-0.8341	6.0653	0.21758	4.0	4.3	4.4	4.9	5.3	6.1	7.1	7.8	9.3	10.0	11.7
47	-0.8402	6.0661	0.21876	4.0	4.3	4.4	4.9	5.3	6.1	7.1	7.8	9.3	10.0	11.8
48	-0.8462	6.0669	0.21993	4.0	4.3	4.4	4.9	5.3	6.1	7.1	7.8	9.3	10.1	11.9
49	-0.852	6.0679	0.22109	4.0	4.3	4.4	4.9	5.3	6.1	7.1	7.8	9.4	10.1	11.9
50	-0.8578	6.069	0.22223	4.0	4.2	4.4	4.9	5.3	6.1	7.1	7.8	9.4	10.2	12.0
51	-0.8634	6.0703	0.22335	4.0	4.2	4.4	4.9	5.3	6.1	7.1	7.9	9.4	10.2	12.1
52	-0.869	6.0717	0.22447	3.9	4.2	4.4	4.9	5.3	6.1	7.1	7.9	9.5	10.3	12.2
53	-0.8745	6.0732	0.22556	3.9	4.2	4.4	4.9	5.3	6.1	7.2	7.9	9.5	10.3	12.3
54	-0.8799	6.0748	0.22664	3.9	4.2	4.4	4.9	5.3	6.1	7.2	7.9	9.5	10.4	12.3
55	-0.8852	6.0765	0.22771	3.9	4.2	4.4	4.9	5.3	6.1	7.2	7.9	9.6	10.4	12.4
56	-0.8904	6.0784	0.22876	3.9	4.2	4.4	4.9	5.3	6.1	7.2	7.9	9.6	10.5	12.5
57	-0.8955	6.0803	0.22979	3.9	4.2	4.4	4.9	5.3	6.1	7.2	7.9	9.6	10.5	12.6
58	-0.9006	6.0823	0.23081	3.9	4.2	4.4	4.9	5.3	6.1	7.2	8.0	9.7	10.5	12.7
59	-0.9056	6.0844	0.23182	3.9	4.2	4.4	4.9	5.3	6.1	7.2	8.0	9.7	10.6	12.8
60	-0.9105	6.0865	0.2328	3.9	4.2	4.4	4.9	5.3	6.1	7.2	8.0	9.7	10.6	12.8

LIST OF FIGURES: WHO CHILD GROWTH CHARTS

Source: Figures based upon the tabular data given in the 2nd set of standards of the WHO Child Growth Standards: http://www.who.int/nutrition/topics/childgrowth/en/index.html

Figure V.28. Percentiles of Triceps Skinfold (mm) by Age for Girls Ranging in Age from 3 Months to 5 Years.

Figure V.29. Percentiles of Subscapular Skinfold (mm) by Age for Boys Ranging in Age from 3 Months to 5 Years.

Figure V.30. Percentiles of Subscapular Skinfold (mm) by Age for Girls Ranging in Age from 3 Months to 5 Years.

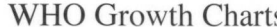

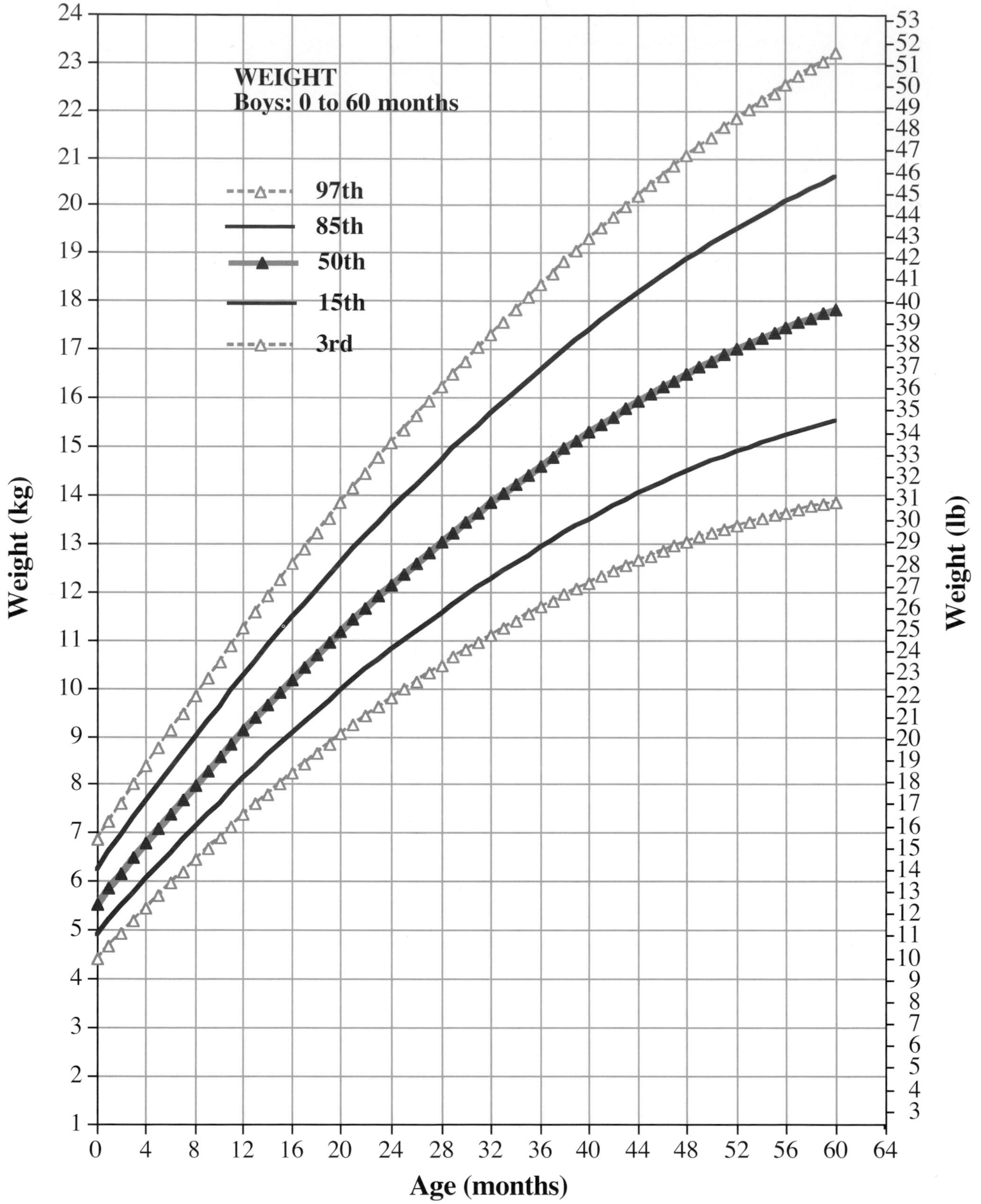

Figure V.15. Percentiles of Weight in Kilograms (kg) and Pounds (lb.) by Age for Boys Ranging in Age from Birth to 5 Years.

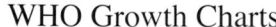

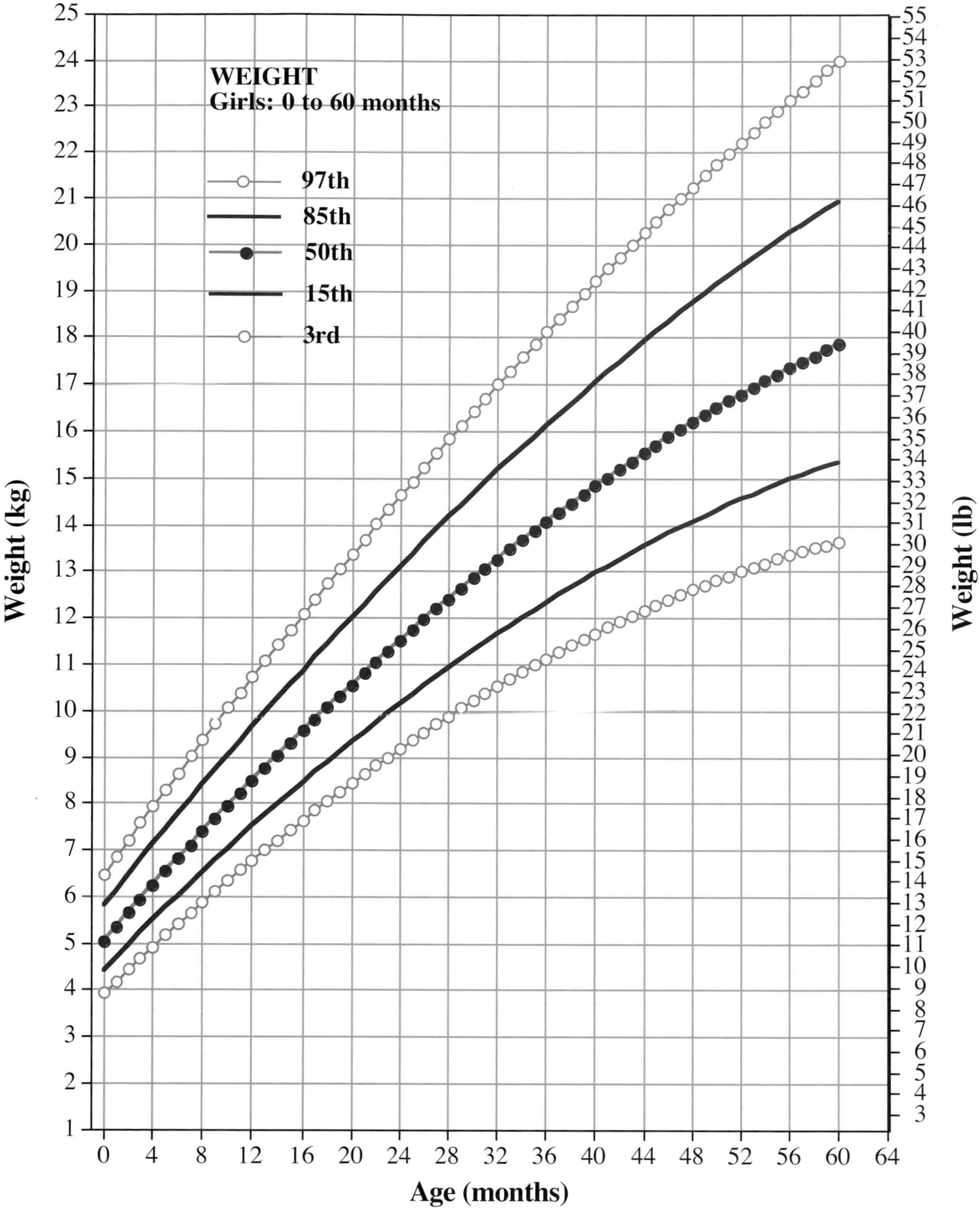

Figure V.16. Percentiles of Weight in Kilograms (kg) and Pounds (lb.) by Age for Girls Ranging in Age from Birth to 5 Years.

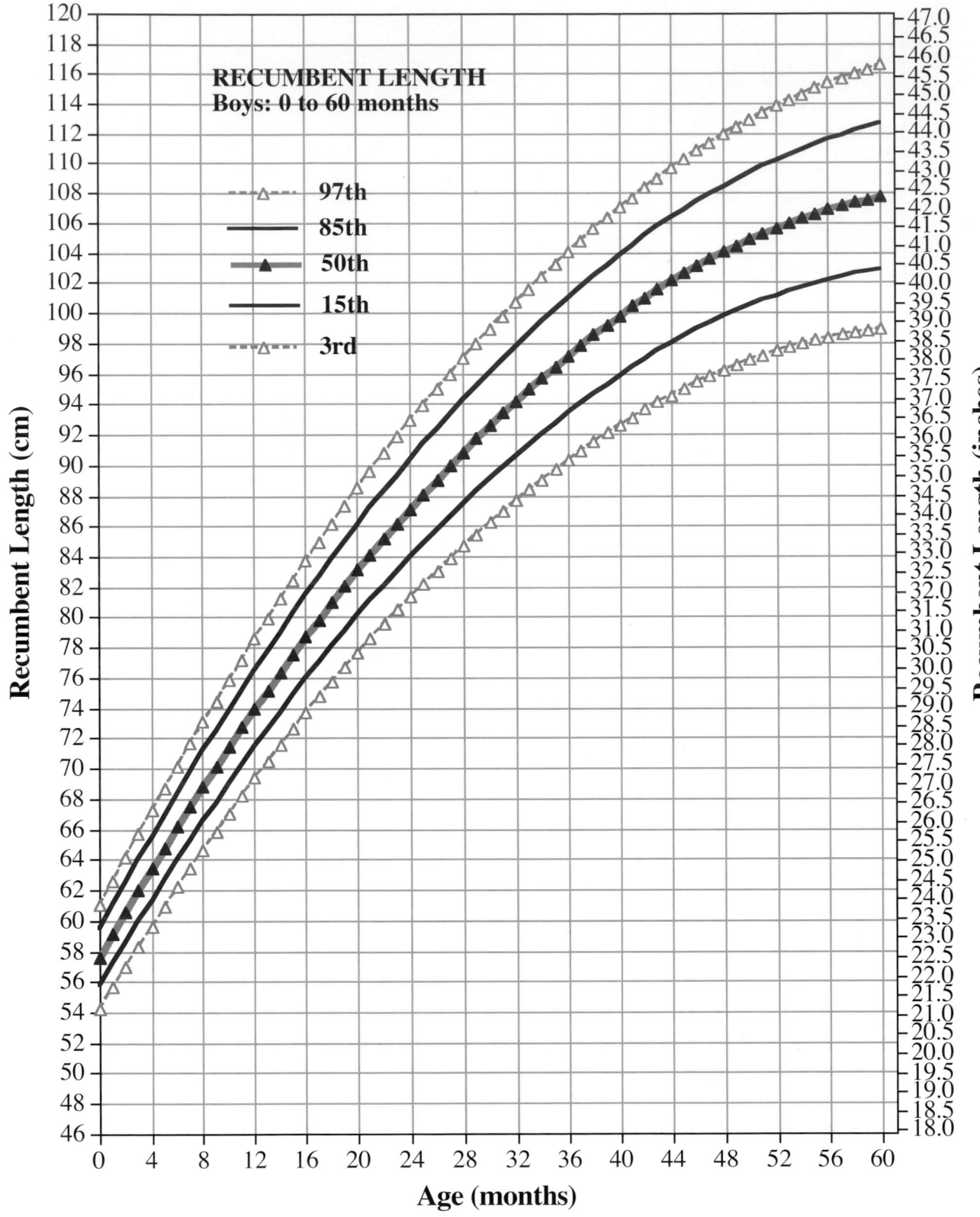

Figure V.17. Percentiles of Length in Centimeters (cm) and Inches (in.) by Age for Boys Ranging in Age from Birth to 5 Years.

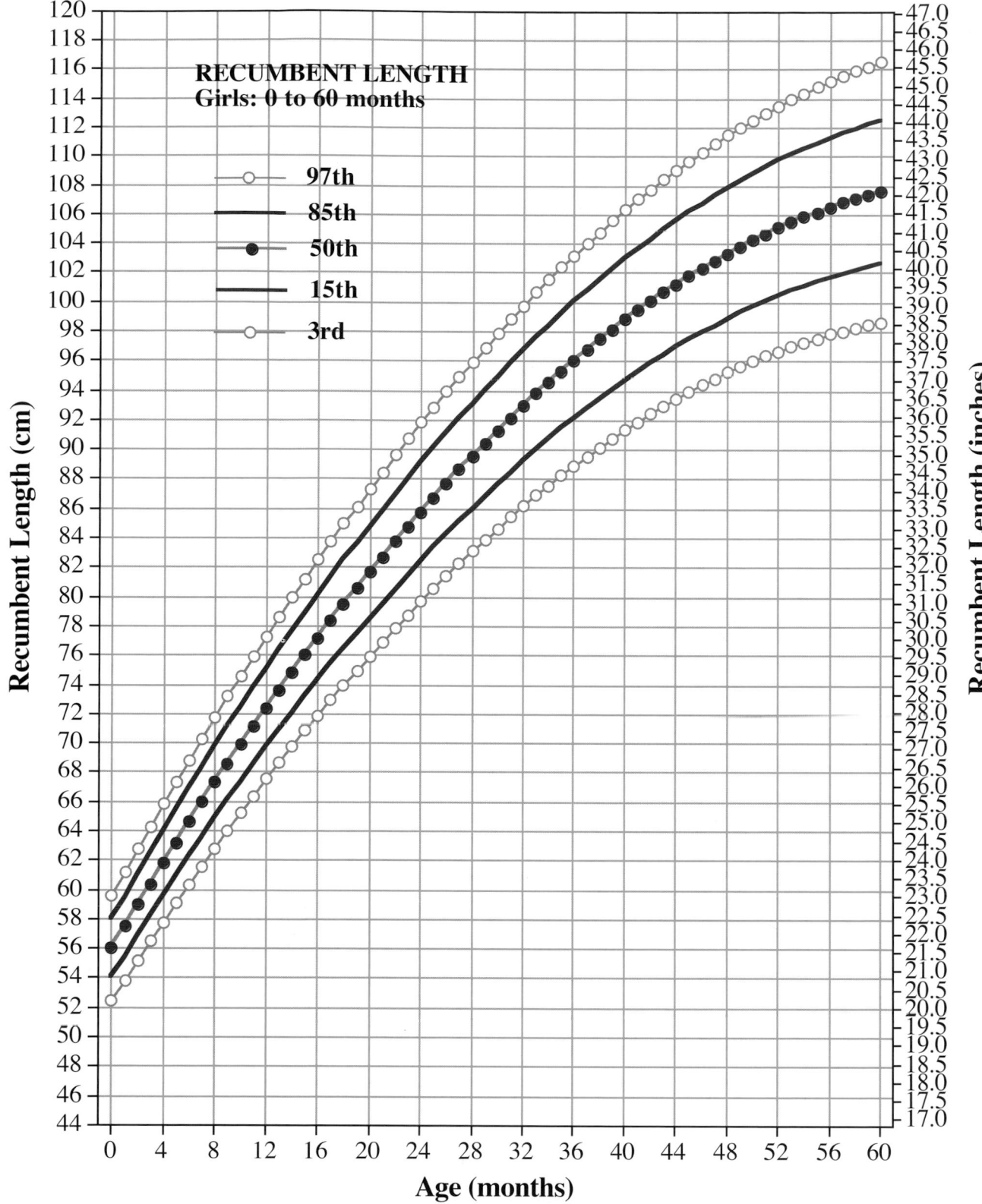

Figure V.18. Percentiles of Length in Centimeters (cm) and Inches (in.) by Age for Girls Ranging in Age from Birth to 5 Years.

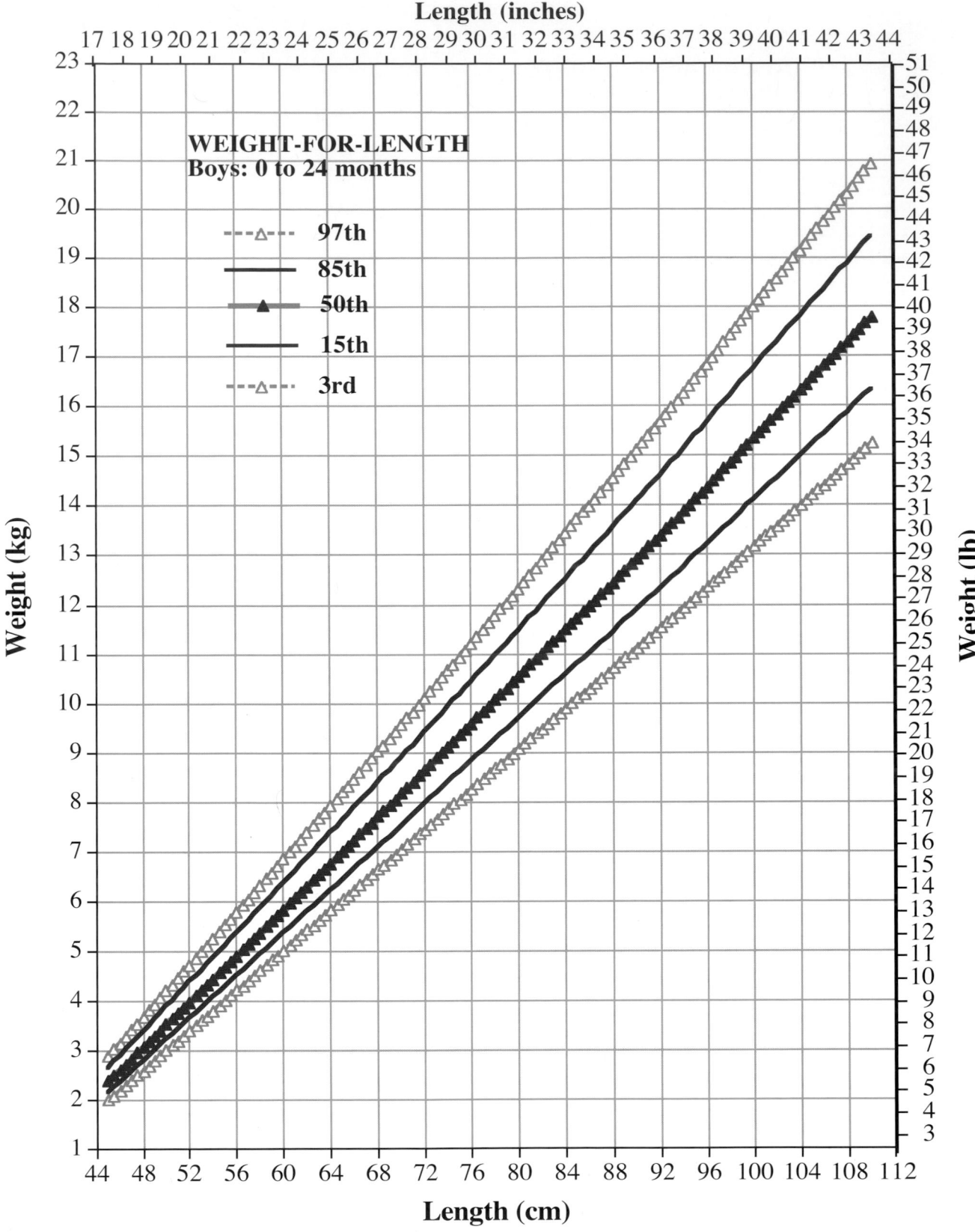

Figure V.19. Percentiles of Weight (kg)-for-Length (cm) by Age for Boys Ranging in Age from Birth to 2 Years.

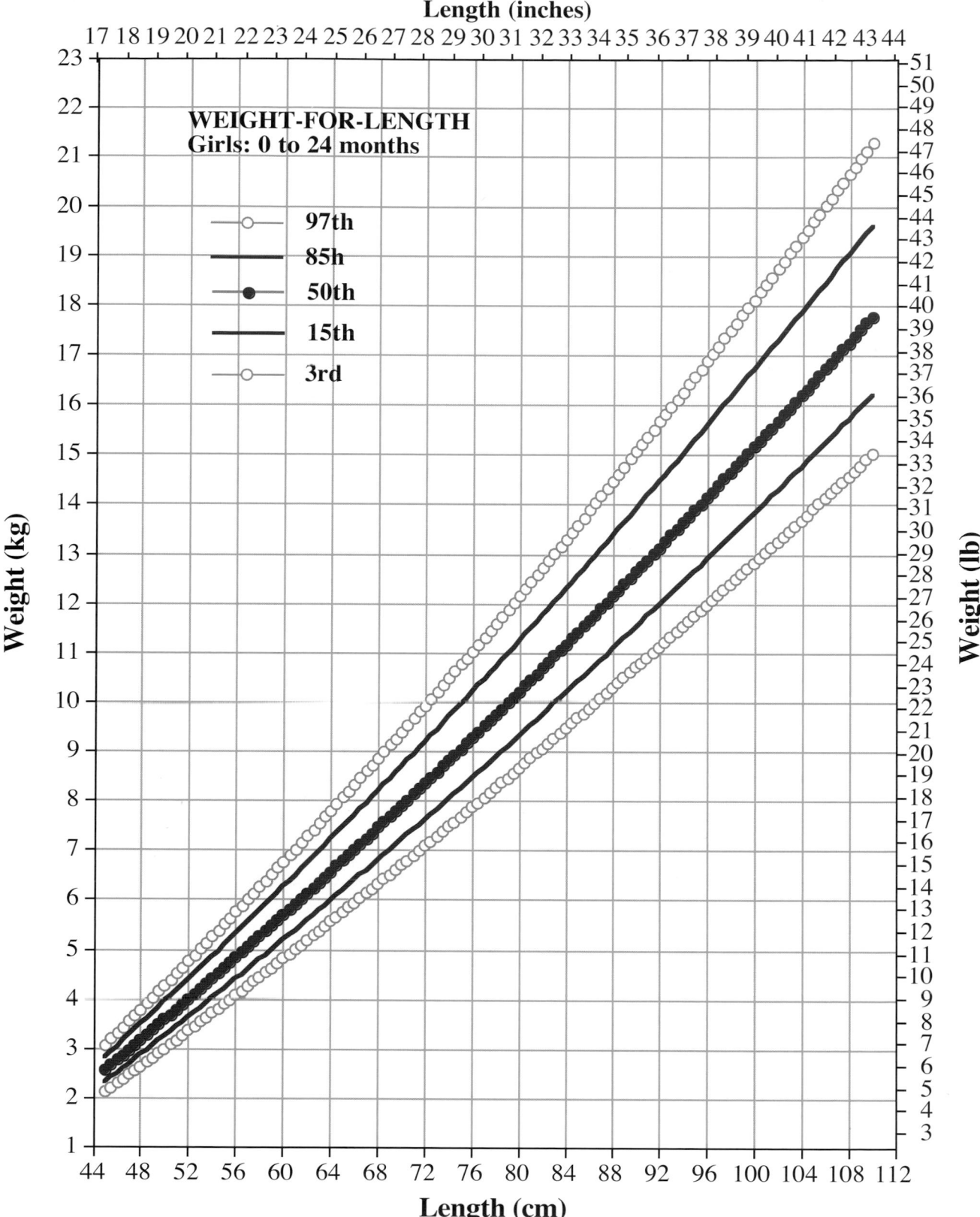

Figure V.20. Percentiles of Weight (kg) for Length (cm) by Age for Girls Ranging in Age from Birth to 2 Years.

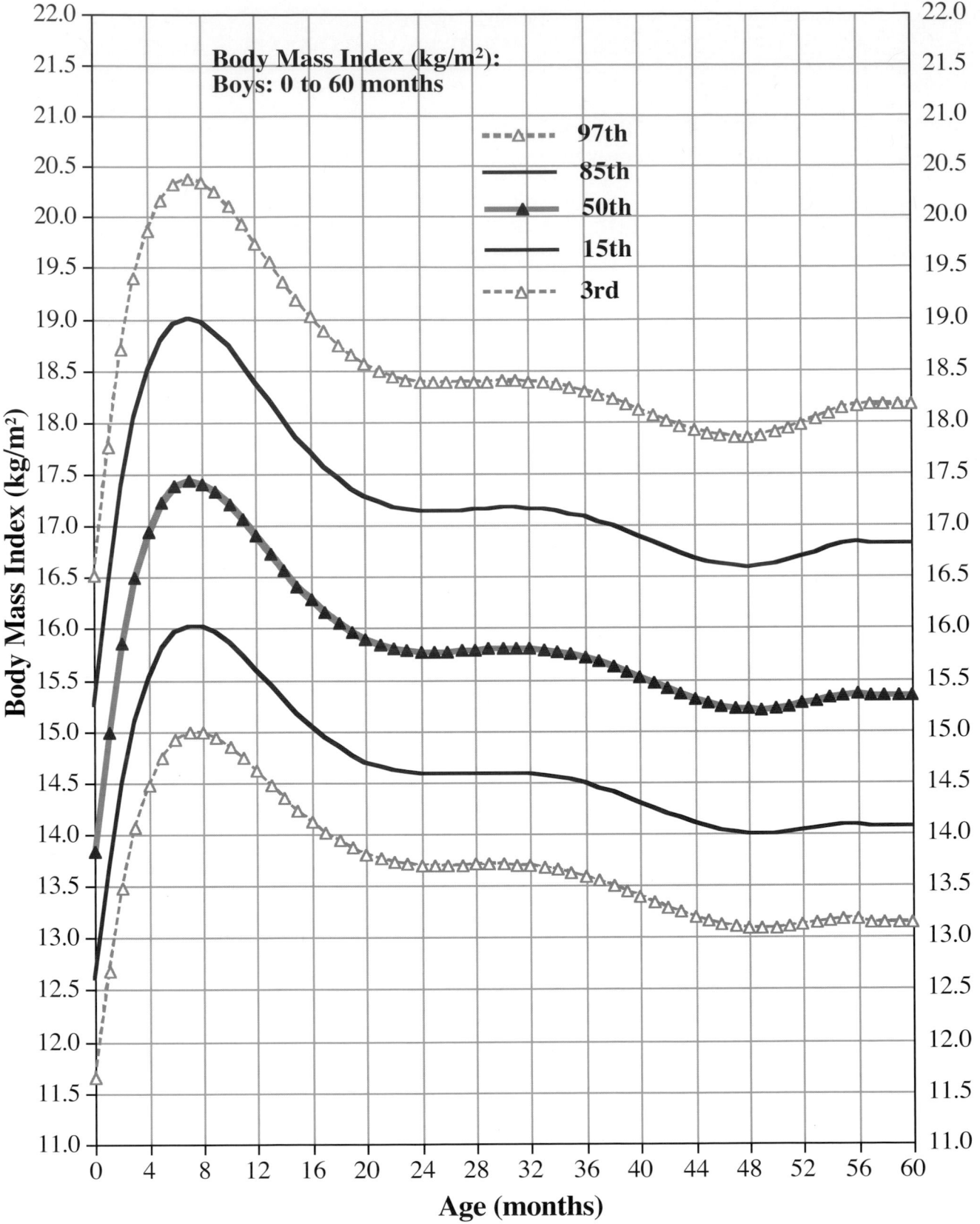

Figure V.21. Percentiles of Body Mass Index (kg/m²) by Age for Boys Ranging in Age from Birth to 5 Years.

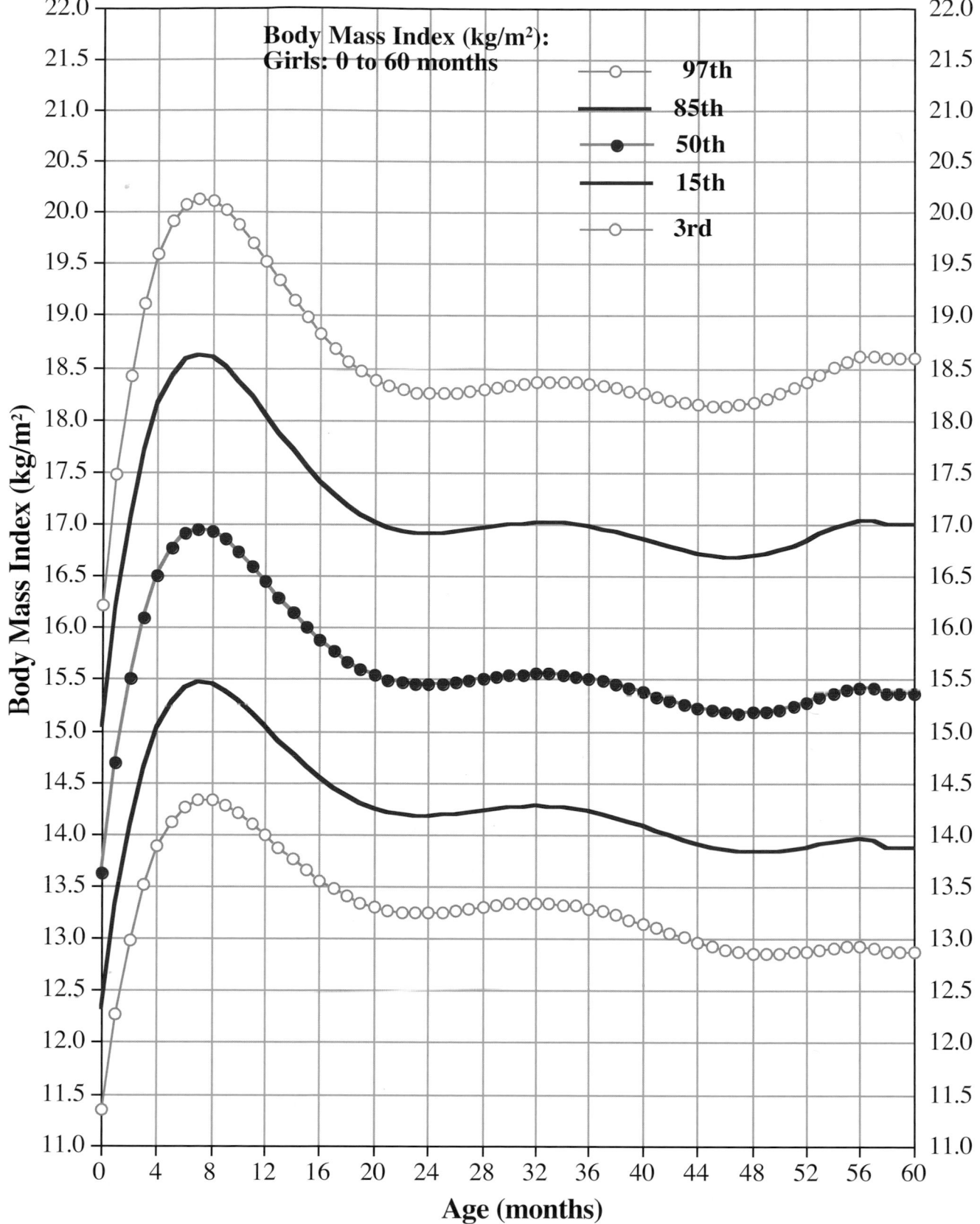

Figure V.22. Percentiles of Body Mass Index (kg/m²) by Age for Girls Ranging in Age from Birth to 5 Years.

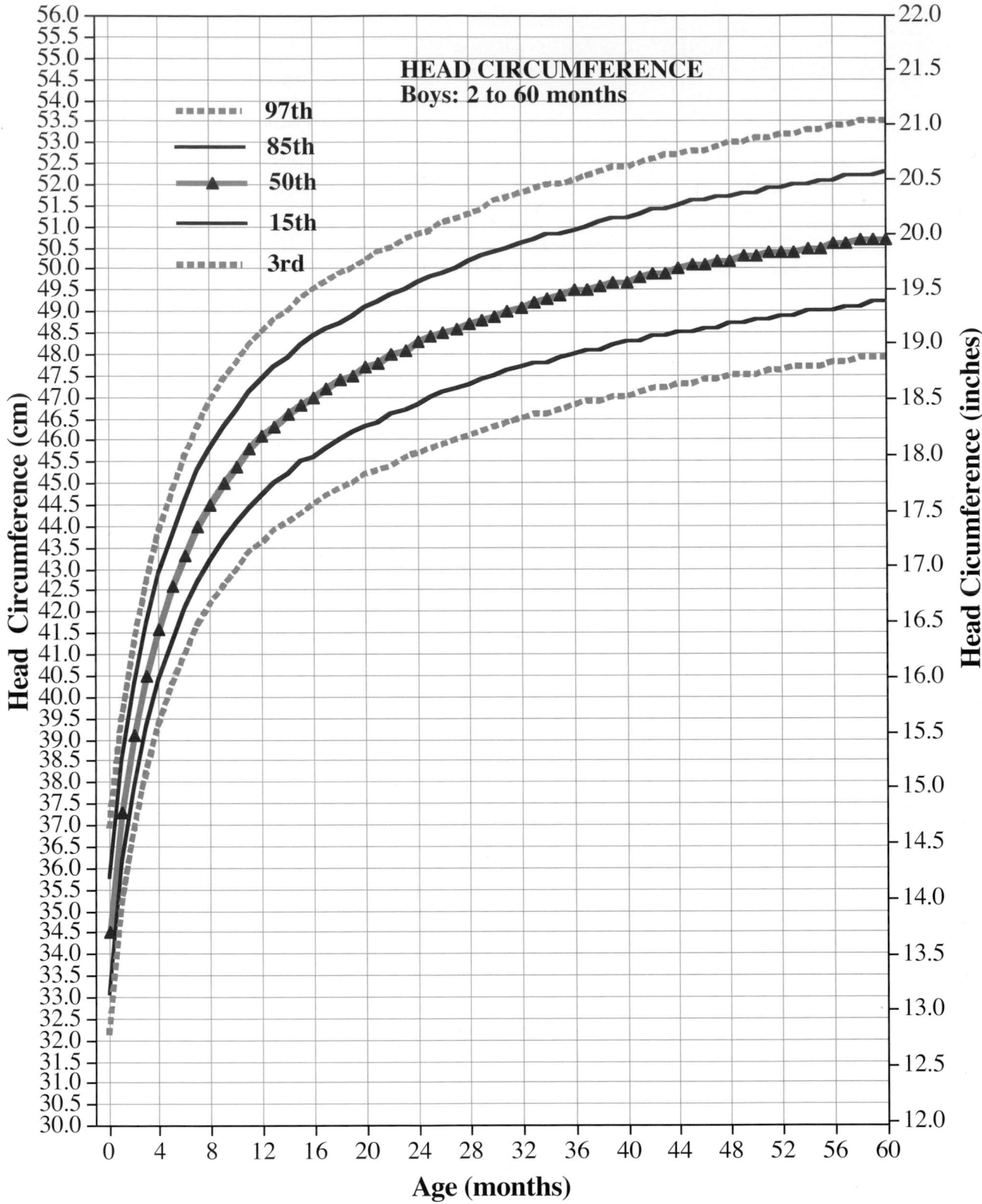

Figure V.23. Percentiles of Head Circumference (cm and in.) by Age for Boys Ranging in Age from Birth to 5 Years.

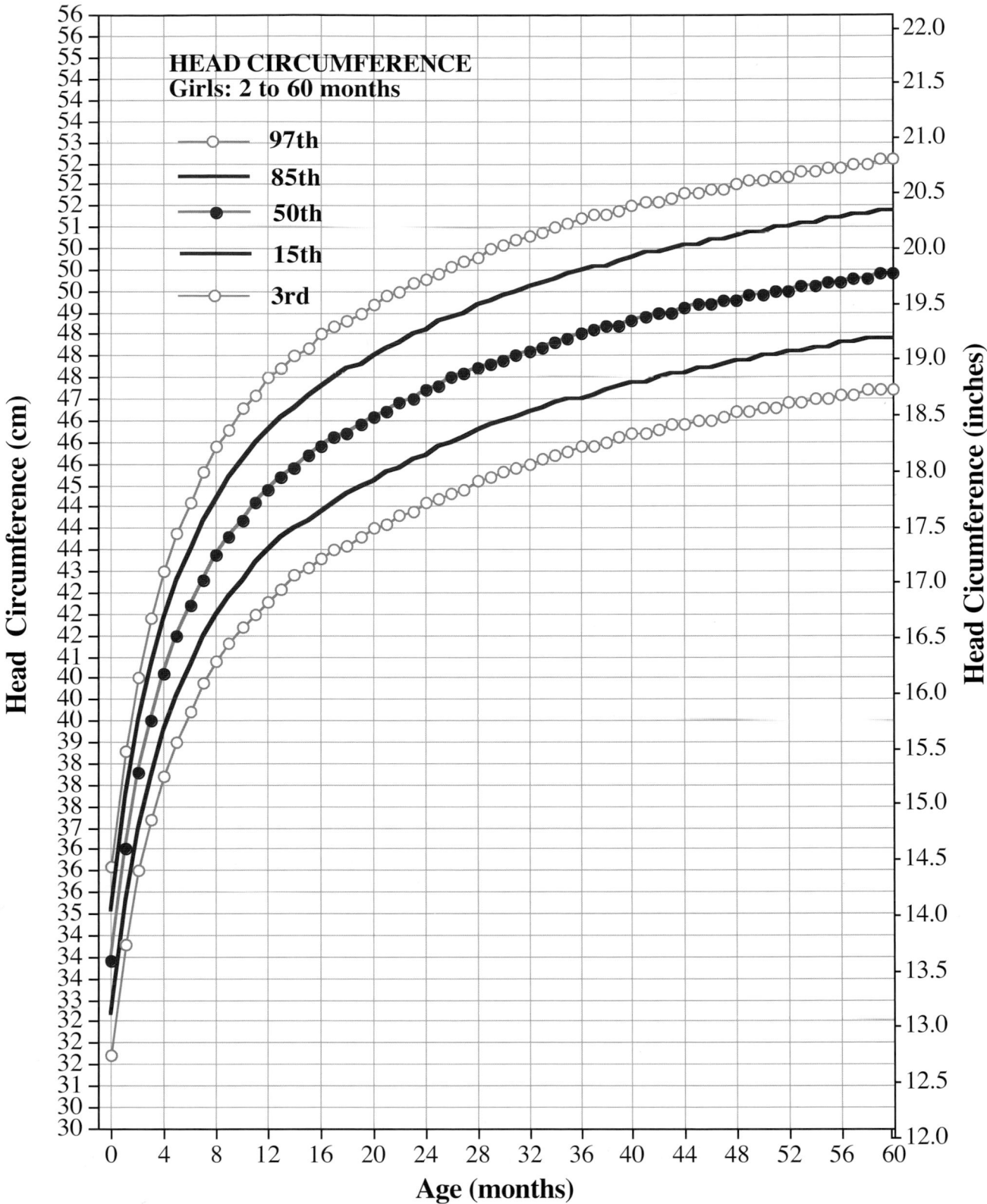

Figure V.24. Percentiles of Head Circumference (cm and in.) by Age for Girls Ranging in Age from Birth to 5 Years.

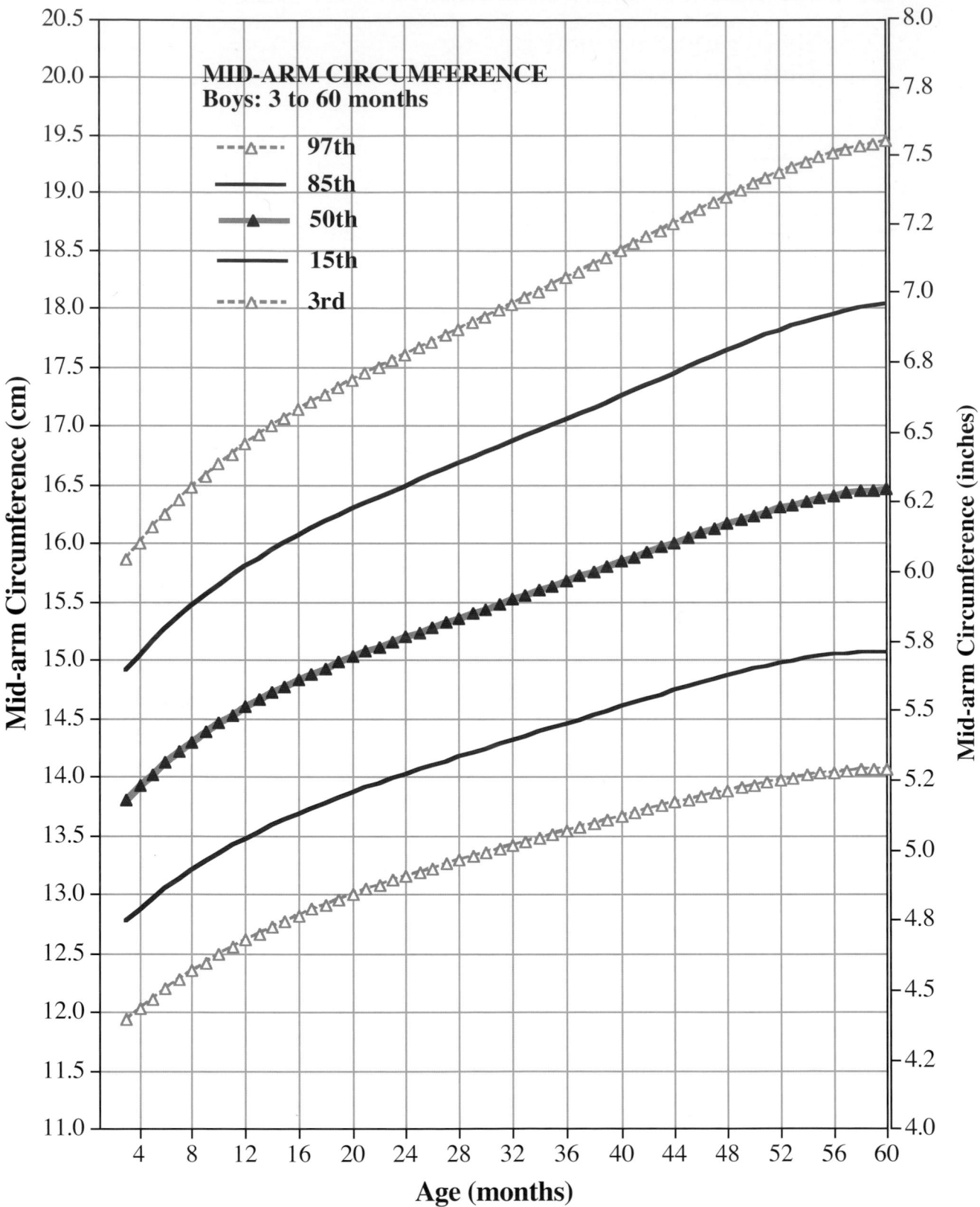

Figure V.25. Percentiles of Mid-Arm Circumference (cm and in.) by Age for Boys Ranging in Age from 3 Months to 5 Years.

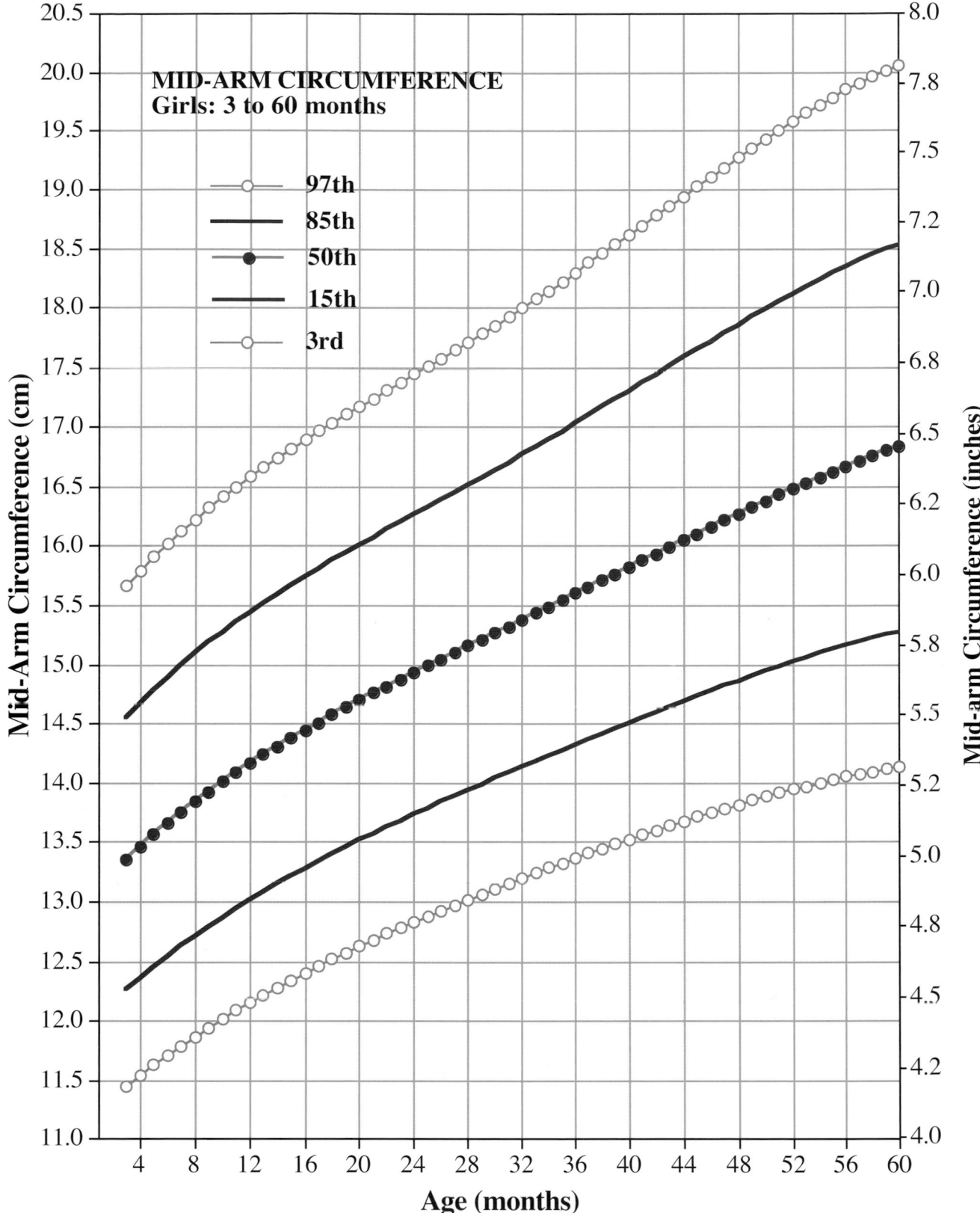

Figure V.26. Percentiles of Mid-Arm Circumference (cm and in.) by Age for Girls Ranging in Age from 3 Months to 5 Years.

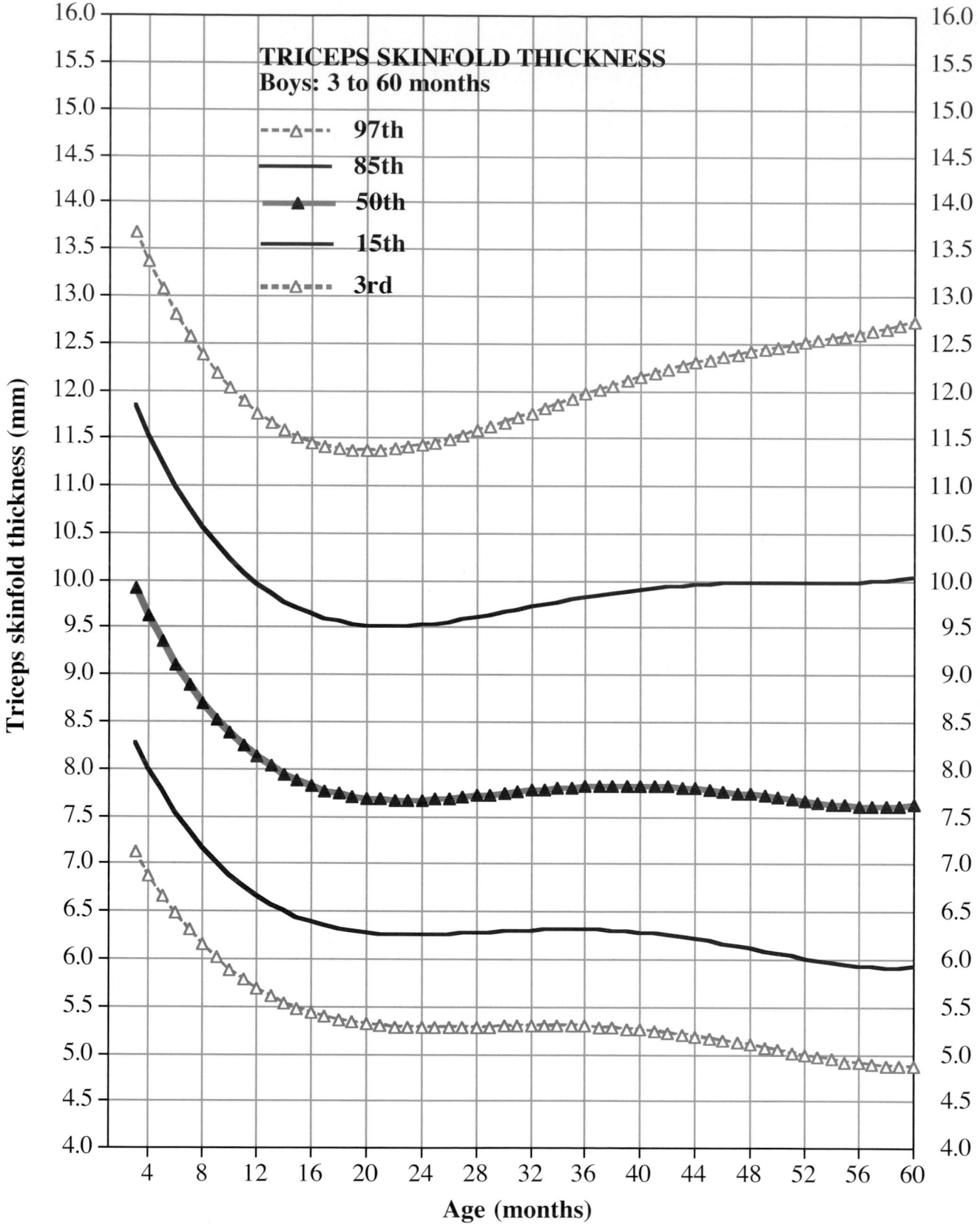

Figure V.27. Percentiles of Triceps Skinfold (mm) by Age for Boys Ranging in Age from 3 Months to 5 Years.

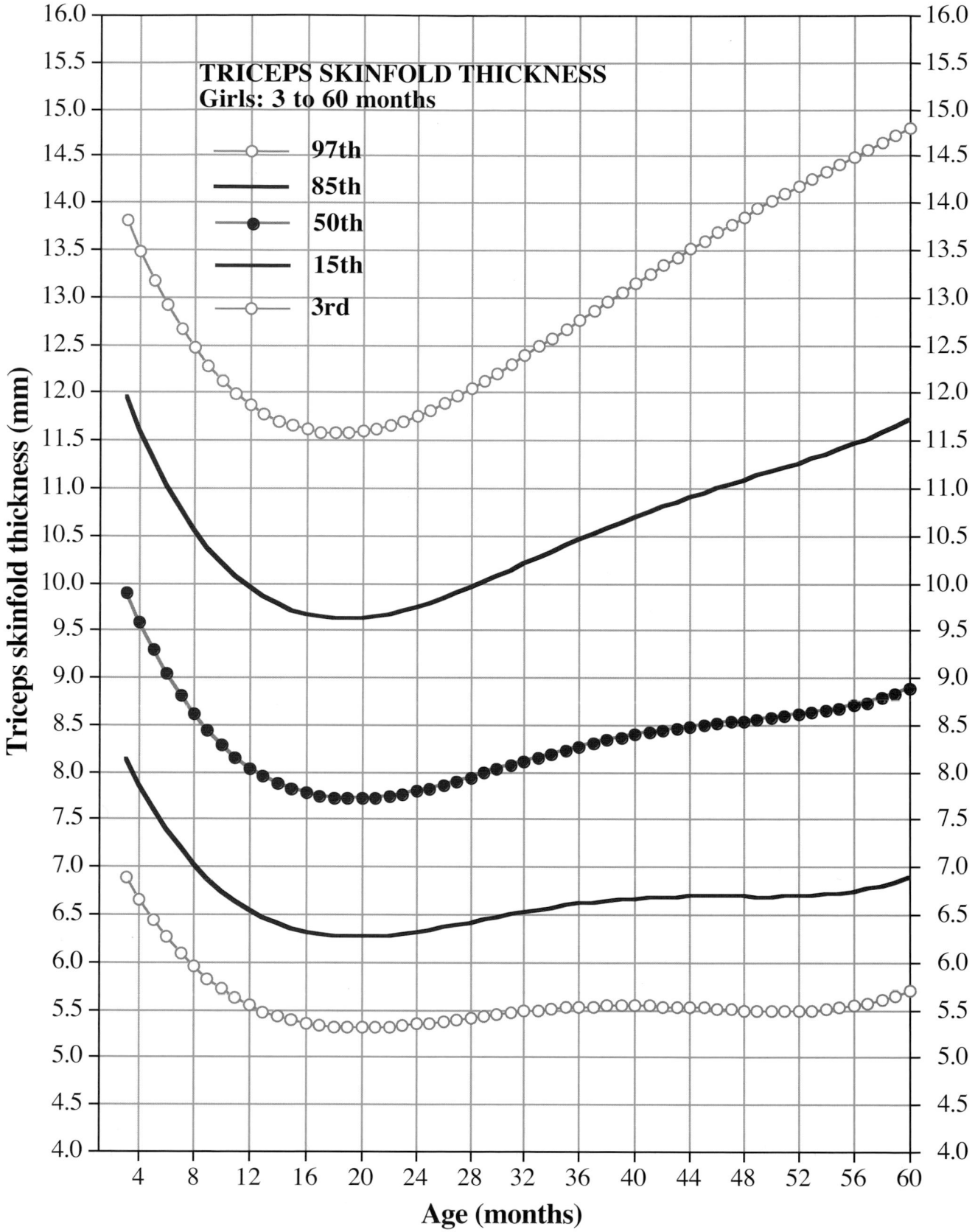

Figure V.28. Percentiles of Triceps Skinfold (mm) by Age for Girls Ranging in Age from 3 Months to 5 Years.

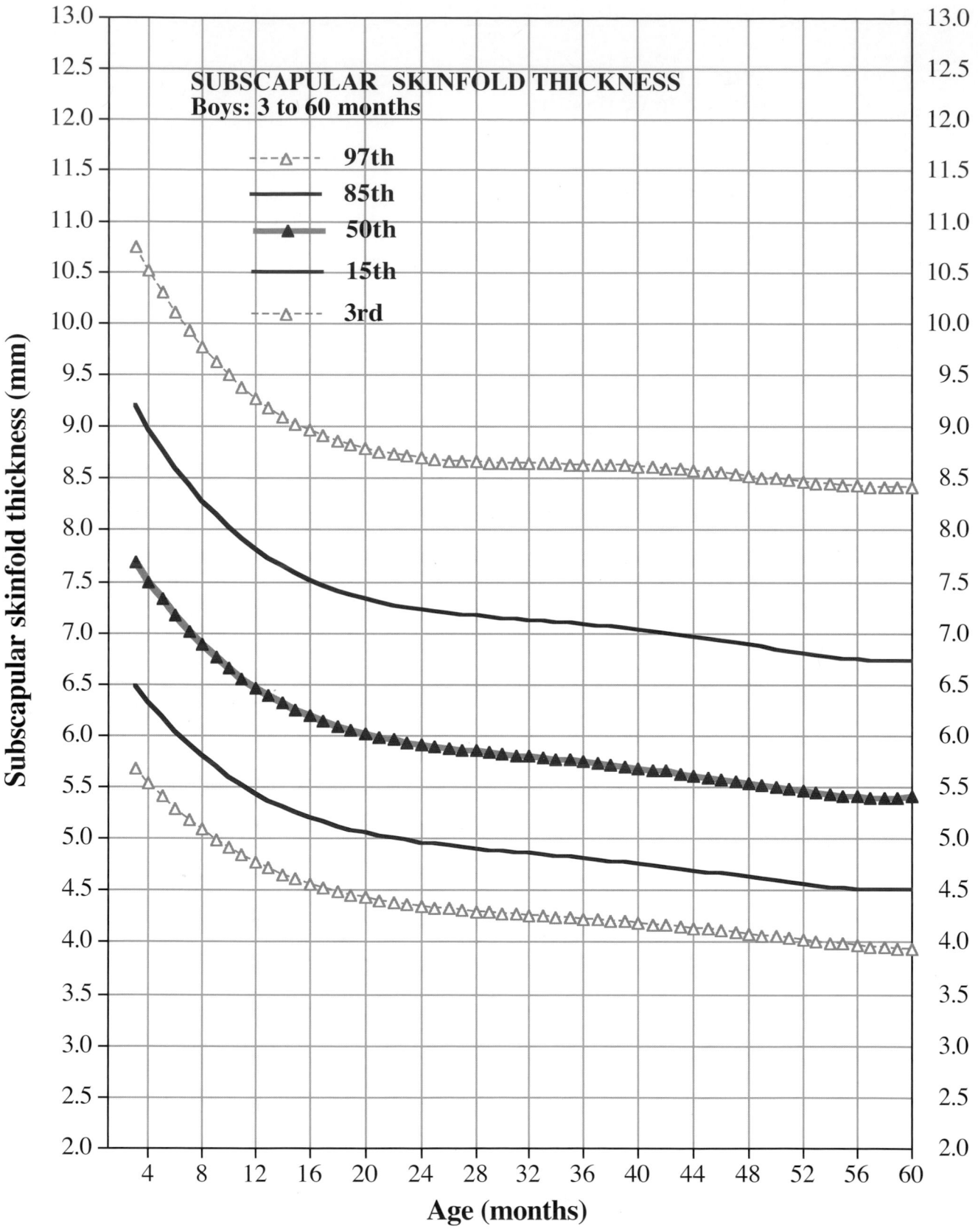

Figure V.29. Percentiles of Subscapular Skinfold (mm) by Age for Boys Ranging in Age from 3 Months to 5 Years.

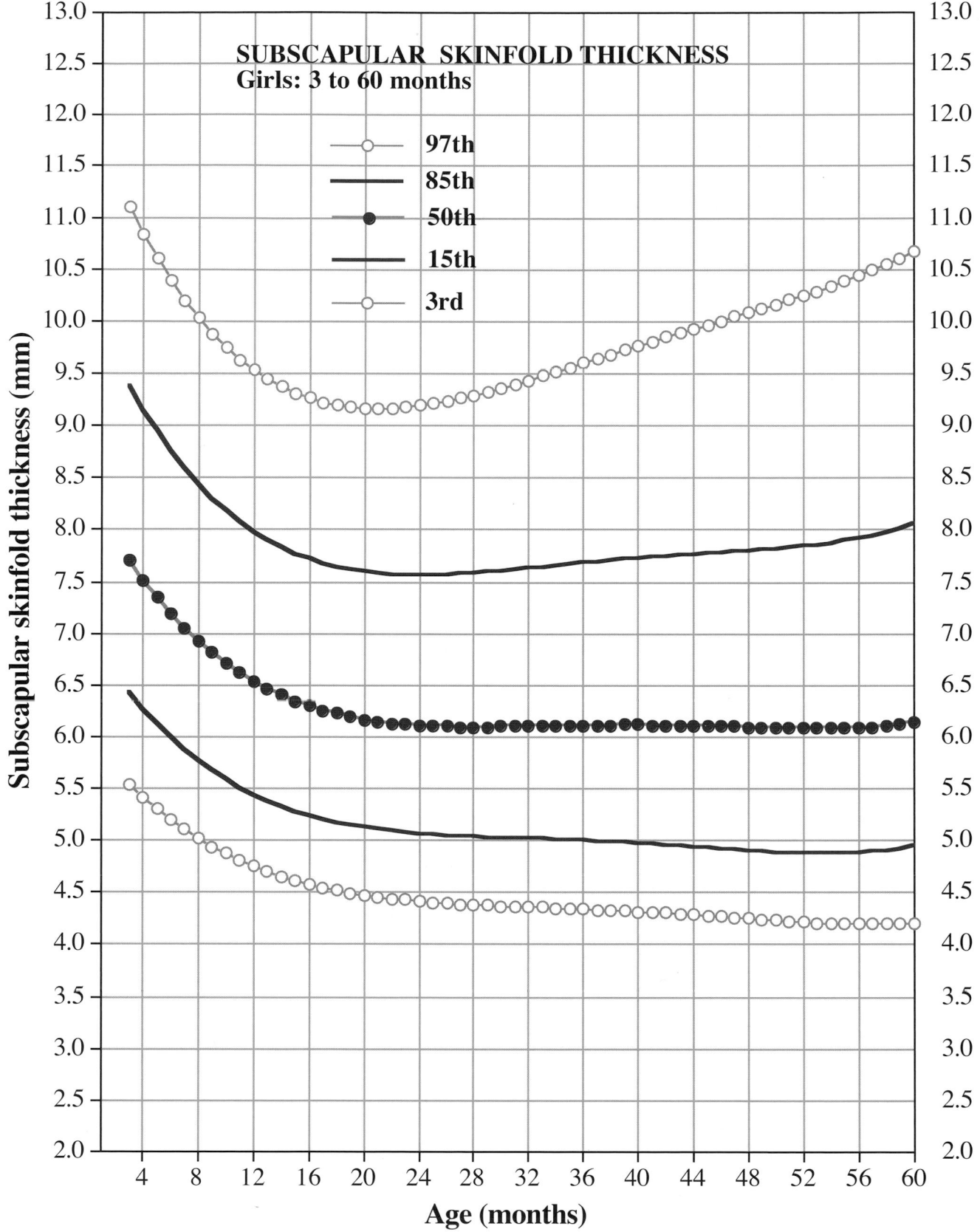

Figure V.30. Percentiles of Subscapular Skinfold (mm) by Age for Girls Ranging in Age from 3 Months to 5 Years.

LIMITATIONS OF THE WHO GROWTH STANDARDS

The goal of the WHO growth standards was to develop a universal *reference or standard* that embodies the concept of a norm. It was based upon a selected sample of children who met rigorous standards of health. These children not only had to be free of debilitating diseases, but also had to come from families that had conformed with health recommendations in areas such as breast-feeding and smoking cessation, recruited from all of the world's major regions to underscore that all children, regardless of ethnic background or regional origin, grow similarly when their needs are met (2). In addition, the primary criterion for inclusion in the study was that the children should be born in cities located at an altitude 1500 m or less above sea level (2). However, it should be indicated that as of 1994 of the total of 5617.5 million inhabitants, 7% live below 1500 m altitude above sea level and the remaining 93% of the world population lives at altitudes higher than 1500 m above sea level (10). However, the distribution of populations that live above 1500 m above sea level is not uniform throughout the world (11). For example, among Andean populations in North and South American countries such as Mexico, Peru, Ecuador and Bolivia, altitudes around 2500 m have higher population density (>1000 people/km^2) than lower altitudes. Likewise, Andean populations and Tibetan populations have a greater density at altitudes above 3500 m than below. Furthermore, previous studies demonstrate that for populations that live above an altitude of 1500 m above sea level, irrespective of socio-economic status and throughout the world, the weight at birth is decreased about 100 to 2500 grams when compared to those that live 1500 m above sea level (12-24). As a consequence of this difference, an undetermined excess fraction of the children born at high altitude would be improperly qualified as "low weight." Conversely, a high proportion of children born at high altitude would be considered as "acceptable" weight, even though they had a birth weight that is above the 95th percentile for high altitude populations.

Hence, the WHO growth standards need to be adjusted to take into account regional differences in birth weight associated with altitude. However, during postnatal development the WHO growth standards may be applicable to all populations without making any modifications because after the first two years of postnatal life growth trajectories of both low and high altitude populations are similar (15, 25-27).

MILESTONES OF MOTOR DEVELOPMENT OF CHILDREN

Because motor behavior is an important aspect of child development the WHO and the MGRS also established the ages of achievement of six gross motor milestones such as sitting without support, hands-and-knees crawling, standing with assistance, walking with assistance, standing alone, and walking alone that are fundamental to acquiring self-sufficient erect locomotion.

Table V.28. MGRS performance criteria for six motor milestones*

Gross motor milestones	MGRS criteria
Sitting without support	Child sits up straight with the head erect for at least 10 seconds. Child does not use arms or hands to balance body or support position.
Hands-and-knees crawling	Child alternately moves forward or backward on hands and knees. The stomach does not touch the ground. There are continuous and consecutive movements, at least three in a row.
Standing with assistance	Child stands in upright position on both feet, holding onto a stable object with both hands without leaning on it for at least 10 seconds. The body does not touch the stable object, and the legs support most of the body weight.
Walking with assistance	Child is in upright position with the back straight. Child makes sideways or forward steps by holding onto a stable object with one or both hands. One leg moves forward while the other supports part of the body weight. Child takes at least five steps in this manner.
Standing alone	Child stands alone for at least 10 seconds. Child stands in upright position on both feet (not on the toes) with the back straight. The legs support 100% of the child's weight. There is no contact with a person or object.
Walking alone	Child takes at least five steps independently in upright position with the back straight. One leg moves forward while the other supports most of the body weight. There is no contact with a person or object.

*Adapted from: ref. #8: Wijnhoven TMA et al. 2004. Assessment of gross motor development in the WHO Multicentre Growth Reference Study. Food and Nutrition Bulletin, Vol. 25, no. 1 (supplement 1).

The assessments were done monthly from 4 until 12 months of age and bimonthly thereafter until children could walk alone or reached 24 months. All milestones were assessed in all the cultural settings using the same standardized criteria and procedures as shown in **Table**

V.28. The results of this study are summarized in **Figure V.31**. These data show that although there is an average age at which the six universal growth milestones are achieved, each milestone has a wide age variability that ranges from 5.7 to 10.7 months. Analysis of the relationships among physical growth indicators and ages of achievement of the six gross motor milestones in the WHO Child Growth Standards population indicate that the attainment of each motor milestone is largely independent of variations in physical growth (9). However, from a practical perspective the observed milestones in motor development serve as a baseline and are expected to be of significant educational value to parents and health-care providers.

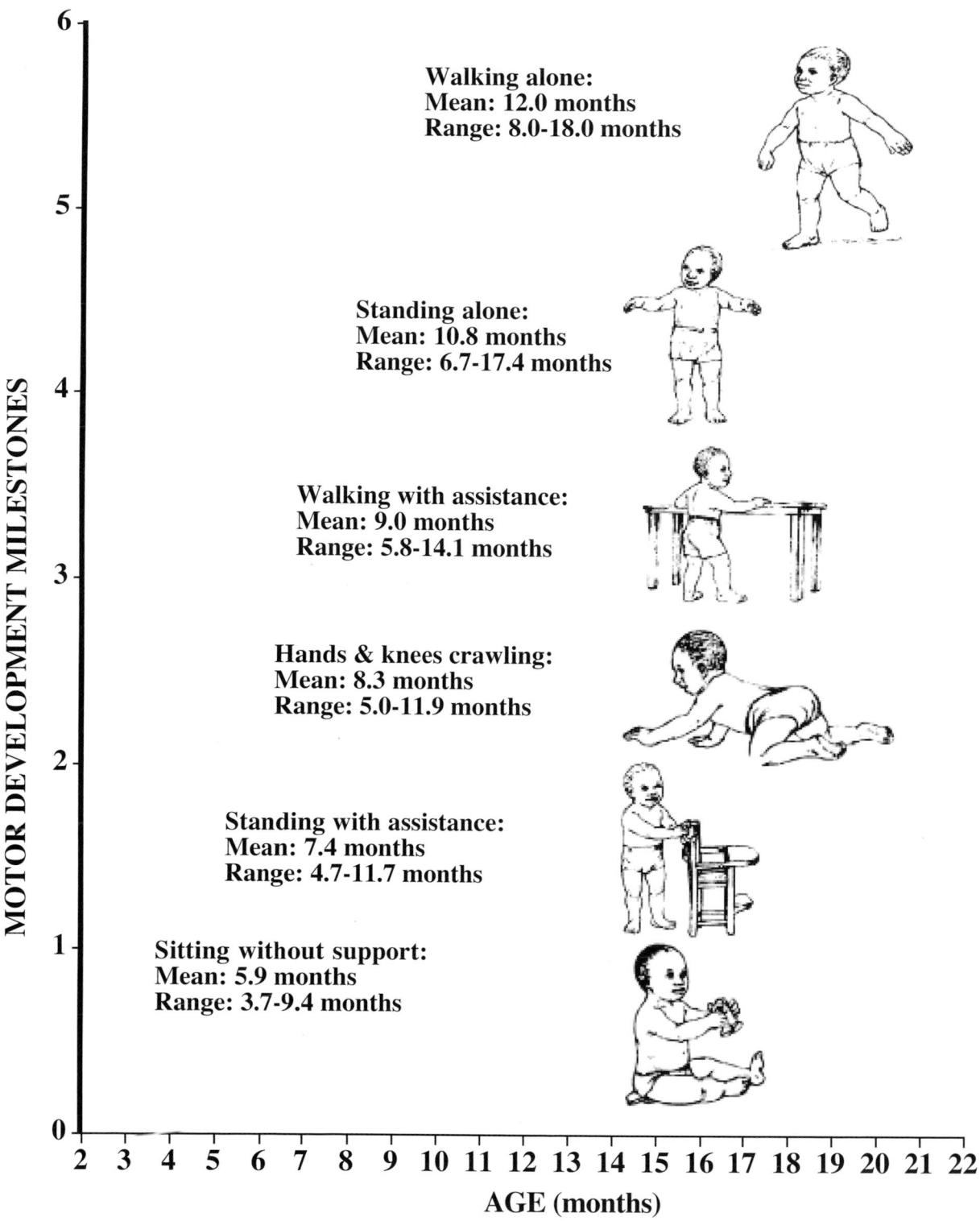

MOTOR DEVELOPMENT MILESTONES

AGE (months)

Walking alone:
Mean: 12.0 months
Range: 8.0-18.0 months

Standing alone:
Mean: 10.8 months
Range: 6.7-17.4 months

Walking with assistance:
Mean: 9.0 months
Range: 5.8-14.1 months

Hands & knees crawling:
Mean: 8.3 months
Range: 5.0-11.9 months

Standing with assistance:
Mean: 7.4 months
Range: 4.7-11.7 months

Sitting without support:
Mean: 5.9 months
Range: 3.7-9.4 months

Figure V.31. Motor Development Milestones of Infant Development. Based upon data from ref. #2: http://www.who.int/nutrition/topics/childgrowth/en/index.html and ref. #8: Wijnhoven TMA et al. 2004. Assessment of gross motor development in the WHO Multicentre Growth Reference Study. Food and Nutrition Bulletin, Vol. 25, no. 1 (supplement 1).

LITERATURE CITED

1. National Health and Nutrition Examination Survey. Anthropometric Reference Data, United States, 1988-1994. Available online at: http://www.cdc.gov/growthcharts/

2. http://www.who.int/nutrition/topics/childgrowth/en/index.html.

3. Garza, C., de Onis, M. 2004. WHO Multicentre Growth Reference Study Group. Rationale for developing a new international growth reference. Food Nutr. Bull. 25: Suppl 1:S5–S14. [Medline]

4. de Onis, M., Garza, C., Victora, C. G., Onyango, A. W., Frongillo, E. A., Martines, J. 2004. WHO Multicentre Growth Reference Study Group. The WHO Multicentre Growth Reference Study: planning, study design and methodology. Food Nutr. Bull. 25: Suppl 1:S15–26.

5. WHO Multicentre Growth Reference Study Group. 2006. Assessment of differences in linear growth among populations in the WHO Multicentre Growth Reference Study. Acta. Paediatr. Suppl 450:56–65.

6. Onyango, A. W., de Onis, M., Caroli, M., Shah, U., Sguassero, Y., Redondo, N., Carroli, B. 2007. Field-testing of the WHO child growth standards in four countries. J. Nutr. 137:149–152.

7. de Onis, M., Garza, C., Onyango, A. W., Borghi, E. 2007. Comparison of the WHO Child Growth Standards and the CDC 2000 Growth Charts. J. Nutr. 137:144-148.

8. Wijnhoven, T. M. A., de Onis, M., Onyango, A. W., Wang, T., Bjoerneboe, G. E. A., Bhandari, N., Lartey, A., Rashidi, B. A. 2004. Assessment of gross motor development in the WHO Multicentre Growth Reference Study. Food Nutr. Bull., 25, no. 1 (supplement 1). The United Nations University.

9. WHO Multicentre Growth Reference Study Group. 2006. Relationship between physical growth and motor development in the WHO Child Growth Standards. Acta Paediatr., Suppl 450:96–101.

10. Cohen J. E., Small, C. 1998. Hypsographic demography: the distribution of human population by altitude. Proc. Natl. Acad. Sci. USA 95:14009–14014.

11. Pérez-Padilla, R. 2002. Population distribution residing at different altitudes: implications for hypoxemia. Arch. Med. Res. 33:162–166.

12. Yip, R. 1987. Altitude and birth weight. J. Pediatr. 111:869–876.

13 Unger, C., Weiser, J. K., McCullough, R. E., Keefer, S., Moore, L. G. 1988. Altitude, low birth weight, and infant mortality in Colorado. JAMA 17;259:3427–3432.

14. Jensen, G. M., Moore, L. G. 1997. The effect of high altitude and other risk factors on birthweight: independent or interactive effects? Am. J. Public Health 87:1003–1007.

15. Frisancho, A. R. 2006. Humankind Evolving. An Exploration on the Origins of Human Diversity. Dubuque, IA: Kendall/Hunt Publishers, Inc.

16. Haas, J. D. 1980. Maternal adaptation and fetal growth at high altitude in Bolivia. In Social and Biological Predictors of Nutritional Status, Physical Growth, and Neurological Development. L. S. Greene, F. E. Johnston, Eds. 257–290. New York/London: Academic.

17. Beall, C. M. 1981. Optimal birth weights in Peruvian populations at high and low altitudes. Am. J. Phys. Anthropol. 56:209–216.

18. Mortola, J. P., Frappell, P. B., Aguero, L., Armstrong, K. 2000. Birth weight and altitude: a study in Peruvian communities. J. Pediatr. 136:324-329.

19. Hartinger, S., Tapia, V., Carrillo, C., Bejarano, L., Gonzales, G. F. 2006. Birth weight at high altitudes in Peru. Int. J. Gynaecol. Obstet. 93:275-278.

20. Giussani, D. A., Seamus Phillips, P., Anstee, S., Barker, D. J. P. 2001. Effects of altitude versus economic status on birth weight and body shape at birth. Pediatr. Res. 49:490–494.

21. Zamudio, S., Palmer, S. K., Dahms, T. E., Berman, J. C., McCullough, R. G., McCullough, R. E., Moore, L. G. 1993. Blood volume expansion, preeclampsia, and infant birth weight at high altitude. J. Appl. Physiol. 75:1566–1573.

22. Moore, L. G., Shriver, M., Bemis, L., Hickler, B., Wilson, M., Brutsaert, T., Parra, E., Vargas, E. 2004. Maternal adaptation to high-altitude pregnancy: an experiment of nature—a review. Placenta. Suppl A:S60-71.

23. Vargas, M., Vargas, E., Julian, C. G., Armaza, J. F., Rodriguez, A., Tellez, W., Niermeyer, S., Wilson, M. J., Parra, E., Shriver, M., Moore, L. G. 2007. Determinants of blood oxygenation during pregnancy in Andean and European residents of high altitude. Am. J. Physiol. Regul. Integr. Comp. Physiol. 2007, July 3.

24. Lopez Camelo, J. S., Campana, H., Santos, R., Poletta, F. A. 2006. Effect of the interaction between high altitude and socioeconomic factors on birth weight in a large sample from South America. Am. J. Phys. Anthropol. 129:305–310.

25. Leonard, W. R. 1989. Nutritional determinants of high altitude growth in Nuñoa, Perú. Am. J. Phys. Anthropol. 80:341–352.

26. Obert, P., Fellman, N., Falgairette, G., Bedu, M., Van Praagh, E., Kemper, H., Post, B., Spielvogel, H., Tellez, V., A. Qintela. 1994. The importance of socioeconomic and nutritional conditions rather than altitude on the physical growth of prepubertal Andean highland boys. Ann. Hum. Biol. 21:145–154.

27. Pawson, I. G., Huicho, L., Muro, M., A. Pacheco. 2001. Growth of children in two economically diverse Peruvian high-altitude communities. Am. J. Hum. Biol. 13:323–340.

CHAPTER VI
EVALUATION OF POSTNATAL GROWTH AND NUTRITIONAL STATUS OF CHILDREN AND ADULTS USING THE NHANES III ANTHROPOMETRIC REFERENCE

GENERAL DESCRIPTIVE STATISTICAL INFORMATION
Z-Score
Percentile
Percentiles and Z-Scores

CATEGORIES OF GROWTH AND NUTRITIONAL STATUS
Weight
Rohrer's Index
Body Mass Index
Body Mass Index and Skinfold Thickness
Height
Adjustment of Children's Height for Parent's Height
Leg Length and Developmental History
Head Circumference
Mid-Upper Arm Muscle Area
Waist Circumference
Fat-Free Mass and Fat-Free Mass Index
Body Fat and Fat Mass Index
Excess Body Fat and the Metabolic Syndrome
Classification of Body Mass Index
Waist Circumference and Body Mass Index

SUMMARY

LITERATURE CITED

CHAPTER VI

EVALUATION OF POSTNATAL GROWTH AND NUTRITIONAL STATUS OF CHILDREN AND ADULTS USING THE NHANES III ANTHROPOMETRIC REFERENCE

GENERAL DESCRIPTIVE STATISTICAL INFORMATION

The present anthropometric reference is applicable to surveys addressed at determining the growth and nutritional status and body composition of children and adults ranging in age from birth to 90 years. This reference is also very applicable to surveys where the age of participants is rounded to the nearest year. On the other hand, for studies where the age of children is rounded to the nearest month the CDC and WHO growth standards given in Chapter V are the appropriate references to evaluate growth and nutritional status from birth to 20 years. Likewise, the evaluation of growth status of very low birth weight (VLBW) infants (birth weights of <1500 grams, or <3.3 lb.) should be done with reference to the growth chart for preterm babies (2,3). However, the following statistical approaches are applicable to all three anthropometric references.

Z-Score

A productive way for determining the individual's or the population's nutritional status is to determine how the measurements compare to an anthropometric reference that is based upon normally distributed variables categories. A Z-score tells the distance in standard deviation units the value is above or below the mean. Since the Z-score and percentile distribution are calculated with regard to age-specific and sex-specific anthropometric references, they provide a common standard for comparison of different measures. In addition, probability values for all sample values are known. For example, in a normal distribution, approximately 68% of values lie within 1 standard deviation of the mean. Approximately 95% of values lie within 2 standard deviations of the mean. Approximately 2.1% of values lie below 2 standard deviations below the mean. Approximately 2.1% of values lie above 2 standard deviations above the mean. Furthermore, because the cutoff points are comparable across anthropometric dimensions and across all ages, Z-scores can be used to classify the anthropometric measurements into categories of nutritional status.

Percentile

A percentile is a value on a scale of one hundred that indicates the percent of a distribution that is equal to or below it. Percentiles range from lowest to highest, with the average equal to 50. A percentile ranks the individual measurement relative to the other individuals used in the reference. For instance, if a child's height is equal to the 15th percentile that means that the child's score is equivalent to that achieved by 15% of children of the same age. Likewise, if the child's height is equivalent to the 95th percentile of height, it implies that 95% of the population for his age and gender is smaller.

Percentiles and Z-Scores

As illustrated in **Figure VI.1** and **Table VI.1**, a value that is less than 1.65 and 1.04 Z-scores from the mean is comparable to a value that is below the 5th and 15th percentile. Conversely, a value that is above the 85th and 95th percentile is comparable to a value that is 1.04 and 1.65 Z-scores above the mean. From this it follows that an individual's anthropometric dimension can be classified into five statistical categories whose upper limit of normality is the 95th percentile, as shown in **Table VI.2**. Therefore the use of Z-scores and percentiles maximizes the diagnostic effectiveness of anthropometric information even when the sample size is small. They can be used to determine the inter-relationship among anthropometric dimensions and their relations to independent and non-independent variables.

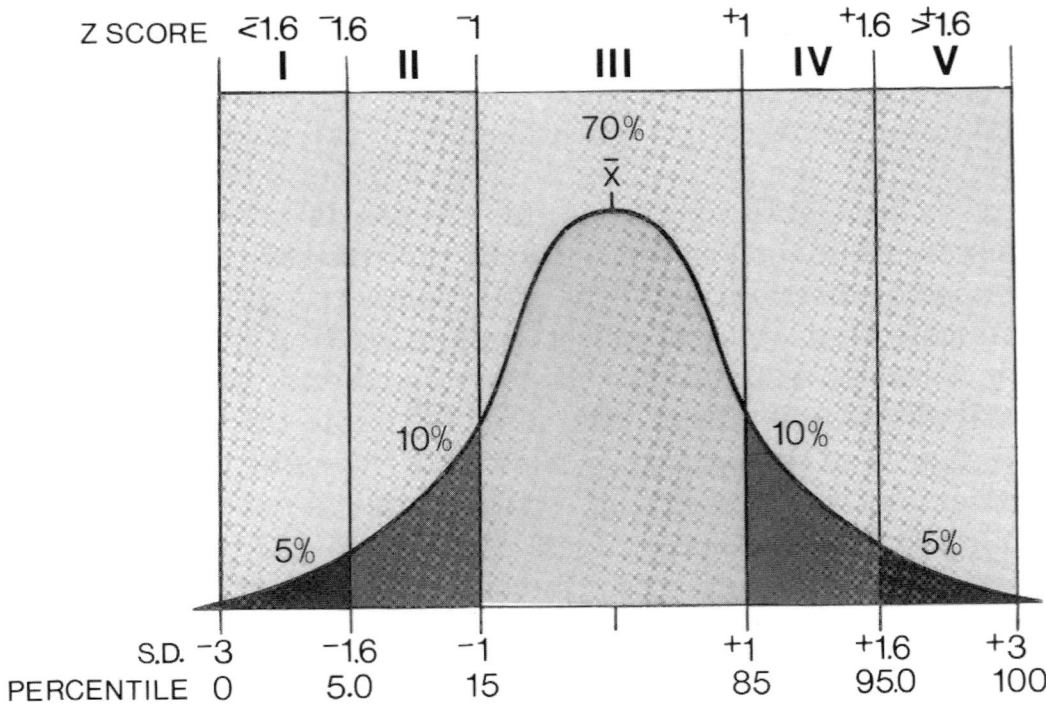

Figure VI.1. Schematization of the Statistical Relationship of Z-Scores, Percentile Ranges, and Standard Deviations. Adapted from refer. #1: Frisancho AR. 1990. Anthropometric Standards for the Assessment of Growth and Nutritional Status. Ann Arbor, MI: University of Michigan Press.

Table VI.1. Equivalents of Percentile and Z-scores in a Normal Distribution

Below Mean		Above Mean	
Percentile	**Z-score**	**Percentile**	**Z-score**
0.0 to 4.9	-3.090 to -1.650	50.0 to 54.9	0.000 to 0.120
5.0 to 9.9	-1.645 to -1.290	55.0 to 59.9	0.126 to 0.250
10.0 to 14.9	-1.282 to -1.040	60.0 to 64.9	0.253 to 0.380
15.0 to 19.9	-1.036 to -0.850	65.0 to 69.9	0.385 to 0.520
20.0 to 24.9	-0.842 to -0.680	70.0 to 74.9	0.524 to 0.670
25.0 to 29.9	-0.675 to -0.530	75.0 to 79.9	0.675 to 0.840
30.0 to 34.9	-0.524 to -0.390	80.0 to 84.9	0.842 to 1.030
35.0 to 39.9	-0.385 to -0.260	85.0 to 89.9	1.036 to 1.280
40.0 to 44.9	-0.253 to -0.130	90.0 to 94.9	1.282 to 1.640
45.0 to 50.0	-0.126 to -0.000	95.0 to 99.9	1.645 to 3.090

Table VI.2. Categories of Anthropometric Nutritional Status Based on Z-scores and Percentile

Statistical Category	Nutritional Anthropometry	Percentile and Z-scores Equivalents
I	Low	Below the 5th percentile or Z-score is less than -1.650.
II	Below Average	5.0 to 15th percentile or Z-score is between -1.645 and -1.040.
III	Healthy Range	15.1 to 85th percentile or Z-score is between -1.036 and +1.030.
IV	Above Average	85.1 to 95th percentile or Z-score is between +1.036 and +1.640.
V	Excessive	Above the 95.1th to 100th percentile or Z-score is equal to or greater than +1.645.

*Adapted from refer. #1: Frisancho AR. 1990. Anthropometric Standards for the Assessment of Growth and Nutritional Status. Ann Arbor, MI: University of Michigan Press.

CATEGORIES OF GROWTH AND NUTRITIONAL STATUS

Weight

The tabular data of means, standard deviations, and percentiles of weight of children and adolescents, by age and sex, is given in **Tables IV.1** and **IV.5**. **Figures IV.7** to **IV.8** and **IV.15** to **IV.16** provide, in graphic form, the age-associated changes in weight of children and adolescents. Body thinness and excess weight of children can be inferred from evaluations of weight-for-age. For example, a child whose weight-for-age is below the 5th percentile (Category I) can be classified as underweight and undernourished, while another whose weight-for-age is above the 85th percentile (Category IV or V) indicates excess weight.

Rohrer's Index

Measurements of Rohrer's index provide information for determining the components of variability in body weight of infants. Thus, a child whose Rohrer's index is below the 5th percentile (Category I) can be classified as underweight and undernourished, while another whose Rohrer's index is above the 85th percentile (Category IV or V) certainly indicates good nutritional status, which is also reflected in high stature by age. The tabular data of means, standard deviations, and percentiles of Rohrer's index of infants by age and sex is given in **Table IV.3. Figures IV.10** and **IV.11** provide, in graphic form, the age-associated changes in Rohrer's index of infants.

Body Mass Index

The International Obesity Task Force (IOTF) and the World Health Organization (WHO) (16,17) recommend that a BMI >85th percentile (specific for age and sex) is indicative of obesity in children and adolescents, while a BMI below the 5th percentile is indicative of underweight. The tabular data of means, standard deviations, and percentiles of body mass index is given in **Table IV.7**. **Figures IV.17** and **IV.18** present the age-associated changes in body mass index. Based upon this information children can be classified into four categories:

1. Undernutrition = <5th percentile
2. Underweight = between 5th and 15th percentile
3. Average weight or healthy range = between 15th and 85th percentile
4. Overweight = ≥85th percentile.

Body Mass Index and Skinfold Thickness

Because BMI is a measure of weight relative to height estimates of excess body fatness for children and adolescents must be made along with the measurement of skinfold thickness (88,89). Analysis of the relationship of percentage of body fat determined by dual-energy radiograph absorptiometry and skinfold measurements at the triceps and subscapular sites indicate that measurements of skinfold thickness provide additional information on excess body fat for pediatric subjects ages 5 to 18 years with BMI-for-age of the 85th to 95th percentiles but not for those with BMI-for-age 95th percentile (90, 91). In other words, once weight is very high the excess weight is associated not only high lean body mass but it is due to high amount of body fat.

Height

The measurements of height are presented in **Table IV.6** and **Figures IV.19** and **IV.20**. Based on this information there are three categories of risk nutritional status applicable to infants and children in general:

1. Stunted or chronic undernutrition = Z-score of ≤-1.645 of height-for-age (or height below 5th percentile for age and sex)

2. Normal or average range = Z-score -1.645 < Z to <+1.640 of height-for-age (or height between 5.1[th] and 95th percentile for age and sex)

3. Tall = Z-score > +1.645 of height-for-age (or height above 95th percentile for age and sex)

Adjustment of Children's Height for Parent's Height

In general, it is assumed that if children are tall for their age, they may be tall because their parents are tall or they may be tall because they grew in a positive environmental condition. On the other hand, if children are short for their age, this could be indicative of environmentally caused delayed growth. However, a child can be short for his age not only due to environmental factors but also because his parents are short (in which case he is probably genetically short). A productive way of taking into account the role of genetic factors is to evaluate growth with reference to parental statures. For this reason, the present standards of stature are incorporated with a reference that permits the adjustment of the child's stature to his or her parents' statures. **Table VI.3** gives the parent-offspring specific regression equations of stature published by Himes et al. (18). With these regression equations one can adjust the child's height for the parent's height. These regression equations were based upon well-nourished samples from the Fels Longitudinal study. This table provides information on age (column 1), median stature (column 2 or 7), standard deviation (SD) (column 3 or 8), a-intercept (column 4 or 9), b slope (column 5 or 10), and standard error (SE) (column 8 or 11). The application of these regression equations given in **Table VI.3** can be best shown by the following examples.

Example 1. 10-year-old girl whose stature (CS) = 126 cm, mother's stature (MS) = 155 cm, father's stature (FS) = 165 cm.

The regression equation for the adjustment of parents' height is as follows:

Adjustment for Parents' Height (As) = (Standard SD/SE) x [CS - (a + (b x MPS))] + (MdS - CS)

where As is the child stature adjusted for mid-parent height; SD, SE, a, b, and MdS correspond to the values given in Table III.1; CS is the child's stature; and MPS is the mid-parent stature,

(1) Calculate the mid-parent's stature (MPS) by adding the father and mother's stature and dividing the total by 2. In this case the MPS = 160 cm (MPS = 165 + 155/2). (When one parent's stature cannot be measured, ask the other parent whether the spouse is tall, medium or short and using **Table VI.3**, determine the corresponding stature to calculate the mid-parent stature.)

(2) Locate the age closest to that of the child, and for that age, use the corresponding values requested by the formula to obtain the adjustment for parent stature (AS):

Adj. for Parent's Height = (5.92/5.51) x [126 – (52.69 + (0.505 x 160))] + (138.3 – 126)

Adj. for Parent's Height = (1.07) x (–7.49) + (12.3) = 4.25 cm

Add the parent-specific adjustment to the child's stature if the adjustment has no sign; subtract the adjustment if it has a minus sign. Thus, in this case, the child's stature adjusted for mid-parents' stature should be 131.02 cm (126.0 + 4.25 = 130.25).

Compared to the standard of stature given in **Table IV.6**, the girl's height (126 cm) is below the 5th percentile, and when adjusted for her parents' heights (130 cm), her height is still between the 5th and 15th percentile. Therefore, the short stature of this girl is probably of genetic origin (or related to her parents' shortness).

Example 2. 8-year-old boy whose stature (CS) = 135 cm, father's stature (FS) = 187.0 cm, mother's stature (MS) = 165 cm, and mid-parent stature (MPS) = 176.0 cm (187 + 165/2). Accordingly, following the same procedure and applying the parent-offspring regression equations for the adjustment for parent stature, we have the following results:

Adj. for Parent's Height = (5.24/4.73) x [135 – (38.05 + (0.525 x 176))] + (127 – 135) = –3.82

Adj. for Parent's Height = (1.10) x (4.55) + (–8) = –2.96 cm

Compared to the standard of stature given in **Table IV.6**, the boy's height (135 cm) is above the 85th percentile, and when adjusted for his parents' heights, he should have been only 132.0 (135 – 2.96 = 132.0 cm). Therefore, the subject is tall for his age and considering his parents' heights, he is taller than expected.

Table VI.3. Medians, Standard Deviations, and Regression Equations for Parent-Specific Adjustments of Recumbent Length (cm) and Stature (cm) by Age for Boys and Girls Ranging in Age from Birth to 18 Years*

Age (years) (1)	Boys: Regression Equation					Girls: Regression Equation				
	Median (2)	SD (3)	a (4)	b (5)	SE (6)	Median (7)	SD (8)	a (9)	b (10)	SE (11)
Recumbent Length (cm), Age = Birth to 3 years										
Birth	50.5	2.37	35.36	0.089	2.35	49.9	1.98	44.04	0.035	1.97
0.08	54.60	2.34	35.53	0.113	2.29	53.50	2.07	42.76	0.063	2.05
0.50	67.80	2.34	40.42	0.162	2.25	65.90	2.32	40.41	0.151	2.23
0.75	72.30	2.49	41.94	0.179	2.37	70.40	2.48	37.93	0.192	2.35
1.00	76.10	2.75	42.59	0.198	2.62	74.30	2.69	36.42	0.224	2.51
1.50	82.40	3.02	44.06	0.226	2.87	80.90	2.88	38.74	0.249	2.64
2.00	87.60	3.26	42.61	0.266	3.06	86.50	3.02	40.12	0.274	2.75
2.50	92.30	3.46	41.26	0.301	3.22	91.30	3.19	40.46	0.300	2.88
3.00	96.50	3.62	41.73	0.323	3.35	95.60	3.39	40.49	0.325	3.06
Stature (cm), Age = 2.5 to 18 years										
2.50	90.40	3.91	25.88	0.381	3.57	90.00	3.08	35.15	0.324	2.76
3.00	94.90	3.90	32.37	0.369	3.57	94.10	3.37	39.37	0.323	3.08
3.50	99.10	3.92	36.56	0.369	3.60	97.90	3.59	42.05	0.330	3.29
4.00	102.90	4.00	39.02	0.377	3.68	101.60	3.78	42.85	0.347	3.44
4.50	106.60	4.16	39.75	0.395	3.81	105.00	3.96	42.53	0.369	3.59
5.00	109.90	4.34	40.24	0.411	3.98	108.40	4.12	42.16	0.391	3.73
5.50	113.10	4.51	40.95	0.426	4.13	111.60	4.27	40.99	0.417	3.86
6.00	116.10	4.66	40.97	0.444	4.25	114.60	4.44	39.40	0.444	4.00
6.50	119.00	4.77	40.38	0.464	4.33	117.60	4.59	39.24	0.463	4.14
7.00	121.70	4.89	39.24	0.487	4.42	120.60	4.72	40.83	0.471	4.26
7.50	124.40	5.05	38.31	0.508	4.56	123.50	4.85	42.76	0.477	4.39
8.00	127.00	5.24	38.05	0.525	4.73	126.40	4.99	44.38	0.484	4.54
8.50	129.60	5.37	38.38	0.539	4.86	129.30	5.14	45.80	0.493	4.69
9.00	132.20	5.46	38.20	0.555	4.93	132.20	5.34	47.40	0.501	4.88
9.50	134.80	5.57	37.14	0.577	5.02	135.20	5.59	49.77	0.504	5.14
10.00	137.50	5.72	36.69	0.595	5.14	138.30	5.92	52.69	0.505	5.51
10.50	140.30	5.88	37.90	0.605	5.29	141.50	6.31	55.44	0.508	5.96
11.00	143.30	6.07	40.56	0.607	5.48	144.80	6.67	57.29	0.517	6.32
11.50	146.40	6.32	43.64	0.607	5.76	148.20	6.88	57.60	0.535	6.49
12.00	149.70	6.63	46.43	0.610	6.10	151.50	6.94	57.92	0.552	6.51
12.50	153.00	7.04	48.01	0.620	6.53	154.60	6.80	59.97	0.559	6.38
13.00	156.50	7.47	48.12	0.640	6.94	157.10	6.40	63.83	0.551	5.99
13.50	159.90	7.70	46.71	0.668	7.11	159.00	5.94	68.42	0.535	5.54
14.00	163.10	7.75	44.20	0.702	7.13	160.40	5.65	71.16	0.527	5.23
14.50	166.20	7.67	40.78	0.740	7.00	161.20	5.53	71.38	0.530	5.07
15.00	169.00	7.40	36.58	0.782	6.58	161.80	5.49	69.90	0.543	5.00
15.50	171.50	7.00	32.69	0.819	6.02	161.10	5.50	66.91	0.562	4.99
16.00	173.50	6.60	30.07	0.847	5.50	162.40	5.53	64.03	0.581	5.01
16.50	175.20	6.30	29.38	0.861	5.11	162.70	5.56	62.42	0.592	5.04
17.00	176.20	6.13	29.53	0.866	4.87	163.10	5.56	62.29	0.595	5.03
17.50	176.70	6.08	28.86	0.873	4.75	163.40	5.46	64.54	0.584	4.94
18.00	176.80	6.12	26.31	0.888	4.72	163.70	5.18	70.70	0.549	4.72

*Adapted from ref. #18: Himes et al. (1981).

Table VI.4. Values of Parental Statures Used in Calculation of Mid-parent Stature When One Parent's Stature Is Reported as Short, Medium, or Tall*

| | Values (cm) of stature categories | | |
Parent	Short	Medium	Tall
Father	156.6	176.3	185.4
Mother	154.9	162.8	170.7

*Adapted from ref. #18: Himes et al. (1981).

Leg Length and Developmental History

Total Leg Length. In general, the pattern of human growth is characterized by a head-to-foot (cephalo-caudal) gradient, whereby the head is more advanced at birth than the trunk and the trunk is more advanced than the legs (1,19-23). This implies that the head is more advanced than the trunk and the trunk, as a whole, is more advanced than the legs. In this context the head grows first and reaches its adult status much earlier than the trunk, and the trunk in turn grows earlier and attains its adult size earlier than the legs. Since the longer the period of growth, the greater the possibility of environmental influence, one would expect that growth in leg length is more susceptible to environmental influences than other body segments that terminate growth earlier. Analysis of the anthropometric and socio-economic data of Mexican-Americans who participated in the Hispanic Health and Nutrition Examination Survey from 1982-1984 shows that the poverty income index is more associated with the leg length index than with the sitting height index (23). Recent studies indicate that adult differences in leg length are associated with significant differences in cardiovascular disease, insulin resistance, and birth weight (24-26). These findings support the hypothesis that adverse environmental circumstances operating during childhood and adolescence influence leg growth and increase variability in leg length (23). Hence, differences in relative leg length can be used to ascertain the individual's developmental history (23). Namely, a relatively long leg length is indicative of positive developmental history. On the other hand, a relatively short leg length suggests that the individual has grown under a negative environment that led to a slow growth and short legs. Based upon percentiles and Z-scores for the measures of relative total leg length and lower leg length (see **Tables IV.10** to **IV.15** and **Figures IV.21** and **IV.22**), the following categories of developmental history can be established:

1. Short legs = Z-score of $\leq$-1.645 of either relative total leg length-for-age or relative lower leg length-for-age (or relative total or relative lower leg length below 5th percentile for age and sex).

2. Normal or average = Z-score of -1.645 < Z to <+1.640 of either relative total leg length-for-age or relative lower leg length-for-age (or relative total or relative lower leg length between 5.1[th] and 95th percentile for age and sex).

3. Long legs = Z-score of > +1.645 of either relative total leg length-for-age or relative lower leg length-for-age (or relative total or relative lower leg length above 95th percentile for age and sex).

Analysis of parent-offspring similarities in anthropometric dimensions among Mexican-Americans (n = 2876 parent-offspring pairs) (29) indicates that the estimates of heritability for absolute measurements of length such as stature, sitting height, and leg length are significantly higher than for relative measurements such as sitting height index and leg length index (**Table VI.5**). These findings suggest that inter-individual differences in relative leg length are probably related more to the operation of environmental factors than to genetic factors. On the other hand, inter-population differences in limb length are probably related to the operation of genetic factors. For example, African-Americans have consistently longer tibiae relative to stature than do Euro-Americans, irrespective of nutritional status. For this reason, evaluations of developmental history must be done taking population differences into account.

Lower Leg Length. Osteometric studies indicate that within human populations, the distal limb segments tend to exhibit more relative variability than the proximal segments, especially in the lower limb (30). Experimental studies with animals indicate that the length of the distal limb segment is phenotypically more plastic than the proximal limb. For example, tibia length is reduced in animals raised in a cold environment, relative to warm-environment controls (31,32). Evaluation of the morphology of Neanderthals and contemporary cold-adapted populations indicates that the lower limb is reduced (33). The relative reduction of the lower limb has been explained as a cold-induced adaptation that reduces surface area. Studies of African-Americans and European-Americans who have over the last 170 years undergone a positive "secular trend" in body size indicate that the lower limb distal limb segments have increased in length more than have the proximal (34). These findings suggest that within human populations, the lower limb distal limb segment is more variable than the proximal. In view of the fact that the lower leg length is more sensitive to environmental influences than the proximal limb, one would expect that the diagnostic efficiency of growth retardation would be greater in the lower leg length and would be more sensitive to environmental influences than the proximal limb. Based on the measures of dispersion (see **Tables IV.12** and **IV.13** and **Figures IV.23** and **IV.24**) of the lower length, a measure below 15% of height would be indicative of a developmental stress associated with growth delay.

Table VI.5. Percent Heritability Estimates (% h²) Derived from Mid-parent-Offspring Correlation Coefficients (R) Adjusted for the Effects of Non-Random Assortative Mating in Anthropometric Dimensions of Mexican-Americans Derived from the Data Sets of Hispanic Health Examination Survey of 1982-1984 (HHANES)*

	Mid-parent-Son N = 572 % h²	Mid-parent-Daughter N = 578 % h²	Mid-parent-Offspring N = 1150 % h²
Stature (cm)	65.1	63.5	65.1
Sitting Height (cm)	66.7	65.0	65.0
Leg Length (cm)	65.0	68.3	66.7
Sitting Height Index (%)	56.7	60.0	58.3
Leg Length Index (%)	56.7	60.0	58.3

*From ref. #27: Frisancho AR. (unpublished manuscript).

Head Circumference

Table IV.4 presents the reference for head circumference for the first 84 months (**Figures IV.13** and **IV.14**). A unique feature of head circumference is that during the first 2 years of postnatal life it is closely related to brain volume (4,5). As such, variability in head circumference has been used to diagnose disease and environmental factors on brain size. Several studies have found that infants of smoking mothers are at an increased risk to have a smaller head circumference (<32 cm) than infants of non-smoking mothers (6-10). On the other hand, various studies indicate that autism in children is associated with large head circumference and hence large brain size (11-14). Recent studies (15) have found that compared with normative data of healthy infants, children that develop autism at birth have a significantly smaller head circumference (below the 5th percentile or less than 32 cm), but after birth the head circumference rapidly increases, reaching above the 84th percentile (or more than 54 cm) by the age of 6 to 14 months (15). From these findings together it appears that excessive growth in brain size (i.e. macrocephaly) is an important component of autism. Therefore, depending upon how they compare with the four categories of head circumference, variability in brain growth and the risk associated with it can be identified:

1. Small head circumference if Z-score of head circumference is ≤-1.645 (or head circumference below 5th percentile for age and sex).

2. Healthy range of head circumference if Z-score of head circumference is between ≤-1.036 and $<+1.036$ (or head circumference between 15.1[th] and 85th percentile for age and sex).

3. Above average head circumference if Z-score of head circumference is $>+1.036$ (or head circumference above 85th percentile for age and sex).

4. Large head circumference if Z-score of head circumference is $>+1.645$ (or head circumference above 95th percentile for age and sex).

Mid-Upper Arm Muscle Area

The skeletal muscle (SM) makes up the largest fraction of body mass and about three-quarters of total-body skeletal muscle exists in the extremities. Although there are several methods (i.e., computed axial tomography, magnetic resonance imaging, and body potassium concentration) to quantify skeletal muscle, anthropometric estimates of mid-upper muscle area (UAMA) have been repeatedly shown to provide useful information on the nutritional status of children, adolescents, and adults (39-47). The advantage of UAMA is that only two anthropometric measures (triceps skinfold thickness and upper arm circumference) are required to quickly yield an index of muscularity. The tabular data of mid-upper arm area, muscle area, and arm fat index of children, adolescents, and adults by age and sex are given in **Tables IV.31 to IV.35**. **Figures IV.29** and **IV.30** present in graphic form the age-associated changes in the estimates of mid-upper arm muscle area for children. Based upon this information the subject's muscle status can be classified into five categories:

1. Low muscle and wasted if Z-score of mid-upper arm muscle area is <-1.645 (or mid-upper arm muscle area is below the 5th percentile for age and sex).

2. Below average if Z-score of mid-upper arm muscle area is $-1.645 < Z < -1.040$ (or mid-upper arm muscle area is between 5.1[th] to 15.0[th] percentile for age and sex).

3. Average if Z-score of mid-upper arm muscle area is between -1.036 < Z < +1.030 (or mid-upper arm muscle area is between 15.1[th] to 85.0[th] percentile for age and sex).

4. Above average if Z-score of mid-upper arm muscle area is between +1.036 < Z < +1.640 (or mid-upper arm muscle area is between 85.1[th] to 95.0[th] percentile for age and sex).

5. High muscle if Z-score of mid-upper arm muscle area is >+1.645 (or mid-upper arm muscle area is above 95.1[th] percentile for age and sex).

Waist Circumference

Recent evidence indicates that a high waist circumference in children and adolescents similar to that of adults (see below) is also associated with the emergence of the metabolic syndrome (48-51). The age- and sex-specific percentiles of waist circumference for children are presented in **Table IV.21** and **Figures IV.31** and **IV.32**. From this data it is evident that a waist circumference above the 85th percentile in males and females approaches the waist cutoff (>90 cm for females and >100 cm for males) of adults associated with increased risk of obesity-related metabolic syndrome. Hence, based on statistical criteria, the following five categories of waist circumference can be established:

1. Low waist circumference if Z-score of waist circumference is <-1.645 (or waist circumference is below the 5th percentile for age and sex).

2. Below average if Z-score of waist circumference is -1.645 < Z < -1.040 (or waist circumference is between 5.1[th] to 15.0[th] percentile for age and sex).

3. Average if Z-score of waist circumference is between -1.036 < Z < +1.030 (or waist circumference is between 15.1[th] to 85.0[th] percentile for age and sex).

4. Above average if Z-score of waist circumference is between +1.036 < Z < +1.640 (or waist circumference is between 85.1[th] to 95.0[th] percentile for age and sex).

5. High waist circumference if Z-score of waist circumference is >+1.645 (or waist circumference is above 95.1[th] percentile for age and sex).

Fat-Free Mass and Fat-Free Mass Index

Traditionally, estimates of fat-free mass (FFM) and fat mass (FM) are expressed either as absolute weights (in kilograms or pounds) or as percentages of body weight. However, expressing body composition in this form does not differentiate individuals who differ in height but have the same body composition. For example, a healthy and well-nourished young man can have similar values of FFM and FM as those of a similarly aged but taller individual who suffers from protein-energy malnutrition (PEM). To overcome this difficulty Van Itallie et al. (78) and others (81-84) recommended that FFM and FM be expressed in terms of kilograms normalized for height in a similar form as BMI. For this reason, the present reference in **Tables IV.36** to **IV.37** and **Figures IV.33** to **IV.36** provides information both as kilograms (kg) of lean body mass and as kilograms per squared meter of height (kg/m^2). Based upon this information the subject's muscle status can be classified into five categories:

1. Low fat-free mass and wasted if Z-score of fat-free mass is <-1.645 (or fat-free mass is below the 5th percentile for age and sex).

2. Below average if Z-score of fat-free mass is -1.645 < Z < -1.040 (or fat-free mass is between 5.1[th] to 15.0[th] percentile for age and sex).

3. Average if Z-score of fat-free mass is between -1.036 < Z < +1.030 (or fat-free mass is between 15.1[th] to 85.0[th] percentile for age and sex).

4. Above average if Z-score of fat-free mass is between +1.036 < Z < +1.640 (or fat-free mass is between 85.1[th] to 95.0[th] percentile for age and sex).

5. High fat-free mass if Z-score of fat-free mass is >+1.645 (or fat-free mass is above 95.1[th] percentile for age and sex).

These classifications can also be applied to identify individuals at risk of sarcopenia and muscle hypertrophy. Sarcopenia is characterized by a decrease in resting metabolic rate, decrease in physical activity, decrease in body muscle, and a high percentage of body fat (71-77). Based upon the present reference, sarcopenic obesity can be identified when the FFMI is below the 15th percentile and is associated with FMI that is above the 85th percentile. Likewise, a high FFMI (above the 85th percentile) and a low FMI (below the 15th percentile) can be identified as evidence of muscle hypertrophy.

Body Fat and Fat Mass Index

In most studies the normal amount of body fat for young adult males ranges between 15% and 25%. Similarly, the normal amount of body fat for young adult females ranges between 20% and 30%. Researchers have pointed out that in physically active females and athletes in specific sports, such as ballet dancers, a percentage of body fat below 15% to 17% is associated with a delayed onset of menstruation, irregular menstrual cycles, and a complete cessation of the menses (67-69). Experimental studies, such as those of the Minnesota starvation (79) and US

Army Rangers (80), of individuals exposed to cycles of restricted energy intakes indicate that the lower limit of percent body fat compatible with survival for males is about 5%. This value corresponds to about 2 kg of fat mass and a FMI of 0.8 k/m^2. Based upon the information presented in **Tables IV.39** to **IV.40** and **Figures IV.37** to **IV.40** the subject's fat status can be classified into five categories:

1. Low fat mass if Z-score of fat mass is <-1.645 (or fat mass is below the 5th percentile for age and sex).

2. Below average if Z-score of fat mass is -1.645 < Z < -1.040 (or fat mass is between 5.1th to 15.0th percentile for age and sex).

3. Average if Z-score of fat mass is between -1.036 < Z < +1.030 (or fat mass is between 15.1th to 85.0th percentile for age and sex).

4. Above average if Z-score of fat mass is between +1.036 < Z < +1.640 (or fat mass is between 85.1th to 95.0th percentile for age and sex).

5. High fat mass if Z-score of fat mass is >+1.645 (or fat mass is above 95.1th percentile for age and sex).

These classifications can also be applied to identify fat loss even when there is no change in percent body fat. In many cases, a person loses weight but this reduction is not reflected in the measurements of percent body fat. However, the loss of weight can be quantified with the FMI (kg/m^2). For example, if a participant of 80 kg loses 8 kg (i.e., 10% of his body weight), but does not show change in percent body fat, he will also drop his FMI (and FFMI) by 10%. In other words, identification of the FMI value will allow a more appropriate comparison of the decrease in fatness with other persons of different heights who have lost the same amount of weight but have a different initial BMI.

Excess Body Fat and the Metabolic Syndrome

The metabolic syndrome is a clustering of cardiovascular risk factors associated with having one or more of the following three risk factors associated with cardiovascular disease (52): (1) a high glucose concentration [plasma glucose concentration >125 mg/dL (>6.94 mmol/L) or current use of medication for diabetes],

(2) high blood pressure (diastolic blood pressure ≥90 mmHg, systolic blood pressure ≥140 mmHg, or current use of medication for hypertension), and

(3) dyslipidemia [LDL concentration ≥160 mg/dL (≥4.14 mmol/L), HDL concentration <35 mg/dL (<0.91 mmol/L) for men, and <45 mg/dL (<1.17 mmol/L) for women, or current use of medication for hypercholesterolemia].

There is agreement that overweight and obese individuals are more likely to be associated with the metabolic syndrome than those with normal weight (52-55). For this reason, current studies are addressed at determining the role of anthropometric variables such as body mass index, waist circumference, etc., on the risk of obesity.

Classification of Body Mass Index

Traditionally, a body mass index >30.0 kg/m^2 has been used as an indicator of excess body fat and a BMI <18.50 kg/m^2 as an expression of low body fat stores (1). However, in 1998 the National Institutes of Health (NIH) and the World Health Organization (WHO) changed the BMI cutoff for diagnosing normal weight from >25.0-29.9 kg/m^2 to 18.5-25.0 kg/m^2 and established six categories of BMI (56,57), which are given in **Table VI.6**. Although the BMI-based classification system has become a proxy for identifying individuals at risk of obesity, several studies have questioned its applicability. This is because the BMI is a ratio of weight over height, and weight is the sum of fat, muscle, bone, and water, and as such, it does not differentiate the components that contribute to the excess in weight or underweight. Analysis of the NHANES III data sets shows that individuals with high BMIs (referred to as overweight, Obesity Class I) not only have large quantities of body fat, but also have higher amounts of muscle fat-free mass than those with low BMI. Therefore, a subject with a high amount of muscle and large skeletal mass can have a high body mass index and be falsely identified as obese. Conversely, an individual can have a low BMI and still have a high amount of body fat. In other words, body mass index alone cannot be used to identify deficiency or excess in body fat.

Waist Circumference and Body Mass Index

Clinical studies indicate that in men and women, waist circumference (WC) is directly related to intra-abdominal fat (whether measured by skinfold thickness, computer tomography, or dual x-ray energy absorptionmetry). These studies have shown that WC and hip or thigh circumference have independent and opposite effects on the risk of developing the obesity-associated risk factors (58-66). While WC is positively associated with health risk, hip and thigh circumferences are negatively associated with health risks (63-66). The majority of studies support the hypothesis that a high WC is more important than a high BMI in predicting the risk of cardiovascular disease. The reason for the greater role of WC is related to the fact that WC is a surrogate for abdominal fat. In fact, WC in combination with BMI is a better predictor of abdominal fat than is BMI alone. These observations support the recommendations that the combined use of BMI and WC values can substantially increase the diagnostic effectiveness of obesity. Analysis of the NHANES III data sets (86) indicates that the distribution of BMI becomes less skewed at better health levels. Specifically, in this analysis the distributions of BMI were based upon participants with low blood pressure (systolic blood pressure at or below 140 mmHg or having a diastolic blood pressure at or below 90 mmHg), low blood cholesterol [serum cholesterol level of 6.22 mmol/l (240 mg/dl or lower)], high HDL-cholesterol (HDL-cholesterol level above 40 mg/dl for men and above 50 mg/dl for women), low LDL-cholesterol (less than 160 mg/dl), and normal glucose tolerance (morning fasting plasma glucose level below 110 mg/dl). Results of this analysis indicate that the distribution of BMI for healthy men and women was approximately 19.5-30 kg/m^2 for men and 18-30 kg/m^2 for women. Studies of Asian populations indicate that the cutoff of waist circumference and BMI associated with high risk of cardiovascular risk factor(s) occurs at lower levels than those of Western populations (87).

Table VI.6. Classification of Body Mass Index (kg/m^2) for Defining Underweight and Overweight Adults*

BMI Cutoffs	Classification
(1) <18.49 kg/m^2	Underweight
(2) 18.50 to 24.99 kg/m^2	Normal weight
(3) 25.0 to 29.9 kg/m^2	Overweight
(4) 30.00 to 34.99 kg/m^2	Obesity class I
(5) 35.00 to 39.99 kg/m^2	Obesity class II
(6) ≥40.00 kg/m^2	Obesity class III

*From ref. #56: World Health Organization. 1998. Obesity: preventing and managing the global epidemic. Report of a WHO consultation on obesity. Geneva: World Health Organization.
*From ref. #57: National Institutes of Health, National Heart, Lung, and Blood Institute. 1998. Clinical guidelines on the identification, evaluation, and treatment of overweight and obesity in adults: the evidence report. Obes Res 6 [Suppl 2]:51-210.

The NIH guidelines (57) recommended that the identifications of obesity be done using as reference both BMI and waist circumference (WC). These guidelines recommend that a single

WC threshold: >102 cm (>40 in.) for men and >88 cm (>34 in.) for women be used to denote a high WC, regardless of BMI category. Thresholds were designed to be used in place of BMI as an alternative way to identify those in need of weight management. However, several studies indicate that these single WC thresholds are insufficient to discriminate health risks within all BMI categories. To overcome this difficulty, new health risk-related waist circumference thresholds within BMI categories have been established (66). As shown in **Table VI.7**, in both males and females the waist circumference cutoffs increase in direct proportion to the four-BMI cutoffs. Furthermore, analyses of the NHANES III data set show that within each BMI category (normal weight, overweight, and class I obese), the percent of body fat increases incrementally with the increase in WC category (85). This association implies that within each BMI category, those with high WC also have a higher body fat (%) than those with low WC and body fat. Hence, males with a BMI between 18.5-25.9 km/m^2 can be considered to be of normal weight if their waist circumference is less than 90 cm (<35 in.), but if their waist circumference is greater than 90 cm (≥35.4 in.) they can be considered to be overweight. Likewise, males with a BMI between 25.0-29.9 km/m^2 can also be considered to be of normal weight if their waist circumference is below 100 cm (<39 in.), but if their waist circumference is greater than 100 cm (≥39.4 in.) they can be considered to be overweight. Similarly, females with a BMI between 18.5-25.9 km/m^2 can be considered overweight if their waist circumference is greater than 80 cm (≥31.5 in.), but if waist circumference is less than 80 cm (<31.0 in.) they can be considered to be of normal weight. Females with a BMI between 25.0-29.9 km/m^2 can still be considered to be of normal weight if their weight circumference is below 90 cm (≤35.4 in.).

SUMMARY

The present anthropometric reference permits the investigator to determine whether the child's growth is adequate or below that expected for his/her age. For example, it is usually assumed that a child whose height is below the 5th percentile is considered to be short for his age. The child could be short either because his parents are short (in which case he is probably genetically short), or because of environmental and/or genetic reasons. Adjusting the child's height for his/her parent's height permits the determination whether the short stature of a participant is due to either environmental or familial factors. Another way of ascertaining whether the short stature of a participant is due to environmental factors is to determine the proportion of leg length. At present, if the leg length in children is below the 5th percentile, and if in adults it accounts for less than 45% of the total height, the short stature is due to the effect of negative environmental factors. On the other hand, if in children the leg length is above the 85th percentile, and if in adults it accounts for more than 51% of total height, the tall stature is due to the effect of positive environmental factors. For this reason, the present standards also include references of total and lower leg lengths.

Table VI.7. Waist Circumference (WC) Corresponding to the Four BMI Cutoffs and Its Association with Percent Body Fat (%)†

BMI kg/m²	Weight Classification*	Waist Circumference Threshold cm (in.)*	Associate with Body Fat (%)†
Males			
18.5-24.9	Normal weight	≤90 cm (≤35.4 in)	≤26.0
18.5-24.9	Overweight	≥90 cm (≥35.4 in)	≥26.0
25.0-29.9	Normal weight	≤100 cm (≤39.4 in)	≤31.0
25.0-29.9	Overweight	≥100 cm (≥39.4 in)	≥31.0
30.0-34.9	Obesity class I	≥110 cm (≥43.3 in)	≥35.0
≥35.0	Obesity class II	≥125 cm (≥49.0 in)	≥39.0
Females			
18.5-24.9	Normal weight	≤80 cm (≤31.5 in)	≤34.0
18.5-24.9	Overweight	≥80 cm (≥31.5 in)	≥34.0
25.0-29.9	Normal weight	≤90 cm (≤35.4 in)	≤39.5
25.0-29.9	Overweight	≥90 cm (≥35.4 in)	≥39.5
30.0-34.9	Obesity class I	≥105 cm (≥41.3 in)	≥43.0
≥35.	Obesity class II	≥115 cm (≥45.2 in)	≥50.0

* From ref. #66: Ardern CI, Janssen I, Ross R, and Katzmarzyk PT. 2004. Development of Health-Related Waist Circumference Thresholds Within BMI Categories. Obes Res 12: 1094-1103.
† The percents body fat were calculated using the measurements of bio-impedance of the NHANES III data sets. (From ref. #85: Frisancho AR. Unpublished.)

The references of body mass index and composition permit the determination of whether a child is heavy or underweight for his/her height. For example, if a child's body mass index, upper arm muscle area, and subcutaneous fat are below the 5th percentile, this suggests that this child has been suffering from severe acute undernutrition. If in terms of stature he or she approaches the average, the malnutrition is probably of recent origin, and if this condition continues it will become chronic and the subject's growth will be stunted. On the other hand, if the body mass index is above the 85th percentile (is heavy) for his/her age and for his/her height, the high weight is associated with an excess of body fat.

In adults, evaluation of nutritional status must be done with reference to body mass index and waist circumference, along with direct and indirect measurements of body composition. The estimates of muscle area, along with measurements of fat mass and fat-free mass, expressed as kg and as kg/m^2 of height, have been shown to be useful for identifying the risk of excess fat and deficit of muscle mass, such as in wasting disease and sarcopenia, as well as muscle hypertrophy. Now that many of the conditions associated with the metabolic syndrome have been linked as a co-morbid condition associated with the childhood obesity epidemic, the need for an anthropometric reference to quantify changes in body composition of children becomes critical. Within this context, until more precise field techniques are available, the present anthropometric references provide valuable research strategies for assessing and interpreting the nutritional status of children and adults in both clinical and research settings.

LITERATURE CITED

1. Frisancho, A. R. 1990. Anthropometric Standards for the Assessment of Growth and Nutritional Status. Ann Arbor, MI: University of Michigan Press.

2. Babson, S. G., Benda, G. I. 1976. Growth graphs for the clinical assessment of infants of varying gestational age. J. Pediatr. 89:814-20.

3. Fenton, T. R. 2003. A new growth chart for preterm babies: Babson and Benda's chart updated with recent data and a new format. BMC Pediatr. 3:13-23.

4. Bartholomeusz, H. H., Courchesne, E., Karns, C. M. 2002. Relationship between head circumference and brain volume in healthy normal toddlers, children, and adults. Neuropediatrics 33:239-41.

5. Lindley, A. A., Benson, J. E., Grimes, C., Cole, T. M. III, Herman, A.A. 1999. The relationship in neonates between clinically measured head circumference and brain volume estimated from head CT-scans. Early Hum. Dev. 56:17-29.

6. Kallen, K. 2000. Maternal smoking during pregnancy and infant head circumference at birth. Early Hum. Dev. 58:197-204.

7. Lindley, A. A., Becker, S., Gray, R. H., Herman, A. A. 2000. Effect of continuing or stopping smoking during pregnancy on infant birth weight, crown-heel length, head circumference, ponderal index, and brain: body weight ratio. Am. J. Epidemiol. 152:219-25.

8. Ong, K. K., Preece, M. A., Emmett, P. M., Ahmed, M. L., Dunger, D. B. 2002. Size at birth and early childhood growth in relation to maternal smoking, parity and infant breast-feeding: longitudinal birth cohort study and analysis. Pediatr. Res. 52:863-67.

9. Berlanga, Mdel. R., Salazar, G., Garcia, C., Hernandez, J. 2002. Maternal smoking effects on infant growth. Food. Nutr. Bull. 23 [Suppl]:142-45.

10. Miles, J. H., Hadden, L. L., Takahashi, T. N., Hillman, R. E. 2000. Head circumference is an independent clinical finding associated with autism. Am. J. Med. Genet. 95:339-50.

11. Eriksson, M., Jonsson, B., Zetterstrom, R. 2000. Children of mothers abusing amphetamine: head circumference during infancy and psychosocial development until 14 years of age. Acta. Paediatr. 12:1474-78.

12. Aylward, E. H., Minshew, N. J., Field, K., Sparks, B. F., Singh, N. 2002. Effects of age on brain volume and head circumference in autism. Neurology 59:175-83.

13. Gillberg, C., de Souza L. 2002. Head circumference in autism, Asperger syndrome, and ADHD: a comparative study. Dev. Med. Child Neurol. 44:296-300.

14. Sparks, B. F., Friedman, S. D., Shaw, D. W., et al. 2002. Brain structural abnormalities in young children with autism spectrum disorder. Neurology 59:184-92.

15. Courchesne, E., Carper, R., Akshoomoff, N. 2003. Evidence of brain overgrowth in the first year of life in autism. JAMA 290:337-44.

16. WHO Expert Consultation. 2004. Appropriate body-mass index for Asian populations and its implications for policy and intervention strategies. Lancet 363:157-63.

17. Cole, T. J., Bellizzi, M. C., Flegal, K. M., Dietz, W. H. 2000. Establishing a standard definition for child overweight and obesity worldwide: international survey. BMJ 320:1240-43.

18. Himes, J. H., Roche, A. F., Thissen, D., Moore, W. M. 1981. Parent-specific adjustments of recumbent length and stature. Monographs in Paediatrics, vol. 13. Basel, Switzerland: S. Karger.

19. Scammon, R. E. 1930. The ponderal growth of the extremities of the human fetus. Am. J. Phys. Anthropol. 15:111-21.

20. Krogman, W. M. 1972. Child Growth. Ann Arbor, MI: The University of Michigan Press.

21. Tanner, J. M. 1978. Fetus into Man. Physical Growth from Conception to Maturity. Cambridge, MA: Harvard University Press.

22. Bogin, B. 1988. Patterns of Human Growth. Cambridge: Cambridge University Press.

23. Frisancho, A. R., Guilding, N., Tanner, S. 2001. Growth of leg length is reflected in socio-economic differences. Acta Med. Auxol. 33:47-50.

24. Smith, G. D., Gunnell, D., Sweetnam, P., Yarnell, J., Elwood, P. 2001. Leg length, insulin resistance and coronary heart disease risk: the Caerphilly study. J. Epidemiol. Commun. H. 55:867-72.

25. Wadsworth, M. E. J., Hardy, R. J., Paul, A. A., Marshall, S. F., Cole, T. J. 2002. Leg and trunk length at 43 years in relation to childhood health, diet and family circumstances; evidence from the 1946 national birth cohort. Int. J. of Epidemiol. 31:383-90.

26. Gunnell, D. 2002. Can adult anthropometry be used as a "biomarker" for prenatal and childhood exposures? Int. J. of Epidemiol. 31:65-75.

27. Lawlor, D. A., Ebrahim, S., Davey Smith, G. 2002. The association between components of adult height and type II diabetes and insulin resistance: British Women's Heart and Health Study. Diabetologia 45:1097-1106.

28. Langenberg, C., Hardy, R., Kuh, D., Wadsworth, M.E. 2003. Influence of height, leg and trunk length on pulse pressure, systolic and diastolic blood pressure. J. Hypertens. 21:537-43.

29. Frisancho, A. R. Heritability estimates of sitting height and percent leg length. (Unpublished manuscript.)

30. Holliday, T. W., Ruff, C. B. 2001. Relative variation in human proximal and distal limb segment lengths. Am. J. Phys. Anthropol. 116:26-33.

31. Weaver, M. E., Ingram, D. L. 1969. Morphological changes in swine associated with environmental temperature. Ecology 50:710-13.

32. Lee, M. M. C., Chu, P. C., Chan, H. C. 1969. Effects of cold on the skeletal growth of albino rats. Am. J. Anat. 124:239-50.

33. Ruff, C. B. 1994. Morphological adaptation to climate in modern and fossil hominids. Yrbk. Phys. Anthropol. 37:65-107.

34. Jantz, L. M., Jantz, R. L. 1999. Secular change in long bone length and proportion in the United States, 1800–1970. Am. J. Phys. Anthropol. 110:57-67.

35. Sarria, A., Garcia-Llop, L. A., Moreno, L. A., Fleta, J., Morellon, M. P., Bueno, M. 1998. Skinfold thickness measurements are better predictors of body fat percentage than body mass index in male Spanish children and adolescents. Eur. J. Clin. Nutr. 52:573-76.

36. King, S., Wilson, J., Kotsimbos, T., Bailey, M., Nyulasi, I. 2005. Body composition assessment in adults with cystic fibrosis: comparison of dual-energy X-ray absorptiometry with skinfolds and bioelectrical impedance analysis. Nutrition 21:1087-94.

37. Steinberger, J., Jacobs, D. R., Raatz, S., Moran, A., Hong, C. P., Sinaiko, A. R. 2005. Comparison of body fatness measurements by BMI and skinfolds vs. dual energy X-ray absorptiometry and their relation to cardiovascular risk factors in adolescents. Int. J. Obes. 29:1346-52.

38. Hollander, F. M., De Roos, N. M., De Vries, J. H., Van Berkhout, F. T. 2005. Assessment of nutritional status in adult patients with cystic fibrosis: whole-body bioimpedance vs. body mass index, skinfolds, and leg-to-leg bioimpedance. J. Am. Diet. Assoc. 105:549-55.

39. Frisancho. A. R. 1981. New norms of upper limb fat and muscle areas for assessment of nutritional status. Am. J. Clin. Nutr. 34:2540-45.

40. Katch, F. I., Hortobagyi, T. 1990. Validity of surface anthropometry to estimate upper-arm muscularity, including changes with body mass loss. Am. J. Clin. Nutr. 52:591-95.

41. Leonard, M. B., Zemel, B. S., Kawchak, D. A., Ohene-Frempong, K., Stalling, V. A. 1998. Plasma zinc status, growth, and maturation in children with sickle cell disease. J. Pediatr. 132:467-71.

42. Bolzan, A., Guimarey, L., Frisancho, A. R. 1999. Study of growth in rural school children from Buenos Aires, Argentina using upper arm muscle area by height and other anthropometric dimensions of body composition. Ann. Hum. Biol. 26:185-93.

43. Grinspoon, S., Corcoran, C., Rosenthal, D., et al. 1999. Quantitative assessment of cross-sectional muscle area, functional status, and muscle strength in men with the acquired immunodeficiency wasting syndrome. J. Clin. Endocrinol. Metab. 84:201-6.

44. Becque, M. D., Lochman, J. D., Melrose, D. R. 2000. Effects of oral creatine supplementation on muscular strength and body composition. Med. Sci. Sports. Exerc. 32:654-58.

45. Trowbridge, F. L., Hiner, C. D., Robertson, A. D. 1982. Arm muscle indicators and creatinine excretion in children. Am. J. Clin. Nutr. 36:691-96.

46. Boye, K. R., Dimitriou, T., Manz, F., Schoenau, E., Neu, C., Wudy, S., Remer, T. 2002. Anthropometric assessment of muscularity during growth: estimating fat-free mass with 2 skinfold-thickness measurements is superior to measuring midupper arm muscle area in healthy prepubertal children. Am. J. Clin. Nutr. 76:628-32.

47. Hediger, M. L., Overpeck, M. D., Kuczmarski, R. J., McGlynn, A., Maurer, K. R., Davis, W. W. 1998. Muscularity and fatness of infants and young children born small- or large-for-gestational-age. Pediatrics 102:E60.

48. Savva, S. C., Tornaritis, M., Savva, M. E., Kourides, Y., Panagi, A., Silikiotou, N., Georgiou, C., Kafatos, A. 2000. Waist circumference and waist-to-height ratio are better predictors of cardiovascular disease risk factors in children than body mass index. Int. J. Obes. Relat. Metab. Disord. 24:1453-58.

49. Eisenmann, J. C., Wickel, E. E., Welk, G. J., Blair, S. N. 2005. Association between cardiorespiratory fitness and fatness during adolescence and cardiovascular disease risk factors in adulthood: the Aerobics Center Longitudinal Study. Am. Heart J. 149:46-53.

50. Janssen, I., Katzmarzyk, P. T., Srinivasan, S. R., Chen, W., Malina, R. M., Bouchard, C., Berenson, G. S. 2005. Combined influence of body mass index and waist circumference on coronary artery disease risk factors among children and adolescents. Pediatrics 115:1623-30.

51. Fernandez, J. R., Redden, D. T., Pietrobelli, A., Allison, D. B. 2004. Waist circumference percentiles in nationally representative samples of African-American, European-American, and Mexican-American children and adolescents. J. Pediatr. 145:439-44.

52. Expert Panel on Detection, Evaluation, and Treatment of High Blood Cholesterol in Adults: Executive Summary of the Third Report of the National Cholesterol Education Program (NCEP) Expert Panel on Detection, Evaluation, and Treatment of High Blood Cholesterol in Adults (Adult Treatment Panel III). 2001. JAMA 285:2486-97.

53. DeFronzo, R. A., Ferranini, E. 1991. Insulin resistance. A multifaceted syndrome responsible for NIDDM, obesity, hypertension, dyslipidemia and atherosclerotic cardiovascular disease. Diabetes Care 14:173-94.

54. Laaksonen, D. E., Niskanen, L., Lakka, H. M., Lakka, T. A., Uusitupa, M. 2004. Epidemiology and treatment of the metabolic syndrome. Ann. Med. 36:332-46.

55. Alexander, C. M., Landsman, P. B., Teutsch, S. M., Haffner, S. M. 2003. NCEP defined metabolic syndrome, diabetes, and prevalence of coronary heart disease among NHANES III participants age 50 years and older. Diabetes 52:1210–14.

56. World Health Organization. Obesity: preventing and managing the global epidemic. Report of a WHO consultation on obesity, Geneva. June 3-5, 1998. Geneva: World Health Organization, 9-14.

57. National Institutes of Health. 1998. Clinical guidelines on the identification, evaluation, and treatment of overweight and obesity in adults—the evidence report. Obes. Res. 6 [Suppl 2]:51-209.

58. Han, T. S., Leer, E. M., Seidell, J. C., Lean, M. E. J. 1995. Waist circumference action levels in the identification of cardiovascular risk factors: prevalence study in a random sample. BMJ 311:1401-5.

59. Pouliot, M. C., Despres, J. P., Lemieux, S., et al. 1994. Waist circumference and abdominal sagittal diameter: best simple anthropometric indexes of abdominal visceral adipose tissue accumulation and related cardiovascular risk in men and women. Am. J. Cardiol. 73:460-68.

60. Ross, R., Leger, L., Morris, D., de Guise, J., Guardo, R. 1992. Quantification of adipose tissue by MRI: relationship with anthropometric variables. J. Appl. Physiol. 72:787-95.

61. Han, T. S., Seidell, J. C., Currall, J. E., Morrison, C. E., Deurenberg, P., Lean, M. E. 1997. The influences of height and age on waist circumferences as an index of adiposity in adults. Int. J. Obes. Relat. Metab. Disord. 12:83-89.

62. Gallagher, D., Heymsfield, S., Heo, M., Jebb, S. A., Murgatroyd, P. R., Sakamoto, Y. 2000. Healthy percentage body fat ranges: an approach for developing guideline based on body mass index. Am. J. Clin. Nutr. 72:694-701.

63. Onat, A. 1999. Waist circumference and waist-to-hip in Turkish adults: interrelation with other risk factors and association with cardiovascular disease. Int. J. Cardiol. 70:43-50.

64. Lean, M. E. J., Han, T. S., Morrison, C. E. 1995. Waist circumference as a measure for indicating need for weight management. BMJ 311:158-61.

65. Zhu, S., Heymsfield, S. B., Toyoshima, H., Wang, Z., Pietrobelli, A., Heshka, S. 2005. Race-ethnicity-specific waist circumference cutoffs for identifying cardiovascular disease risk factors. Am. J. Clin. Nutr. 81:409-15.

66. Ardern, C. I., Janssen, I., Ross, R., Katzmarzyk, P. T. 2004. Development of health-related waist circumference thresholds within BMI categories. Obes. Res. 12:1094-103.

67. Frisch R. E., et al. 1980. Delayed menarche and amenorrhea in ballet dancers. N. Engl. Med. 303:17.

68. Warren, M. P. 1980. The effects of exercise on pubertal progression and reproductive function. Clin. Endocrinol. Metab. 51:1150.

69. Loucks, A. B. 1990. Effects of exercise training on the menstrual cycle: existence and mechanisms. Med. Sci. Sports Exerc. 22:275.

70. Expert Subcommittee on the Use and Interpretation of Anthropometry in the Elderly. Uses and interpretation of anthropometry in the elderly for the assessment of physical status: report to the nutrition unit of the World Health Organization. J. Nutr. Health Aging 2:5-17.

71. Chumlea, W. C., Quo, S. S., Glasser, R. M., Vellas, B. J. Sarcopenia, function and health. J. Nutr. Health Aging 1:7-12.

72. Heber, D., Ingles, S., Ashley, J. M., Maxwell, M. H., Lyons, R. F., Elashoff, R. M. 1996. Clinical detection of sarcopenic obesity by bioelectrical impedance analysis. Am. J. Clin. Nutr. [Suppl] 64:472-77.

73. Baumgartner, R. N., Koehler, K. M., Gallagher, D., et al. 1998. Epidemiology of sarcopenia among the elderly in New Mexico. Am. J. Epidemiol. 147:755-63.

74. Castaneda, C., Janssen, I. 2005. Ethnic comparisons of sarcopenia and obesity in diabetes. Ethn. Dis. 15:664-70.

75. Karakelides, H., Sreekumaran, Nair K. 2005. Sarcopenia of aging and its metabolic impact. Curr. Top. Dev. Biol. 68:123-48.

76. Frontera, W. R., Hughes, V. A., Fielding, R. A., Fiatarone, M. A., Evans, W. J., Roubenoff, R. 2000. Aging of skeletal muscle: a 12-yr longitudinal study. J. Appl. Physiol. 88:1321-26.

77. Sowers, M. R., Crutchfield, M., Richards, K., Wilkin, M. K., Furniss, A., Jannausch, M., Zhang, D., Gross, M. 2005. Sarcopenia is related to physical functioning and leg strength in middle-aged women. J. Gerontol. A. Biol. Sci. Med. Sci. 60:486-90.

78. Van Itallie, T. B., Yang, M. U., Heymsfield, S. B., Funk, R. C., Boileau, R. A. 1990. Height-normalized indices of the body's fat-free mass and fat mass: potentially useful indicators of nutritional status. Am. J. Clin. Nutr. 52:953-59.

79. Keys, A., Brozek, J., Henschel, A., Mickelsen, O., Taylor, H. L. 1950. The biology of human starvation. Minneapolis: University of Minnesota Press.

80. Friedl, K. E., Moore, R. J., Martinez-Lopez, L. E., et al. 1994. Lower limits of body fat in healthy active men. J. Appl. Physiol. 77:933-40.

81. Bartlett, H. L., Puhl, S. M., Hodgson, J. L., Buskirk, E. R. 1991. Fat-free mass in relation to stature: ratios of fat-free mass to height in children, adults, and elderly subjects. Am. J. Clin. Nutr. 53:1112-16.

82. Hattori, K., Tatsumi, N., Tanaka, S. 1997. Assessment of body composition by using a new chart method. Am. J. Hum. Biol. 9:573-78.

83. Schutz, Y., Kyle, U. U. G., Pichard, C. 2002. Fat-free mass index and fat Caucasians aged 18–98 years. Int. J. Obes. 26:953-60.

84. Freedman, D. S., Wang, J., Maynard, L. M., Thornton, J. C., Mei1, Z., Pierson, R. N. Jr., Dietz, W. H., Horlick, M. 2005. Relation of BMI to fat and fat-free mass among children and adolescents. Int. J. Obes. 29:1-8.

85. Frisancho, A. R. 2005. Anthropometric Reference for the Identification Components of Excess Weight and Obesity in Adults. (Unpublished manuscript.)

86. Flegal, K. M. 2006. Body mass index of healthy men compared with healthy women in the United States. Int. J. Obes. Relat. Metab. Disord. 30:374-79.

87. Misra, A., Vikram, N. K., Gupta, R., Pandey, R. M., Wasir, J. S., Gupta, V. P. 2006. Waist circumference cutoff points and action levels for Asian Indians for identification of abdominal obesity. Int. J. Obes. Relat. Metab. Disord. 30:106-11.

88. Himes, J. H., Dietz, W. H. 1994. Guidelines for overweight in adolescent preventive services: recommendations from an expert committee. Am. J. Clin. Nutr. 59:307–316.

89. Barlow, S. E., Dietz, W. H. 1998. Obesity evaluation and treatment: expert committee recommendations. Pediatrics 102(3). Available at: www.pediatrics.org/cgi/content/full/102/3/e29.

90. Freedman, D. S., Wang, J., Ogden, C. L., Thornton, J. C., Mei, Z., Pierson, R. N., Dietz, W. H., Horlick, M. 2007. The prediction of body fatness by BMI and skinfold thicknesses among children and adolescents. Ann. Hum. Biol. 34:183-94.

91. Mei, Z., Grummer-Strawn, L. M., Wang, J., Thornton, J. C., Freedman, D. S., Pierson, R. N. Jr., Dietz, W. H., Horlick, M. 2007. Do skinfold measurements provide additional information to body mass index in the assessment of body fatness among children and adolescents? Pediatrics 119:e1306-13.

SUBJECT INDEX